Nutrition Management of Patients with Inherited Metabolic Disorders

Edited by
Phyllis B. Acosta, MS, DrPH, RD

Nutrition Consultant
Southeastern Regional Genetics Group
Division of Medical Genetics
Emory University
School of Medicine
Atlanta, Georgia

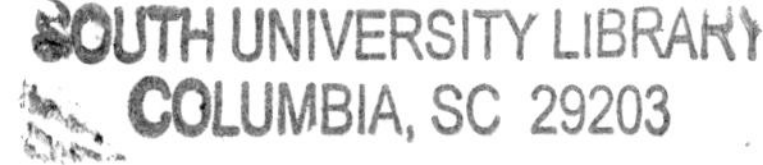

JONES AND BARTLETT PUBLISHERS
Sudbury, Massachusetts
BOSTON TORONTO LONDON SINGAPORE

World Headquarters
Jones and Bartlett Publishers
40 Tall Pine Drive
Sudbury, MA 01776
978-443-5000
info@jbpub.com
www.jbpub.com

Jones and Bartlett Publishers
Canada
6339 Ormindale Way
Mississauga, Ontario L5V 1J2
Canada

Jones and Bartlett Publishers
International
Barb House, Barb Mews
London W6 7PA
United Kingdom

Jones and Bartlett's books and products are available through most bookstores and online booksellers. To contact Jones and Bartlett Publishers directly, call 800-832-0034, fax 978-443-8000, or visit our website, www.jbpub.com.

Substantial discounts on bulk quantities of Jones and Bartlett's publications are available to corporations, professional associations, and other qualified organizations. For details and specific discount information, contact the special sales department at Jones and Bartlett via the above contact information or send an email to specialsales@jbpub.com.

Production Credits
Publisher: David Cella
Acquisitions Editor: Katey Birtcher
Editorial Assistant: Catie Heverling
Editorial Assistant: Teresa Reilly
Senior Production Editor: Tracey Chapman
Associate Production Editor: Kate Stein
Senior Marketing Manager: Sophie Fleck
Marketing Manager: Grace Richards
Manufacturing and Inventory Control Supervisor: Amy Bacus
Composition and Art: Cape Cod Compositors, Inc.
Cover Design: Scott Moden
Cover Image: © Kirsty Pargeter/Dreamstime.com
Printing and Binding: Malloy, Inc.
Cover Printing: Malloy, Inc.

Library of Congress Cataloging-in-Publication Data
Nutrition management of patients with inherited metabolic disorders / [edited by] Phyllis Acosta.
p. ; cm.
Includes bibliographical references and index.
ISBN-13: 978-0-7637-5777-9 (hardcover)
ISBN-10: 0-7637-5777-2 (hardcover)
1. Metabolism, Inborn errors of Patients—Nutrition. I. Acosta, Phyllis B.
[DNLM: 1. Metabolism, Inborn Errors—therapy. 2. Nutrigenomics. 3. Nutrition Therapy—methods. WD 205 N9756 2010]
RC627.8.N88 2010
616.3'9042—dc22

2009019490

6048

Printed in the United States of America
13 12 11 10 09 10 9 8 7 6 5 4 3 2 1

Contents

Acknowledgments

Without the many people who shared their knowledge with me over the last 50-plus years, preparation of this book would not have been possible. Three persons in particular aroused my interest in the field of inherited metabolic disorders such that they became the focus of my professional life. Willard Centerwall, MD, of the White Memorial Medical Center, Los Angeles, California, was the first person to develop an approach to screening of infants for phenylketonuria. He introduced me to the difference nutrition management could make in the long-term outcomes of these patients. Later, Richard Koch, MD, of the Los Angeles Children's Hospital, expanded my vision to the beneficial effects of nutrition management on many other patients with inherited metabolic disorders. Subsequently, Louis J. Elsas II, MD, of the Emory University School of Medicine, Atlanta, Georgia, helped broaden my knowledge of the field by requesting justification of the nutrition management prescriptions I wrote, resulting in increased professional confidence in my knowledge and expertise in the expanding field of inherited metabolic disorders.

At the same time, the several hundreds of families who trusted me to provide guidance for the nutrition management of their children with inherited metabolic disorders supported my desire to increase my knowledge in the field in order to be able to provide further help to them. Much appreciation is extended to the contributors of the chapters in this book. Without their experience, knowledge, time, and contributions, this book would not have been completed. The editors at Jones and Bartlett were so very kind in guiding this "greenhorn" through all the work in editing a book. The great help of Christine Downs, of Columbus, Ohio, was essential to the outcome, and the financial support of Rick Finkel, President of Applied Nutrition Corp., Cedar Knoll, New Jersey, helped defray the cost of word processing. Thank you all very, very much.

Preface

Nutrition Management of Patients with Inherited Metabolic Disorders is the first book dedicated to nutrition management of patients with inherited metabolic disorders (IMDs) for which newborn screening and diagnoses are routinely practiced. The aim of this book is to supply information that will enhance the knowledge and skills needed by nutritionists, dietitians, and other healthcare professionals who provide these services to patients with IMDs. Newborn screening, followed by diagnosis, has demonstrated that about 1 of every 1000 to 3000 infants born yearly in the United States suffers from an IMD that results in mental retardation or death if untreated, and most are treatable with nutrition management.

Patients with galactosemia (galactose-1-phosphate uridyl transferase deficiency) were some of the first who were managed by diet over a century ago. Since that time, many disorders that are disastrous to patients have been diagnosed and managed by diet, improving neurological and physical outcomes. Over the years, knowledge has also accrued that has improved medical foods and nutrition management. However, nutrition problems still occur, whether due to the quality of the medical foods, inadequate prescription by healthcare providers, or poor diet adherence by the patient. It is hoped that this book will adequately describe these problems and supply appropriate knowledge to encourage medical food manufacturers, medical geneticists, nutritionists/dietitians, and other healthcare providers to search further and to conduct the research needed to find alternative forms of nutrients that would provide optimal nutrition and health for the patients. It is anticipated that nutrition management and other therapies of many disorders will continue to improve in the future. This book should be helpful in promoting nutrition management.

Phyllis B. Acosta

Contributors

Dianne M. Frazier, MPH, PhD, RD
Professor of Pediatrics
Division of Genetics and Metabolism
University of North Carolina
Chapel Hill, North Carolina

Melanie B. Gillingham, PhD, RD
Assistant Professor
Molecular and Medical Genetics
Oregon Health and Science University
Portland, Oregon

Barbara Marriage, PhD, RD
Senior Research Scientist
Abbott Nutrition
Columbus, Ohio

Kimberlee Michals Matalon, PhD, RD
Associate Professor
Department of Health and Human Performance
University of Houston
Houston, Texas

Rani H. Singh, PhD, RD
Associate Professor
Department of Human Genetics
Emory University School of Medicine
Atlanta, Georgia

Sandra van Calcar, PhD, RD
Senior Metabolic Dietitian
Biochemical Genetics Program
Waisman Center, University of Wisconsin
Madison, Wisconsin

Steven Yannicelli, PhD, RD
Director of Science and Education
Nutricia North America
Valencia, California

Chapter 1

Introduction to Genetics and Genetics of Inherited Metabolic Disorders

Kimberlee Michals Matalon

INTRODUCTION

Normal metabolism encompasses all the biochemical reactions in tissues that keep an organism alive and in a state of health. The concept of inborn error of metabolism (IEM) or inherited metabolic disorder (IMD) was introduced by Sir Archibald E. Garrod in 1902.[1] He suggested that a block in the metabolic process that caused disease led to the accumulation of intermediary metabolites that could not be processed further. He published his findings in 1908[2] and summarized these findings in a book that included the autosomal recessive inheritance of alkaptonuria, albinism, cystinuria, and pentosuria.[3] Garrod is considered the "grandfather" of biochemical genetics, where identification of intermediary metabolites from IMDs led to the discovery of enzyme defects causing these diseases. Intermediary metabolites are usually present in trace amounts and not normally detected; however, in IMDs such metabolites are present in large quantities due to the specific enzyme defect.

Advances in the field of genetics include the introduction of the concept of the gene as the unit of inheritance by Johannsen.[4] Later, Beadle and Tatum introduced the idea of "one gene, one enzyme."[5,6] Pauling and Ingram conceived of the molecular disease concept. Pauling worked on sickle-cell anemia and demonstrated that mutation of genes could alter protein structure.[7] Ingram showed that an alteration in a gene is responsible for an amino acid change in the protein, and that sickle-cell disease was caused by valine substituted for glutamic acid in the β-globin chain; thus the concept of molecular disease was established.[8] The understanding that deoxyribonucleic acid (DNA) is the basis of inheritance and the discovery of the double helix by Watson and Crick created tremendous scientific excitement, ushering in a new era of molecular genetics.[9]

Discoveries of gene defects and improved methods of diagnosis have led to the discovery of inherited diseases that are summarized in the ever-expanding volumes of texts of general genetics, biochemical genetics, and neurological diseases.[10-13] Many IMDs are treatable, often by nutrition management of the patient. For many diseases early detection is important, so that treatment can begin before damage occurs. The success of early detection and treatment of phenylketonuria (PKU) led to the expanded newborn screening of today.[14,15] The technology of tandem mass spectrometry with the ability to screen newborns for more than 40 different IMDs using a blood spot on Guthrie cards has resulted in new challenges of diagnosis verification, treatment and counseling, and follow up.[16] Many of the IMDs can also be genotyped from the same newborn blood sample. The genotype is determined by the type of mutations on a gene. Biochemical geneticists can often predict how much residual enzyme activity will occur with each genotype. The clinical expression of the genotype is called the phenotype. It is useful for the treating centers' dietitians and other experts to know the genotypes of their patients so that treatment can be more reliably tailored to the patients' needs. In general this concept is true for many diseases; however, individual variations of genotype/phenotype will be encountered and treatment has to be individualized.

Human Genome

Inherited metabolic disorders are genetic diseases caused by defects in specific genes. The human genome contains all the human genes, which are estimated to number between 30,000 and 70,000.[17,18]

Genes are made of DNA, found mainly in the cell nucleus packaged in chromosomes, and referred to as nuclear DNA (nDNA). The entire human genome is located in the 46 chromosomes, 22 pairs of autosomes, and one pair of sex chromosomes, XY for males and XX for females. Only a small percentage (1.5% of the entire genome) of the DNA in the human genome are genes that transcribe and code for specific proteins.[19] These coding sequences in each gene are called exons and are interspersed in a specific order in the DNA of the gene. The bulk of DNA in each gene that is not translated resides in introns. Why the human genome contains so much DNA that does not code for proteins is unclear. It has been suggested that the functions of the noncoding DNA are regulatory and protective elements for the functioning genes.[20,21] Each gene contains a specific number of exons that are located in a specific order between the introns. The mitochondrial DNA (mDNA), while small, is also part of the human genome.[22] Mitochondrial DNA contains no introns, so the number of base pairs is very small.

DNA Structure

The structure of DNA consists of four bases: two purine bases, adenine (A) and guanine (G); and two pyrimidine bases, thymine (T) and cytosine (C).[9,23,24] Each base is bound to a pentose sugar and a phosphate group. Deoxyribose is the pentose sugar found in DNA, while ribose is the pentose sugar found in ribonucleic acid (RNA). The RNA uses the base uracil (U) instead of thymine (T). The DNA structure is a twisted double helix as described by Watson and Crick.[9] The side chains are made up of the sugar and phosphate groups. The pairing by hydrogen bonds of the corresponding bases creates the "stairs" of the helix. One purine is paired with one pyrimidine: A with T and C with G. The sequence of the bases is varied for each gene, and three bases in each gene code for a single amino acid, called a triplet code. The DNA of a gene that codes for a specific protein is made up of several exons, interrupted by noncoding DNA called introns. The message in the exons is transcribed to a messenger RNA (mRNA), and in the process, the introns are excised. The coding exons of a gene usually contain a small number of base pairs, about 25,000, while the entire gene with the introns can be 25×10^6 base pairs. The translation of the message leads to the synthesis of the specific protein.

The first codon to be identified in mRNA was UUU, which codes for phenylalanine.[25] In DNA the base uracil (U) is replaced with thymine (T), so that in DNA TTT codes for phenylalanine. The first amino acid in every polypeptide chain is methionine with a specific code, ATG in the DNA triplet and AUG in the RNA. Considering three bases in each codon, the four bases should result in 64 triplets. However, there are 61 triplets that code for amino acids and three triplets that are stop codons: T(U)AG, T(U)GA, and T(U)AA. The stop codon triplets are read by release proteins that release the completed polypeptide chain. Only methionine has one codon (AUG). Other amino acids have more than one triplet. For example, six different triplets code for leucine. The fact that more than one triplet codes for one amino acid is termed degeneracy of the code. The degeneracy of the code serves for protection against deleterious mutations.

The initiation of peptide synthesis is rather complex and requires certain DNA elements, although not translated, that are critical to the regulation of gene expression. The synthesis of protein involves ribosomes that attach transfer RNA (tRNA) which carry the amino acid to match the specific triplet in the RNA message. Each tRNA is specific for the amino acid that it carries to the site of synthesis, and each amino acid is attached to the coding triplet with the help of ribosomes that advance along the mRNA until the synthesis of the protein is halted by a triplet that is called a stop codon.

Mitochondrial Genome

The mitochondria are small subcellular organelles that produce energy for the cell through oxidative phosphorylation. The mitochondria have their own DNA. This extra chromosomal DNA is part of the human genome. The mitochondrial genome is a double-stranded circle with 16,569 base pairs.[26] There are 37 genes encoded by the mitochondrial DNA and only 13 encode for polypeptides. There are no introns in these genes. The 13 polypeptides join other nuclear polypeptides to form a complete enzyme. All of these enzymes are important in electron transport and energy generation and are located in the mitochondrial membrane.[22,27]

Mitochondrial DNA, which originates in the egg, is maternally inherited. Therefore, mitochondria are inherited as sex linked. Because mitochondrial polypeptides function together with nuclear proteins to give a complete enzyme, mitochondrial diseases can be recessive, sex linked, or dominant depending on the defective polypeptide.[22,27,28]

The inheritance of mitochondrial alleles is different than nuclear alleles where there are two for each gene. Because cells contain many mitochondria, there are many alleles for one gene and if some alleles are mutated, then the cells become "heteroplasmic;" that is, they contain normal and mutated mitochondrial genes, and diseases with the same mutations can have different expressivity, depending on the number of mutated mitochondria in that cell or that tissue.[22,27,29]

Mitochondria are important in energy metabolism. Mitochondrial defects can be caused not only by mutations of the genes encoding the 13 polypeptides, but also by the mutations affecting the 22 tRNA. These specific tRNA diseases lead to severe disorders causing stroke, acidosis, blindness, and muscle weakness.[27,30,31]

Nutrition management of mitochondrial diseases has not been very successful. Such treatment involves antioxidants, docosahexaenoic acid (DHA), and mitochondrial "cocktails" containing riboflavin, coenzyme Q_{10}, vitamin K, vitamin C, and vitamin E.

Mutations

The basis of genetic variation is mutations or changes in DNA sequence.[32,33] Any error in the coding sequence of a gene may result in an abnormal protein or enzyme. Many mutations are silent or benign while others lead to variable severity of a defect. There are several types of mutations. A point mutation involves a single base pair change, and if there is no change in the amino acid code, it is a silent mutation. If one amino acid changes, it is a "missense" mutation. A point mutation could also produce a stop codon that terminates the code prematurely, leading to a "nonsense" mutation. Mutations that border an exon are called intervening sequence (IVS) mutations and can also affect the translation of the exon. In some IVS mutations, part of the message is translated by "skipping" that area, and the result can be a severe or mild mutation.[11,34,35]

Other types of mutations are deletions or insertions of one or more base pairs. Deletions or insertions usually disrupt the normal codes and synthesis of protein. If the deletion or insertion is not a multiple of three, a frameshift occurs. This means that all downstream codons are altered and the protein changes greatly. Even deletion of a single triplet can lead to a severe disease. For example, deletion of phenylalanine, ΔF508, in cystic fibrosis where phenylalanine is deleted results in a protein with severely reduced function.[36]

Another type of mutation can change the tandem repeat DNA sequences.[37,38] Some genes contain a long series of identical triplet repeats before the coding area of the gene. The number of repeats can expand during meiosis, with a higher number of expanded repeats correlating to a more severe phenotype. In fragile X the noncoding repeats are associated with hypermethylation. The hypermethylation is associated with loss of function. In other diseases, the loss of function can be attributed to different mechanisms, such as toxic effect or interference with transcription. Friedreich's ataxia is an example of a loss of function through transcriptional interference. Some mutations can be classified as causing gain of function. In such mutations the mutant enzyme abnormally increases the normal function or may lead to a gene that can perform more than one function. The new function interferes with the normal enzyme activity. This in turn can lead to over expression or inappropriate expression of a gene product. Such proteins may interfere with folding, transport, or degradation of proteins.[39]

Some mutations can cause a novel property to the synthesized protein without altering the function. For example, in sickle-cell anemia the protein still carries oxygen, but the mutation leads to deformed red cells caused by altered solubility of hemoglobin S.

Finally, some mutations can cause abnormal expression over time. These include cancer-causing genes, oncogenes, which normally regulate cell proliferation. If these genes are expressed in adults or in cells in which they are not supposed to be expressed, they may lead to cancer.

It is important to realize that a single gene does not function independently, but it interacts with other genes. A phenotype is a result of such interaction.

Polymorphism

The human genome is derived from a small number of persons and it is not expected to be identical for all individuals. Different copies of a gene are called alleles. Approximately 2% of the population have polymorphic alleles. Such alleles differ by a single nucleotide polymorphism (SNP).[21,40,41,42] The SNP usually does not change the overall activity of protein, but may cause slight differences compared to the normal protein. Such changes in the genome are considered polymorphic. Polymorphism of the enzyme methylene tetrahydrofolate reductase (MTHFR) is an example.[43,44] Certain polymorphic mutations in MTHFR can lead to elevated blood homocysteine concentrations that may lead to the tendency to increase blood coagulation and coronary artery disease, as reviewed by Trabetti.[45] Such a polymorphism is important to recognize, because high folate intake can reduce the risk for coronary heart disease by decreasing plasma homocysteine concentrations in susceptible individuals. MTHFR polymorphism may also be linked to increased incidence of neural tube defects. In susceptible pregnancies with increased risk for neural tube defects, high doses of folate are indicated. Polymorphic genes are important to recognize in prevention of serious diseases such as heart disease, diabetes, and stroke.

Genotype/Phenotype

Genotype is the genetic constitution of an individual cell or organism.[32] There are two alleles for every gene, at a specific location (locus) on a chromosome. If the alleles code for the same amino acids on a gene at a specific site, the person is homozygous, and if the alleles code for different amino acids at a specific site, the person is heterozygous.

The phenotype is the physical and metabolic expression of the genotype and includes the observed structural, biochemical, and physiological characteristics of an individual. In the last decade there has been an increase in the identification of mutations in many IMDs and how they correlate to the phenotype. In most cases genotype gives an idea how the phenotype will respond to a specific treatment, although there are individual variations. There can be gene modifiers that may alter an expected phenotype. Environmental factors and the metabolic make up of the individual play a role in the severity of the disease.

Characterization of mutations is commonly used to determine specific mutations causing disease. Such mutations are important in defining the genotype as it correlates to the phenotype. Some mutations cause total deficiency of an enzyme that leads to severe disease. Milder mutations result in a mildly affected phenotype. It is common to determine the residual activity of a mutant enzyme so that the phenotype can be quantitatively defined. A severe mutation expresses no enzyme activity, an intermediate mutation expresses 1 to 5% of the enzyme activity, and a mild mutation expresses 25% or more enzyme activity. Many patients are heterogeneous for a gene and have combinations of gene mutations; for example, a severe mutation with a mild mutation. There is no need to express the mutant genes and determine residual enzyme activity in all patients. There are data banks that contain information for a large number of diseases and their mutations.[46-51]

Gene defects sometimes involve large deletions that may involve adjacent genes. For example, glycerol kinase deficiency is X-linked and localized on the short arm of the chromosome, in close proximity to Duchenne muscular dystrophy (DMD) and congenital adrenal hypoplasia.[52-54] Sometimes patients with glycerol kinase deficiency also have severe muscular dystrophy. In these cases the genotype gives a clear phenotype.

The genotype/phenotype correlation is also important in predicting response to nutrition or coenzyme treatment in patients with an IMD.

Nomenclature of Mutations

Enzymes are synthesized using the amino acids coded by the exons with the introns excised. The amino acids in the protein are indicated by numbers, starting with methionine as the first amino acid and ending with the number of the last amino acid.[55] The number for each amino acid indicates its position on the polypeptide chain and each amino acid is abbreviated as a single letter (see Table 1.1).[23] When reading mutations, the first letter denotes the amino acid in the original protein and the last letter indicates the amino acid in the mutant protein. Using examples from PKU,[56,57] a common severe mutation is R408W, which means that arginine (R) in position 408 changed to tryptophan (W). A mild PKU mutation is Y414C. This means that tyrosine (Y) at amino acid 414 changed to cysteine (C). Mutations in the intronic regions of the gene are noted as IVS, for intervening sequence or intron. These types of mutations are named by the number of the intron, such as IVS12 meaning intron number 12. Minor deletions are usually 1 to 4 base pairs. For example, P211fsdel(c) is a frameshift mutation that occurs following the triplet coding for proline at amino acid number 211 of the polypeptide. In this case the base pair cytosine in the next triplet is deleted and the triplet concensus is disrupted, causing a frameshift (fs). After one base pair is deleted, the "reading frame" changes and amino acids after the proline will be different from the original protein. Another type of mutation involves stopping the code. For example, R111X means that arginine (R) at amino acid number 111 changed to a termination codon (X), which stops the production of the enzyme prematurely. The nomenclature for other diseases follows a similar pattern.

Table 1.1 ***Abbreviations Used for Amino Acids***

A	Alanine	N	Asparagine
B	Asparagine or aspartic acid	O	Glutamine
C	Cysteine	P	Proline
D	Aspartic acid	Q	Glutamine
E	Glutamic acid	R	Arginine
F	Phenylalanine	S	Serine
G	Glycine	T	Threonine
H	Histidine	V	Valine
I	Isoleucine	W	Tryptophan
K	Lysine	X	Termination codon
L	Leucine	Y	Tyrosine
M	Methionine	Z	Glutamine or glutamic acid

Determining the genotype in patients with an IMD is a common practice. There are data banks containing the mutations for various disorders with the predicted phenotype. In diseases such as galactosemia experience shows that the mild Duarte mutation N314D, where asparagine (N) is substituted by aspartic acid (D), is more prevalent than any of the classic galactosemia mutations. Similar situations have been found with biotinidase and ornithine transcarbamylase deficiency (OTC). Therefore, it is recommended to genotype inborn errors of metabolism when possible.

Chromosomal Disorders

Humans have 46 chromosomes, 22 pairs of each autosome, and 1 pair of sex chromosomes: XY for males and XX for females.[35] Chromosomes are long sequences of DNA containing hundreds or thousands of genes. Each chromosome carries a number of specific genes, and together with the mitochondrial DNA make up the human genome. Chromosomal defects involve many genes, and so the phenotype is rather complex. Examples include an extra chromosome, such as trisomy 21, Down's syndrome, or deletion of a chromosome in Turner syndrome, XO. However, there are some small chromosomal changes that yield interesting phenotypes. Such chromosomal defects include missing a piece or pieces of a chromosome, translocation of one piece of a chromosome to another chromosome, and ring formation or mosaicism, where only some of the cells are affected. Many of these changes are sporadic, but some can be inherited.

The smaller defects in chromosomes can be determined using fluorescent in situ hybridization (FISH). Copies of genes that are affected light up and can be counted under the microscope, such that small deletions or duplications can be detected.

Some of the genetic material may be imprinted depending on whether it comes from the mother or father. Prader–Willi syndrome is caused by paternal imprinting, while the same area on the chromosome when imprinted by the mother causes Angelman syndrome.[58] In such cases if the chromosome's origin is the father, the baby will have Prader–Willi syndrome. However, if the same chromosome comes from the mother, the baby will have Angelman syndrome.

Patterns of Inheritance

There are three patterns of inheritance: autosomal recessive, autosomal dominant, and X-linked. Common inborn errors of metabolism are usually single gene defects, inherited as an autosomal recessive condition.[35] A few are inherited as X-linked conditions such as OTC deficiency. Autosomal dominant inborn errors often involve structural proteins such as osteogenesis imperfecta.

Autosomal defects are on chromosomes other than the sex chromosome. In order to have an autosomal recessive disease, two defective copies of the mutant gene need to be inherited for the disease to be expressed. The affected person gets one mutant gene from the mother and one from the father. The parents are obligate heterozygotes (carriers) for the condition. Affected offspring can be homozygous for the recessive mutant allele or compound heterozygote for two different mutant alleles. Couples who are carriers for the mutant allele have a 25% risk of an affected offspring with each pregnancy. Unaffected siblings have a 66% chance of carrying the mutant allele.

In autosomal dominant disorders, only one copy of the mutant allele is needed to inherit a disorder. The mutant allele could come from either the mother or the father. There is a 50% chance of an affected offspring with each pregnancy. The pedigree shows vertical transmission with about half of the individuals being affected in each generation. Male-to-male transmission rules out X-linked inheritance.[35] Unaffected individuals do not carry the mutant allele. Occasionally an autosomal dominant mutation is the result of a germ line mutation. In such cases both parents have normal phenotypes and one of the parents has a mutation in his or her reproductive system (germ line). Dominant mutations may also occur spontaneously with both parents being normal.

Autosomal dominant diseases in a homozygous state can be severe or lethal. Hypercholesterolemia is autosomal dominant and the heterozygous individual is symptomatic, but homozygous individuals have more severe disease and often die from myocardial infarction in early adult life.

X-linked disorders occur due to mutations of genes on the X sex chromosome. Females have two X chromosomes and males have one X and one Y chromosome. X-linked recessive single gene defects affect men, while women are carriers of the mutant allele. Males who inherit the mutant allele are affected. The pedigree shows only affected males and no male-to-male transmission. All females from an affected male are obligate carriers of the mutant allele.[35]

X-linked recessive disorders can sometimes be found in females because of the Lyon hypothesis.[59,60] Early in embryogenesis one of the X chromosomes is inactivated and the other forms a Barr body. The process is random, but once a cell inactivates one X chromosome all the descendants from that cell have the same inactive X chromosome. The process of X-inactivation follows a pattern of a bell-shaped curve. At the top of the curve is the X-inactivation of the mutant allele to the X-inactivation of the normal allele of 50:50. As one follows the curve the randomization process can be skewed in as many as 5 to 10% of women, where a pattern of 80:20 or greater means that there is 80% or more of the mutant alleles present. In these cases the X-linked recessive trait will be observed in those females. The phenotype in the females is usually milder than in the affected males because some of the X chromosomes have the normal gene allele.

X-linked dominant conditions occur with one copy of the X chromosome. Women or men can have the disease. In women the normal X chromosome can modify the disease so that the disease is often milder in females than in males. Some X-linked dominant diseases are often lethal in males, such as Aicardi syndrome.[35]

Multigenic and Multifactorial Inheritance

Multigenic diseases are diseases affected by multiple genes and their interaction with environmental factors. There could be two or more single genes that contribute to a phenotype. Various environmental exposures may also affect the phenotype. Most diseases inherited as a Mendelian trait do not show precise genotype/phenotype correlation and are affected by the genome of the entire individual. Even phenylketonuria is a complex monogenic disorder.[61] There is interfamilial variability of diseases with the same genotype.[62] There are modifier genes in an individual that modify the genotype, producing a milder or more severe phenotype.[63]

Congenital defects such as cleft lip and palate, neural tube defects, cardiac defects, and metabolic disorders such as diabetes, coronary artery disease, and other common disorders, are inherited in a multifactorial manner. The genetic factors for these disorders are not clear. The environmental factors are partially known and can be ameliorated. For example, phenylalanine during pregnancy in a woman with PKU can act as a teratogen. Folate may prevent neural tube defects. Control of obesity may reduce the risk of diabetes. Environmental factors may also influence mitochondrial disorders.[33]

Genetics and Inherited Metabolic Disorders

Inborn errors of metabolism are usually diagnosed by excessive amounts of intermediary metabolites caused by an enzyme deficiency. Often patients with an IMD develop symptoms that are not specific to any disease, such as failure to thrive, seizures, or developmental delay. During a medical work up diseases can be identified through abnormal metabolites. The high concentration of metabolites that normally exist in trace amounts indicates a block in the natural flow of metabolic processes, resulting in a disease.

Phenylketonuria was initially recognized by abnormally high concentrations of phenylketones in the urine.[64] It took some time for the enzyme deficiency that causes PKU to be identified.[65] The understanding of the enzyme defect and that the disease was caused by excessive phenylalanine, not the phenylketones, led Dr. H. Bickel in 1953 to treat PKU by restricting the substrate, phenylalanine.[14] In order for nutrition management to prevent mental deterioration in PKU, detection of the disease was needed at an early age. Guthrie developed a bacterial inhibition assay that required a drop of blood on filter paper from newborn infants, which effectively identified babies with elevated plasma phenylalanine concentrations early in life.[15] This was a cost-effective method of diagnosing PKU, and soon testing for other diseases using the same blood spot was developed and used throughout the United States. Currently, all states screen for IMDs, but each state specifies the conditions for which they screen.

Newer technology using automated tandem mass spectroscopy (MS/MS) for mass screening of newborns for diseases was introduced in 1995 for rapid diagnosis of maple syrup urine disease (MSUD).[66] This method was adopted in Europe and the United States, and newborn screening for IMDs using the same blood on filter paper samples was accepted by state newborn screening programs through this country.[66-73] This method analyzes the intermediary metabolites and not the enzyme deficiency. The method is fast and allows screening of many samples in a short period of time. The method is very precise, but the interpretation is complex and may require input from the metabolic clinician.

The amino acid disorders that can be detected by the MS/MS method are shown in Table 1.2.[74] The amino acid disorders are all autosomal recessive. The method is not able to detect with certainty non-ketotic hyperglycinemia. This should be kept in mind for a patient with seizures and a normal newborn screen. The treatment of patients with these amino acid disorders involves nutrition management.

Organic acid disorders that are identified by MS/MS are indicated in Table 1.3. Most of these conditions are inherited as autosomal recessive disorders. Many of the organic acid disorders present with feeding problems, seizures, metabolic acidosis, and lethargy. Some conditions may be mild and could be caused by an asymptomatic mother who is homozygous for a defect such as 3-methylcrotonyl-CoA carboxylase deficiency. If the baby is doing well, it is important to check the mother for this condition. Other diseases can be severe and require prompt attention. A minor illness can cause decompensation in patients with organic acid defects. Most of the organic acid disorders require nutrition management.

Fatty acid oxidation disorders that can be detected by MS/MS are shown in Table 1.4. Most of the fatty acid disorders are inherited as autosomal recessive diseases. In this table the defective enzymes are noted, although the MS/MS analyzes the analytes in the blood. Most fatty acid oxidation defects present with symptoms such as hypoketotic hypoglycemia, muscle weakness, and seizures; some have cardiomyopathy. Most of these conditions require dietary alterations.

Table 1.2 ***Amino Acid Disorders That Can Be Detected Using Tandem Mass Spectroscopy (MS/MS) for Newborn Screening***

Argininemia
Argininosuccinic aciduria (ASA)
Citrullinemia
Homocystinuria (HCY)
Hypermethioninemia (HCY/MET)
Maple syrup urine disease (MSUD)
Phenylketonuria (PKU)
Tetrahydrobiopterin (BH_4) defects
Tyrosinemia

Table 1.3 ***Organic Acid Disorders Detected by Tandem Mass Spectrometry (MS/MS) in Newborn Screening Programs***

2-methyl-3-hydroxybutyric aciduria
2-methyl butyryl-CoA dehydrogenase deficiency
3-methylcrotonyl-CoA carboxylase deficiency
3-methylglutaconic aciduria
3-OH-3-CH_3 glutaric aciduria
β-ketothiolase deficiency
Glutaric acidemia type I
Isobutyryl-CoA dehydrogenase deficiency
Isovaleric acidemia
Malonic acidemia
Methylmalonic acidemia, mutase, Cbl A, B, C, D
Multiple carboxylase deficiency
Propionic acidemia

Table 1.4 ***Fatty Acid Oxidation Disorders Detected in Newborn Screening With Tandem Mass Spectrometry (MS/MS)***

Carnitine acylcarnitine translocase deficiency
Carnitine palmitoyltransferase IA deficiency
Carnitine palmitoyltransferase II deficiency
Carnitine uptake defect
Dienoyl-CoA reductase deficiency
Glutaric acidemia type II
Long-chain L-3-OH-acyl-CoA dehydrogenase deficiency
Medium-chain acyl-CoA dehydrogenase deficiency (MCAD)
Medium-chain ketoacyl-CoA thiolase deficiency
Medium/short-chain L-3-OH acyl-CoA dehydrogenase deficiency
Short-chain acyl-CoA dehydrogenase deficiency
Trifunctional protein deficiency
Very long-chain acyl-CoA dehydrogenase deficiency

Other disorders that are screened for in the newborn period by methods other than MS/MS are shown in Table 1.5. Patients with galactosemia, biotinidase deficiency, and cystic fibrosis all require nutrition management.

Infants who have abnormal newborn screening are referred to a medical specialist who confirms the diagnosis and begins proper therapy.[75] Treatment strategies vary with each disease and include: (1) restriction of substrate, (2) vitamin or coenzyme supplementation to enhance residual enzyme activity or supply a missing coenzyme caused by recycling failure, (3) supplementation of a deficient product, or (4) conjugation of a toxic metabolite.

Mutations causing IMDs appear in different frequency in different populations. For example, PKU is more common among Northern Europeans, Irish, Scots, and also among those from Turkey and Iran.[11,76] Ethnic background and migration patterns influence the gene pool. Sometimes certain mutations can be assigned to different ethnic groups. The IMDs are rare, occurring from 1 in 10,000 births to 1 in 300,000 births. Most IMDs are inherited as autosomal recessive traits. It is estimated that everyone has several defective genes; however, in order to produce an affected offspring both parents must carry the same gene defect and both parents would need to pass the affected gene to the offspring.

Genetic defects on the X chromosome can be inherited as dominant or recessive disorders. An example of an X-linked dominant disorder is OTC deficiency. This disease is a urea cycle defect and leads to a deficiency of compounds needed to keep the urea cycle recirculating, and blood ammonia builds up to toxic concentrations. This disease is often lethal for males, while females have milder expressivity of the disease because they have one normal X chromosome. The treatment of this disease involves restriction of substrate by limiting protein. In addition, replacement of deficient end products are given in the form of citrulline and arginine. Finally, conjugation of toxic end products is used by giving sodium benzoate to bind glycine and phenylacetic or phenylbutyric acids to bind glutamine for elimination of nitrogen waste products.

Table 1.5 ***Other IMDs Screened by Newborn Screening Programs With Methods Other Than Tandem Mass Spectrometry (MS/MS)***

Hemoglobin disorders	• Sickle-cell anemia • β-thalassemia
Endocrine disorders	• Congenital adrenal hyperplasia • Congenital hypothyroidism
Other disorders	• Galactosemia (GALT) • Biotinidase deficiency • Cystic fibrosis (CF)

There is interest in IMDs that respond to vitamin supplementation. They are usually coenzymes for the enzyme that is impaired in an IMD. The vitamin or coenzyme acts as a chaperone in most cases to increase the activity of the defective enzyme. The enzyme biotinidase recycles biotin and responds to pharmacological doses of biotin. In cases of multiple carboxylase deficiency, biotin improves the activity of the deficient enzyme. Tetrahydrobiopterin (BH_4), a coenzyme in the hydroxylation reaction of phenylalanine to tyrosine, is sometimes used as an adjunct to dietary treatment for PKU. In some patients BH_4 results in a decline in blood phenylalanine concentration. The genotype of a patient can be helpful in predicting which patients with PKU will respond to BH_4 favorably.

Many patients with an IMD receive treatment that involves dietary alterations or supplementation. Most of the treatable IMDs are followed by measuring the response of affected intermediary metabolites. In this volume there is a detailed description of many categories of IMDs that includes approaches for diagnosis, treatment, and follow up of the condition.

CONCLUSION

The field of IMDs has expanded remarkably in the last two decades because of improved technology in testing for analytes and genotyping. Many diseases are well characterized at the enzyme and gene level. The new, improved methods for detection of IMDs have led to a better understanding of many IMDs and their spectrum of expression. The technology of detection is improving, and the number of diseases detected is rising. Ideas of gene, stem cell, and enzyme therapy are entering the field of IMDs. Newborn screening programs can help establish protocols for new treatments as the diagnoses of IMDs advance.

REFERENCES

1. Garrod AE. The incidence of alkaptonuria: a study in chemical individuality. *Lancet*. 1902;2:1616–1620.
2. Garrod AE. The Croonian lectures on inborn errors of metabolism. *Lancet*. 1908; 2:73–79.
3. Garrod AE. *Inborn Errors of Metabolism*. 2nd ed. London, England: Oxford University Press; 1923.
4. Johannsen W. The genotype concept of heredity. *Am Nat*. 1911;45:129–159.
5. Beadle GW, Tatum EL. Genetic control of biochemical reactions in *Neurospora*. *Proc Natl Acad Sci USA*. 1941;27:499–506.
6. Tatum EL. A case history of biological research. *Science*. 1959;129:1711–1715.
7. Pauling L, Itano HA, Singer SJ, Wells IC. Sickle cell anemia: a molecular disease. *Science*. 1949;110:543–548.

8. Ingram VM. A specific chemical difference between globins of normal human and sickle cell anemia haemoglobin. *Nature*. 1957;178:792–794.
9. Watson JD, Crick FH. Molecular structure of nucleic acids; a structure for deoxyribose nucleic acid. *Nature*. 1953;171:737–738.
10. McCusick VA, Francomano CA, Antonarakis SE, et al. *McCusick's Mendelian Inheritance in Man: A Catalog of Human Genes and Genetic Disorders*. Baltimore, MD: Johns Hopkins University Press; 1998.
11. Beaudet AL, Scriver CR, Sly WS, et al. Genetics and biochemisty of variant human phenotypes. In: Scriver CR, Beaudet AL, Sly WS, Valle D, eds. *The Metabolic and Molecular Bases of Inherited Disease*. 6th ed. New York, NY: McGraw-Hill; 1989:3–163.
12. Scriver CR, Beaudet AL, Sly WS, Valle D, eds. *The Metabolic and Molecular Bases of Inherited Disease*. 8th ed. New York, NY: McGraw-Hill; 2001.
13. Rosenberg RN, Prusiner SB, DiMauro S, Barchi RL, Nestler EJ, eds. *The Molecular and Genetic Basis of Neurologic and Psychiatric Disease*. 3rd ed. Philadelphia, PA: Butterworth-Heinemann; 2003:91–100.
14. Bickel H, Gerrard AJ, Hickman EM. Influence of phenylalanine intake on phenylketonuria. *Lancet*. 1953;265:812–813.
15. Guthrie R, Susi A. A simple phenylalanine method for determining phenylketonuria in large populations of newborn infants. *Pediatrics*. 1963;14:338–343.
16. Chace DH, Naylor EW. Expansion of newborn screening programs using automated tandem mass spectrometry. *MRDD Research Reviews*. 1999;5:150–154.
17. Lander ES, Linton LM, Birren B, et al. Initial sequencing and analysis of the human genome. *Nature*. 2001;409:860–921.
18. Collins FS, Patrinos A, Jordan E, Chakravarti A, Geteland R, Walters L. New goals for the U.S. Human Genome project: 1998–2003. *Science*. 1998;282:682–689.
19. Gottgens B, Barton LM, Chapman MA, et al. Transcriptional regulation of the stem cell leukemia gene (SCL)—comparative analysis of five vertebrate SCL loci. *Genome Res*. 2002;12:749–759.
20. Pennacchio LA, Rubin EM. Genomic strategies to identify mammalian regulatory sequences. *Nat Rev Genet*. 2001;2:100–109.
21. Nussbaum RL. The human genome project. In: Rosenberg RN, Prusiner SB, DiMauro S, Barchi RL, Nestler EJ, eds. *The Molecular and Genetic Basis of Neurologic and Psychiatric Disease*. 3rd ed. Philadelphia, PA: Butterworth-Heinemann; 2003: 91–100.
22. Schon EA. The mitochondrial genome. In: Rosenberg RN, Prusiner SB, DiMauro S, Barchi RL, Nestler EJ, eds. *The Molecular and Genetic Basis of Neurologic and Psychiatric Disease*. 3rd ed. Philadelphia, PA: Butterworth-Heinemann; 2003: 179–187.
23. Stryer L. *Biochemistry*. 3rd ed. New York, NY: W. H. Freeman; 1988.
24. Watkins JD, Hopkins NH, Roberts JW, Steitz JA, Weiner AM. *Molecular Biology of the Gene*. Menlo Park, CA: Benjamin/Cummings; 1987.
25. Nirenberg M. Historical review: deciphering the genetic code—a personal account. *Trends Biochem Sci*. 2004;29:46–54.
26. Anderson S, Bankier AT, Barrell BG, et al. Sequence and organization of the human mitochondrial genome. *Nature*. 1981;290:457–465.
27. DiMauro S, Bonilla E. Mitochondrial disorders due to mutations in the mitochondrial genome. In: Rosenberg RN, Prusiner SB, DiMauro S, Barchi RL, Nestler EJ, eds. *The Molecular and Genetic Basis of Neurologic and Psychiatric Disease*. 3rd ed. Philadelphia, PA: Butterworth-Heinemann; 2003:189–195.

28. Hirano M. Mitochondrial disorders due to mutations in the nuclear genome. In: Rosenberg RN, Prusiner SB, DiMauro S, Barchi RL, Nestler EJ, eds. *The Molecular and Genetic Basis of Neurologic and Psychiatric Disease*. 3rd ed. Philadelphia, PA: Butterworth-Heinemann; 2003:197–204.
29. Wallace DC. Pathophysiology of mitochondrial disease as illuminated by animal models. In: Schapira AHV, DiMauro S, eds. *Mitochondrial Disorders in Neurology*. Boston, MA: Butterworth-Heinemann; 2002:175–212.
30. Servidei S. Mitochondrial encephalomyopathies: gene mutation. *Neuromusc Disord*. 2002;12:101–110.
31. Smeitick J, van den Heuvel L, DiMauro S. The genetics and pathology of oxidative phosphorylation. *Nat Rev Genet*. 2001;2:342–352.
32. Hoyme HE. The molecular basis of genetic disorders. In: Behrman RE, Kliegman RM, Jenson HB, eds. *Nelson Textbook of Pediatrics*. 17th ed. Philadelphia, PA: Saunders; 2004:367–371.
33. Lupski JR, Zoghbi HY. Molecular genetics and neurological disease: an introduction. In: Rosenbeg RN, Prusiner SB, DiMauro S, Barchi RL, eds. *The Molecular and Genetic Basis of Neurological Disease*. 2nd ed. Boston, MA: Butterworth-Heinemann; 1997:3–22.
34. Lanpher B, Brunetti-Pierri N, Lee B. Inborn errors of metabolism: the flux from Mendelian to complex diseases. *Nat Rev Genet*. 2006;7:449–460.
35. Inoue K, Lupski JR. Mendelian, nonmendelian multigenic inheritance and complex traits. In: Rosenberg RN, Prusiner SB, DiMauro S, Barchi RL, Nestler EJ, eds. *The Molecular and Genetic Basis of Neurologic and Psychiatric Disease*. 3rd ed. Philadelphia, PA: Butterworth-Heinemann; 2003:33–50.
36. The CF Genotype-Phenotype Consortium. Correlation between genotype and phenotype in patients with cystic fibrosis. *N Engl J Med*. 1993;329:1308–1313.
37. Brandt VL, Zoghbi HY. Triplet repeat disease: general concepts and mechanisms of disease. In: Rosenberg RN, Prusiner SB, DiMauro S, Barchi RL, Nestler EJ, eds. *The Molecular and Genetic Basis of Neurologic and Psychiatric Disease*. 3rd ed. Philadelphia, PA: Butterworth-Heinemann; 2003:3–11.
38. Pearson CF, Sinden RR. Trinucleotide repeat DNA structures: dynamic mutations from dynamic DNA. *Curr Opin Struct Biol*. 1998;8:321–330.
39. Liquori CL, Ricker K, Moseley ML, et al. Myotonic dystrophy type 2 caused by a CCTG expansion in intron 1 of ZNF9. *Science*. 2001;293(5531):864–867.
40. Stoneking M. Single nucleotide polymorphism: from the evolutionary past. *Nature*. 2001;409:821–822.
41. Sachidanandam R, Weissman D, Schmidt SC, et al. A map of human genome sequence variation containing 1.42 million single nucleotide polymorphisms. *Nature*. 2001;409:928–933.
42. Holden AL. The SNP consortium: summary of a private consortium effort to develop an applied map of the human genome. *Biotechniques*. 2002;26:S22–S24.
43. Rady PL, Szucs S, Grady J, et al. Genetic polymorphisms of methylenetetrahydrofolate reductase (MTHFR) and methionine synthase reductase (MTRR) in ethnic populations in Texas; a report of a novel MTHFR polymorphic site, G1793A. *Am J Med Genet*. 2002;107:162–168.
44. Rady PL, Tyring SK, Hudnall SD, et al. Methylenetetrahydrofolate reductase (MTHFR): the incidence of mutations C677T and A1298C in the Ashkenazi Jewish population. *Am J Med Genet*. 1999;86:380–384.
45. Trabetti E. Homocysteine, MTHFR gene polymorphisms, and cardio-cerebrovascular risk. *J Appl Genet*. 2008;49:267–282.

46. National Center for Biotechnology Information (NCBI). U.S. National Library of Medicine. Available at http://www.ncbi.nlm.nih.gov/Genbank/index.html. Accessed August 7, 2008.
47. Basic Local Alignment Search Tool (Blast) NCBI. Available at http://blast.ncbi.nlm.nih.gov/Blast.cgi. Accessed August 7, 2008.
48. Hamosh A. McKusick's Online Mendelian Inheritance in Man. OMIM. 2002. Available at http://www.ncbi.nlm.gov/OMIM. Accessed August 7, 2008.
49. Layla J. The Frequency of Inherited Disorders Database (FIDD). University of Wales College of Medicine, Cardiff. Available at http://archive.uwcm.ac.uk/uwcm/mg/fidd/index.html. Accessed August 7, 2008.
50. HUGO, Human Genome Organisation. Available at http://www.hugo-international.org. Accessed August 7, 2008.
51. Scriver CR, Waters PJ, Sarkissian C, et al. PAHdb: a locus-specific knowledgebase. *Hum Mutat* 2000;15:99–104.
52. McCabe ER, Seltzer WK. Glycerol kinase deficiency: compartmental considerations regarding pathogenesis and clinical heterogeneity. *Adv Exp Med Biol.* 1986; 194:481–493.
53. Wise JE, Matalon R, Morgan AM, McCabe ERB. Phenotypic features of patients with congenital adrenal hypoplasia and glycerol kinase deficiency. *Am J Dis Child.* 1987;141:744–747.
54. Renier WO, Nabben FAE, Hustinx TWJ, et al. Congenital adrenal hypoplasia, progressive muscular dystrophy and severe mental retardation, in association with glycerol kinase deficiency, in male sibs. *Clin Genet.* 1983;24:243–251.
55. Anronarakis SE. Recommendations for a nomenclature system for human gene mutations. Nomenclature Working Group. *Hum Mutat.* 1998;11:1–3.
56. Eisensmith RC, Woo SLC. Molecular basis of phenylketonuria and related hyperphenylalaninemias: mutations and polymorphisms in the human phenylalanine hydroxylase gene. *Hum Mutat.* 1992;1:13–23.
57. Guldberg P, Levy HL, Hanley WB, et al. Phenylalanine hydroxylase gene mutations in the United States: report from the Maternal PKU Collaborative Study. *Am J Hum Genet.* 1996;59:84–94.
58. Hall J. Genetic imprinting: review and relevance to human diseases. *Am J Hum Genet.* 1990;46:857–873.
59. Lyon MF. Lyonisation of the X chromosome. *Lancet.* 1963;2:1120–1121.
60. Lyon MF. Gene action in the X-chromosome of the mouse. *Nature.* 1961;190: 372–373.
61. Scriver CR, Waters PJ. Monogenic traits are not simple: lessons from phenylketonuria. *Trends Genet.* 1999;15:267–272.
62. Dipple KM, McCabe ER. Phenotypes of patients with "simple" Mendelian disorders are complex traits: thresholds, modifiers, and systems dynamics. *Am J Hum Genet.* 2000;66:1729–1735.
63. Dipple KM, McCabe ER. Modifier genes convert "simple" Mendelian disorders to complex traits. *Mol Genet Metab.* 2000;71:43–50.
64. Folling A. The original detection of phenylketonuria. In: Bickel H, Hudson FP, Woolf LI, eds. *Phenylketonuria and Some Other Inborn Errors of Amino Acid Metabolism.* Stuttgart, Germany: Georg Thieme Verlag; 1971:1–3.
65. Jervis GA. Phenylpyruvic oligophrenia deficiency of phenylalanine-oxidizing system. *Proc Soc Exp Biol Med.* 1953; 82[3]:514–515.

66. Chace DH, Hillman SL, Millington DS, Kahler SG, Roe CR, Naylor EW. Rapid diagnosis of maple syrup urine disease in blood spots from newborns by tandem mass spectrometry. *Clin Chem.* 1995;41:62–68.
67. Naylor EW, Chace DH. Automated tandem mass spectroscopy for mass newborn screening for disorders in fatty acid, organic acid and amino acid metabolism. *J Child Neurol.* 1999;14:S4–S8.
68. Simonsen H. Screening of newborns for inborn errors of metabolism by tandem mass spectrometry. *Ugeskr Laeger.* 2002;164:5607–5612.
69. Wilcken B, Wiley V, Hammond J, Carpenter K. Screening newborns for inborn errors of metabolism by tandem mass spectrometry. *N Engl J Med.* 2003;348: 2304–2312.
70. Schulze A, Linder M, Kohlmuller D, Olgemoller K, Mayatepek E, Hoffmann GF. Expanded newborn screening for inborn errors of metabolism by electrospray ionization-tandem mass spectrometry: results, outcome and implications. *Pediatr.* 2003;111:1399–1406.
71. Pandor A, Eastham J, Beverley C, Chilcott J, Paisley S. Clinical effectiveness and cost-effectiveness of neonatal screening for inborn errors of metabolism using tandem mass spectrometry: a systematic review. *Health Technol Assess.* 2004;12:1–121.
72. Frazier DM, Millington DS, McCandless SE, et al. The tandem mass spectrometry newborn screening experience in North Carolina: 1997–2005. *J Inherit Metab Dis.* 2006;29:76–85.
73. McCabe LL, McCabe ER. Expanded newborn screening: implications for genomic medicine. *Annu Rev Med.* 2008;59:163–75.
74. Michigan Department of Community Health. Newborn Screening Program. April 22, 2008. Available from: mdch-newbornscreening@michigan.gov. Accessed August 7, 2008.
75. American College of Medical Genetics (ACMG). Newborn Screening Act Sheets and Confirmatory Algorithms. March 22, 2006. Available from: Maternal and Child Health Bureau of the Health Resources and Services Administration. Available at: http://www.acmg.net/resources/policies/NBS/NBS-sections.htm. Accessed August 7, 2008.
76. Scriver CR, Kaufman S. Hyperphenylalaninemias: phenylalanine hydroxylase deficiency. In: Scriver CR, Beaudet AL, Sly WS, Valle D, eds. *The Metabolic and Molecular Bases of Inherited Disease*. 8th ed. New York, NY: McGraw-Hill; 2001:1667–1724.

Chapter 2

Newborn Screening by Mass Spectrometry

Dianne M. Frazier

INTRODUCTION

The contributions of several individuals, over the span of nearly three decades, have been recognized as dramatically improving the outcome of those patients born with phenylketonuria (PKU). They include Asbjörn Fölling, credited with discovering PKU in 1934,[1] George Jervis with describing the enzyme defect,[2] Horst Bickel with synthesizing the first phenylalanine (PHE)-free formula,[3] and Willard Centerwall with developing the ferric chloride diaper test.[4] It wasn't until Robert Guthrie developed a test that allowed presymptomatic screening of all newborns[4] that a significant impact on the devastation of untreated patients with PKU was realized. It is not surprising that many still erroneously refer to the much-expanded and complex newborn screening panel simply as the "the PKU test."

Guthrie's research began in an attempt to find a means to monitor the blood PHE concentrations in patients with PKU ingesting a PHE-restricted diet. He spotted serum from a venous blood sample on a filter paper disk and placed this on an agar culture gel embedded with a strain of bacteria that required PHE for growth. The zone of growth around the disk was proportional to the amount of PHE in the sample and could be quantified by comparing to controls of known concentrations.[5]

Although the PHE test Guthrie developed was simple and specific, his greatest contribution was the realization that the test could be done on blood that was spotted directly from a heel prick, placed on filter paper, and allowed to dry. Using a simple paper punch, he then had a small disk of dried whole blood that could be used in the same manner as the earlier serum samples. He next went on to determine if blood concentrations of PHE were sufficiently high in newborns with PKU to use this as a screening tool. In 1962, the U.S. Children's Bureau supported a pilot study utilizing Guthrie's technique. Test kits, each containing enough materials and directions for 500 tests, were prepared under Guthrie's supervision. It was hoped that by screening 400,000 infants approximately 40 patients with PKU would be detected. Within 2 years, 400,000 infants had been tested and 39 patients with PKU were detected and confirmed.[6] There were no known missed cases during this period. The majority of the infants screened in this pilot study were from Massachusetts because of the enthusiastic support of Dr. Robert MacCready, the State Laboratory Director.[7] In 1963, Massachusetts became the first state to mandate PKU screening for all newborns. By 1973, there were formal statutes in 34 states that mandated screening for PKU.[8,9]

After Guthrie's successful use of dried blood spots in the bacterial inhibition assay for PHE, he and other researchers developed similar assays to be used to screen for galactosemia and maple syrup urine disease (MSUD). The blood spots were also found to be suitable for newborn screening (NBS) using other testing modalities. The automated fluorometric assay for PHE, perfected for NBS by Hill et al.,[10] was followed by similar fluorometric tests for other analytes.[11] The dried blood spots also proved suitable for measuring other biological components (e.g., enzyme activity for galactose-1-PO_4 uridyltransferase-deficient galactosemia,[12] hormone levels for hypothyroidism,[13] hemoglobin variants for sickle-cell disease,[14] and DNA mutation analysis for cystic fibrosis[15]).

The most recent application using the dried blood spot sample in NBS is tandem mass spectrometry (MS/MS). The remainder of this chapter is devoted largely to MS/MS NBS: theoretical and technical issues of the methodology, interpretation of results, integration into the NBS paradigm, impact on the clinical outcome of newborns identified, and impact on the metabolic treatment team.

Tandem Mass Spectrometry

Mass Spectrometry

To be able to evaluate MS/MS as an appropriate tool for NBS, one needs to have a basic understanding of the technology. Mass spectrometry, the underlying technique for MS/MS, began as an analytical tool used by the petroleum industry in the 1940s. Its application to biological fluids was not appreciated until the mid-1980s. In the early 1990s, Millington and others were able to demonstrate that it could be used with blood spotted on filter paper.[16-18] In 1997, North Carolina became the first state to use the mass spectrometry technology in a statewide NBS program.[19]

A mass spectrometer identifies molecules by their characteristic mass-to-charge ratio (m/z). It does this by ionizing the compounds and separating them using a combination of magnetic and electric fields. The resulting spectrograph, produced by the detection system, displays the m/z on the x-axis and the relative abundance on the y-axis. Radio-labeled internal standards enable accurate interpretation by a trained spectrometrist or a sophisticated computer program. When a mass spectrometer is used in combination with methodologies that allow prior separation of the compounds being analyzed—such as gas chromatography—it can be a very powerful tool for determining both structure and molecular weight.

MS/MS utilizes two mass spectrometers, in tandem, to eliminate the necessity of having prior separation or purification steps when trying to identify compounds in complex biological specimens. A simple diagram is shown in Figure 2.1. Ionized molecules, created by a "soft ionization" method such as electrospray (that produces charged un-fragmented molecules) pass into the first mass spectrometer (MS1). There, these "parent ions" are separated by passing sequentially, based on their m/z ratio, through the electrical and magnetic fields into the reaction/collision cell. Within the reaction cell, these parent ions collide with an inert gas that causes them to fragment into their "daughter ions." The fragmentation pattern is unique for individual parent ions and is dependent on its molecular structure. The second mass spectrometer (MS2) separates the charged fragments, and the detection system records the spectrograph. Figure 2.2 shows the mass spectrograph for a simple molecule of water (parent ion) after fragmentation into its characteristic daughter ions.

The majority of molecules, or analytes, targeted in MS/MS NBS for inherited metabolic disorders (IMDs) are substrates that accumulate in abnormally high concentrations behind a blocked or partially blocked enzymatic

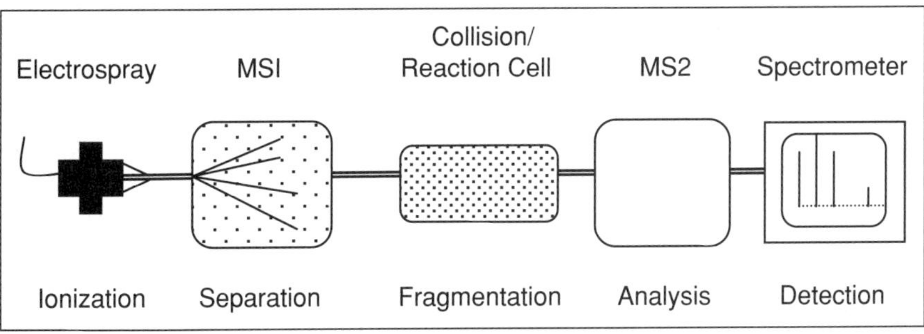

Figure 2.1 *Diagram of the Tandem Mass Spectrometry System as Used in Newborn Screening*

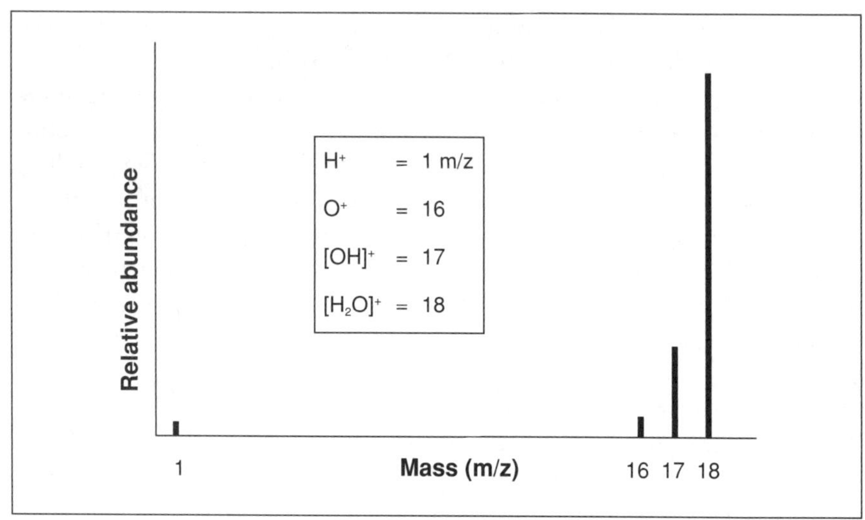

Figure 2.2 *Mass Spectrum of a Molecule of Water After Soft Ionization and Fragmentation*

step. For the aminoacidopathies, it may be the specific amino acid substrate of the nonfunctioning enzyme, such as PHE in PKU or an amino acid several enzymatic steps before the block such as methionine in cystathionine-β-synthase deficiency (homocystinuria or HCY). For the fatty acid oxidation disorders and organic acidemias, the analytes targeted are the acylcarnitine adjuncts of the accumulated respective fatty acid and organic acid intermediates. An example of the formation of the acylcarnitine intermediate in the organic acidemia, 3-methylcrotonyl-CoA carboxylase (3-MCC) deficiency is seen in Figure 2.3. A few analytes targeted for their abnormally low concentrations as poorly made products of a blocked enzymatic step occur. An example is an abnormally low concentration of free carnitine in carnitine plasma membrane transporter deficiency (also known as carnitine uptake deficiency or CUD).[20]

Laboratories differ in the exact protocols they use for processing their NBS samples for MS/MS analysis. A typical procedure begins with punching a one-eighth-inch circle from the blood spotted on the filter paper NBS card. Methanol is most often used to elute the blood from the paper. This eluate is dried, and then mixed with a solution containing both radio-labeled internal standards and a derivitizing agent to convert both acylcarnitines and amino acids to their butyl esters. Multi-well trays allow many samples, along with appropriate controls, to be processed at one time.

The electrospray ionization of the analytes in the sample produces charged ions that sequentially enter the reaction cell from MS1 based on their m/z ratio. In the reaction cell, they are fragmented. Each of the buty-

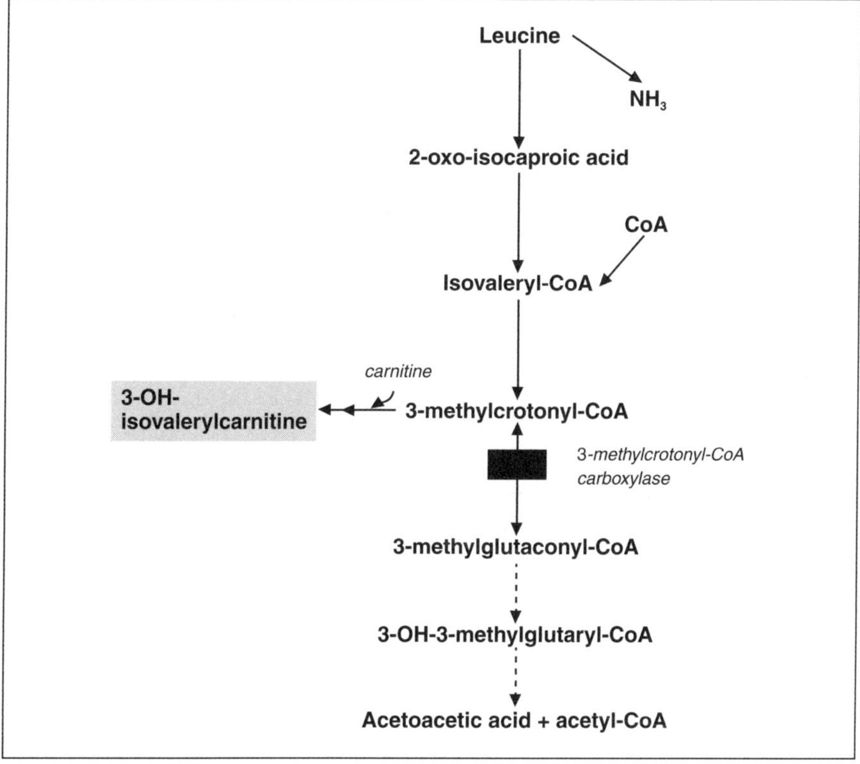

Figure 2.3 *Accumulation of Acylcarnitines in an Inborn Error of Organic Acid Metabolism: Formation of 3-Hydroxyisovaleryl Carnitine in 3-Methylcrotonyl-CoA Carboxylase Deficiency*

lated acylcarnitines produces a common fragment, or daughter ion, with an m/z ratio of 85. This fragment is the marker for carnitine intermediates. The MS2 is programmed to search for the 85 m/z markers. It then scans the charged (parent) molecules coming from MS1 over the range of 200 to 500 m/z, which includes the molecular weight of all the acylcarnitines of interest, and records those that produce the 85 m/z marker. The computer can generate a spectrum of the acylcarnitines that indicates the relative concentration of each. The spectra or "metabolic profiles" produced are suggestive of organic acidemias and fatty acid oxidation disorders where there is an accumulation of carnitine intermediates. The MS/MS spectrum of an NBS sample from a neonate with medium-chain acyl-CoA dehydrogenase deficiency is compared to that from an unaffected newborn in Figure 2.4.

For the butylated amino acids, the reaction cell produces an uncharged marker fragment of butyryl formate that has a neutral mass of 102. As with the acylcarnitines, the computer can generate a spectrum of the molecular

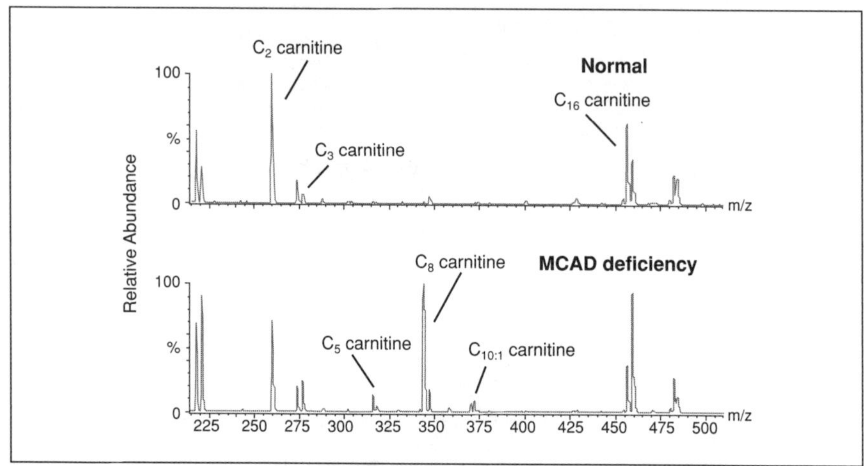

Figure 2.4 *MS/MS Spectrum of a Sample from an Infant With Normal Profile (top) and One From an Infant With Medium-Chain Acyl-CoA Dehydrogenase Deficiency (bottom)*

weight and relative abundance of each of the targeted amino acids along with the internal standards.

The MS/MS methodology analyzes the NBS samples for both amino acids and acylcarnitines from a single punched disk. The total time from sample injection to production of a spectrum is approximately 2 minutes. This time frame is important when one considers the number of newborn samples a centralized laboratory must analyze in a single day. A single MS/MS instrument can handle 30 specimens per hour, and because of advances in automation, it is also possible to run prepared samples overnight.

The computer-generated output from the MS/MS analysis gives the concentration of all the targeted analytes. The NBS report, which may vary in style from program to program, indicates which of these are present in abnormal concentrations. These are the data that the follow-up arm of the NBS program must interpret and upon which it must act.

Targeted Analytes

The analytes that are targeted in most MS/MS NBS programs are listed in Table 2.1 along with the disorders that may be causing their abnormal concentrations. The abbreviations for the disorders are those published by the American College of Medical Genetics (ACMG) in order to have consistency throughout.[21] The accepted abbreviations for the amino acids are straightforward, but the shorthand designations for the acylcarnitines have evolved over time. The carbon chain attached to carnitine is designated as "C" followed by

Table 2.1 *Expected Analyte Profiles for MS/MS Newborn Screening Disorders*

MS/MS analytes	*Possible disorder(s)*	*Acronym*	*McKusick number*
↓ C0	Primary carnitine deficiency (carnitine plasma membrane transporter deficiency/carnitine uptake deficiency)	CUD	212140
↑C3, C3/C2	Methylmalonic acidemia (methylmalonyl-CoA mutase deficiency and cobalamin defects) Cobalamin A Cobalamin B Cobalamin C Cobalamin D Propionic acidemia (propionyl-CoA carboxylase deficiency)	MUT CblA CblB CblC CblD PROP	251000 251100 251110 277410 277400 606054
↑C4	Short-chain acyl-CoA dehydrogenase deficiency Isobutyryl-CoA dehydrogenase deficiency	SCAD IBG	201470 611283
↑C4, C5, C5-DC, C6, C8, C12, C14, C16	Glutaric acidemia type II (multiple acyl-CoA dehydrogenase deficiency)	GA II	231680
↑C5	Isovaleric acidemia (isovaleryl-CoA dehydrogenase deficiency) 2-methylbutyryl-CoA dehydrogenase deficiency/ short-branched-chain CoA dehydrogenase deficiency	IVA 2MBG SBCAD	243500 600006 600301
↑C5:1 (±C5OH)	β-ketothiolase deficiency (acetoacetyl-CoA thiolase deficiency)	BKT	248600
↑C5-DC	Glutaric acidemia type I (glutaryl-CoA dehydrogenase deficiency)	GA I	231670
↑C5-OH	3-methylglutaconyl hydratase deficiency	3MGA	250950
↑C5-OH (±C5:1)	3-methylcrotonyl glycinuria (3 methylcrotonyl-CoA carboxylase deficiency)	3MCC	210200
↑C5-OH (±C6-DC)	3-OH-3-methylglutaryl-CoA lyase deficiency	HMG	246450
↑C5-OH (±C3)	Multiple carboxylase deficiency	MCD	253260
↑C8 and C8/C10 (±C6,C10:1)	Medium-chain acyl-CoA dehydrogenase deficiency	MCAD	201450
↑C14:1 and ↑C14:1/C12:1 (±C14, C16, C18:1)	Very-long-chain-acyl-CoA dehydrogenase deficiency	VLCAD	201475

(continues)

Table 2.1 ***Expected Analyte Profiles for MS/MS Newborn Screening Disorders, Continued***

MS/MS analytes	***Possible disorder(s)***	***Acronym***	***McKusick number***
↑C16, C18:1	Carnitine palmitoyltransferase II deficiency	CPTII	255110
	Carnitine-acylcarnitine translocase deficiency	CACT	212138
↑C16-OH, C18:1-OH	Long-chain hydroxy acyl-CoA dehydrogenase deficiency	LCHAD	609016
	Trifunctional protein deficiency	TFP	609015
↑CIT	Citrullinemia (argininosuccinate synthetase deficiency)	CIT	215700
	Argininosuccinic aciduria (argininosuccinate lyase deficiency)	ASA	207900
	Citrin deficiency	CIT II	603471
↑LEU (± VAL)	Maple syrup urine disease (branched chain α-ketoacid dehydrogenase deficiency)	MSUD	248600
↑MET	Homocystinuria (cystathionine-β-synthase deficiency)	HCY	236200
	Methionine adenosyltransferase deficiency	MET	250850
↑PHE, PHE/TYR	Phenylketonuria (phenylalanine hydroxylase deficiency)	PKU	261600
	Biopterin synthesis defects	BIOPT-BS	261630
	Biopterin regeneration defect		
↑TYR	Tyrosinemia: Fumarylacetoacetic acid hydrolase deficiency	TYR Ia*	276700
	Maleylacetoacetic acid isomerase deficiency	TYR Ib	603758
	Tyrosine aminotransferase deficiency	TYR II	276600
	p-OH phenylpyruvic acid dioxygenase deficiency	TYR III	276710

*TYR 1a and 1b may be missed by MS/MS NBS targeting elevated TYR—see text.
**2MBG and SBCAD are two names for the same disorder.

the number of carbons, as in C3 for propionylcarnitine; the degree of unsaturation is designated with a colon (:) followed by the number of double bonds, as in C10:1 for decenoylcarnitine; and the important side groups of hydroxyl- and dicarboxyl- are OH and DC, respectively.

Amino Acids

Phenylalanine

Although PHE has been successfully measured in blood spots for decades, using either bacterial inhibition or fluorometry, MS/MS has helped to streamline screening for patients with PKU. MS/MS allows the simultaneous measurement of both PHE and tyrosine (TYR). The increased PHE/TYR ratio, combined with the absolute PHE concentration, allows a more predictive screening result.[22] Infants who are being fed parenteral amino acids or are being given breast milk fortified with additional amino acids may have PHE and PHE/TYR ratios that mimic those found in infants with PKU. Usually, but not always, there are elevations in other amino acids as well. Sometimes blood samples in very small infants are erroneously taken from the same line used for intravenous feeding. Repeat NBS samples should be taken after the infant is off the parenteral amino acids for 1 hour. If a newborn has PKU, the repeat NBS sample should have a concentration of PHE that is increased over the initial sample. If a newborn has an elevated blood PHE concentration in the initial sample, is not receiving parenteral or supplemental amino acids, and the PHE returns to normal in the repeat sample, the possibility of maternal PKU should be investigated. Infants with defects in the biopterin synthetic or regeneration pathways may present with elevated concentrations of PHE on their NBS and these disorders should be part of the differential diagnostic testing.[23] Infants who have had no protein or amino acid feedings should not have their screening delayed until they are on full feeds. In newborns with PKU, PHE will begin to accumulate from endogenous protein catabolism even in the absence of exogenous feeds. The same is true for analyte accumulation in other amino acidopathies. Infants with PKU who are poor feeders and are not gaining weight often have very high blood PHE concentrations in the neonatal period. This may lead to the erroneous assumption that their final diet prescription will require severe PHE restriction.

Many metabolic programs are using MS/MS to monitor blood PHE and TYR concentrations for their patients with PKU or tyrosinemia. It is important to examine results by both the MS/MS and previous monitoring tool to ascertain that they are comparable.[24] The healthcare community working with patients with PKU may take some time to be comfortable with expressing PHE concentrations in micromoles per liter (µmol/L) rather than milligrams per deciliter (mg/dL) or mg%.

Tyrosine

Tyrosine (TYR) is included in the MS/MS screening panel because of the rare disorders of TYR metabolism: fumarylacetoacetic acid hydrolase deficiency (TYR Ia), maleylacetoacetic acid isomerase deficiency (TYR Ib), tyrosine aminotransferase deficiency (TYR II), and p-hydroxyphenylpyruvic acid dioxygenase deficiency (4-HPPD; TYR III). Although TYR II has been diagnosed in newborns based solely on elevated blood TYR concentrations on their MS/MS NBS, TYR I has not.[25] Because the enzymatic step blocked in TYR I is several steps down the pathway from TYR, the accumulation of TYR is not significant in the neonatal period. The compound, which does accumulate and has been shown to be present in significant amounts in blood of newborns with TYR I, is succinylacetone. Several NBS programs have attempted to measure blood succinylacetone concentrations on all samples with elevated TYR.[26] However, in the newborn with TYR I, the succinylacetone becomes elevated long before there is any significant elevation of TYR. In order to screen for TYR I in the newborn period, the primary analyte should be succinylacetone. The standard sample preparation for the MS/MS analyses for amino acids and acylcarnitines must be modified to allow detection of succinylacetone.[27,28] At this time, the methodology has not been widely implemented.

Newborns with TYR II have elevations of blood TYR concentrations that, like PHE in patients with PKU, increase over time. Using MS/MS to monitor both TYR and PHE in patients with either TYR I or TYR II is extremely helpful, as it is sometimes difficult to achieve appropriate TYR concentrations with dietary TYR restriction without the patient becoming deficient in PHE.

The most common reason for elevations of TYR concentrations in NBS samples is neonatal tyrosinemia. This is believed to be the result of the inability to completely metabolize either endogenous or exogenous tyrosine because the enzyme 4-HPPD may not be completely expressed at birth.[29] Infants with neonatal tyrosinemia usually normalize TYR concentrations in 4 to 6 weeks after birth. Serial blood spot samples show a steady decline over time. Because 4-HPPD requires ascorbic acid as a coenzyme, some physicians supplement these infants with ascorbic acid for the first month of life.[30] Also, infants with liver disease caused by a number of factors, including classical galactosemia, can have blood TYR concentrations that may exceed 1000 μmol/L.[31]

Methionine

Methionine (MET) accumulates when there is a block in the conversion of homocysteine to cystathionine via cystathionine-β-synthetase, causing HCY. Although MET is not the immediate precursor of the targeted enzyme defect, it will begin to accumulate shortly after birth. As with other aminoacidopathies detected through MS/MS NBS, a continual increase of the analyte should be seen in successive samples. There is some concern that depending on neonatal elevations of MET concentration as a marker analyte for HCY may lead to an unacceptable number of missed cases.[32] MS/MS can also be used to follow the MET concentration while the infant is challenged with pyridoxine during the differential diagnostic testing for vitamin B_6 responsiveness. MET is also elevated in methionine adenosyltransferase (MAT) deficiency. Most cases that have been ascertained during routine screening of newborns for hypermethioninemia or family screening have some residual activity of MAT and are clinically well. Although very rare, complete MAT deficiency can lead to demyelination of the brain.[33] Most elevations of MET seen in MS/MS NBS are secondary to liver disease, immaturity, or parenteral feeding of amino acids. An apparent "epidemic" of hypermethioninemia in newborns was reported in 2003 and found to be due to an elemental formula manufactured between May 1998 and February 2001 that contained an unusually high concentration of MET (778 mg/L).[34]

Citrulline

Citrulline (CIT) is a sensitive marker for certain urea cycle enzyme defects. When NBS samples are taken promptly, and MS/MS analyses results are available soon after, the presence of CIT in the NBS sample can prompt life-saving intervention. In some cases, the newborn may already have hyperammonemia by the time screening results are available. The increased CIT concentration can direct further diagnostic testing and treatment toward a urea cycle enzyme defect rather than other possible causes of hyperammonemia such as organic acidemias or fatty acid oxidation defects. Plasma amino acid analysis allows the differentiation between argininosuccinate synthetase (ASS) and argininosuccinate lyase (AL) deficiencies. Citrin deficiency (CIT II) has recently been recognized as a potential source of elevated CIT concentration in the newborn.[35] Other, seemingly nonspecific elevations may also be seen in concentrations of MET, PHE, or galactose in citrin deficiency.[36] Newborns with CIT II deficiency may have normal or mildly elevated ammonia and this would make the NBS result indistinguishable from a mild ASS or AL deficiency. Confirmatory testing is extremely important because treatment for CIT II deficiency, unlike that for ASS and AL deficiencies, does not involve protein restriction.[37]

Leucine

Leucine (LEU) has been used as a marker for branched-chain α-ketoacid dehydrogenase deficiency, or MSUD, for many years.[38,39] Because LEU has the same molecular weight as its isomers, isoleucine and allo-isoleucine, the combination of all three analytes will appear as a single peak in the MS/MS NBS profile of a newborn with MSUD. Valine (VAL) may or may not be elevated by the time the NBS sample is taken. The most common cause of elevated blood LEU concentration in the newborn is excessive amino acids in parenteral solutions or fortified human milk. These newborns usually have elevated concentrations of other amino acids, and their MS/MS profiles can often be distinguished from the profiles of infants with MSUD by calculating their LEU-to-PHE ratio.[40] Because newborns with MSUD require immediate intervention, all samples with elevated LEU concentrations (regardless of their LEU-to-PHE ratio) should be followed up. Infants with intermediate MSUD may not have sufficient elevation of the concentrations of branched-chain amino acids in the neonatal period to be detected by MS/MS NBS, and those with intermittent MSUD do not have elevated concentrations except during catabolic illness.[41] For that reason, even if an older child had a normal NBS result, MSUD should not be ruled out of the differential diagnosis if the presenting symptoms suggest it. Hydroxyproline also has the same molecular weight as LEU and would be detected by MS/MS analysis. Hydroxyproline is an amino acid normally present in human plasma. It is derived primarily from endogenous collagen turnover and the breakdown of dietary collagen. The finding of an elevated concentration (five-to-tenfold increase from the normal of less than 50 μM) of serum hydroxyproline is thought to be an inherited defect of 4-α-hydroxy-L-proline oxidase in the catabolism of hydroxyproline. Elevated serum hydroxyproline concentration appears not to cause any significant clinical symptoms.[42]

Acylcarnitines

Carnitine 0 (C0)

Both elevated and decreased concentrations of free carnitine (C0) can be markers for defects in the carnitine cycle. Low concentration of free carnitine would be expected in disorders in which the carnitine is unable to be released from the acylcarnitine in forming the expected acyl-CoA intermediates. In carnitine palmitoyltransferase II (CPT II) deficiency there is a significant accumulation of long-chain acylcarnitines (from long-chain fatty acids) and a relative deficiency of the short- and medium-chain acylcarnitines, because the enzymatic block prevents the conversion of the acylcarnitines to acyl-CoA moieties inside the inner mitochondrial membrane. With most of the carnitine bound to these intermediates, the C0 is relatively low. A defect in carnitine/acylcarnitine translocase (CACT) produces a very similar acylcarnitine profile, but the underlying defect is in transporting the acylcarnitines across the inner mitochondrial membrane for further oxidation, rather than a defect in regenerating the acyl-CoA moieties.[20] For a newborn with CPT I deficiency, one would expect the MS/MS profile to be just the opposite of the above. Because the enzyme defect prevents carnitine from replacing the CoA on the acyl group to form the acylcarnitines on the outer mitochondrial membrane, the C0 will be elevated and the long-chain acylcarnitines will be very low. Primary carnitine deficiency (CUD) results from a defect in the active transport of carnitine across membranes in the small intestine, renal tubules, and skeletal muscle. These infants should have very high concentrations of carnitine in the urine and low free carnitine and acylcarnitine in their blood.[43] The relationship of these enzymes to the transport of carnitine is seen in Figure 2.5. An abnormal concentration of C0 alone is not sufficient to suspect one of these carnitine transport disorders; it is necessary to examine the MS/MS profile for abnormal concentrations of the long-chain acylcarnitines as well. C0 deficiency may also be present in newborns whose mothers are carni-

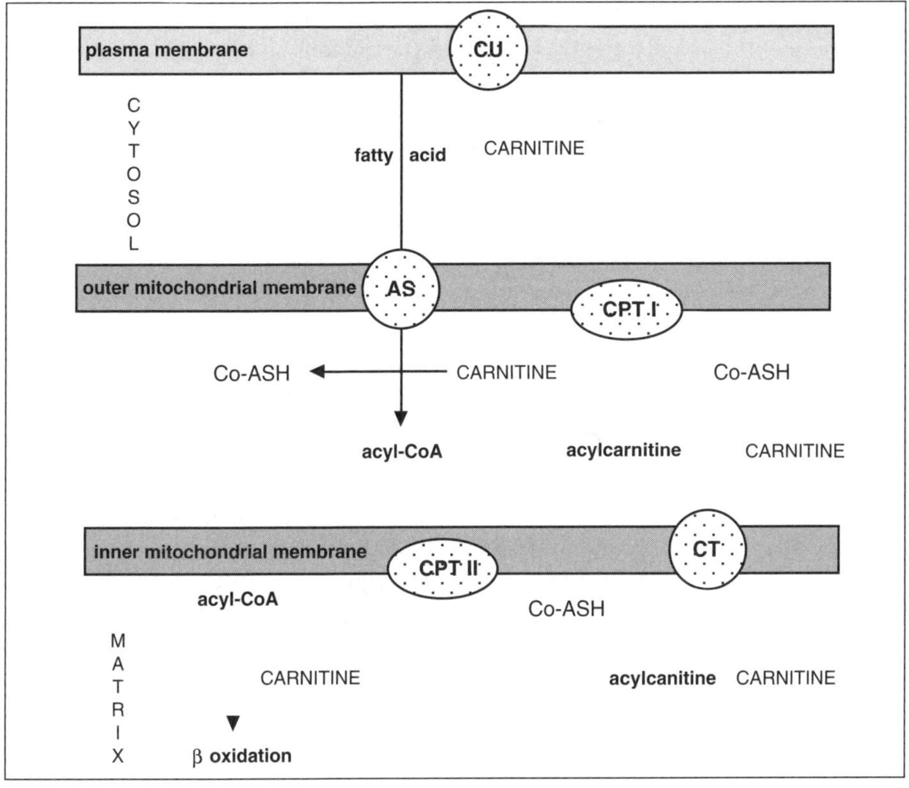

Figure 2.5 *The Carnitine Transport Cycle*

Source: Adapted with permission from Roe CR, Ding J. Mitochondrial fatty acid oxidation disorders. *The Online Metabolic Bases of Inherited Disease.* http://www.ommbid.com/OMMBID. Accessed February 25, 2008.

Notes: CU: carnitine uptake; AS: acyl-CoA synthetase; Co-ASH: coenzyme A; CPT I: carnitine palmitoyltransferase I; CPT II: carnitine palmitoyl transferase II; CT: carnitine acylcarnitine translocase.

tine deficient. Furthermore, C0 deficiency can be expected in some newborns with organic acidemias and fatty acid oxidation defects in which most of their carnitine is bound to the intermediates accumulating behind their specific enzymatic block.

Carnitine 3 (C3)

Propionic acidemia (PROP) and methylmalonic acidemia (MMA) cause an accumulation of propionylcarnitine (C3) that can be used as a marker in MS/MS NBS.[44] Short-chain acylcarnitine concentrations tend to be higher in the neonatal period among many unaffected infants, and so the addition of an elevated C3/C2 ratio to the elevated C3 helps to define potential cases and reduce the number of false positives.[44] Although higher concentrations of the

C3 would be expected in patients with PROP than in patients with MMA, the timing of the sample greatly influences the amount of accumulated analyte.[44] Without urine organic acid analysis, it can be impossible to distinguish PROP from MMA in newborns with elevated concentrations of C3 and C3/C2. There are several forms of MMA. Mutations may occur in the methylmalonyl-CoA mutase (mut^{o} and mut^{-}) gene. Defects in the synthesis of adenosylcobalamin, which is a necessary coenzyme for the mutase, are referred to as cblA and cblB subtypes. These may be responsive to vitamin B_{12} administration. Elevated concentrations of C3 and plasma homocysteine (determined in confirmatory testing) are seen in individuals with defects impairing the synthesis of both adenosylcobalamin and methylcobalamin. These are designated as cblC, D, or F subtypes, and affected individuals are treated for both MMA and HCY.

Carnitine 4 (C4)

Butyryl and isobutyrylcarnitine are both four-carbon isomers that, although they have identical m/z on MS/MS, are analytes that separately accumulate in three very different disorders.[45] Isolated butyrylcarnitine (C4) is a marker for short-chain acyl-CoA dehydrogenase (SCAD) deficiency. This enzymatic step is necessary for the complete beta oxidation of fatty acids. Deficiency of SCAD places individuals at some risk for hypoglycemia when in a catabolic state. A single case of lethal ethylmalonic acid (EMA) encephalopathy has also been described in an infant who had elevated C4 on MS/MS NBS.[46] Isolated isobutyrylcarnitine (C4) accumulates in isobutyryl-CoA dehydrogenase (IBD) deficiency, an enzymatic block in the valine degradative pathway. Individuals with these disorders have unique urine organic acid findings. Only those patients with SCAD deficiency and EMA encephalopathy have elevated urinary ethylmalonic acid, while those with IBD deficiency have elevated or high normal isobutyryl glycine. Most infants with either SCAD or IBD deficiency have a completely benign neonatal course. An algorithm has been proposed for diagnostic testing in infants with elevated C4 concentrations on MS/MS NBS.[46] C4 can also be seen in combination with other markers in medium-chain acyl-CoA dehydrogenase (MCAD) and multiple acyl-CoA dehydrogenase (MAD) deficiencies (see below), in infants on carnitine therapy and in postmortem samples.[47]

Carnitine 5 (C5)

Two isomers of five-carbon acylcarnitines (C5) appear identical in the MS/MS NBS output. Isovalerylcarnitine is elevated in isovaleryl-CoA dehydrogenase deficiency (IVA). Some newborns with IVA may have metabolic decompensation soon after birth, and so immediate follow up for MS/MS NBS samples with elevated C5 is extremely important. Short-branched-chain acyl-CoA dehydrogenase (SBCAD) deficiency, also known as

2-methylbutyryl-CoA dehydrogenase (2MBD) deficiency, results in an accumulation of the isomer, 2-methylbutyrylcarnitine. This disorder was first described in 2000 and determined to be a defect in the degradation of isoleucine.[48] Although there have been patients with 2MBD deficiency with significant neurological sequelae, there have also been affected siblings who were asymptomatic.[49] A fairly high incidence of seemingly benign 2MBD deficiency in infants born to Hmong parents has been reported.[50] Urine organic acid analysis can clearly distinguish between IVA and 2MBD deficiency.

Carnitine 5:1 (C5:1)

Acetoacetyl-CoA thiolase deficiency, also known as β-ketothiolase (BKT) deficiency, results in an accumulation of tiglylcarnitine (C5:1) due to a block in the degradative pathway of isoleucine. There may also be an accumulation of C5OH (see below). While C5:1 is considered a primary marker for BKT, it is often seen as a secondary marker in 3-methylcrotonyl-CoA carboxylase deficiency. As with IVA, newborns with BKT deficiency may present seriously ill, have no symptoms, or have acute intermittent ketoacidosis.[51] Infants with BKT deficiency should have tiglylglycine, and may also have 2-methyl-3-hydroxybutyric acid, 2-methylacetoacetic acid, and 2-butanone in their urine.

Carnitine 5DC (C5DC)

Glutarylcarnitine (C5DC) accumulates in glutaryl-CoA dehydrogenase deficiency (glutaric acidemia type I or GA I).[52] In the absence of GA I, there is very little natural accumulation of C5DC in the blood, such that any elevations should be treated with suspicion, and confirmatory testing ordered. In healthy newborns with GA I, the C5DC concentrations will be highest in the immediate neonatal period, probably secondary to the catabolic stress of labor and delivery. A repeat newborn screen with C5DC in the normal range should not rule out the possibility of GA I. It is also possible that no C5DC accumulation will be detected in infants with GA I who are "low excretors," and some cases of GA I may be missed by MS/MS NBS.[53] Another analyte, hydroxyoctanoylcarnitine, with the same m/z 388 signal as C5DC, may be seen in MS/MS screening profiles of some infants with medium-chain acyl-CoA dehydrogenase deficiency (MCADD) or infants being fed medium-chain triglyceride (MCT)-containing formulas.[54]

Carnitine 5-OH (C5OH)

The analyte 3-hydroxyisovalerylcarnitine (C5OH) accumulates in blood in several enzyme defects in the branched-chain amino acid catabolic pathway. The most common cause of the elevated concentrations of C5OH is 3-methylcrotonyl-CoA carboxylase (3-MCC) deficiency. The presence of

3-methylcrotonyl glycine (and possibly also 3-methylcrotonic acid and 3-OH-isovaleric acid) in the urine distinguishes 3-MCC deficiency from BKT deficiency (see above), 3-OH-3-methylglutaryl-CoA lyase (HMG-CoA lysase) deficiency, and 3-methylglutaconylhydratase (3-MGA) deficiency. Infants with multiple carboxylase deficiency are expected to have elevated concentrations of urinary lactate, 3-OH-propionate, methylcitrate, tiglylglycine, and 3-OH isovaleric acid as well as 3-methylcrotonylglycine. Unaffected infants born to mothers with 3-MCC deficiency will often have an accumulation of C5OH in their newborn's blood sample that is even higher than that found in infants affected with 3-MCC deficiency.[55] These unaffected infants may also have a urine organic acid profile and low free carnitine concentrations in the newborn period that mimic those of an affected infant. For this reason, it is becoming standard protocol to test the mothers of all infants with elevated blood concentrations of C5OH as part of the confirmatory testing for 3-MCC deficiency.[56]

Carnitine 8 (C8)

The presence of octanoylcarnitine (C8) together with an elevated ratio of C8/C10 (decanoylcarnitine) in blood is a significant marker for medium-chain acyl-CoA dehydrogenase (MCAD) deficiency. Other concentrations of medium-chain acylcarnitines, C4, C6, C10, and C10:1, are often elevated as well. In MCADD, as with other fatty acid oxidation disorders, the accumulation of these intermediates in blood may be highest in the first days after birth.[57] As with all fatty acid oxidation disorders, prevention of fasting should be a primary concern even before the diagnostic testing is completed. A repeat newborn screen, with lower (or normal) concentrations of medium-chain acylcarnitines should not rule out a diagnosis. Studies have indicated that the concentration of C8 on the MS/MS NBS can be a fairly accurate predictor of residual MCAD activity with the "severe" mutations resulting in the highest neonatal C8.[58]

The greatest contributor to non-MCAD blood elevations of the medium-chain acylcarnitines is MCT-containing formulas. These formulas are most often used for premature and ill infants in the neonatal intensive care units (NICU). Because of its ease of absorption, MCT oil is widely utilized as a fat source in hyperalimentation solutions, breast milk fortifiers, and proprietary formulas for infants in the NICU. In the NICU, these infants who have their NBS samples taken in the first 24 to 48 hours of life are not usually on significant amounts of these oral MCT-containing formulas, and do not show elevated concentrations of their medium-chain acylcarnitines.[25] Repeat NBS samples are often taken from these infants because of abnormalities found in other NBS tests, or as part of the NICU protocol.[37] When elevated medium-chain acylcarnitines are detected only in the repeat NBS testing, the possibility of dietary

MCT should be investigated. Elevated concentrations of medium-chain acylcarnitines may also be part of the blood profile for infants with GA II (see below).

Carnitine C14:1 (C14:1)

Tetradecenoylcarnitine (C14:1) accumulates in very-long-chain acyl-CoA dehydrogenase (VLCAD) deficiency. Elevated concentrations of both tetradecanoylcarnitine (C14) and the ratio of C14:1 to C12:1 are usually seen in infants with VLCAD deficiency. In addition, other long-chain species (C16, C18:1) may have also accumulated in the blood by the time the MS/MS NBS sample is taken. As with other fatty acid oxidation disorders, the marker analytes may normalize on a repeat MS/MS NBS.[59] Since this MS/MS profile is fairly specific to VLCAD deficiency, instruction to avoid fasting and ordering of diagnostic testing should be immediate. Diet changes, to provide MCT as an energy source, can wait until diagnostic testing is complete in non-symptomatic infants.

Carnitine 16OH (C16-OH)

3-hydroxyhexadecenoylcarnitine (C16-OH) and 3-hydroxyoctadecanoylcarnitine (C18-OH) accumulate in long-chain hydroxyacyl-CoA dehydrogenase (LCHAD) and trifunctional protein (TFP) deficiencies. The TFP consists of long-chain enoyl-CoA hydratase and long-chain ketoacylthiolase activities in addition to the LCHAD. Although the two disorders can be distinguished by differences in the urine organic acid analysis and the finding of a common mutation in one of the TFP subunits, the treatment is the same.[60] As with the medium- and very-long-chain disorders, immediate follow up with avoidance of fasting and diagnostic testing is essential. Dietary considerations are similar to those with VLCAD deficiency. If there is a history of maternal HELLP (hemolysis, elevated liver enzymes, and low platelet count) syndrome, a high suspicion of LCHAD deficiency should be raised.[61]

Multiple Elevated Acylcarnitines

Multiple acyl-CoA dehydrogenase deficiency, also known as glutaric acidemia type II (GA II) can present with an MS/MS NBS profile that is quite variable.[62] Caused by defects of the electron transport system, GA II can result in accumulation of short-, medium-, and/or long-chain acylcarnitine intermediates. Elevated blood concentrations of C5DC may or may not be present in the MS/MS NBS profile. Infants, especially those in the NICU, who are on high doses of carnitine often accumulate acylcarnitine intermediates in a nonspecific pattern that may be similar to that for an infant with GA II. An infant without GA II, born to a riboflavin-deficient mother, was reported to have an MS/MS NBS profile and clinical findings consistent with GA II.[63] For symptomatic infants with GA II, the MS/MS NBS blood profile may help direct intervention, as well as diagnostic testing. Counseling the families of non-symptomatic infants about avoidance of fasting and awareness of symptoms can be done before diagnostic testing is complete and dietary intervention initiated.

Newborn Screening

Definitions

MS/MS testing represents a paradigm shift in newborn screening. Unlike measuring the electrophoretic pattern of hemoglobin molecules when screening for sickle-cell disease, MS/MS screening does not fit a "one test, one disorder" model. An abnormal concentration of a particular analyte, or a pattern of several analytes, may be suggestive of a particular disorder. However, it could also be due to feeding, medication, or a different disorder with accumulation of another analyte that has the same m/z ratio. MS/MS NBS, like all newborn screening technologies, requires confirmatory testing and clinical evaluation before a diagnosis can be made. Newborn screening is not limited to laboratory testing, but is a large, interactive, and multifaceted program. A widely accepted definition of newborn screening was published in 2000 by the American Academy of Pediatrics:[9]

> Newborn screening in the United States is a public health program aimed at the early identification of conditions for which early and timely intervention can prevent or reduce associated mortality and morbidity. (p. 389)

Criteria

For a newborn screening program to be successful, it must meet criteria for each of its components.[64,65] The components are the panel of disorders to be included, the testing methodology to be employed, and the clinical follow up for confirmation, management, and program evaluation. These are outlined in Table 2.2.

Disorders that are potential candidates for the newborn screening panel need to be well-defined. The questions that must be asked are: Is the abnormal concentration of a particular analyte a true marker of an inborn error of

Table 2.2 ***Criteria for a Successful Newborn Screening Program***

The **conditions** included in the panel:

1. Are biochemically and clinically definable
2. Manifest early
3. Have proven early interventions that are accessible to all newborns
4. Are interventions that can decrease morbidity/mortality
5. Have a reasonable incidence
6. Can be confirmed with tests beyond screening
7. Can be changed when evidence supports addition or elimination from the panel

The **test**(s), or assay, used in the screening program:

1. Can be done on a small, noninvasive sample
2. Can be done on the samples collected for other newborn screening tests
3. Can be done with a very short turnaround time
4. Has a reasonable cost when applied to all newborns
5. Is valid in samples taken at 24 hours after birth
6. Has a very high specificity and sensitivity, allowing very few false positives and virtually no false negatives for the analytes being measured
7. Uses control samples
8. Is being done in a laboratory with tight quality control oversight by a professional accreditation organization

The **follow up**:

1. Has established protocols for contacting care providers, disseminating information, and facilitating clinical follow up
2. Has defined procedures for confirmatory testing
3. Has accredited clinical professionals and facilities for management and monitoring the long-term follow up
4. Has identified resources for medical food, medications, and supplements required for treatment
5. Has data management capability to report false positive and false negative rates, and negative and positive predictive values
6. Has data management capability for long-term outcome surveillance

metabolism? Does identifying this metabolic disorder change its course (i.e., is there a successful intervention)? Is it imperative that the intervention begin in the newborn period, or is this an adult-onset disorder? Is the metabolic disorder so rare that the financial burden of screening all newborns would not be cost-beneficial? The second set of criteria is related to the test itself: Can the test be done on a small, easily obtainable sample? Can the test be done quickly with a very short turnaround time? Is the test precise and accurate, with minimal false positives and negligible false negatives? Is the cost of the test reasonable? Lastly, criteria are also applied to the newborn screening program as a whole: Is the short-term follow up prompt and well organized? Is a system in place that will allow a definitive diagnosis through confirmatory testing? Are there adequate staff, facilities, and financial means to support both short- and long-term treatment? Is a program evaluation component in place?

MS/MS in Newborn Screening

The Panel of Disorders

When mass spectrometry was added as a tool to NBS programs, the total number of disorders that could potentially be detected appeared to be limitless. MS/MS technology allows screening for multiple very rare disorders, for which separate screening tests would not be cost-effective. This has led to questions about the accepted criteria for adding certain types of disorders to the screening panel. Because the technique will identify any analyte having an m/z ratio within the chosen spectrum range, it is not, strictly speaking, disorder-specific testing. If an analyte pattern is abnormal, further diagnostic testing may be undertaken, even if it is not the pattern of one of the targeted disorders. For this reason, disorders may be detected for which there is, as yet, no treatment or for which the exact molecular mechanism is as yet unknown.

Most screening programs have adopted the "uniform" or "core" panel of 29 primary conditions recommended by the ACMG in 2006.[21] Of the 29, there are 20 that are detected using the MS/MS technology for acylcarnitines, amino acids, and appropriate ratios. The College also lists an additional 25 "secondary" conditions of which 22 can be targeted by MS/MS. Most of the secondary conditions are part of the differential diagnosis for the primary conditions in the core panel. The ACMG report was commissioned through the Maternal and Child Health Bureau of the Health Resources and Services Administration (HRSA) with the goals of providing guidance for state NBS programs as they expanded and examining the possibility of having national oversight for quality assurance. For conditions to be included in the core panel, they were scored based on the clinical characteristics of the disease, the characteristics of the screening test, and the availability of specific and effective diagnostic testing, treatment, and management.[21]

The core panel is viewed by many as a significant starting point.[66] It is recognized that there are additional conditions detectable using the same MS/MS analyte markers as those used for detecting the core conditions. Furthermore, conditions originally designated as secondary conditions may be elevated to primary, and new conditions may be added to the secondary list. The 42 disorders presently recommended by ACMG for inclusion in NBS programs, and their designation as primary or secondary conditions, are listed in Table 2.3.

Table 2.3 ***ACMG Recommended Core Panel and Secondary Target Disorders Detectable by MS/MS Newborn Screening***

Organic acidemias	*Fatty acid oxidation disorders*	*Aminoacidopathies*
Core Panel		
3MCC 3-methylcrotonyl-CoA carboxylase deficiency	CUD Carnitine uptake deficiency	ASA Argininosuccinic acidemia
BKT β-ketothiolase deficiency	LCHAD Long-chain OH-acyl-CoA dehydrogenase deficiency	CIT Citrullinemia
Cbl A, B Cobalamin types A and B defects	MCAD Medium-chain acyl-CoA dehydrogenase deficiency	HCY Homocystinuria
GA I Glutaric acidemia type I	TFP Trifunctional protein deficiency	MSUD Maple syrup urine disease
HMG HMG-CoA reductase deficiency	VLCAD Very-long-chain acyl-CoA dehydrogenase deficiency	PKU Phenylketonuria
IVA Isovaleric acidemia		TYR I Tyrosinema type I
MCD Multiple carboxylase deficiency		
PROP Propionic acidemia		

(continues)

Table 2.3 ***ACMG Recommended Core Panel and Secondary Target Disorders Detectable by MS/MS Newborn Screening, Continued***

Organic acidemias	*Fatty acid oxidation disorders*	*Aminoacidopathies*
Secondary Targets		
2M3HBA 2Methyl 3-OH-butyric acidemia	CACT Carnitine acylcarnitine transporter deficiency	ARG Argininemia
2MBG 2Methylbutyryl-CoA dehydrogenase deficiency	CPT IA Carnitine palmitoyltransferase I	BIOPT (REG) Biopterin regeneration deficiency
3MGA 3Methylglutaconyl hydratase deficiency	CPT II Carnitine palmitoyltransferase II	BIOPT (BS) Biopterin synthetic defect
Cbl C, D Cobalamin types C and D defects	DE RED 2,4,Dienoyl-CoA reductase deficiency	CIT II Citrin deficiency
IBG Isobutyryl-CoA dehydrogenase deficiency	GA II Glutaric acidemia type II	HYPER-PHE Hyperphenylalaninemia
MAL Malonic acidemia	MCKAT Medium-chain ketoacyl-CoA thiolase deficiency	MET Hypermethioninemia
	M/SCHAD Medium-/short-chain OH acyl-CoA dehydrogenase deficiency	TYR II Tyrosinemia type II
	SCAD Short-chain acyl-CoA dehydrogenase deficiency	TYR III Tyrosinemia type III

Source: American College of Medical Genetics. Newborn screening: toward a uniform screening panel and system. *Genet Med.* 2006;851:1S–252S.

The Test

When it was determined that the MS/MS technology could be applied to blood spots dried on filter paper, the possibilities for application to NBS became a reality.[17,18] The amount of whole blood in a one-eighth-inch punch from the spot is approximately 3.4 microliters. This leaves a significant sample for testing for other disorders that use methodologies other than MS/MS.

The same care taken for all newborn screening samples applies to those for MS/MS. This includes accurate identification of the newborn, avoidance of contaminating the filter paper either before or after the sample application, proper drying of the sample, and prompt delivery of the sample to the screening laboratory.

The blood samples collected on Guthrie cards permit rapid and nearly noninvasive sampling of newborns 24 to 72 hours after birth. Once air-dried, these samples can be mailed without any special handling to a centralized newborn screening laboratory. Along with the blood specimen, the Guthrie card contains a form that allows pertinent information to be recorded. The newborn screening card used in North Carolina is shown in Figure 2.6 as an example of the information collected. The completed card contains data, such as type of feeding, birth weight, age when sample was taken, and transfusion status, which help in the interpretation of the results of the screening tests. Additional information aids in locating the infant and the primary care provider once the testing is complete. As more tests have been added to the screening panels, the amount of information about the newborn, necessary for accurate interpretation of results,

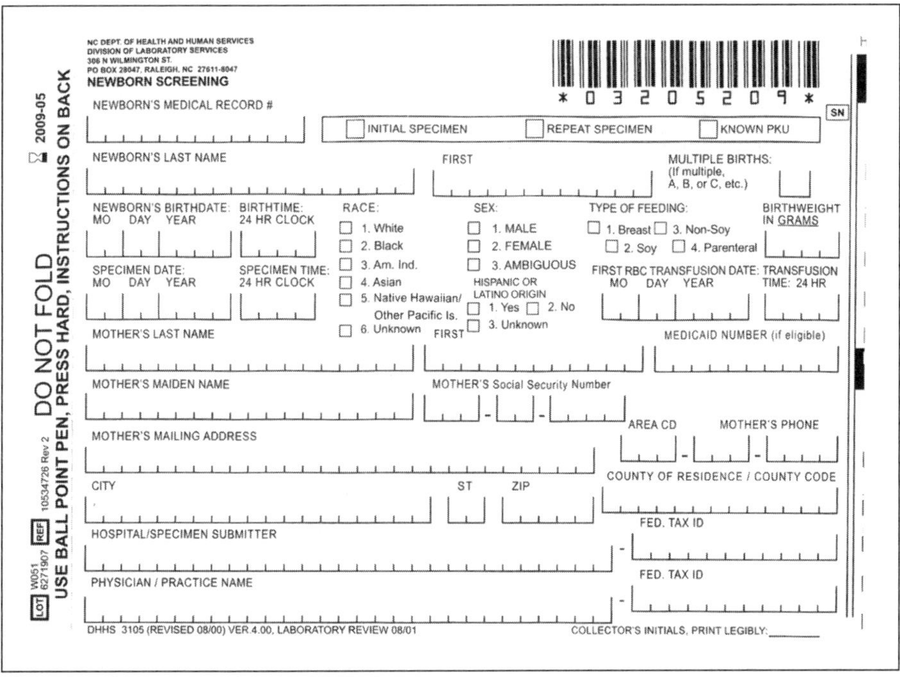

USE BALL POINT PEN, PRESS HARD, INSTRUCTIONS ON BACK

DO NOT FOLD

LOT W051 6271907 REF 10534726 Rev 2 2009-05

NC DEPT. OF HEALTH AND HUMAN SERVICES
DIVISION OF LABORATORY SERVICES
306 N WILMINGTON ST.
PO BOX 28047, RALEIGH, NC 27611-8047
NEWBORN SCREENING

* 0 3 2 0 5 2 0 9 *

SN

NEWBORN'S MEDICAL RECORD #

☐ INITIAL SPECIMEN ☐ REPEAT SPECIMEN ☐ KNOWN PKU

NEWBORN'S LAST NAME — FIRST — MULTIPLE BIRTHS: (If multiple, A, B, or C, etc.)

NEWBORN'S BIRTHDATE: MO DAY YEAR — BIRTHTIME: 24 HR CLOCK

RACE: ☐ 1. White ☐ 2. Black ☐ 3. Am. Ind. ☐ 4. Asian ☐ 5. Native Hawaiian/ Other Pacific Is. ☐ 6. Unknown

SEX: ☐ 1. MALE ☐ 2. FEMALE ☐ 3. AMBIGUOUS

HISPANIC OR LATINO ORIGIN ☐ 1. Yes ☐ 2. No ☐ 3. Unknown

TYPE OF FEEDING: ☐ 1. Breast ☐ 3. Non-Soy ☐ 2. Soy ☐ 4. Parenteral

BIRTHWEIGHT IN GRAMS

SPECIMEN DATE: MO DAY YEAR — SPECIMEN TIME: 24 HR CLOCK

FIRST RBC TRANSFUSION DATE: MO DAY YEAR — TRANSFUSION TIME: 24 HR

MOTHER'S LAST NAME — FIRST — MEDICAID NUMBER (if eligible)

MOTHER'S MAIDEN NAME — MOTHER'S Social Security Number

MOTHER'S MAILING ADDRESS — AREA CD — MOTHER'S PHONE

CITY — ST — ZIP — COUNTY OF RESIDENCE / COUNTY CODE

HOSPITAL/SPECIMEN SUBMITTER — FED. TAX ID

PHYSICIAN / PRACTICE NAME — FED. TAX ID

DHHS 3105 (REVISED 08/00) VER.4.00, LABORATORY REVIEW 08/01

COLLECTOR'S INITIALS, PRINT LEGIBLY: ________

Figure 2.6 *Typical Newborn Screening Card Showing the Data Collection Portion*

Notes: Information about the infant includes infant's medical record number, name, birth order (for multiple births), birth date and time, date of sample collection and time, race, ethnicity, sex, type of feeding, birth weight, and date of transfusion and time. Further information includes mother's name and maiden name, Medicaid number, mother's mailing address and telephone number, and county of birth. Health care provider information includes birthing facility that collected and submitted the sample, physician from whom the infant will be receiving his or her ongoing care, and initials of the person who drew the sample.

increases. For example, when measuring galactose analytes in screening for galactosemia, it is essential to know if the infant has received feedings containing lactose. Information about ethnicity contributes to the growing knowledge about the incidence of certain disorders among different population groups.

The analytes detected by MS/MS were described in earlier sections. The methodology is accurate in its ability to detect and quantify the analytes; however, it cannot be expected to be as accurate in its ability to predict a given disorder. Analyte concentrations may be abnormal due to other disorders with elevated analytes that have the same m/z. Results are also influenced by the infant's type of feeding and medication (e.g., MCT oil and carnitine), or analytes of maternal origin (e.g., 3-OH isovaleryl carnitine in maternal 3-MCC deficiency). Analyte concentrations are also dependent on the clinical condition of the infant at the time the sample was taken and the number of days after birth the sample was drawn. Affected newborns with some partial enzyme activity may not have significantly elevated concentrations of analytes until they are stressed with their first catabolic illness.

Cutoffs

While many factors need to be taken into consideration, the most important aspect in evaluating MS/MS NBS results is having appropriate cutoffs. If the cutoff is too low, a large number of unaffected newborns (false positives) will be identified as having a presumptive positive NBS. These can lead to unnecessary and expensive diagnostic testing, anxiety on the part of the families, and lack of confidence in the screening program by health professionals.[67] If the cutoff is too high, affected newborns (false negatives) will not be identified. If the NBS result is reported as normal due to inappropriate cutoffs, a false sense of security could possibly delay targeted diagnostic testing at the onset of clinical symptoms. In order to set the appropriate cutoffs, a profile of the analyte concentration in all screened newborns (i.e., the normal population) must be determined. Initially, cutoffs are set at a given number of standard deviations above the mean. By examining the number of unaffected newborns (false positives) that would require follow up and the analyte concentrations of true positives, adjustments can then be made. Rinaldo has demonstrated the effectiveness of setting the cutoffs between the 99th percentile of the normal population and the 5th percentile of the affected infants.[68]

The appropriate cutoffs are dependent on the time after birth that the sample is obtained. Many of the acylcarnitine markers for fatty acid oxidation defects will begin to decrease after the immediate neonatal period, while the markers for the aminoacidopathies will continue to increase. A certain number of false positives is inevitable, and even desirable, as there often is overlap between the analyte concentration of a small percentage of unaffected

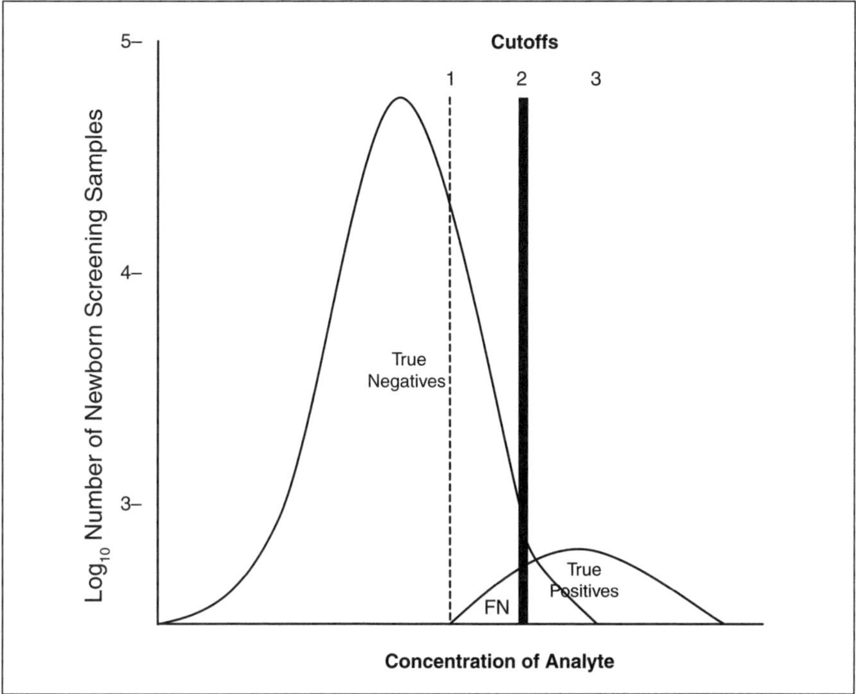

Figure 2.7 *Establishing Cutoffs in NBS to Minimize Both False Positives (FP) and False Negatives (FN)*

Note: Cutoff 1 is too low and results in a very high number of unaffected newborns having a positive NBS (FP). Cutoff 3 is too high and results in affected newborns having a normal NBS (FN).

newborns and those who are true positives. The goal is to keep the false-positive rate as low as possible while trying to eliminate the possibility of false negatives. These relationships can be seen in Figure 2.7.

In any given NBS program, the cutoffs are evaluated and adjusted over time as more data about analyte concentrations of the total newborn population, and of the affected newborns, become available.

Stratification

Many programs stratify cutoffs. There may be a so-called "borderline" analyte cutoff concentration that will prompt a request for a repeat newborn screening sample. No clinical intervention or diagnostic testing will be done unless the repeat sample is also elevated. A higher cutoff concentration than that for the borderline may be referred to as the "abnormal" cutoff and will prompt immediate clinical evaluation. Both the borderline and abnormal cutoff concentrations are "out of range" and require some kind of further testing. In North Carolina, between 2003 and 2004, 33% of samples with concentrations in the borderline range on both the initial and repeat NBS were identified as true positives through confirmatory testing.[25]

Stratification of cutoff concentrations is also being done in some programs for infants who are premature, low birth weight, or have other reasons to be in the NICU. Policies are being developed that will address the impact of certain interventions on NBS results of the infant in the NICU. One recommendation is to take an initial blood sample before any NICU interventions, to repeat the screen at the end of the first week, and then again when the feeding status is stable.[69] As acylcarnitine profiles change in the several days after birth,[70] stratification of analyte cutoff concentrations, based on the age of the newborn when the NBS sample is taken, has been explored.

Since analyte cutoffs are population-based, there are some differences among the state NBS programs. However, there are ongoing HRSA data collection and analysis efforts to establish guidelines based on each state's own profiles.[68] This is especially helpful for smaller NBS programs where the number of affected newborns is proportionately small. The study is also looking at analyte ratios that may be predictive and help reduce the number of false positives.[68]

Second-Tier Testing

Second-tier testing is additional testing, done within the NBS laboratory and applied to initial presumptive positive NBS samples to help reduce the false-positive rate. The premise is that an analyte may be elevated due to causes other than accumulation from the targeted IMD.

Second-tier testing is not a new concept in newborn screening. It is already being widely used in testing for cystic fibrosis and galactosemia. The second-tier tests are usually more specific, but more complex, costly, and not feasible for application to all NBS samples. Because they are applied to only the presumptive positive samples, they are an excellent means to reduce both the monetary and emotional costs of follow-up testing.

In MS/MS NBS laboratories, methodologies are being perfected to test for homocysteine in initial screening samples with elevated concentrations of MET, alloisoleucine in those with elevated LEU, and methylmalonic and 3-OH propionic acids in those with elevated C3.[27,71]

Routine Second Screening

Routine second screening is part of NBS programs in several states.[72] The timing of this testing is important if data are to be compared. Many presumptive positive results found on initial tests will be normal on repeat. If obtaining a second sample at 1 to 2 weeks of age is automatically done at the first well-child checkup or at a specific time for hospitalized infants, the difficulty in trying to find these infants for retesting is minimized. This procedure may also capture those newborns who did not get an initial screen because of early discharge, home birth, or transfer to a critical care center. Routine second screening also has the potential for finding cases among the false negatives. Oregon reported that 31 of 130 cases detected through MS/MS NBS were identified only on the second screen. However, nearly half of these 31 infants had their initial blood samples obtained prior to 24 hours of age.[73]

Neither stratification, second-tier testing, nor routine repeat testing replaces confirmatory testing of infants with positive results. The MS/MS NBS laboratory remains a screening laboratory, and infants identified as presumptive positive require both clinical evaluation and further confirmatory testing.

Follow Up

Follow up encompasses all post-analytical tasks in a newborn screening program, from interpretation of results to long-term treatment of those identified through screening. NBS programs differ widely in how and by whom the follow-up tasks are accomplished. However, the ultimate goals are the same: to reduce mortality and morbidity by providing meaningful screening results within days of birth, expedite confirmation, initiate treatment, and provide long-term intervention and monitoring. Because NBS programs are within the states' public health systems, they must operate within the constraints of the personnel and fiscal policies of their particular state.

The steps included in the typical protocol for the follow up of newborn screening results are shown in Table 2.4. If the result of the MS/MS analysis of the initial specimen is out of range, usually another sample punch is taken from the same blood spot. If the mean of the two results is within range, no further action is required and it is reported as normal; if out of range, it is categorized as either borderline or abnormal. When the result is in the borderline range, a repeat screening sample from the infant is requested from the primary care provider (PCP) or the birthing facility. When the result is in the abnormal range, the newborn is at higher risk of being a true positive and immediate clinical and biochemical evaluations by a genetic/metabolic specialist are recommended. When diagnostic testing confirms the diagnosis, appropriate short- and long-term intervention is initiated. The NBS laboratory is notified of these confirmatory/diagnostic test results, so they can be added to the database to aid in the program's self-evaluation for continuous improvement.

Table 2.4 *Steps for the Follow Up Within an NBS Program*

I. Pre-analytical
   A. Newborn's blood and identification data collected on NBS card
   B. NBS card transported to the NBS laboratory
   C. NBS data logged into the laboratory database

II. Analytical
   A. Laboratory analyses performed
   B. Results interpreted and recorded
   C. Laboratory quality control maintained

III. Post-analytical
   A. Short-term follow up
      1. Out-of-range results communicated immediately to the follow-up staff.
      2. Written/web-based reports on all samples (normal as well as out-of-range) made available to the primary care physician (PCP) and birthing centers.
      3. Follow-up contacts PCP and/or birthing centers. Procedures may differ if the NBS program uses a two-tiered cutoff. A borderline value may require only a request for a repeat NBS sample.
      4. Follow-up requests that PCP ascertain the infant's clinical condition.
      5. Follow-up makes recommendation for immediate transport to a tertiary center if infant is symptomatic, or refers infant to the genetic center if non-symptomatic.
      6. Follow-up gives confirmation testing recommendations to either center. For some disorders, the PCP may order confirmatory testing for asymptomatic newborns in lieu of immediate referral to the genetic center.
      7. Symptomatic infants given emergency treatment with disorder-specific treatment initiated when confirmatory laboratory test results and clinical presentation support the diagnosis.
      8. Non-symptomatic infants begin disorder-specific treatment when confirmatory laboratory tests support the diagnosis.
      9. Follow-up confirms with the genetic center that the confirmatory testing is completed, diagnoses and false positives are recorded, and long-term follow up is initiated.
   B. Long-term follow up
      1. The genetic center counsels the patients, enables access to medical foods, necessary medications and supplements, monitors patients, makes dietary and medical prescription changes as needed, and communicates with the PCP.
      2. The genetic center records outcome data and reports back any false negatives in symptomatic patients who had normal newborn screens.
   C. Evaluation
      1. The NBS laboratory, follow up, and genetic center personnel meet periodically to update patient and laboratory data. Evidence-based decisions are made about procedural changes, cutoff adjustments, or treatment modifications.
      2. Reports are given to the NBS Advisory Board.
      3. The NBS Advisory Board also hears recommendations for changes in the disorders included in the screening panel.

Short-Term Follow Up

When an out-of-range analyte concentration is received by the follow-up coordinator, the immediate task is to locate the infant through the PCP or birthing facility. It may be that the PCP, identified on the newborn screening form, has not yet seen the infant or is not the provider that the family ultimately chose. In the latter case, the birthing facility often has further information about the infant that may enable the infant to be located. No child with an out-of-range NBS should be lost to follow up. Name changes are routine and out-of-state moves are not uncommon. Occasionally, extraordinary means are needed to locate an infant, including law enforcement and social service assistance or an Internet search for nearby addresses or similar names.

It is unlikely that the PCP will be familiar with all the very rare disorders in the screening panel and so may need guidance in how to proceed. Since the PCP will have the first contact with the family, it is important that he or she receive accurate information about the results (including false-positive rates) and the potential risks in the newborn period. It is important that the infant be seen immediately so that the clinical status and the possible need for immediate intervention and stabilization can be determined. If confirmatory tests are to be done on samples taken locally, complete and accurate directions for collection of specimens and ordering of tests must be relayed. A series of web-based Action (ACT) sheets have been developed by the ACMG that some NBS programs find useful for communicating this information to the PCP.[74] These are broad-based and may not accurately address the procedures followed in every NBS program. They can be used as a starting point for developing program-specific procedures.

If the infant is to be referred to a genetic center, every effort should be made to have this referral within the next 24 to 36 hours or immediate transport if the infant is symptomatic. Two quotes from a French NBS task force, which included parents of affected infants with abnormal screens, reflect the emotional impact of that first contact:[75]

> The period elapsing between the first alarm signal and the actual onset of care remains permanently engraved in the parents' memory, and blunders committed in word or deed will never be forgotten. (p. 738)

> The worse possible . . . scenario . . . is when the announcement is made by telephone, by a person with little knowledge of the disease, who asks the parents to make an appointment, or offers them an appointment several days hence. (p. 738)

Confirmatory Testing

Laboratory Testing

Confirmatory or diagnostic testing is essential for every newborn who has an initial abnormal result, or two borderline results on the MS/MS newborn screen. Diet modifications, except in symptomatic infants, may be delayed until the diagnosis is confirmed. The confirmatory testing should include analytical procedures that are different from the newborn screen testing and should involve additional specimens, often including urine, plasma, and/or skin fibroblasts. These confirmatory tests are more costly than the NBS and turnaround times are often longer. Some tests for very rare disorders are offered only at one or two laboratories in the world. Each NBS program and their genetic centers must have access to this testing as part of their follow up and should follow an accepted protocol for confirmatory testing so that all reported confirmed cases meet the same diagnostic criteria. At this time, most state NBS programs do not have adequate funding to include the confirmatory testing within their budgets; therefore, coverage is through third-party payers.[76]

Clinical Evaluation

In addition to the laboratory testing, clinical evaluation is an essential part of the differential diagnosis. Newborns identified through MS/MS newborn screening may not manifest symptoms in the first few days of life and may not become symptomatic until there is sufficient accumulation of the substrate, or until there is catabolic stress from an intercurrent illness. While presymptomatic newborn screening can save lives, it sometimes makes it difficult to explain to caregivers the potential seriousness of a disorder in a newborn who appears robust. Other newborns, especially some with organic acidemias or urea cycle disorders, may manifest metabolic decompensation within hours of birth. These infants will need routine laboratory tests and adequate fluid, electrolyte, and energy support even if the final diagnosis has not been made. Obtaining MS/MS NBS results rapidly can help direct further intervention even before confirmatory testing is complete.

Long-Term Follow Up

A newborn screening program cannot be successful without expertise to interpret MS/MS screening and confirmatory testing results, a coordinated metabolic team to manage identified newborns for both the short and long term, and access to appropriate medical food, special supplements, and/or medical equipment.

Access to Treatment

There is great concern about the access to treatment for newborns identified through MS/MS NBS programs. More professionals with expertise to treat and manage patients with an IMD, more laboratories accredited to do confirmatory testing, and more clinics to increase the physical access to care for families are needed.[77] Even if all this could be accomplished, there remains one very large barrier: lack of access to the medical foods essential for the management of these disorders. In 1992, Buist and Tuerck stated that in the United States, the weakest link in NBS programs was lack of unified access to treatment.[78] Little has changed in the intervening years. Even proposed national mandates to create a uniform approach to expanded screening do not include provisions for medical foods. Buist and Huntington estimate that 1:3000 newborns screened each year require nutrition management that includes use of medical foods and/or special supplements. The yearly cost in Oregon is estimated to be approximately $5000 per patient.[79] With successful nutrition management, the cost of institutional care, which may range up to $100,000 per year, can be avoided. Even though the Orphan Drug Act Amendments of 1988 defined medical foods as "requiring prescription and supervision by a physician,"[80] most insurance companies deny coverage. Some states have passed legislation mandating insurance coverage. The amount of coverage, the items covered, and the interpretation of coverage varies from state to state. Families who change employers or move to another state may lose coverage, and treatment for their child may be jeopardized. A concerted effort to establish a national mandate requiring third-party payment for medical foods is underway.

Natural History and Treatment Options

In the late 1950s and early 1960s, many viewed PKU as a genetic disorder in which mental retardation or disability was an inevitable outcome.[4] Even when a special metabolic formula and lists of low PHE foods became available, many patients with PKU were not able to lead normal lives because the PHE restriction had not begun until they were symptomatic. After newborn screening began, there was a nationwide awareness of PKU. Government-funded longitudinal studies led to an understanding of the importance of presymptomatic diagnosis and the possibility of a normal, productive life when an appropriate diet was followed.[81] History has been repeating itself over the last decade with the presymptomatic diagnosis of other rare disorders, detected through MS/MS newborn screening. Early descriptions of

MCAD deficiency described long-term neurological sequelae in many infants and behavioral issues in later childhood.[82] Some early treatment modalities included strict round-the-clock carbohydrate intake and fat restriction. With the accumulated data from many centers that have followed patients with MCAD deficiency since their detection by MS/MS NBS, the current message to new parents of infants with MCAD deficiency is quite different.[83] These parents can expect their infant to reach his or her full intellectual potential, and need be concerned about short-term fasting only in times of physiological stress. A web-based guide for treatment of MCAD deficiency was developed by the Genetic Metabolic Dietitians International (GMDI).[84]

Because many of the disorders detected through MS/MS newborn screening are very rare, cooperative data sharing among programs is allowing natural history information to be available as more and more infants are screened and identified presymptomatically.

Mutation analyses contribute to the accumulated data about these disorders. It is hoped that genotype/phenotype correlations can predict the potential severity of these disorders. Although environmental factors, epigenetic considerations, and intercurrent illnesses can greatly impact clinical outcome, it has been possible to identify some so-called "mild" mutations among newborns identified through MS/MS NBS.[85]

Questions have also been raised about whether certain disorders, now identified through MS/MS NBS, require medical intervention at all. Germany has decided to remove 3-MCC deficiency from its list of screened disorders.[86] They feel that the potential stigma attached to being given the diagnosis and the relatively mild course in most patients with 3-MCC deficiency does not warrant its being included. Others have documented cases with mild-to-severe problems with 3-MCC deficiency that seem to validate its inclusion.[55,56]

Evaluation

For affected newborns who are subsequently managed by the metabolic team, careful documentation regarding symptoms, laboratory test results, interventions, and monitoring is extremely helpful in evaluating the MS/MS NBS program. This information should be documented at the treatment centers and collected by the NBS program's follow-up coordinator. Nationwide data collection and evaluation are being done by the Centers for Disease Control, the Newborn Screening and Genetic Testing Resource Center,[87] and the Region 4 Genetics Collaborative,[88] which is collecting data from screening programs outside the United States as well.

Outcome

Incidence

In the past decade, MS/MS has been implemented in NBS programs around the globe. The incidence of disorders detected has been calculated to be approximately 1 in every 3000 newborns screened.[25,68] Comparison studies have looked at the higher incidence for disorders detected through MS/MS NBS than the prevalence of the same disorders that had been symptomatically diagnosed prior to screening.[89,90] These differences represent both ends of the severity spectrum of given disorders. Some of the newborns identified through MS/MS NBS represent milder forms of the disorder, and they may never have come to clinical attention.[86,91] Others represent newborns who may have had an early demise without a diagnosis and would have been missed cases, if they had been born prior to MS/MS NBS.

Clinical Outcome

Several studies have included MS/MS NBS outcome data. Schulze and colleagues evaluated the outcome data for 250,000 infants screened over a period of 42 months.[92] Of the 106 newborns receiving a diagnosis after having been detected by MS/MS NBS, 70 required treatment/intervention, while 36 were judged to have mild disorders or milder variants. Nine infants became symptomatic in the newborn period; six of these before screening results were available. In total, 58% of the newborns detected through MS/MS NBS who needed treatment remained asymptomatic over the observation period of 5 to 38 months of the study.

Another study compared outcomes of infants born with inborn errors of metabolism in two areas of Germany with similar populations, only one of which had an established MS/MS NBS program for presymptomatic diagnoses.[93] No clinically symptomatic cases were reported in the 46 infants diagnosed through MS/MS NBS, while 22 of the 33 infants among the unscreened infants had an acute metabolic crisis, 5 of which were fatal.

Many of the studies on clinical outcome have focused on a single disorder, MCAD deficiency (MCADD). A study in Australia compared outcomes in 35 unscreened patients with MCADD with 24 who had been screened. There were 23 episodes of severe metabolic decompensation and 5 deaths in the unscreened cohort, and only 3 episodes and 1 (neonatal) death in the screened population. To make the two cohorts comparable, only events between birth and 4 years of age were compared. The calculated relative risk (screened vs unscreened) for an adverse event before the age of 2 years was

0.26. Neuropsychological testing did not show a significant difference between the cognitive ability of the two groups.[94,95]

One study looked at published adverse outcomes from newborn screening, specifically inappropriate treatment of infants with false-positive results from NBS programs since 1980. The authors concluded that although there may be some bias against publishing accounts of medical error, they were unable to find any documented evidence of harm.[96] Some infants may be erroneously started on a restrictive diet as soon as NBS results are known, but standards of care dictate that clinical evaluation and confirmatory testing are necessary before a disease-specific intervention is initiated. The role of a comprehensive follow-up program that includes the metabolic team cannot be overstated.

Benefit and Effectiveness

Another parameter used to evaluate MS/MS NBS is economic analyses.[97] Cost-benefit analysis (CBA) can be used to make direct comparison of the costs of MS/MS NBS to the costs of making the diagnosis using other technologies to achieve the same benefit. Assessing outcomes/consequences in monetary terms is required when comparing the costs and benefits of one type of program to another. For example, this type of analysis might include such nonmonetary parameters as reassurance or anxiety to families (caused by receiving NBS results).

Cost-effectiveness analysis (CEA) is the technique most often used in evaluating MS/MS NBS programs. CEA expresses benefits in terms of "natural units" such as life-years saved, cases detected, and so on. CEA is sometimes difficult to use as a tool in this context because often there is no common denominator that would allow complete health gains to be compared between MS/MS NBS and other technologies. For example, it is difficult to evaluate the quality of life for a newborn detected through MS/MS NBS who remains on a complex restricted diet for life. And, although early diagnosis and initiation of treatment may be life-saving, the lifetime cost of treatment may be staggering. Cost-effectiveness is not the same as cost saving. An expensive screening test can be cost-effective. Cost-utility analysis (CUA) is a subset of CEA that allows comparisons of health interventions that improve quality of life. This allows alternative programs to be evaluated in terms of "quality-adjusted life-years" when quality of life is the desired outcome measure. Analyses of this kind allowed Venditti et al. to estimate that over the first 20 years of life, the cost of MS/MS NBS for MCADD was $11,000 per life-year saved, or $5600 per quality-adjusted life-years saved. When they projected over a life span of 70 years, these numbers became $300 and $100, respectively.[98]

Cost-effectiveness has also been used by policy makers when deciding whether to implement or expand MS/MS NBS in a given region. A study from Ontario, Canada, concluded that in order for MS/MS NBS to be cost-effective, one must "bundle" together only those diseases that individually cost less than $100,000 per life-year gained. This would suggest including PKU and 14 other disorders, but not the full ACMG panel.[99] Expansion of MS/MS NBS for MCADD in The Netherlands was based on a comparison of infants with MCADD who were diagnosed symptomatically between 1985 and 2003 with those detected presymptomatically in one region of the country due to MS/MS NBS. They reported an incremental cost-effectiveness ratio (ICER) of $1653 per life-year gained.[100] It is often difficult to include all possible factors in such analyses. Rarely is there an estimate of the cost of false positives or the cost of treatment for individuals who may have remained asymptomatic even without treatment. Equally rare is inclusion of the benefit of MS/MS NBS in helping to provide a diagnosis even if there is no effective treatment. Some feel that in these cases the knowledge gained can guide further family planning, or lessen the time and cost involved in searching for a diagnosis.[101-107] With limited healthcare dollars, the results of these types of economic analyses and their limitations are often quoted by both the proponents and detractors of expanded screening.

Future

Expansion

Active research and pilot studies are underway to determine the efficacy of NBS for disorders such as lysosomal storage diseases,[101,102] severe combined immunodeficiency disease,[103] type I diabetes,[104] Duchene muscular dystrophy,[105,106] fragile X,[107] and others. While these specific disorders do not presently have interventions that would involve the metabolic team, they do represent the development of more advanced laboratory and program methodologies. These same methodologies may find application to metabolic disorders in the future. They will also be subjected to the same type of scrutiny (i.e., criteria for inclusion) faced by the panel of disorders in the current ACMG recommended panel.[108]

Since blood samples are collected from every newborn, there is a great deal of interest in population-based screening for disorders not traditionally considered appropriate for NBS. For some, the hope is that by identifying individuals early, the diagnostic odyssey will be shortened even if there is no cure or effective treatment at this time.[109] The accepted guidelines for inclusion into the NBS panel now exclude adult-onset disorders, but some hope that early detection will lead to monitoring and gathering of natural history data that may lead to successful intervention in the future. Ethical considerations include the testing of minors for adult-onset disorders, the identification of carriers, the need for informed consent for certain genetic tests, and the possible stigma attached to carrying a diagnosis for a mild disorder throughout life.[110]

Toward Uniform Guidelines

Uniform national guidelines are being proposed for each step of the NBS program from collection of samples to long-term management protocols. The HRSA grants given to the Regional Genetic Collaboratives have provided the opportunity for groups of states within a particular geographic region to explore evidence-based guidelines.[111] A guide, *Program Evaluation and Assessment Scheme* (PEAS), to help individual states evaluate their own NBS program, is available and provides a uniform set of questions that can be used as a self-assessment tool in evaluating the way the various parts of individual screening systems function.[112] The ACT sheets and screening algorithms provide a starting point for follow up of newborn screening results.[74] And, there have been a few evidence-based guidelines for the long-term management of specific disorders detected through MS/MS NBS.[56]

Education

Each NBS program should have a defined education plan to provide newborn screening information to all public health professionals, healthcare providers, birthing facilities, parents, and state policy makers.[112] The means to disseminate this information should include in-service programs, written materials, web-based information, media spots, and so on. Information should be presented at regular intervals and always when there are announcements about changes to the program. Information for families needs to be prepared in several formats that address their cultural, language, and educational diversity.[112] All materials should be reviewed and updated on a regular basis. An evidence-based evaluation of the educational/informational arm of the NBS program is essential. Although there are some excellent materials available explaining newborn screening to parents and professionals, these may not address all the needs of any specific state's NBS programs. States differ in the time that the blood sample is obtained, whether a mandatory second screen is required, the disorders included in the screening panel, how the screening results are reported, and so on. Although there is a drive to standardize all aspects of NBS, each state needs to prepare or modify an educational plan that is appropriate for their program and their consumers.

Manpower

Training of more health professions, especially metabolic specialists, is seen as a pressing need for the future if MS/MS newborn screening *is* to be successful. The professional educators who evaluate the curricula for U.S. medical school education have long recommended genetics within the didactic portion of training.[113] Discussion of the management of patients with metabolic disorders is often limited to PKU, but needs to be expanded. There are medical genetics fellowships available to medical school graduates.[114] It is important that medical students and residents be attracted to these opportunities in order to be educated as the metabolic specialists of the future.

The emerging role of the genetic metabolic dietitian with expertise in the nutrition management of patients with rare inborn errors of metabolism must be recognized.[115] Beyond their traditional roles of dietary intervention and case management, genetic metabolic dietitians hold positions as state MS/MS follow-up coordinators, they are on national newborn screening and genetic policy boards, and are actively engaged in metabolic disease research as principal investigators. Although at the present time there is no accreditation board for metabolic dietitians, there is an active professional organization working toward that goal.[116] There have been a number of postgraduate educational opportunities offered for genetic metabolic dietitians and an ongoing listserve (PNO-METAB-L@listserv.cc.emory.edu) that promotes immediate access to shared expertise.

Financial Constraints

In the United States, individual state programs charge NBS fees that range from $0 to $139 per newborn.[76] For many programs, this fee is used to fund not only laboratory costs, but also program administrative costs, follow-up services, genetic services, medical foods, or educational programs.[76] This means that the budgets for any one of these services may be limited, even when other funding sources are sought. And, although many hardworking and talented people are involved in the screening programs, their hands are tied without funding to initiate new projects or improve established programs.[117,118] For a newborn detected through the NBS program, the extent of comprehensive care and follow up is dependent on the state in which the infant is born, rather than the diagnosis.

Within the tertiary medical centers, highly qualified metabolic specialists spend hours researching, counseling, and managing very complex patients without being fully reimbursed by third-party payers for the time involved. Vockley advises metabolic professionals that they need to work closely with insurance companies to help them understand the uniqueness of this patient population and their needs, with parent advocacy groups to help pass appropriate national mandates, and with the medical establishment to make them aware of the expertise of the metabolic professionals.[119]

CONCLUSION

Widespread incorporation of MS/MS technology in newborn screening is less than a decade old. The potential to detect many more than the previously detected metabolic disorders presymptomatically has already been realized. Outcome data have shown a drop in both morbidity and mortality among patients with disorders in the screening panel. While the metabolic specialists are struggling to keep up with the increased patient numbers as a result of MS/MS NBS, the wider medical community has shown a keen interest in expanding newborn screening to include many other disorders.

The lessons learned in the past 10 years strongly suggest that establishment of strict criteria for inclusion of disorders in an NBS panel, adequate personnel and financial resources, evidence-based interventions, and uniform performance-based guidelines should precede unbridled expansion.

REFERENCES

1. Fölling I. The discovery of phenylketonuria. *Acta Paediatr.* 1994;407(Suppl 1): 4–10.
2. Jervis GA. Phenylpyruvic oligophrenia deficiency of phenylalanine-oxidizing system. *Proc Soc Exp Biol Med.* 1953;82:514–515.
3. Bickel H, Gerrard E, Hickmans M. Influence of phenylalanine intake on phenylketonuria. *Lancet.* 1953;265:812–813.
4. Koch JH. *Robert Guthrie: The PKU Story*. Pasadena, CA: Hope Publishing House; 1997:24.
5. Guthrie R, Susi R. A simple phenylalanine method for detecting phenylketonuria in large populations of newborn infants. *Pediatrics.* 1963;32:338–343.
6. Guthrie R, Whitney S. *Phenylketonuria Detection in the Newborn Infant as a Routine Hospital Procedure: A Trial of the Phenylalanine Screening Method in 400,000 Infants*. Washington, DC: US Government Printing Office; 1964.
7. MacCready R. Phenylketonuria screening program. *N Engl J Med.* 1963;9:52–56.
8. Paul DB. The history of newborn screeing in the U.S. In: Holtzman NA, Watson MS, eds. *Promoting Safe and Effective Genetic Testing in the United States: Final Report of the Task Force on Genetic Testing*. Bethesda, MD: National Institutes of Health; 1997:137–160.
9. Health Resources and Services Administration and American Academy of Pediatrics. Serving the family from birth to the medical home: a report from the Newborn Screening Task Force convened in Washington DC, May 10–11, 1999. *Pediatrics.* 2000;106:383–427.

10. Hill JB, Summer GK, Pender MW, Roszel NO. An automated procedure for blood phenylalanine. *Clin Chem.* 1965;11:541–546.
11. Frazier PD, Summer GK. An automated fluorometric method for analysis of glycine in biological fluids. *Anal Biochem.* 1971;44:66–76.
12. Beutler E, Baluda MC. A simple spot screening test for galactosemia. *J Lab Clin Med.* 1966;68:137–141.
13. Dussault JH, Morissette J, Letarte J, Guyda H, Laberge C. Modification of a screening program for neonatal hypothyroidism. *J Pediatr.* 1978;92:274–277.
14. Jacobs S, Peterson L, Thompson L, et al. Newborn screening for hemoglobin abnormalities: a comparison of methods. *Am J Clin Pathol.* 1986;85:713–715.
15. Raskin S, Phillips JA III, Kaplan G, McClure M, Vnencak-Jones C. Cystic fibrosis genotyping by direct PCR analysis of Guthrie blood spots. *PCR Methods Appl.* 1992;2:154–156.
16. Millington DS, Kodo N, Norwood DL, Roe CR. Tandem mass spectrometry: a new method for acylcarnitine profiling with potential for neonatal screening for inborn errors of metabolism. *J Inherit Metab Dis.* 1990;13:321–324.
17. Chace DH, Millington DS, Terada N, Kahler SG, Roe CR, Hofman LF. Rapid diagnosis of phenylketonuria by quantitative analysis for phenylalanine and tyrosine in neonatal blood spots by tandem mass spectrometry. *Clin Chem.* 1993;39: 66–71.
18. Rashed MS, Bucknall MP, Little D, et al. Screening blood spots for inborn errors of metabolism by electrospray tandem mass spectrometry with a microplate batch process and a computer algorithm for automated flagging of abnormal profiles. *Clin Chem.* 1997;43:1129–1141.
19. Muenzer J, Frazier D, Weavil SD. Incidence of metabolic disorders detected by newborn screening in North Carolina using tandem mass spectrometry. *Am J Human Genet.* 2000;67:36.
20. Wilcken B, Wiley V, Sim KG, Carpenter K. Carnitine transporter defect diagnosed by newborn screening with electrospray tandem mass spectrometry. *J Pediatr.* 2001;138:581–584.
21. American College of Medical Genetics. Newborn screening: toward a uniform screening panel and system. *Genet Med* 2006;8(Suppl 1):1S–252S.
22. Chace DH, Sherwin JE, Hillman SL, Lorey F, Cunningham GC. Use of phenylalanine-to-tyrosine ratio determined by tandem mass spectrometry to improve newborn screening for phenylketonuria of early discharge specimens collected in the first 24 hours. *Clin Chem.* 1998;44:2405–2409.
23. Thony B, Blau N. Mutations in the BH4-metabolizing genes GTP cyclohydrolase I, 6-pyruvoyl-tetrahydropterin synthase, sepiapterin reductase, carbinolamine-4a-dehydratase, and dihydropteridine reductase. *Hum Mutat.* 2006;27:870–878.
24. Gregory CO, Yu C, Singh RH. Blood phenylalanine monitoring for dietary compliance among patients with phenylketonuria: comparison of methods. *Genet Med.* 2007;9:761–765.
25. Frazier DM, Millington DS, McCandless SE, et al. The tandem mass spectrometry newborn screening experience in North Carolina: 1997–2005. *J Inherit Metab Dis.* 2006;29:76–85.
26. Magera MJ, Gunawardena ND, Hahn SH, et al. Quantitative determination of succinylacetone in dried blood spots for newborn screening of tyrosinemia type I. *Mol Genet Metab.* 2006;88:16–21.

27. Matern D, Tortorelli S, Oglesbee D, Gavrilov D, Rinaldo P. Reduction of the false-positive rate in newborn screening by implementation of MS/MS-based second-tier tests: the Mayo Clinic experience (2004–2007). *J Inherit Metab Dis*. 2007;30: 585–592.
28. Al Dirbashi OY, Rashed MS, Brink HJ, et al. Determination of succinylacetone in dried blood spots and liquid urine as a dansylhydrazone by liquid chromatography tandem mass spectrometry. *J Chromat B Analyt Technol Biomed Life Sci*. 2006; 831:274–280.
29. Mitchell GA, Grompe M, Lambert M, Tanguay RM. Hypertyrosinemia. In: Scriver CR, Beaudet AL, Sly WS, Valle D, eds. *The Metabolic and Molecular Bases of Inherited Disease*. 8th ed. New York, NY: McGraw-Hill; 2001:1777–1805.
30. Vitamin C for prophylaxis of tyrosinemia in the newborn. Statement by the Nutrition Committee of the Canadian Paediatric Society. *Can Med Assoc J*. 1976; 114:447.
31. David M, Michel M, Collombel C, Dutruge J, Cotte J, Jeune M. Transient hypertyrosinemia secondary to hepatic involvement: 2 cases of different etiologies (galactosemia, hepatitis). *Pediatrie*. 1970;25:459–466.
32. Sokolova J, Janosikova B, Terwilliger JD, Freiberger T, Kraus JP, Kozich V. Cystathionine beta-synthase deficiency in Central Europe: discrepancy between biochemical and molecular genetic screening for homocystinuric alleles. *Hum Mutat*. 2001;18:548–549.
33. Surtees R, Leonard J, Austin S. Association of demyelination with deficiency of cerebrospinal-fluid S-adenosylmethionine in inborn errors of methyl-transfer pathway. *Lancet*. 1991;338:1550–1554.
34. Harvey MS, Braverman N, Pomper M, et al. Infantile hypermethioninemia and hyperhomocysteinemia due to high methionine intake: a diagnostic trap. *Mol Genet Metab*. 2003;79:6–16.
35. Ohura T, Kobayashi K, Tazawa Y, et al. Neonatal presentation of adult-onset type II citrullinemia. *Hum Genet*. 2001;108:87–90.
36. Ohura T, Kobayashi K, Abukawa D, et al. A novel inborn error of metabolism detected by elevated methionine and/or galactose in newborn screening: neonatal intrahepatic cholestasis caused by citrin deficiency. *Eur J Pediatr*. 2003;162: 317–322.
37. Saheki T, Kobayashi K. Mitochondrial aspartate glutamate carrier (citrin) deficiency as the cause of adult-onset type II citrullinemia (CTLN2) and idiopathic neonatal hepatitis (NICCD). *J Hum Genet*. 2002;47:333–341.
38. Naylor EW, Guthrie R. Newborn screening for maple syrup urine disease (branched-chain ketoaciduria). *Pediatrics*. 1978;61:262–266.
39. Levy HL. Genetic screening. *Adv Hum Genet*. 1973;4:1–104.
40. Chace DH, Kalas TA, Naylor EW. The application of tandem mass spectrometry to neonatal screening for inherited disorders of intermediary metabolism. *Annu Rev Genomics Hum Genet*. 2002;3:17–45.
41. Bhattacharya K, Khalili V, Wiley V, Carpenter K, Wilcken B. Newborn screening may fail to identify intermediate forms of maple syrup urine disease. *J Inherit Metab Dis*. 2006;29:586.
42. Kim SZ, Varvogli L, Waisbren SE, Levy HL. Hydroxyprolinemia: comparison of a patient and her unaffected twin sister. *J Pediatr*. 1997;130:437–441.
43. Nezu J, Tamai I, Oku A, et al. Primary systemic carnitine deficiency is caused by mutations in a gene encoding sodium ion-dependent carnitine transporter. *Nat Genet*. 1999;21:91–94.

44. Chace DH, DiPerna JC, Kalas TA, Johnson RW, Naylor EW. Rapid diagnosis of methylmalonic and propionic acidemias: quantitative tandem mass spectrometric analysis of propionylcarnitine in filter-paper blood specimens obtained from newborns. *Clin Chem.* 2001;47:2040–2044.
45. Koeberl DD, Young SP, Gregersen NS, et al. Rare disorders of metabolism with elevated butyryl- and isobutyryl-carnitine detected by tandem mass spectrometry newborn screening. *Pediatr Res.* 2003;54:219–223.
46. Oglesbee D, He M, Majumder N, et al. Development of a newborn screening follow-up algorithm for the diagnosis of isobutyryl-CoA dehydrogenase deficiency. *Genet Med.* 2007;9:108–116.
47. Chace DH, DiPerna JC, Mitchell BL, Sgroi B, Hofman LF, Naylor EW. Electrospray tandem mass spectrometry for analysis of acylcarnitines in dried postmortem blood specimens collected at autopsy from infants with unexplained cause of death. *Clin Chem.* 2001;47:1166–1182.
48. Gibson KM, Burlingame TG, Hogema B, et al. 2-Methylbutyryl-coenzyme A dehydrogenase deficiency: a new inborn error of L-isoleucine metabolism. *Pediatr Res.* 2000;47:830–833.
49. Korman SH. Inborn errors of isoleucine degradation: a review. *Mol Genet Metab.* 2006;89:289–299.
50. van Calcar SC, Gleason LA, Lindh H, et al. 2-methylbutyryl-CoA dehydrogenase deficiency in Hmong infants identified by expanded newborn screen. *WMJ.* 2007; 106:12–15.
51. Daum RS, Scriver CR, Mamer OA, Delvin E, Lamm P, Goldman H. An inherited disorder of isoleucine catabolism causing accumulation of alpha-methylacetoacetate and alpha-methyl-beta-hydroxybutyrate, and intermittent metabolic acidosis. *Pediatr Res.* 1973;7:149–160.
52. Hedlund GL, Longo N, Pasquali M. Glutaric acidemia type 1. *Am J Med Genet C Semin Med Genet.* 2006;142C:86–94.
53. Lindner M, Ho S, Fang-Hoffmann J, Hoffmann GF, Kolker S. Neonatal screening for glutaric aciduria type I: strategies to proceed. *J Inherit Metab Dis.* 2006;29: 378–382.
54. Napolitano N, Wiley V, Pitt JJ. Pseudo-glutarylcarnitinaemia in medium-chain acyl-CoA dehydrogenase deficiency detected by tandem mass spectrometry newborn screening. *J Inherit Metab Dis.* 2004;27:465–471.
55. Frazier DM. Maternal 3-MCC deficiency diagnosed secondary to elevated 3-OH isovaleryl carnitine on tandem mass spectrometry newborn screening in NC. Available at http://www.aphl.org/conference/2005_conferences/newborn_screening_genetics_ 2005. Accessed February 27, 2008.
56. Arnold GL, Koeberl DD, Matern D, et al. A Delphi-based consensus clinical practice protocol for the diagnosis and management of 3-methylcrotonyl CoA carboxylase deficiency. *Mol Genet Metab.* 2008;93:363–370.
57. Clayton PT, Doig M, Ghafari S, et al. Screening for medium-chain acyl-CoA dehydrogenase deficiency using electrospray ionisation tandem mass spectrometry. *Arch Dis Child.* 1998;79:109–115.
58. Blois B, Riddell C, Dooley K, Dyack S. Newborns with C8-acylcarnitine level over the 90th percentile have an increased frequency of the common MCAD 985A>G mutation. *J Inherit Metab Dis.* 2005;28:551–556.
59. Schymik I, Liebig M, Mueller M, et al. Pitfalls of neonatal screening for very-long-chain acyl-CoA dehydrogenase deficiency using tandem mass spectrometry. *J Pediatr.* 2006;149:128–130.

60. Gregersen N, Andresen BS, Bross P. Prevalent mutations in fatty acid oxidation disorders: diagnostic considerations. *Eur J Pediatr*. 2000;159(Suppl 3):S213–S218.
61. Levy HL. Reproductive effects of maternal metabolic disorders: implications for pediatrics and obstetrics. *Turk J Pediatr*. 1996;38:335–344.
62. Singla M, Guzman G, Griffin AJ, Bharati S. Cardiomyopathy in multiple Acyl-CoA dehydrogenase deficiency: a clinico-pathological correlation and review of literature. *Pediatr Cardiol*. 2008;29:446–451.
63. Chiong MA, Sim KG, Carpenter K, et al. Transient multiple acyl-CoA dehydrogenation deficiency in a newborn female caused by maternal riboflavin deficiency. *Mol Genet Metab*. 2007;92:109–114.
64. Khoury MJ, McCabe LL, McCabe ER. Population screening in the age of genomic medicine. *N Engl J Med*. 2003;348:50–58.
65. Dhondt JL. Neonatal screening: from the "Guthrie age" to the "genetic age." *J Inherit Metab Dis*. 2007;30:418–422.
66. Sweetman L, Millington DS, Therrell BL, et al. Naming and counting disorders (conditions) included in newborn screening panels. *Pediatrics*. 2006;117:S308–S314.
67. Hewlett J, Waisbren SE. A review of the psychosocial effects of false-positive results on parents and current communication practices in newborn screening. *J Inherit Metab Dis*. 2006;29:677–682.
68. Rinaldo P, Zafari S, Tortorelli S, Matern D. Making the case for objective performance metrics in newborn screening by tandem mass spectrometry. *Ment Retard Dev Disabil Res Rev*. 2006;12:255–261.
69. Balk KG. Recommended newborn screening policy change for the NICU infant. *Policy Polit Nurs Pract*. 2007;8:210–219.
70. Meyburg J, Schulze A, Kohlmueller D, Linderkamp O, Mayatepek E. Postnatal changes in neonatal acylcarnitine profile. *Pediatr Res*. 2001;49:125–129.
71. la Marca G, Malvagia S, Pasquini E, Innocenti M, Donati MA, Zammarchi E. Rapid 2nd-tier test for measurement of 3-OH-propionic and methylmalonic acids on dried blood spots: reducing the false-positive rate for propionylcarnitine during expanded newborn screening by liquid chromatography-tandem mass spectrometry. *Clin Chem*. 2007;53:1364–1369.
72. National Newborn Screening Information System. Criteria for second screens. Available at: http://www2.uthscsa.edu/nnsis/. Accessed March 14, 2008.
73. Hermerath C. APHL 2005 Newborn Screening and Genetics Testing Symposium. Tandem mass spectrometry and second newborn screening specimens. Available at: http://www.aphl.org/conference/2005_conferences/newborn_screening_genetics_2005. Accessed February 27, 2008.
74. American College of Medical Genetics. Newborn screening ACT sheets and confirmatory algorithms. Available at: http://www.acmg.net/resources/policies/ACT/condition-analyte-links.htm. Accessed February 27, 2008.
75. Farriaux JP, Vidailhet M, Briard ML, Belot V, Dhondt JL. Neonatal screening for cystic fibrosis: France rises to the challenge. *J Inherit Metab Dis*. 2003;26:729–744.
76. National Newborn Screening Information System. Summation of fees charged for newborn screening. Available at: http:www2.uthscsa.edu/nnsis. Accessed March 9, 2008.
77. Hoff T, Hoyt A. Practices and perceptions of long-term follow-up among state newborn screening programs. *Pediatrics*. 2006;117:1922–1929.
78. Buist NR, Tuerck JM. The practitioner's role in newborn screening. *Pediatr Clin North Am*. 1992;39:199–211.

79. Buist NR, Huntington K. Scene from the USA: the illogic of mandating screening without also providing for treatment. *J Inherit Metab Dis*. 2007;30:445–446.
80. Orphan Drug Amendments of 1988. Pub L No. 100–290. Available at: http://www.cfsan.fda.gov/%7Edms/medfguid.html#q7. Accessed March 26, 2009.
81. Michals K, Azen C, Acosta P, Koch R, Matalon R. Blood phenylalanine levels and intelligence of 10-year-old children with PKU in the National Collaborative Study. *J Am Diet Assoc*. 1988;88:1226–1229.
82. Iafolla AK, Thompson RJ Jr, Roe CR. Medium-chain acyl-coenzyme A dehydrogenase deficiency: clinical course in 120 affected children. *J Pediatr*. 1994;124:409–415.
83. Andresen BS, Dobrowolski SF, O'Reilly L, et al. Medium-chain acyl-CoA dehydrogenase (MCAD) mutations identified by MS/MS-based prospective screening of newborns differ from those observed in patients with clinical symptoms: identification and characterization of a new, prevalent mutation that results in mild MCAD deficiency. *Am J Hum Genet*. 2001;68:1408–1418.
84. Genetic Metabolic Dietitians International. Nutrition Guidelines. Available at: http://gmdi.org./guidelines/index.php. Accessed February 27, 2008.
85. Waddell L, Wiley V, Carpenter K, et al. Medium-chain acyl-CoA dehydrogenase deficiency: genotype-biochemical phenotype correlations. *Mol Genet Metab*. 2006;87:32–39.
86. Stadler SC, Polanetz R, Maier EM, et al. Newborn screening for 3-methylcrotonyl-CoA carboxylase deficiency: population heterogeneity of MCCA and MCCB mutations and impact on risk assessment. *Hum Mutat*. 2006;27:748–759.
87. National Newborn Screening and Genetics Resource Center. Individual state overviews. Available at: http://genes-r-us.uthscsa.edu. Accessed February 27, 2008.
88. Region 4 Genetics Collaborative. Role of newborn screening by MS/MS cluster. Available at: http://www.region4genetics.org/cluster1-information.aspx. Accessed February 27, 2008.
89. Grosse SD, Khoury MJ, Greene CL, Crider KS, Pollitt RJ. The epidemiology of medium-chain acyl-CoA dehydrogenase deficiency: an update. *Genet Med*. 2006;8:205–212.
90. Rhead WJ. Newborn screening for medium-chain acyl-CoA dehydrogenase deficiency: a global perspective. *J Inherit Metab Dis*. 2006;29:370–377.
91. Wilcken B. Recent advances in newborn screening. *J Inherit Metab Dis*. 2007;30:129–133.
92. Schulze A, Lindner M, Kohlmuller D, Olgemoller K, Mayatepek E, Hoffmann GF. Expanded newborn screening for inborn errors of metabolism by electrospray ionization-tandem mass spectrometry: results, outcome, and implications. *Pediatrics*. 2003;111:1399–1406.
93. Hoffmann GF, von Kries R, Klose D, et al. Frequencies of inherited organic acidurias and disorders of mitochondrial fatty acid transport and oxidation in Germany. *Eur J Pediatr*. 2004;163:76–80.
94. Wilcken B, Haas M, Joy P, et al. Outcome of neonatal screening for medium-chain acyl-CoA dehydrogenase deficiency in Australia: a cohort study. *Lancet*. 2007;369:37–42.
95. Haas M, Chaplin M, Joy P, Wiley V, Black C, Wilcken B. Healthcare use and costs of medium-chain acyl-CoA dehydrogenase deficiency in Australia: screening versus no screening. *J Pediatr*. 2007;151:121–126.

96. Brosco JP, Seider MI, Dunn AC. Universal newborn screening and adverse medical outcomes: a historical note. *Ment Retard Dev Disabil Res Rev*. 2006;12:262–269.
97. Feuchtbaum L, Cunningham G. Economic evaluation of tandem mass spectrometry screening in California. *Pediatrics*. 2006;117:S280–S286.
98. Venditti LN, Venditti CP, Berry GT, et al. Newborn screening by tandem mass spectrometry for medium-chain Acyl-CoA dehydrogenase deficiency: a cost-effectiveness analysis. *Pediatrics*. 2003;112:1005–1015.
99. Cipriano LE, Rupar CA, Zaric GS. The cost-effectiveness of expanding newborn screening for up to 21 inherited metabolic disorders using tandem mass spectrometry: results from a decision-analytic model. *Value Health*. 2007;10:83–97.
100. van der Hilst CS, Derks TG, Reijngoud DJ, Smit GP, TenVergert EM. Cost-effectiveness of neonatal screening for medium chain acyl-CoA dehydrogenase deficiency: the homogeneous population of The Netherlands. *J Pediatr*. 2007;151: 115–120.
101. Gelb MH, Turecek F, Scott CR, Chamoles NA. Direct multiplex assay of enzymes in dried blood spots by tandem mass spectrometry for the newborn screening of lysosomal storage disorders. *J Inherit Metab Dis*. 2006;29:397–404.
102. Meikle PJ, Grasby DJ, Dean CJ, et al. Newborn screening for lysosomal storage disorders. *Mol Genet Metab*. 2006;88:307–314.
103. Puck JM. Population-based newborn screening for severe combined immunodeficiency: steps toward implementation. *J Allergy Clin Immunol*. 2007;120:760–768.
104. Eising S, Svensson J, Skogstrand K, et al. Type 1 diabetes risk analysis on dried blood spot samples from population-based newborns: design and feasibility of an unselected case-control study. *Paediatr Perinat Epidemiol*. 2007;21:507–517.
105. Kemper AR, Wake MA. Duchenne muscular dystrophy: issues in expanding newborn screening. *Curr Opin Pediatr*. 2007;19:700–704.
106. Ross LF. Screening for conditions that do not meet the Wilson and Jungner criteria: the case of Duchenne muscular dystrophy. *Am J Med Genet A*. 2006;140:914–922.
107. Bailey DB Jr. Newborn screening for fragile X syndrome. *Ment Retard Dev Disabil Res Rev*. 2004;10:3–10.
108. Green NS, Rinaldo P, Brower A, et al. Committee report: advancing the current recommended panel of conditions for newborn screening. *Genet Med*. 2007;9:792–796.
109. Bailey DB Jr, Beskow LM, Davis AM, Skinner D. Changing perspectives on the benefits of newborn screening. *Ment Retard Dev Disabil Res Rev*. 2006;12:270–279.
110. Nelson RM, Botkjin JR, Kodish ED, et al. Ethical issues with genetic testing in pediatrics. *Pediatrics*. 2001;107:1451–1455.
111. Puryear M, Weissman G, Watson M, Mann M, Strickland B, van Dyck PC. The regional genetic and newborn screening service collaboratives: the first two years. *Ment Retard Dev Disabil Res Rev*. 2006;12:288–292.
112. National Newborn Screening and Genetics Resource Center. Performance evaluation and assessment scheme (PEAS) for newborn screening systems. Available at: http://genes-r-us.uthscsa.edu/NBS_PEAS.htm. Accessed February 27, 2008.
113. Robinson DM, Fong CT. Genetics in medical school curriculum: a look at the University of Rochester School of Medicine and Dentistry. *J Zhejiang Univ Sci B*. 2008;9:10–15.
114. Accreditation Council for Graduate Medical Education. List of ACMGE accredited programs and sponsoring institution. Available at: http://www.abng.org/adspublic/reports/accreditede-programs.asp. Accessed March 9, 2008.

115. Acosta PB, Ryan AS. Functions of dietitians providing nutrition support to patients with inherited metabolic disorders. *J Am Diet Assoc*. 1997;97:783–786.
116. Genetic Metabolic Dietitians International. Mission. Available at: http://gmdi.org/index.php?page=about%20us. Accessed February 27, 2008.
117. Wang G, Watts C. The role of genetics in the provision of essential public health services. *Am J Public Health*. 2007;97:620–625.
118. Therrell BL, Williams D, Johnson K, Lloyd-Puryear MA, Mann MY, Ramos LR. Financing newborn screening: sources, issues, and future considerations. *J Public Health Manag Pract*. 2007;13:207–213.
119. Vockley J. Newborn screening: after the thrill is gone. *Mol Genet Metab*. 2007;92:6–12.

Chapter 3

Evaluation of Nutrition Status

Phyllis B. Acosta

INTRODUCTION

Several components are involved in the assessment of nutrition status, among which are nutrient intakes, growth, laboratory analyses, clinical signs, and health history. Because patients with inherited disorders of amino acid metabolism must ingest much of their diet in the elemental form and because no fat, minerals, or vitamins are included in some of the medical foods used, frequent evaluation of the patient's nutrition status by several parameters is essential.

Nutrient Intake Assessment

In order to determine if nutrient intakes are adequate in patients with inherited metabolic disorders (IMDs), one must first know the approximate requirement for each nutrient at different ages. Several factors influence the need for and use of nutrients by patients with IMDs that are not present in normal persons. These factors include forms in which nutrients are ingested, other nutrients consumed concomitantly with elemental foods, heat treatment of specific nutrients, and in the patient, presence of normal and abnormal metabolites in greater than normal concentrations, as well as elevated body temperature. Thus, many nutrients are required in larger amounts than described in Recommended Dietary Allowances (RDAs).[1]

Energy

Early studies to determine which amino acids are essential for humans and in what amounts indicated that when free amino acids (FAAs) supplied the entire protein requirement, energy needs were increased, both in infants[2] and adults.[3] Pratt et al.[2] reported that when all nitrogen (N) was supplied as FAAs to infants, in order for growth to proceed normally, energy intake often had to be increased from 125/kcal/kg body weight (BW) to 150 kcal/kg BW, a 20% increase. Rose[3] found that to maintain N balance in normal adult males ingesting 10.03 to 10.08 g N (62 to 63 g protein equivalent) daily from FAAs, energy intake had to be increased by about 28%; that is, from 35 kcal/kg BW to 45 kcal/kg BW.

Other factors that influence energy requirements are physical activity; protein intake; body composition, including lean body mass, gender, age, growth rate; and health status, including body temperature. Humans appear to be able to adapt to low energy intakes by decreasing growth rate or maintaining a low body weight, decreasing activity, and decreasing basal metabolic rate.[4] Otten et al.[1] provided equations to estimate individual energy requirements of normal persons to which it may be necessary to add 20 to 28% more energy if the patient is ingesting a diet in which FAAs provide a high percentage of N intake. See Table 3.1 for the suggested range of energy intakes for patients ingesting FAAs.

Excess weight gain by a child with an IMD is to be avoided because weight loss leads to elevated concentrations of toxic metabolites. Weight gain and linear growth within the normal range are good indicators of adequate intake of macronutrients.

Protein/Protein Equivalent

Amino acids are used to manufacture the structure of the body as well as to synthesize the enzymes, hormones, and other proteins that direct the functions of the body.[1] Proteins consist, on average, of 16% N. Except for glycine, the 20 α-amino acids that are used in human protein synthesis and metabolism are in the L-form. The L-configuration refers to the isomeric form of the amino acid. On all 20 amino acids, except glycine, the amino group is to the left when the carboxyl group is at the top and all are considered levarotatory. Thus, all elemental medical foods for human consumption contain all FAAs, except glycine, in the L-form.

The biologic value or nutrient quality of a protein has been historically defined by its digestibility, essential amino acid content, and use for body protein synthesis. However, a number of other factors are now known to influence amino acid utilization for body protein synthesis and the sites in the body where protein synthesis occurs.[5-13] These factors include digestion rate of the protein that determines the rapidity of availability of amino acids; diet composition,[14,15] including energy and protein intake;[16-18] and heat treatment of protein and amino acids that renders some amino acids and

Table 3.1 ***Recommended Daily Intakes (RDIs) for Patients Ingesting Elemental Diets***

	Recommended intake at age							
Nutrient	***0 < 6 mos***	***6 < 12 mos***	***1 < 4 yr***	***4 < 7 yr***	***7 < 11 yr***	***11 < 19 yr***	***Adult***	***Pregnant***
Protein[†], g	4.5 to 3.0/ 100 kcal	4.5 to 3.0/ 100 kcal	≥ 35	≥ 40	≥ 50	≥ 65	≥ 70	1st trim 70 2nd trim 85 3rd trim 100
Fat, g	6.0 to 3.3/ 100 kcal	6.0 to 3.3/ 100 kcal	> 30	45	55	60	60 to 70	75
Linoleic acid, g	4.4	4.6	7.0	10.0	12.0	16.0	17.0	14.0
α-linolenic acid, g	0.5	0.5	0.7	0.9	1.2	1.6	1.6	1.5
Energy[‡], kcal	120/kg	110/kg	900 to 1800	1300 to 2300	1650 to 3300	1500 to 1900	2000 to 3300	1700 to 2700
Fluid, mL	1.5/kcal	1.5 to 1.0/kcal	900 to 1800	1300 to 2300	1650 to 3300	1500 to 1900	2000 to 3300	1700 to 2700
Minerals								
Calcium, mg	400	600	800	800	1300	1300	1200	1300
Chloride								
mg	55 to 150/ 100 kcal	55 to 150/ 100 kcal	1500	1900	2300	2300	2300	2300
mEq	1.55 to 4.2/ 100 kcal	1.55 to 4.2/ 100 kcal	42.3	54	65	65	65	65
Chromium, μg	0.2	5.5	11	15	25	35	30	3.0
Copper, mg	0.60	0.80	1.5	2.0	2.5	3.0	3.0	3.5
Iodine, μg	25 to 75/100 kcal		90	90	120	150	150	220
Iron[§,¶], mg	10	15	15	15	15	18	18	48
Magnesium, mg	50	75	150	200	250	420	420	430

(continues)

Table 3.1 ***Recommended Daily Intakes (RDIs) for Patients ingesting Elemental Diets,*** *Continued*

	Recommended intake at age							
Nutrient	***0 < 6 mos***	***6 < 12 mos***	***1 < 4 yr***	***4 < 7 yr***	***7 < 11 yr***	***11 < 19 yr***	***Adult***	***Pregnant***
Manganese, mg	0.3	0.6	1.5	2.0	2.0	2.5	2.5	3.0
Molybdenum, μg	2.0	3.0	17	22	34	45	45	50
Phosphorus, mg	350	500	800	800	1250	1250	1000	1250
Potassium								
mg	80 to 200/ 100 kcal	80 to 200/ 100 kcal	117	149	176	184	184	184
mEq	2.0 to 5.1/ 100 kcal	2.0 to 5.1/ 100 kcal	3.0	3.8	4.5	4.7	4.7	4.7
Selenium, μg	20	25	30	40	50	65	65	70
Sodium								
mg	20 to 60/ 100 kcal	20 to 60/ 100 kcal	1000	1200	1500	1500	1500	1500
mEq	0.87 to 2.61/ 100 kcal	0.87 to 2.61/ 100 kcal	43	52	65	65	65	65
Zinc, mg	5	5	10	10	15	15	15	20
Vitamins								
A								
IU	250 to 750/ 100 kcal	250 to 750/ 100 kcal	400	500	700	900	900	1000
μg RAE	75 to 225/ 100 kcal	75 to 225/ 100 kcal	120	150	210	270	270	300
D								
IU	40 to 100/ 100 kcal	40 to 100/ 100 kcal	400	400	400	400	400	480
μg	1.0 to 2.5/ 100 kcal	1.0 to 2.5/ 100 kcal	10	10	10	10	10	12

(continues)

Table 3.1 ***Recommended Daily Intakes (RDIs) for Patients Ingesting Elemental Diets,*** *Continued*

	Recommended intake at age							
Nutrient	***0 < 6 mos***	***6 < 12 mos***	***1 < 4 yr***	***4 < 7 yr***	***7 < 11 yr***	***11 < 19 yr***	***Adult***	***Pregnant***
E, mg	6	7	6	7	11	15	15	12
K, μg	5	10	30	55	60	75	90	90
Ascorbic acid, mg	40	50	45	45	45	75	60	60
Biotin, μg	35	50	50	50	50	50	50	50
B_6, mg	0.3	0.6	0.9	1.3	1.6	1.8	2.0	2.2
B_{12}, μg	0.6 to 0.9	0.9 to 1.8	2.0	2.5	3.0	3.0	3.0	3.0
Choline, mg	125	150	200	250	375	550	550	450
Folate, μg	65	80	150	200	300	400	400	800
Inositol, mg	4/100 kcal	4/100 kcal	60	80	100	120	130	140 to 200
Niacin Equivalent**,††, mg	6	8	9	11	16	18	19	20
Pantothenic acid, mg	2.0	3.0	2.0	3.0	4.0	5.0	5.0	6.0
Riboflavin, mg	0.4	0.6	0.8	1.0	1.4	1.6	1.7	1.7
Thiamin, mg	0.3	0.5	0.7	0.9	1.2	1.4	1.5	1.6

Sources:

Acosta PB, Michals-Matalon K, Austin V, et al. Nutrition findings and requirements in pregnant women with phenylketonuria. In: Platt LD, Koch R, de la Cruz F, eds. *Genetic Disorders and Pregnancy Outcome*. New York, NY: Parthenon; 1997:21–32.

Acosta PB, Trahms C, Wellman NS, Williamson M. Phenylalanine intakes of 1- to 6-year-old children with phenylketonuria undergoing therapy. *Am J Clin Nutr*. 1983;38:694–700.

Acosta PB, Wenz E, Williamson M. Nutrient intake of treated infants with phenylketonuria. *Am J Clin Nutr*. 1977;30:198–208.

Acosta PB, Yannicelli S. Protein intake affects phenylalanine requirements and growth of infants with phenylketonuria. *Acta Paediatr Suppl*. 1994;407:66–67.

Acosta PB, Yannicelli S, Singh R, et al. Nutrient intakes and physical growth of children with phenylketonuria undergoing nutrition therapy. *J Am Diet Assoc*. 2003;103:1167–1173.

(continues)

Table 3.1 ***Recommended Daily Intakes (RDIs) for Patients Ingesting Elemental Diets**, Continued*

Allen JR, Baur LA, Waters DL, et al. Body protein in prepubertal children with phenylketonuria. *Eur J Clin Nutr*. 1996;50:178–186.

Boirie Y, Dangin M, Gachon P, Vasson MP, Maubois JL, Beaufrere B. Slow and fast dietary proteins differently modulate postprandial protein accretion. *Proc Natl Acad Sci USA*. 1997;94:14930–14935.

Bujko J, Schreurs VV, Nolles JA, Verreijen AM, Koopmanschap RE, Verstegen MW. Application of a ($^{13}CO_2$) breath test to study short-term amino acid catabolism during the postprandial phase of a meal. *Br J Nutr*. 2007;97:891–897.

Daenzer M, Petzke KJ, Bequette BJ, Metges CC. Whole-body nitrogen and splanchnic amino acid metabolism differ in rats fed mixed diets containing casein or its corresponding amino acid mixture. *J Nutr*. 2001;131:1965–1972.

Dangin M, Boirie Y, Garcia-Rodenas C, et al. The digestion rate of protein is an independent regulating factor of postprandial protein retention. *Am J Physiol Endocrinol Metab*. 2001;280:E340–E348.

Food and Drug Administration Rules and Regulations: Nutrient requirements for infant formulas (21 CFR Part 107). *Fed Regist*. 1985;50:45106–45108.

Fouillet H, Mariotti F, Gaudichon C, Bos C, Tome D. Peripheral and splanchnic metabolism of dietary nitrogen are differently affected by the protein source in humans as assessed by compartmental modeling. *J Nutr*. 2002;132:125–133.

Jones BJ, Lees R, Andrews J, Frost P, Silk DB. Comparison of an elemental and polymeric enteral diet in patients with normal gastrointestinal function. *Gut*. 1983;24:78–84.

Kindt E, Motzfeldt K, Halvorsen S, Lie SO. Is phenylalanine requirement in infants and children related to protein intake? *Br J Nutr*. 1984;51:435–442.

Lacroix M, Bos C, Leonil J, et al. Compared with casein or total milk protein, digestion of milk soluble proteins is too rapid to sustain the anabolic postprandial amino acid requirement. *Am J Clin Nutr*. 2006;84:1070–1079.

MacDonald A, Chakrapani A, Hendriksz C, et al. Protein substitute dosage in PKU: how much do young patients need? *Arch Dis Child*. 2006;91:588–593.

Monchi M, Rerat AA. Comparison of net protein utilization of milk protein mild enzymatic hydrolysates and free amino acid mixtures with a close pattern in the rat. *JPEN J Parenter Enteral Nutr*. 1993;17:355–363.

Williamson M, Koch R, Clair T, et al. Treatment effects on physical growth and intelligence among phenylketonuria children. In: Bickel H, Hudson FP, Woolf LI, eds. *Phenylketonuria and Some Other Inborn Errors of Amino Acid Metabolism*. Stuttgart, Germany: Georg Thieme Verlag; 1971:199–207.

†Fifteen percent of energy should be supplied as protein equivalent for protein to be the same as ingested by normal children and adults.

‡Energy needs of males are usually greater than of females.

§Copper, iron, and zinc needs of patients ingesting elemental diets are greater than RDA.

¶Recommended iron intake for men ≥ 19 years of age on elemental diets is 10 to 12 mg/day.

**Niacin needs of patients with PKU are greater than RDA.

Sources: LaDu BN, Zannoni VG. Basic biochemical disturbances in aromatic amino acid metabolism. In: Bickel H, Hudson FP, Woolf LI, eds. *Phenylketonuria and Some Other Inborn Errors of Amino Acid Metabolism*. Stuttgart, Germany: Georg Thieme Verlag; 1971:6–13.

Lewis JS, Loskill S, Bunker ML, Acosta PB, Kim R. N-methylnicotinamide excretion of phenylketonuric children and a child with Hartnup disease before and after phenylalanine and tryptophan load. *Fed Proc*. 1974;33:666A.

††60 mg of tryptophan = 1 mg niacin equivalent. *Source:* Otten JJ, Hellwig JP, Meyers LD. *Dietary Reference Intakes: The Essential Guide to Nutrient Requirements*. Washington, DC: National Academies Press; 2006.

carbohydrates indigestible (Maillard reaction).[19-21] Using an 11-compartment model, Fouillet et al.[5] assessed the fate of amino acids from a meal consisting of 100 g sucrose plus 30 g protein from either slowly digested cow's milk or more rapidly digested soy protein during an 8-hour period in normal subjects. Both proteins were labeled with ^{15}N, and the appearance of ^{15}N was determined in ileal effluents, plasma FAAs, body and urinary urea, and ammonia. All dietary N recovered from accumulated ileal effluents; plasma-free amino acids, body urea, urinary urea, and urinary ammonia were expressed for each as a percentage of ingested N. Intestinal absorption of ^{15}N was, on average, 33% faster from the more rapidly digested soy protein than from the more slowly digested milk protein. During this same period, approximately 33% more ^{15}N was found in urea and ammonia of subjects who ingested the rapidly digested protein than in those who ingested the slowly digested milk protein. Of particular importance were the splanchnic (visceral) and peripheral protein syntheses efficiencies predicted from the rate of appearance of dietary ^{15}N in the free amino acid pool incorporated into protein at 8 and 12 hours after ingestion of the two labeled meals. Protein synthesis efficiency (PSE) was significantly greater in the splanchnic bed than in the peripheral area at both time periods after the ingestion of the slowly digested protein, while PSE in the peripheral area was greater from the slowly digested protein (see Table 3.2).

Boirie et al.[6] reported that 16 healthy subjects 24 ± 4 years old, fed for 3 days either casein (slowly digested protein) or whey (rapidly digested protein)

Table 3.2 ***Source of Amino Acids Influences Their Use***

	Slowly digested protein	***Rapidly digested protein***
Diet	^{15}N-labeled milk with sucrose[†]	^{15}N-labeled soy protein with sucrose[‡]
Number of subjects	9	10
Data collected after meal (hrs)	8	8
Protein synthesis efficiency (%)		
Splanchnic bed	23	30
Peripheral area	32	24

Source: Fouillet H, Mariotti F, Gaudichon C, Bos C, Tome D. Peripheral and splanchnic metabolism of dietary nitrogen are differently affected by the protein source in humans as assessed by compartmental modeling. *J Nutr*. 2002;132:125–133.

[†]30 g labeled milk protein with 100 g sucrose.
[‡]30 g labeled soy protein with 100 g sucrose.

in which leucine was labeled with ^{13}C or $^{2}H_3$ and 38 kcal/kg BW/day, were studied for 7 hours to determine effects on protein accretion by evaluation of leucine disposal. Total leucine oxidation was significantly greater ($p<0.05$) in the whey-protein-fed subjects than in the casein-fed subjects. The conclusion drawn by the investigators was that the speed of amino acid absorption after protein ingestion has a major impact on the metabolic response to a single protein meal. The slowly absorbed amino acids from casein promoted postprandial protein deposition by an inhibition of protein breakdown while the rapidly absorbed amino acids from whey stimulated both protein synthesis and oxidation. Subsequently, Dangin et al.[7] reported leucine oxidation and non-oxidative leucine disposal (NOLD = protein synthesis) in 22 healthy young male volunteers fed one of three meals in which the L-leucine was labeled with ^{13}C-free amino acids simulating the composition of casein. Casein and whey, each yielding 30 g protein, were fed in one meal and whey was also administered in 13 meals every 20 minutes, for a yield of 30 g of protein.

The height of plasma amino acid concentrations after feeding has been considered important in protein synthesis. Gropper and Acosta[22] reported that free amino acids (75% of protein-simulating casein) and casein (25%) to supply 18.9 g protein resulted in higher concentrations of plasma amino acids than casein alone at 30, 60, 90, and 120 minutes than at 150, 180, and 240 minutes. Plasma essential and total amino acid concentrations were described at 120 minutes and 240 minutes by Dangin et al.[7] as a percentage change from baseline. Subjects fed FAAs or whey protein had a greater increase in plasma essential amino acids (EAAs) at 120 minutes than subjects fed casein, and casein-fed subjects had the highest increase in EAAs at 240 minutes. Total plasma amino acid concentrations mimicked the changes found with EAAs and whey protein given in one feed. The subjects fed whey protein every 20 minutes in 13 meals had somewhat lower increases in concentrations of plasma EAAs and total amino acids. Leucine oxidation after the FAA meal was significantly greater ($p<0.001$) than at baseline shortly after meal ingestion to about 2 hours after feeding than found after the casein meal. The subjects fed the whey protein in 13 feeds had significantly lower ($p<0.001$) oxidation of leucine than subjects fed the whey in one feed. When protein synthesis was measured by non-oxidative leucine disposal (NOLD) over 7 hours, it was significantly less ($p<0.01$) in the FAA-fed subjects than in the casein-fed subjects, -12 ± 11 μmol/kg BW in the FAA-fed and $+38 \pm 13$ μmol/kg BW in the casein-fed subjects. Subjects fed the whey protein meal had a leucine balance of $+6 \pm 19$ μmol/kg BW; however, the subjects fed 30 g whey protein in 13 divided doses had a leucine balance of $+87 \pm 25$ μmol/kg BW.

Lacroix et al.[8] reported that the rapidity of protein digestion influenced its ability to sustain the anabolic postprandial amino acid requirement. The macronutrient intake of 23 healthy volunteers was standardized for 1 week after which subjects ingested a meal containing 22.6 to 23.3 g protein as micellar casein (MC), total milk protein (TMP), or micellar soluble milk protein isolate (MSPI). Micellar casein is slowly digested since it precipitates due to the acidic gastric pH, which delays amino acid delivery to the intestine, whereas MSPI is rapidly emptied from the stomach. Urinary N excretion was significantly greater ($p<0.05$) for up to 8 hours after meal ingestion by subjects fed the most rapidly digested protein (14.65 ± 2.84%) than for the two groups of subjects fed the more slowly digested proteins (8.00 ± 2.08%, 8.76 ± 1.38% (mean ± SD)).

Stoll et al.[23] reported that catabolism dominated the first pass of EAAs in the intestine of milk-fed piglets. Animals fed FAAs that simulate hydrolysate of protein have been shown to have less weight gain, lower body N, and poorer net protein utilization than animals fed intact protein. Monchi et al.[9] found that hydrolysate-fed rats had a weight gain during 10 days of feeding while the FAA-fed rats lost weight. Net protein utilization, defined as the ratio of protein gain to protein ingested during the experimental period, was significantly less ($p<0.01$) in the FAA-fed rats as compared to that of the hydrolysate-fed rats (see Table 3.3). Body N content of the FAA-fed rats was 85% of that found in the hydrolysate-fed rats. Weight gain and urinary N excretion of casein- vs FAA-fed rats was found to also differ by Daenzer et al.[10] (see Table 3.4). Further, the weights of stomach and small intestine were greater in the FAA-fed than in the casein-fed rats, supporting Fouillet et al. in sites of use of amino acids by source.[5] Bujko et al.[11] reported that rats fed

Table 3.3 ***Net Protein Utilization in Rats Fed Mild Casein Hydrolysate or Free Amino Acids***

	Hydrolysate-fed	***Free amino acid-fed***	***P value***
Weight change (g)	+11.1 ± 2.2[a]	–4.6 ± 1.8[a]	> 0.001
Net protein utilization[†]	0.277 ± 0.024[a]	0.144 ± 0.011[a]	> 0.001
Body N (g)	2.755 ± 0.070[a]	2.329 ± 0.038[a]	> 0.001

Source: Monchi M, Rerat AA. Comparison of net protein utilization of mild protein mild enzymatic hydrolysates and free amino acid mixtures with a close pattern in the rat. *JPEN J Parenter Enteral Nutr*. 1993;17:355–363.

[†]Net protein utilization = ratio of protein gain to protein ingested during the experimental period.
Note: [a]All values = mean ± SEM.

Table 3.4 ***Weight Gain and 24-Hour Urinary Nitrogen Excretion of Rats Fed Casein or Free Amino Acids of Casein Composition With Identical Nitrogen Intakes***

	Casein-fed (g)	*Free amino acid-fed (g)*	*P value*
Weight gain	20.6 ± 20.0	12.7 ± 7.4	< 0.05
Stomach	1.34 ± 0.27	1.41 ± 0.15	NS
Liver	7.53 ± 1.08	7.17 ±1.10	NS
Small intestine	3.93 ± 0.34	4.15 ± 0.39	NS
24-hour urinary nitrogen excretion	154.1 ± 55.0	204.5 ± 49.5 (↑ 1.33%)	< 0.05

Source: Daenzer M, Petzke KJ, Bequette BJ, Metges CC. Whole-body nitrogen and splanchnic amino acid metabolism differ in rats fed mixed diets containing casein or its corresponding amino acid mixture. *J Nutr*. 2001;131:1965–1972.

Notes: All values = mean ± SD; NS = not significant.

either 1-^{13}C-labeled leucine bound in egg white or in FAAs expired more labeled CO_2 from the FAAs for 2 hours after meal onset than from egg white protein.

Carbohydrate, but not fat, in the diet has been found to significantly decrease the postprandial transfer of labeled protein to urea.[12,13] Carbohydrate halved the oxidative peak of dietary N during the first 2 hours after a meal. Net postprandial protein utilization was improved by about 5% and N retention by about 14% when carbohydrate rather than fat was ingested with protein. When postabsorptive leucine flux, which is an index of proteolysis, was measured using 1-^{13}C leucine as a tracer, overfeeding carbohydrate by 400 g/day without additional protein was found to increase leucine flux by 13 ± 2% compared with values after 10 days on a weight maintenance diet.[14] According to the authors, these data suggest that excess carbohydrate intake without an increase in protein intake stimulates postabsorptive proteolysis.[14] Protein synthesis increased less than proteolysis.

Energy restriction in normal-weight men also changes protein metabolism.[15] Nitrogen loss was several grams daily during the 21-day study period while leucine oxidation during exercise was high even at day 18 of energy restriction.[15] Patients with PKU fed higher protein intakes had lower plasma phenylalanine concentrations[16-18] and better linear growth than patients fed lower protein intakes (see Chapter 5, Table 5.7).

Stoll et al.[23] reported that in piglets fed milk proteins, on average, 56% of EAA intake appeared in the portal blood, but portal amounts of methionine (48% of intake) and threonine (38% of intake) were lower than that of the other EAAs. The conclusion reached was that approximately one-third of dietary intake of EAAs is consumed in first-pass metabolism by the intestine, and amino acid catabolism by the mucosal cells is greater than incorporation into mucosal protein.

Nitrogen retention in patients was found to be less in adults with normal gastrointestinal function fed an elemental diet made with FAAs versus intact protein[24] (see Table 3.5). Mean total body N and height z-score were found to be significantly greater in normal subjects ingesting the same amount of protein as children with phenylketonuria (PKU) fed a high percentage of their protein intake as FAAs[25] (see Table 3.6). Height Z-score was +0.17 ± 0.94 in control subjects and –0.42 ± 0.89 in children with PKU, while total body N was 23% greater in the normal children than in children with PKU.

Table 3.5 ***Nitrogen Retention in Adults With Normal Gastrointestinal Function Fed Intact Protein or Free Amino Acids***

	Intact protein	*Free amino acids*	*P value*
Number	36	34	
Age (years)	56.1 ± 3.1	55.1 ± 3.1	NS
Days of feeding	20.3 ± 2.8	16.0 ± 1.6	NS
N intake (g)	10.2 ± 0.4	10.4 ± 0.5	NS
N retention (g)	+2.6 ± 0.6	–0.64 ± 0.8	NS

Source: Jones BJ, Lees R, Andrews J, Frost P, Silk DB. Comparison of an elemental and polymeric enteral diet in patients with normal gastrointestinal function. *Gut.* 1983;24:78–84.

Notes: All values = mean ± SEM; NS = not significant.

Table 3.6 ***Height Z-Score and Total Body Nitrogen of Normal Children and Children With PKU***

	Control	*PKU*	*P value*
Number	27	37	
Age (years)	4.0–11.5	3.9–11.0	NS
Z-score	+0.17 ± 0.94	–0.42 ± 0.89	< 0.02
Total body nitrogen (g)	710 ± 215	575 ±200	< 0.02
Protein intake	Same	Same	—

Source: Allen JR, Baur LA, Waters DL, et al. Body protein in prepubertal children with phenylketonuria. *Eur J Clin Nutr.* 1996;50:178–186.

Notes: All values = mean ± SD; NS = not significant.

Free amino acids, as well as amino acids in intact proteins, are susceptible to the Maillard reaction between amino acids and carbohydrates that form enzyme-resistant cross-links. The especially highly reactive amino acids are lysine, tryptophan, methionine, cystine, and threonine.[19] The Maillard reaction is affected by pH, heat, liquid, and carbohydrates. Even in a mildly processed food, Maillard reaction products may be noted by a light-brown color, followed by buff yellow, and in the intermediate and final stages by a dark-brown color.[20] Roller-dried skim milk was found to have a 6% decrease in digestibility of lysine, phenylalanine, cystine, aspartic acid, glycine, and total amino acids. Net galactose absorption within 12 hours was about 46%, while lysine absorption was decreased by 50% of that found in pigs fed lyophilized skim milk. Plasma amino acid concentrations were significantly decreased ($p<0.05$) in the pigs fed roller-dried skim milk compared to pigs fed lyophilized skim milk, and fecal excretion as a percentage of intake was significantly greater ($p<0.05$) for lysine, phenylalanine, valine, cystine, aspartic acid, and the sum of essential amino acids by the roller-dried skim milk-fed pigs.[21]

Patients with inherited metabolic disorders, especially those with an organic acidemia, who are treated with one or more restricted EAAs, are often reported to have little or no appetite. Whether this appetite suppression is due to the metabolic acidosis or deficiency of one or more EAAs is unclear. However, Gietzen et al.[26] reported that rats fed a diet deficient in even one essential amino acid stopped growing because they refused to eat the diet. Food refusal began a very short time after feeding the EAA-deficient diet.

In addition to the ability to adapt to low energy intakes,[27] Waterlow[4] reported that the human is capable of adapting to low protein intakes while still maintaining N balance. This adaptation occurs by a decrease in urinary N loss due to reutilization of some urea, a decrease in activity of enzymes that oxidize amino acids, decreased synthesis and degradation of splanchnic (visceral) proteins, decreased weight gain in children, and a fall in lean body mass. Growth in height is thought to be particularly sensitive to protein supply and stunting in height may be a manifestation of protein deficiency.[4]

The abundance of reported studies on better amino acid utilization and N retention with proteins that slowly release amino acids for absorption over the use from rapidly digested proteins or FAAs has led to the recommendation for greater protein intakes (30 to 35% above RDAs[1]) for all patients who ingest a major portion of protein as FAAs.[16-18,22] To maintain normal N retention by patients fed a major portion of protein as FAAs, either a greater protein equivalent must be fed than recommended for normal persons of the same age and gender, or feeding must be more frequent than three to four times daily. Infants are fed more frequently than older individuals. Consequently, recommended intakes of protein and other nutrients for infants in Table 3.1

are similar to those given in the Infant Formula Act per 100 kcal.[28] Since hourly feeding of the school-age child, adolescent, or working adult is not practical, protein-equivalent intake must be greater than RDAs[1] (see Table 3.1) by patients with IMDs. Treated patients with PKU grew normally in length/height when fed the protein noted in Table 3.1.[29-33] Protein provided as FAAs (all in the L-form, except glycine) is called "protein equivalent" (i.e., N, g $\times$ 6.25 = g protein equivalent).

Fats

Fats, essential fatty acids (EFAs), and cholesterol have several important functions in the body. In the infant and young child, fat, which supplies 9 kcal/g, is necessary to supply energy since the stomach is too small to ingest all the energy that is needed as protein and carbohydrate, which supply only 4 kcal/g. Fats also aid in the absorption of the fat-soluble vitamins A, D, E, and K, and carotenoids. Fatty acids are structural components of cell membranes and nervous tissue myelin. Linoleic (C18 2:n-6) and α-linolenic acids (C18 3:n-3) are EFAs and are required for normal epithelial cell function, as components of membrane structural lipids. These are also precursors of eicosanoids, eicosapentenoic acid, and docosahexaenoic acid and are involved in the regulation of genes.[1] Table 3.1 suggests the amounts of fat and EFAs to feed by age.[1] Human milk-fed infants ingest over 50% of total energy as fat since 100 mL may contain up to 5.5 g fat and 65 to 70 kcal. Human mature milk, on average, contains about 0.05 g α-linolenic and 0.39 g linoleic acid per 100 mL.[34]

Cholesterol is essential for the biosynthesis of cell membranes, steroid hormones, bile acids,[1] and other compounds in the human body. For individuals who ingest cholesterol in the diet, about half of the intake is absorbed. No intake has been recommended for cholesterol because of synthesis by all tissues of the human body. However, some patients do not have the enzyme capable of completing the last step in cholesterol synthesis,[35] while others[36] may excrete compounds in the urine used in cholesterol and EFA synthesis as part of a metabolite of phenylalanine.

Minerals and Vitamins

Intakes of most minerals and some vitamins by patients with inherited metabolic disorders must be greater than RDAs by age for normal persons to prevent plasma/serum concentrations below reference ranges. Alexander et al.[37] found greater fecal losses than intakes of copper, iron, and zinc by patients with PKU and branched-chain ketoaciduria who were undergoing nutrition management.

Few studies have been reported on plasma or serum concentrations of minerals or vitamins except in patients undergoing nutrition management for PKU because the incidence of the other IMDs is much less than for PKU. For this reason, the studies reported on patients with PKU (Chapter 5) are used as a basis for recommending increased mineral and vitamin intakes. Table 3.1 suggests recommended mineral and vitamin intakes by patients with IMDs ingesting FAA-containing diets. Metabolism of niacin, biotin, and vitamin A have been reported to be affected by PKU and homocystinuria, respectively.[38-42]

Evaluation of nutrient intake requires information on both quantity and quality of food ingested. Many dietitians in genetic metabolic centers require that parents/caregivers and, later, patients, record complete food and beverage intakes for 3 days immediately prior to each blood drawing. The 3-day mean intake is then evaluated by comparing to Recommended Dietary Intakes (RDIs) (see Table 3.1) rather than to RDAs.[1] However, ingestion of 100% of RDIs does not ensure that growth and all biochemical indices will be within reference ranges and growth, laboratory indices, clinical status, and health history must all be considered together.

Assessment of Growth

Growth in recumbent or supine length or height, head circumference, and weight helps provide visible information of the adequacy of nutrient intake. Growth is described by accurate measurements of supine length/height, head circumference to 3 years of age, weight, and bone mineral content.[43,44] Recumbent or supine length is usually measured until the child can stand, and may be as much as 2 cm greater than standing height.[45]

Length/Stature

Methods of measuring supine length, stature, and weight are described by Chumlea.[43] These measures should be carefully collected at each clinic visit and plotted on Centers for Disease Control, National Center for Health Statistics (NCHS) growth charts.[46] The child who deviates significantly from his or her plotted position on the growth chart may be malnourished or have had a recent infectious illness. Height of both biologic parents, if they were not malnourished in childhood, is helpful in assessing the growth potential of the child.

Height for age that is 90 to 94% of the 50th percentile on the NCHS growth chart is considered mild protein-energy malnutrition, while height for age of 85 to 89% is moderate, and < 85% is severe.[47-49] Length/height standard deviation (SD) scores for age of –2.0 to –3.0 are considered indicative of moderate malnutrition and of more than –3.0 of severe malnutrition.[48,49] An SD or Z-score is defined as units of deviation from the median of that measure for a large group of normal subjects of the same age.[47]

Long-term nutrition status may be assessed by a measure of stature. Recumbent length is measured by two persons, with one person positioning the infant straight on the measuring board with the head flush against the headboard. The infant's knees are held flat to the board and the second person moves the footboard until it is flat against the infant's heels.[43] Children and adults who are cooperative and can stand erect without support with feet together and heels, buttocks, and back of head touching the stadiometer are measured to the nearest 0.1 cm. Since height growth may be stunted in patients with an IMD[50,51] ingesting FAAs, three measurements are essential at each assessment, and the two closest measures are averaged and recorded. Stunting is defined as a slowing in skeletal growth and height.[49]

Height growth is significantly affected by growth of long bones, which, as they grow, store calcium. If calcium stores are low, growth of long bones may be affected and those children with a low bone mass may develop osteoporosis.[43] Dual energy x-ray absorptiometry (DXA) is used to measure the amount of bone mineral content in children and adults with IMDs that may be compared to that of normal children or adults.[52] Z-scores of –1.0 to –2.0 are considered low normal and should be repeated every 1 to 2 years. If the Z-score is –2.0 to –3.0, it is considered reduced and should be repeated annually, while a Z-score of –3.0 or less is significantly reduced and DXA should be repeated every 6 to 12 months.[52]

Head Circumference

The frontal occipital circumference or head circumference should be measured to 3 years of age and beyond in children with an IMD because late diagnosis, inadequate dietary control, malnutrition, and the disorder may all contribute to head size. For example, children with PKU if late diagnosed or if plasma phenylalanine (PHE) concentrations are above treatment range, often have microcephaly.[53] On the other hand, infants and children with glutaric aciduria type I often have macrocephaly.[54]

A flexible metal tape measure is used to measure head circumference. The tape is placed above the supraorbital ridge and extended around the occiput at the maximum distance. The tape measure should be parallel on both sides and flat against the head. At least three measures should be recorded to the nearest 0.1 cm and the two closest averaged, recorded, and charted on NCHS growth charts.[55]

Weight

Weight, which responds rapidly to over- or undernutrition, provides a short-term indication of nutrition status and is reported as weight for age, weight for height, percentile weight for age, and Z-score. Infant weight should be obtained using a digital beam balance pan scale. The infant should be unclothed and without a diaper, while the child and adult should be weighed wearing light clothing and no shoes after emptying the bladder. Infant weight should be recorded to the nearest 0.01 kg and weights of children and adults to 0.1 kg.[55] The scale must be calibrated monthly and zeroed before each measurement.

NCHS growth charts[46] allow comparison of the measure to the reference population. Plotting of a patient's weight on a weight for age, gender, and height growth chart provides information on the nutrition status of the patient and may indicate wasting or obesity. Wasting is defined as a deficit in tissue and fat mass compared with the amount expected in a child of the same height or length.[49]

Mild protein-energy malnutrition (PEM) is defined as weight for age 75 to 89% of the 50th percentile standard for age, moderate malnutrition as 60 to 74% of the 50th percentile standard, and severe malnutrition as a weight < 60% of the 50th percentile standard. When weight for height is used to assess PEM, mild malnutrition is defined as 80 to 89%, moderate 70 to 79%, and severe ≤ 70% of the 50th percentile standard.[47] Z-scores indicating mild malnutrition are –2.0 to –3.0 and severe malnutrition below –3.0.[48] Most often in patients with an IMD, overweight or obesity is found while supine length or stature is depressed (see Chapter 5, Table 5.7).

Pregnant women who are underweight with a body mass index (BMI) at conception of less than or equal to 19.8 should gain at least 2.3 kg the first trimester and 12.5 to 18.0 kg during the entire pregnancy. Normal weight women who, at conception, have a BMI between 19.8 and 26.0, should gain 1.6 kg during the first trimester and 15.5 to 16.0 kg during all of gestation. Women who are overweight at conception (BMI greater than 26.0) should gain only 0.9 kg during the first trimester and a total of 7.0 to 11.5 kg during pregnancy.[56]

Biochemical Assessment

Proteins and Amino Acids

Several different serum proteins are used for assessment of protein-energy nutrition. Among these are concentrations of albumin, transferrin, transthyretin (prealbumin), retinol binding protein (RBP), and the EAAs. Each of the proteins has its own set of limitations and all suffer from the fact that with PEM, both synthesis and degradation (catabolism) are decreased.[4,27,57] Whether rapidly absorbed amino acids (as found when FAAs are the primary protein equivalent source) influence the synthesis and degradation of the liver-synthesized proteins, and lead to the conclusion that protein status is normal when peripheral protein synthesis is decreased, is unclear.[10] This may mislead the dietitian to believe that protein status is normal when height growth and muscle mass are faltering.

A number of other factors are known to influence serum concentrations of proteins, among which are liver disease, renal loss, trauma, infection, neoplasia, or dehydration of the patient.[58-60] Iron status also impacts transferrin concentration, while vitamin A and zinc deficiency influence the concentration of RBP. The half-life of the proteins differ, with those with the shorter half-life responding the most rapidly to PEM. Albumin, with a long half-life of 18 to 20 days, is slow to respond, whereas transferrin has a half-life of 8 to 9 days. Serum proteins that respond the most rapidly to PEM are transthyretin with a half-life of 2 to 3 days and RPB with a half-life of 12 hours.[58,59] Albumin and transthyretin concentrations are those usually assessed in clinical practice. Transthyretin concentrations have been reported to decline with energy deficiency alone.[61] However, whether this results from the use of protein for energy purposes or directly to the inadequate energy is unclear.

Laboratory reference ranges or intervals for assessment of nutrition status are based on age, gender, and state of health and may vary depending on the methods used in the sample preparation and analyses.[60,62] Table 3.7 gives guidelines for assessing concentrations obtained for serum proteins. All plasma or serum amino acid concentrations in patients with an inherited disorder of amino acid metabolism who are treated by restriction of specific amino acids are routinely analyzed and compared to reference ranges found in normal populations[62] of the same age and gender and to established treatment ranges. Large neutral amino acids compete for the same protein carriers across the intestinal mucosa.[63] Thus, in patients with PKU, in whom plasma PHE concentrations are elevated, plasma tyrosine (TYR) concentrations are often reported to be below the lower limit of the reference ranges.[64-66] Plasma cystine concentrations in patients with homocystinuria are often below normal reference ranges.[67] L-cystine is practically insoluble in water.[68] Consequently, the more soluble L-cystine dihyrochloride is often added to medical foods for homocystinuria, but the chloride must be considered in the formulation. Plasma EAA concentrations of normal women studied as controls in the Maternal PKU Collaborative Study are given by trimester of pregnancy 2 to 5 hours postprandially[69] in Table 3.8. Low plasma carnitine concentrations have been reported in untreated patients with PKU.[70] The low

Table 3.7 *Acceptable Laboratory Standards for Assessing Nutrition Status*

Analyte	*Age*	*Minimum standard*
PROTEIN		
Albumin (plasma) g/L		
	3 mo–1 yr	23
	1 < 4 yrs	34
	4 < 7 yrs	35
	7 < 20 yrs	37
	Adult	35
	Pregnant	35
Retinol binding protein (plasma), μmol/L (mg/dL)		
	1 mo < 19 yrs	0.52 (1.09)
Transthyretin (plasma), mg/L		
	0 < 10 yrs	200
	10 < 13 yrs	220
	14 < 20 yrs	240
	Adult and pregnant	230
Total protein (plasma), g/L		
	6 mo < 1 yr	45
	1 < 20 yrs	60
	Adult and pregnant	65
ESSENTIAL FATTY ACIDS (plasma), μg/mL		
Linoleic acid		13.29
Docosahexaenoic acid		38.05
MINERALS		
Calcium, total, (plasma/serum) mmol/L (mg/dL)		
	3 mos–1 yr	2.17 (8.7)
		2.19 (8.8)
Chloride (plasma/serum) mmol/L		
	0–1 yr	96
	1 < 18 yrs	102
	Adult	100
Copper (plasma/serum), μmol/L (μg/dL)		
	0 < 2 yrs	12.6 (80)
	2 < 19 yrs	13.7 (87)
	Adult	10.0 (63)
	Pregnant	26.2 (165)
Iron (plasma/serum), μmol/L (μg/dL)		
	Birth < 20 yrs	5.7 (32)
	Adult	10.0 (63)
Ferritin (plasma), ng/mL		
	Birth < 19 yrs	20
	Adult	20
	Pregnant	20
Hematocrit (whole blood), %		
	0 < 2 yrs	33
	2 < 5 yrs	34
	5 < 8 yrs	35
	8 < 18 yrs	36
	≥ 18 yrs	37
	Pregnant	36

(continues)

Table 3.7 *Acceptable Laboratory Standards for Assessing Nutrition Status, Continued*

Analyte	***Age***	***Minimum standard***
Hemoglobin (whole blood), g/L		
All	0 < 5 yrs	110
	5 < 8 yrs	115
	8 < 12 yrs	120
Females	≥ 12 yrs	120
	Pregnant	120
Males	12 < 15 yrs	125
	15 < 18 yrs	130
	≥ 18 yrs	140
Magnesium (plasma/serum), mmol/L (mg/dL)		
	91 d < 4 yrs	0.65 (1.59)
	4 < 16 yrs	0.61 (1.60)
	16 < 19 yrs	0.64 (1.55)
	Adult	0.76 (NA)
Manganese (whole blood), μg/L (nmol/L)		
	All ages	4.0 (73–274)
Phosphorus (plasma/serum), mmol/L (mg/dL)		
	All ages	1.00 (3.10)
Potassium (plasma/serum), mmol/L		
	Birth < 20 yrs	3.3
	Adult	3.5
Selenium (serum), μmol/L (μg/L)		
	Birth < 1 yr	0.72 (60)
	1 < 20 yrs	1.31 (100)
	Adult	1.31 (100)
	Pregnant	NA (80)
Erythrocyte selenium dependent glutathione peroxidase, nmol/min/mg Hgb		
	Adult	10.5
Sodium (plasma/serum), mmol/L		
	All ages	133
Zinc (plasma/serum), μmol/L (μg/dL)		
	Birth < 1 yr	10.2 (67)
	1 < 19 yrs	12.1 (79)
	Adult	12.2 (60)
	Pregnant	NA (75)
VITAMINS		
Retinol (plasma/serum), μmol/L (μg/dL)		
	3 mos < 1 yr	0.5 (14.8)
	1 < 7 yrs	0.7 (20.0)
	7 < 19 yrs	0.9 (20.0)
	Adults	1.5 (43.0)
25-hydroxvitamin D (serum), μmol/L (μg/dL)		
	1 mo < 4 yrs	12 (17)
	4 < 18 yrs	9 (14)
	Adult	40 (NA)

(continues)

Table 3.7 *Acceptable Laboratory Standards for Assessing Nutrition Status, Continued*

Analyte	*Age*	*Minimum standard*
α-tocopherol (serum), μmol/L (μg/mL)		
	0 < 1 yr	14 (2.3)
	1 < 7 yrs	7 (3)
	7 < 13 yrs	10 (4)
	13 < 20 yrs	13 (6)
	Adult	20 (2.3)
C (plasma), μmol/L (mg/dL)		
	All ages and pregnant	> 23 (0.4)
B_6-pyridoxal phosphate (plasma), nmol/L		
	All ages	> 30
B_{12} (plasma), pmol/L		
	0 < 2 yrs	216
	2 < 10 yrs	182
	10 < 19 yrs	158
	Adult	220
	Pregnant	220 (200 ng/L)
Folate (plasma), nmol/L		
	0 < 2 yrs	16.3
	2 < 7 yrs	6.1
	7 < 10 yrs	5.4
	13 < 20 yrs	2.7
	Adult	NA
	Pregnant (erythrocyte)	450
Niacin (urinary N-methylnicotinamide), mg/24 hrs		
	Adult	> 0.8
Pantothenic acid (erythrocyte), μmol/L		
	All ages	> 1.5
Thiamine (erythrocyte transketolase), % activation assay		
	All ages	15
Riboflavin (erythrocyte glutathione reductase activity coefficient)		
	All ages	< 1.2

Sources:

Ances IG, Granados J, Baltazar M. Serum ferritin as an early determinant of decreased iron stores in pregnant women. *South Med J*. 1979;72:591–592, 604.

Benjamin DR. Laboratory tests and nutritional assessment: protein-energy status. *Pediatr Clin North Am*. 1989;36:139–161.

Gillingham M, van Calcar S, Ney D, Wolff J, Harding C. Dietary management of long-chain 3-hydroxyacyl-CoA dehydrogenase deficiency (LCHADD). A case report and survey. *J Inherit Metab Dis*. 1999;22:123–131.

Hambidge KM, Walravens PA, Casey CE, Brown RM, Bender C. Plasma zinc concentrations of breast-fed infants. *J Pediatr*. 1979;94:607–608.

Pleban PA, Munyani A, Beachum J. Determination of selenium concentration and glutathione peroxidase activity in plasma and erythrocytes. *Clin Chem*. 1982;28:311–316.

Sauberlich HE. *Laboratory Tests for the Assessment of Nutritional Status*. 2nd ed. Boca Raton, FL: CRC Press; 1999;447–467.

Shank JS, Dorsey JL, Anderson K, Cooper WT, Acosta PB. Plasma vitamin E concentrations of older infants fed cow's milk or infant formula. *J Pediatr Gastroenterol Nutr*. 1992;15:375–381.

Soldin SJ, Brugnara C, Wong EC. *Pediatric Reference Intervals*. 6th ed. Washington, DC: AACC Press; 2007.

*Laboratory concentrations vary based on method of sample preparation and analysis. Local laboratory standards based on age, gender, state of health, and method of sample preparation and analysis should be developed.

Table 3.8 ***Essential Plasma Amino Acid Concentrations (Mean ± SD) During Pregnancy in Normal Women****

	Week of pregnancy		
Amino acid	***< 20***	***20 < 30***	***> 30***
Number	34	59	61
Histidine			
µmol/L	84 ± 19	90 ± 13	97 ± 26
mg/dL	1.3 ± 0.3	1.4 ± 0.2	1.5 ± 0.4
Isoleucine			
µmol/L	53 ± 23	53 ± 15	46 ± 15
mg/dL	0.7 ± 0.3	0.7 ± 0.2	0.6 ± 0.2
Leucine			
µmol/L	114 ± 38	107 ± 30	91 ± 23
mg/dL	1.5 ± 0.5	1.4 ± 0.4	1.2 ± 0.3
Lysine			
µmol/L	171 ± 48	178 ± 41	171 ± 41
mg/dL	2.5 ± 0.7	2.6 ± 0.6	2.5 ± 0.6
Methionine			
µmol/L	34 ± 54	20 ± 7	27 ± 7
mg/dL	0.5 ± 0.8	0.3 ± 0.1	0.4 ± 0.1
Phenylalanine			
µmol/L	67 ± 30	60 ± 18	54 ± 12
mg/dL	1.1 ± 0.5	1.0 ± 0.3	0.9 ± 0.2
Threonine			
µmol/L	118 ± 34	168 ± 42	193 ± 50
mg/dL	1.4 ± 0.4	2.0 ± 0.5	2.3 ± 0.6
Tyrosine			
µmol/L	55 ± 22	50 ± 11	50 ± 17
mg/dL	1.0 ± 0.4	0.9 ± 0.2	0.9 ± 0.3
Valine			
µmol/L	196 ± 60	179 ± 43	163 ± 43
mg/dL	2.3 ± 0.7	2.1 ± 0.5	1.9 ± 0.5

Source: Matalon K, Acosta PB, Castiglioni L, et al. *Protocol for Nutrition Support of Maternal PKU*. Bethesda, MD: The National Institute of Child Health and Human Development. 1998;1–51.

Note: All values = mean ±SD.

*Blood drawn 2 to 5 hours postptrandially and analyzed by ion exchange chromatography.

concentrations have been attributed to decreased liver synthesis of carnitine by phenylacetic acid and by increased urinary excretion of carnitine as phenylacetyl-carnitine.

A number of medical foods used in nutrition management of patients with an IMD do not contain fat, minerals, or vitamins, and minerals in elemental diets are poorly absorbed.[37] Further, patients of all ages often fail to adhere to prescribed intake of medications for very serious situations.[71-73] Thus, to expect the patient to remember to take mineral and vitamin tablets daily may lead to malnutrition.

Many factors influence absorption of nutrients,[74,75] among which are competition of nutrients for protein carriers.[63,76] Thus, large amounts of any one nutrient given in one dose may be less well absorbed than the same nutrient given in three or more smaller doses. Consequently, patients with an IMD ingesting medical foods free of fats, minerals, and vitamins require frequent evaluation of essential fatty acid, mineral, and vitamin status.

Essential Fatty Acids

As early as 1960, Holman suggested the ratio of trienoic acids to tetraenoic acids in tissue lipids as a measure of EFA requirement[77] and reported that a ratio of C20:3n-9/C20:4n-6 greater than or equal to 0.2 was indicative of deficiency. Plasma and erythrocyte fatty acids are now assessed and reported as grams per 100 g fatty acids (weight percent) or as micromoles per liter (μmol/L) of serum or erythrocytes. Age,[78] diet,[79] disease,[80] and drugs[81] all influence plasma and erythrocyte fatty acid concentrations. Since many patients with an IMD often have seizures, especially if diagnosis and treatment are delayed, seizure medication may influence concentrations of fatty acids in plasma and erythrocytes. Further, even when the medical food contains fat, total fat and EFA intakes may be less in patients than in their normal siblings.[82,83] Plasma and erythrocyte concentrations of fatty acids may be more useful if reported as μmol/L. Table 3.7 suggests normal plasma concentrations of EFAs.[84]

Minerals and Vitamins

Plasma/serum concentrations below reference ranges have been reported for copper, iron, selenium, and zinc in patients undergoing nutrition management for various IMDs.[22,85-94] Serum ferritin concentrations were found to support the data suggesting iron deficiency,[95,96] along with transferrin receptors.[97] As indicated previously, patients ingesting medical foods free of trace and ultratrace minerals should be assessed routinely for all these minerals. See Table 3.7 for normal reference ranges.[62,98-102]

Prior to 1963, medical foods used in nutrition management of patients with an IMD were very low in vitamins and vitamin supplements and often contained only vitamins A, C, D, thiamine, riboflavin, niacin, and pyridoxine. Vitamins E and K, biotin, choline, folate, vitamin B_{12}, inositol, and pantothenic acid were not added. A number of these infants developed severe skin rashes and failure to thrive, and two infants died.[103,104] The characteristic skin rash completely cleared when the patients were given a complete vitamin supplement.

Well-treated children with PKU in Greece were found to have lower serum concentrations of folate, pyridoxine, and vitamin B_{12} than the group of children who did not comply with diet.[105] Patients with untreated homocystinuria failed to metabolize vitamin A alcohol and folic acid normally, resulting in lower than normal serum concentrations.[41,42] Vitamin B_{12} deficiency has been reported in patients with PKU in Denmark, the United States, United Kingdom, and Canada who failed to ingest animal protein or their prescribed medical food.[106-109] Mild riboflavin deficiency was found in patients with PKU in Poland who were undergoing nutrition management of PKU.[110] Thiamine deficiency, resulting in lactic acidosis, was reported in two patients with propionic acidemia who had inadequate intake and increased need during metabolic stress.[111] Thus, due to increased vitamin needs in some patients with an IMD and no minerals or vitamins in some medical foods, biochemical evaluation of mineral and vitamin status should routinely be conducted. See Table 3.7 for acceptable reference ranges.

Clinical Assessment

Clinical manifestations of nutrient deficiencies have long been known, and examination for their presence is essential to assessment of the patient. Severe nutrient deficiency, such as skin lesions seen in isoleucine deficiency in organic acidemias[112-115] and TYR deficiency in PKU,[64-66] or unusual hair texture and hypopigmentation in a selenium-deficient patient with propionic acidemia, are easily found,[93] while milder signs of malnutrition are more difficult to detect. When milder forms of malnutrition are suspected, evaluation of nutrient intake and biochemical assessment is helpful in verifying the diagnosis; however, any of the signs reported in Table 3.9 may be seen in the patient whose prescription is inadequate, who fails to comply with the diet prescription, refuses medical food, or ingests medical food containing only FAAs with no minerals or vitamins.[116-118]

Table 3.9 *Clinical Symptoms Associated With Nutrient Deficiencies*

Clinical symptom	*Suspected nutrient deficiency*
Appetite poor	Essential amino acids, zinc
Linear growth poor	Protein, essential amino acids, zinc
Eyes	
Bitot spots	Vitamin A
Dry conjunctiva	Vitamin A
Keratomalacia	Vitamin A
Night blindness	Vitamin A
Pale conjunctiva	Copper, iron, folate, vitamins A, B12
Xerosis	Vitamin A
Gums	
Bleed easily	Vitamin C
Loose teeth	Vitamin C
Spongy	Vitamin C
Hair	
Depigmented	Protein, selenium, zinc
Dull, dry, thin	Protein
Easily pluckable	Protein
Loss	Protein, B12, folate
Lips	
Angular stomatitis	B complex, iron, protein
Cheilosis	B complex
Musculoskeletal	
Costachondral beading	Vitamin D
Crainotabes	Vitamin D
Decreased muscle mass	Protein, energy
Epiphyseal enlargement	Vitamin D
Frontal bossing	Vitamin D
Nails	
Brittle	Iron, protein
Koilonychia	Iron, protein
Ridged	Iron, protein

(continues)

Table 3.9 *Clinical Symptoms Associated With Nutrient Deficiencies, Continued*

Clinical symptom	*Suspected nutrient deficiency*
Skin	
Acne-like lesions	Vitamin A
Dermatitis	Essential fatty acids, isoleucine, zinc
Desquamation	Riboflavin
Follicular keratosis	Vitamin A
Peripheral edema	Protein, thiamine
Petachiae	Vitamin C
Xerosis	Vitamin A
Tongue	
Inflammation (glossitis)	Pyridoxine, niacin, riboflavin, folate

Sources:

Bessler S. Nutritional assessment. In: Samour PQ, King K, eds. *Handbook of Pediatric Nutrition*. 3rd ed. Sudbury, MA: Jones and Bartlett; 2005:11–33.

Collier SB, Hendricks KM. Nutrition assessment. In: Baker RD, Baker SB, Davis AM, eds. *Pediatric Nutrition Support*. New York, NY: Chapman and Hall; 1997.

Heimburger DC, McLaren DS, Shils ME. Clinical manifestations of nutrient deficiencies and toxicities. In: Shils ME, Shike M, Olson J, Ross AC, eds. *Modern Nutrition in Health and Disease*. Philadelphia, PA: Lippincott Williams and Wilkins; 2005:595–612.

Hubbard VA, Hubbard LR. Clinical assessment of nutritional status. In: Walker WA, Watkins JB, eds. *Nutrition in Pediatrics, Basic Science and Clinical Applications*. Hamilton, ON: BC Decker; 1997:7–28.

Jensen GL, Binkley J. Clinical manifestations of nutrient deficiency. *JPEN J Parenter Enteral Nutr*. 2002;26:S29–S33.

Health history will not be addressed here because it should be a part of the medical record obtained at each routine visit to the medical geneticist for evaluation of status of the patient with an IMD.

CONCLUSION

Protein equivalent, minerals, and some vitamins must be ingested in amounts greater than those recommended for normal individuals by patients ingesting an elemental diet to support normal growth and prevent nutrient deficiencies. In addition to routine assessment of nutrient intake, biochemical assessment of the restricted nutrient(s), as well as poorly absorbed nutrients, and clinical evaluation of the patient should occur, especially if the patient is ingesting a medical food free of fat, minerals, and vitamins.

REFERENCES

1. Otten JJ, Hellwig JP, Meyers LD. *Dietary Reference Intakes: The Essential Guide to Nutrient Requirements*. Washington, DC: National Academies Press; 2006.
2. Pratt EL, Snyderman SE, Cheung MW, et al. The threonine requirement of the normal infant. *J Nutr*. 1955;56:231–251.
3. Rose WC. Amino acid requirements of man. *Fed Proc*. 1949;8:546–552.
4. Waterlow JC. Metabolic adaptation to low intakes of energy and protein. *Annu Rev Nutr*. 1986;6:495–526.
5. Fouillet H, Mariotti F, Gaudichon C, Bos C, Tome D. Peripheral and splanchnic metabolism of dietary nitrogen are differently affected by the protein source in humans as assessed by compartmental modeling. *J Nutr*. 2002;132:125–133.
6. Boirie Y, Dangin M, Gachon P, Vasson MP, Maubois JL, Beaufrere B. Slow and fast dietary proteins differently modulate postprandial protein accretion. *Proc Natl Acad Sci USA*. 1997;94:14930–14935.
7. Dangin M, Boirie Y, Garcia-Rodenas C, et al. The digestion rate of protein is an independent regulating factor of postprandial protein retention. *Am J Physiol Endocrinol Metab*. 2001;280:E340–E348.
8. Lacroix M, Bos C, Leonil J, et al. Compared with casein or total milk protein, digestion of milk soluble proteins is too rapid to sustain the anabolic postprandial amino acid requirement. *Am J Clin Nutr*. 2006;84:1070–1079.
9. Monchi M, Rerat AA. Comparison of net protein utilization of milk protein mild enzymatic hydrolysates and free amino acid mixtures with a close pattern in the rat. *JPEN J Parenter Enteral Nutr*. 1993;17:355–363.
10. Daenzer M, Petzke KJ, Bequette BJ, Metges CC. Whole-body nitrogen and splanchnic amino acid metabolism differ in rats fed mixed diets containing casein or its corresponding amino acid mixture. *J Nutr*. 2001;131:1965–1972.
11. Bujko J, Schreurs VV, Nolles JA, Verreijen AM, Koopmanschap RE, Verstegen MW. Application of a (13CO2) breath test to study short-term amino acid catabolism during the postprandial phase of a meal. *Br J Nutr*. 2007;97:891–897.
12. Mariotti F, Mahe S, Luengo C, Benamouzig R, Tome D. Postprandial modulation of dietary and whole-body nitrogen utilization by carbohydrates in humans. *Am J Clin Nutr*. 2000;72:954–962.
13. Gaudichon C, Mahe S, Benamouzig R, et al. Net postprandial utilization of (15N)-labeled milk protein nitrogen is influenced by diet composition in humans. *J Nutr*. 1999;129:890–895.
14. Welle S, Matthews DE, Campbell RG, Nair KS. Stimulation of protein turnover by carbohydrate overfeeding in men. *Am J Physiol*. 1989;257:E413–E417.
15. Friedlander AL, Braun B, Pollack M, et al. Three weeks of caloric restriction alters protein metabolism in normal-weight, young men. *Am J Physiol Endocrinol Metab*. 2005;289:E446–E455.
16. Kindt E, Motzfeldt K, Halvorsen S, Lie SO. Is phenylalanine requirement in infants and children related to protein intake? *Br J Nutr*. 1984;51:435–442.
17. Acosta PB, Yannicelli S. Protein intake affects phenylalanine requirements and growth of infants with phenylketonuria. *Acta Paediatr Suppl*. 1994;407:66–67.
18. MacDonald A, Chakrapani A, Hendriksz C, et al. Protein substitute dosage in PKU: how much do young patients need? *Arch Dis Child*. 2006;91:588–593.
19. Dworschak E. Nonenzyme browning and its effect on protein nutrition. *Crit Rev Food Sci Nutr*. 1980;13:1–40.

20. Erbersdobler HF, Somoza V. Forty years of furosine—forty years of using Maillard reaction products as indicators of the nutritional quality of foods. *Mol Nutr Food Res*. 2007;51:423–430.
21. Rerat A, Calmes R, Vaissade P, Finot PA. Nutritional and metabolic consequences of the early Maillard reaction of heat treated milk in the pig: significance for man. *Eur J Nutr*. 2002;41:1–11.
22. Gropper SS, Acosta PB. Effect of simultaneous ingestion of L-amino acids and whole protein on plasma amino acid and urea nitrogen concentrations in humans. *JPEN J Parenter Enteral Nutr*. 1991;15:48–53.
23. Stoll B, Henry J, Reeds PJ, Yu H, Jahoor F, Burrin DG. Catabolism dominates the first-pass intestinal metabolism of dietary essential amino acids in milk protein-fed piglets. *J Nutr*. 1998;128:606–614.
24. Jones BJ, Lees R, Andrews J, Frost P, Silk DB. Comparison of an elemental and polymeric enteral diet in patients with normal gastrointestinal function. *Gut*. 1983;24:78–84.
25. Allen JR, Baur LA, Waters DL, et al. Body protein in prepubertal children with phenylketonuria. *Eur J Clin Nutr*. 1996;50:178–186.
26. Gietzen DW, Hao S, Anthony TG. Mechanisms of food intake repression in indispensable amino acid deficiency. *Annu Rev Nutr*. 2007;27:63–78.
27. Soares MJ, Piers LS, Shetty PS, Jackson AA, Waterlow JC. Whole body protein turnover in chronically undernourished individuals. *Clin Sci (Lond)*. 1994;86:441–446.
28. Food and Drug Administration Rules and Regulations: Nutrient requirements for infant formulas (21 CFR Part 107). *Fed Regist*. 1985;50:45106–45108.
29. Acosta PB, Wenz E, Williamson M. Nutrient intake of treated infants with phenylketonuria. *Am J Clin Nutr*. 1977;30:198–208.
30. Acosta PB, Trahms C, Wellman NS, Williamson M. Phenylalanine intakes of 1- to 6-year-old children with phenylketonuria undergoing therapy. *Am J Clin Nutr*. 1983;38:694–700.
31. Williamson M, Koch R, Clair T, et al. Treatment effects on physical growth and intelligence among phenylketonuria children. In: Bickel H, Hudson FP, Woolf LI, eds. *Phenylketonuria and Some Other Inborn Errors of Amino Acid Metabolism*. Stuttgart, Germany: Georg Thieme Verlag; 1971:199–207.
32. Acosta PB, Michals-Matalon K, Austin V, et al. Nutrition findings and requirements in pregnant women with phenylketonuria. In: Platt LD, Koch R, de la Cruz F, eds. *Genetic Disorders and Pregnancy Outcome*. New York, NY: Parthenon; 1997: 21–32.
33. Acosta PB, Yannicelli S, Singh R, et al. Nutrient intakes and physical growth of children with phenylketonuria undergoing nutrition therapy. *J Am Diet Assoc*. 2003;103:1167–1173.
34. Picciano MF, McDonald SS. Lactation. In: Shils ME, Shike M, Olson J, Ross AC, eds. *Modern Nutrition in Health and Disease*. 10th ed. Philadelphia, PA: Lippincott Williams & Wilkins; 2005:784–796.
35. Tint GS, Irons M, Elias ER, et al. Defective cholesterol biosynthesis associated with the Smith-Lemli-Opitz syndrome. *N Engl J Med*. 1994;330:107–113.
36. Woolf LI. Excretion of conjugated phenylacetic acid in phenylketonuria. *Biochem J*. 1951;49:ix–x.
37. Alexander JW, Clayton BE, Delves HT. Mineral and trace-metal balances in children receiving normal and synthetic diets. *Q J Med*. 1974;169:80–111.

38. LaDu BN, Zannoni VG. Basic biochemical disturbance in aromatic amino acid metabolism. In: Bickel H, Hudson FP, Woolf LI, eds. *Phenylketonuria and Some Other Inborn Errors of Amino Acid Metabolism*. Stuttgart, Germany: Georg Thieme Verlag; 1971:6–13.
39. Lewis JS, Loskill S, Bunker ML, Acosta PB, Kim R. N-methylnicotinamide excretion of phenylketonuric children and a child with Hartnup disease before and after phenylalanine and tryptophan load. *Fed Proc*. 1974;33:666A.
40. Schulpis KH, Nyalala JO, Papakonstantinou ED, et al. Biotin recycling impairment in phenylketonuric children with seborrheic dermatitis. *Int J Dermatol*. 1998;37: 918–921.
41. Carey MC, Donovan DE, Fitzgerald O, McAuley FD. Homocystinuria. I. A clinical and pathological study of nine subjects in six families. *Am J Med*. 1968;45:7–25.
42. Carey MC, Fennelly JJ, Fitzgerald O. Homocystinuria. II. Subnormal serum folate levels, increased folate clearance and effects of folic acid therapy. *Am J Med*. 1968;45:26–31.
43. Chumlea WC. Physical growth and maturation. In: Samour PQ, King K, eds. *Handbook of Pediatric Nutrition*. 3rd ed. Sudbury, MA: Jones & Bartlett; 2005:1–10.
44. Physical status: The use and interpretation of anthropometry. Report of a WHO Expert Committee. *World Health Organ Tech Rep Ser*. 1995;854:1–452.
45. Hamill PV, Drizd TA, Johnson CL, Reed RB, Roche AF, Moore WM. Physical growth: National Center for Health Statistics percentiles. *Am J Clin Nutr*. 1979;32:607–629.
46. National Center for Health Statistics. 2000 CDC Growth Charts: United States. Available at: http://www.cdc.gov/growthcharts/. Accessed January 4, 2008.
47. Bessler S. Nutritional assessment. In: Samour PQ, King K, eds. *Handbook of Pediatric Nutrition*. 3rd ed. Sudbury, MA: Jones & Bartlett; 2005:11–33.
48. Penny ME. Protein-energy malnutrition: pathophysiology, clinical consequences, and treatment. In: Walker WA, Watkins JB, Duggan C, eds. *Nutrition in Pediatrics*. London, England: BC Decker; 2003:174–194.
49. WHO Working Group. Use and interpretation of anthropometric indicators of nutritional status. *Bull World Health Organ*. 1986;64(suppl 1):929–941.
50. Schaefer F, Burgard P, Batzler U, et al. Growth and skeletal maturation in children with phenylketonuria. *Acta Paediatr*. 1994;83:534–541.
51. Dobbelaere D, Michaud L, Debrabander A, et al. Evaluation of nutritional status and pathophysiology of growth retardation in patients with phenylketonuria. *J Inherit Metab Dis*. 2003;26:1–11.
52. Maynard LM, Guo SS, Chumlea WC, et al. Total-body and regional bone mineral content and areal bone mineral density in children aged 8–18 y: the Fels Longitudinal Study. *Am J Clin Nutr*. 1998;68:1111–1117.
53. Michals-Matalon K, Acosta PB, Azen C. Five year postnatal growth of offspring of women with phenylketonuria in the Maternal PKU Collaborative Study. *J Inherit Metab Dis*. 2007;30:19A.
54. Superti-Furga A, Hoffmann GF. Glutaric aciduria type 1 (glutaryl-CoA-dehydrogenase deficiency): advances and unanswered questions. Report from an international meeting. *Eur J Pediatr*. 1997;156:821–828.
55. Olsen IE, Mascarenhas MR, Stallings VA. Clinical assessment of nutritional status. In: Walker WA, Watkins JB, Duggan C, eds. *Nutrition in Pediatrics*. 3rd ed. London, England: BC Decker; 2003:6–16.

56. Subcommittee on Nutritional Status and Weight Gain During Pregnancy. Part 1. Weight Gain. Washington, DC: National Academy Press; 1990.
57. Morlese JF, Forrester T, Del Rosario M, Frazer M, Jahoor F. Transferrin kinetics are altered in children with severe protein-energy malnutrition. *J Nutr*. 1997;127: 1469–1474.
58. Benjamin DR. Laboratory tests and nutritional assessment. Protein-energy status. *Pediatr Clin North Am*. 1989;36:139–161.
59. Collier SB, Hendricks KM. Nutrition assessment. In: Baker RD, Baker SB, Davis AM, eds. *Pediatric Nutrition Support*. New York, NY: Chapman & Hall; 1997:42–63.
60. Sauberlich HE. *Laboratory Tests for the Assessment of Nutritional Status*. 2nd ed. Boca Raton, FL: CRC Press; 1999:447–467.
61. Fletcher JP, Little JM, Guest PK. A comparison of serum transferrin and serum prealbumin as nutritional parameters. *JPEN J Parenter Enteral Nutr*. 1987;11: 144–147.
62. Soldin SJ, Brugnara C, Wong EC. *Pediatric Reference Intervals*. 6th ed. Washington, DC: AACC Press; 2007.
63. Hidalgo IJ, Borchardt RT. Transport of a large neutral amino acid (phenylalanine) in a human intestinal epithelial cell line: Caco-2. *Biochim Biophys Acta*. 1990;1028:25–30.
64. Brouwer M, de Bree PK, van Sprang FJ, Wadman SK. Low serum-tyrosine in patients with phenylketonuria on dietary treatment. *Lancet*. 1977;1:1162.
65. Hanley WB, Lee AW, Hanley AJ, et al. "Hypotyrosinemia" in phenylketonuria. *Mol Genet Metab*. 2000;69:286–294.
66. Francois B, Diels M, de la Brassinne M. Iatrogenic skin lesions in phenylketonuric children due to a low tyrosine intake. *J Inherit Metab Dis*. 1989;12(Suppl 2):332–334.
67. Sansaricq C, Garg S, Norton PM, Phansalkar SV, Snyderman SE. Cystine deficiency during dietotherapy of homocystinemia. *Acta Paediatr Scand*. 1975;64: 215–218.
68. Ajinomoto. *Amino Acids*. 8th ed. Teaneck, NJ: Ajinomoto, USA; 1997:132–133.
69. Matalon K, Acosta PB, Castiglioni L, et al. *Protocol for Nutrition Support of Maternal PKU*. Bethesda, MD: The National Institute of Child Health and Human Development. 1998;1–51.
70. Fischer GM, Nemeti B, Farkas V, et al. Metabolism of carnitine in phenylacetic acid-treated rats and in patients with phenylketonuria. *Biochim Biophys Acta*. 2000;1501:200–210.
71. Matsui D. Current issues in pediatric medication adherence. *Paediatr Drugs*. 2007;9:283–288.
72. Bullington P, Pawola L, Walker R, Valenta A, Briars L, John E. Identification of medication non-adherence factors in adolescent transplant patients: the patient's viewpoint. *Pediatr Transplant*. 2007;11:914–921.
73. Wu JR, Moser DK, Lennie TA, Burkhart PV. Medication adherence in patients who have heart failure: a review of the literature. *Nurs Clin North Am*. 2008;43: 133–153.
74. Krebs NF. Bioavailability of dietary supplements and impact of physiologic state: infants, children and adolescents. *J Nutr*. 2001;131:1351S–1354S.
75. Gibson RS. The role of diet- and host-related factors in nutrient bioavailability and thus in nutrient-based dietary requirement estimates. *Food Nutr Bull*. 2007;28: S77–S100.

76. Pardridge WM. Kinetics of competitive inhibition of neutral amino acid transport across the blood-brain barrier. *J Neurochem*. 1977;28:103–108.
77. Holman RT. The ratio of trienoic: tetraenoic acids in tissue lipids as a measure of essential fatty acid requirement. *J Nutr*. 1960;70:405–410.
78. Holman RT, Smythe L, Johnson S. Effect of sex and age on fatty acid composition of human serum lipids. *Am J Clin Nutr*. 1979;32:2390–2399.
79. Rise P, Eligini S, Ghezzi S, Colli S, Galli C. Fatty acid composition of plasma, blood cells and whole blood: relevance for the assessment of the fatty acid status in humans. *Prostaglandins Leukot Essent Fatty Acids*. 2007;76:363–369.
80. Pazirandeh S, Ling PR, Ollero M, Gordon F, Burns DL, Bistrian BR. Supplementation of arachidonic acid plus docosahexaenoic acid in cirrhotic patients awaiting liver transplantation: a preliminary study. *JPEN J Parenter Enteral Nutr*. 2007;31:511–516.
81. Yuen AW, Sander JW, Flugel D, et al. Erythrocyte and plasma fatty acid profiles in patients with epilepsy: does carbamazepine affect omega-3 fatty acid concentrations? *Epilepsy Behav*. 2008;12:317–323.
82. Acosta PB, Yannicelli S, Singh R, et al. Intake and blood levels of fatty acids in treated patients with phenylketonuria. *J Pediatr Gastroenterol Nutr*. 2001;33: 253–259.
83. Rose HJ, White F, MacDonald A, Rutherford PJ, Favre E. Fat intakes of children with PKU on low phenylalanine diets. *J Hum Nutr Diet*. 2005;18:395–400.
84. Gillingham M, van Calcar S, Ney D, Wolff J, Harding C. Dietary management of long-chain 3-hydroxyacyl-CoA dehydrogenase deficiency (LCHADD): a case report and survey. *J Inherit Metab Dis*. 1999;22:123–131.
85. Lombeck I, Kasperek K, Harbisch HD, et al. The selenium state of children. II. Selenium content of serum, whole blood, hair and the activity of erythrocyte glutathione peroxidase in dietetically treated patients with phenylketonuria and maple-syrup-urine disease. *Eur J Pediatr*. 1978;128:213–223.
86. Acosta PB, Fernhoff PM, Warshaw HS, et al. Zinc and copper status of treated children with phenylketonuria. *JPEN J Parenter Enteral Nutr*. 1981;5:406–409.
87. Taylor CJ, Moore G, Davidson DC. The effect of treatment on zinc, copper and calcium status in children with phenylketonuria. *J Inherit Metab Dis*. 1984;7:160–164.
88. Spooner RJ, Fell GS, Halls DJ, Taitz LS, Worthy E. Selenium depletion and its correction in a child with homocystinuria. *Clin Nutr*. 1986;5:29–32.
89. McCabe ER, McCabe L. Issues in the dietary management of phenylketonuria: breast-feeding and trace-metal nutriture. *Ann NY Acad Sci*. 1986;477:215–222.
90. Acosta PB, Stepnick-Gropper S, Clarke-Sheehan N, et al. Trace element status of PKU children ingesting an elemental diet. *JPEN J Parenter Enteral Nutr*. 1987;11:287–292.
91. Reilly C, Barrett JE, Patterson CM, Tinggi U, Latham SL, Marrinan A. Trace element nutrition status and dietary intake of children with phenylketonuria. *Am J Clin Nutr*. 1990;52:159–165.
92. Bodley JL, Austin VJ, Hanley WB, Clarke JT, Zlotkin S. Low iron stores in infants and children with treated phenylketonuria: a population at risk for iron-deficiency anaemia and associated cognitive deficits. *Eur J Pediatr*. 1993;152:140–143.
93. Yannicelli S, Hambidge KM, Picciano MF. Decreased selenium intake and low plasma selenium concentrations leading to clinical symptoms in a child with propionic acidaemia. *J Inherit Metab Dis*. 1992;15:261–268.

94. Miranda da Cruz BD, Seidler H, Widhalm K. Iron status and iron supplementation in children with classical phenylketonuria. *J Am Coll Nutr*. 1993;12:531–536.
95. Scaglioni S, Zuccotti G, Vedovello M, et al. Study of serum ferritin in 58 children with classic phenylketonuria and persistent hyperphenylalaninaemia. *J Inherit Metab Dis*. 1985;8:160.
96. Acosta PB, Greene C, Yannicelli S. Nutrition studies in treated infants with phenylketonuria. *Int Pediatr*. 1993;8:6–16.
97. Acosta PB, Yannicelli S, Singh RH, Elsas LJ, Mofidi S, Steiner RD. Iron status of children with phenylketonuria undergoing nutrition therapy assessed by transferrin receptors. *Genet Med*. 2004;6:96–101.
98. Ances IG, Granados J, Baltazar M. Serum ferritin as an early determinant of decreased iron stores in pregnant women. *South Med J*. 1979;72:591–592, 604.
99. Hambidge KM, Walravens PA, Casey CE, Brown RM, Bender C. Plasma zinc concentrations of breast-fed infants. *J Pediatr*. 1979;94:607–608.
100. Pleban PA, Munyani A, Beachum J. Determination of selenium concentration and glutathione peroxidase activity in plasma and erythrocytes. *Clin Chem*. 1982;28: 311–316.
101. Shank JS, Dorsey JL, Anderson K, Cooper WT, Acosta PB. Plasma vitamin E concentrations of older infants fed cow's milk or infant formula. *J Pediatr Gastroenterol Nutr*. 1992;15:375–381.
102. Lockitch G. *Handbook of Diagnostic Biochemistry and Hematology in Normal Pregnancy*. Boca Raton, FL: CRC Press; 1993.
103. Wilson KM, Clayton BE. Importance of choline during growth, with particular reference to synthetic diets in phenylketonuria. *Arch Dis Child*. 1962;37: 565–577.
104. Report to the Medical Research Council of a Conference on Phenylketonuria. Treatment of Phenylketonuria. *Br Med J*. 1963;1:1691–1967.
105. Schulpis KH, Karikas GA, Papakonstantinou E. Homocysteine and other vascular risk factors in patients with phenylketonuria on a diet. *Acta Paediatr*. 2002;91:905–909.
106. Hanley WB, Feigenbaum AS, Clarke JT, Schoonheyt WE, Austin VJ. Vitamin B12 deficiency in adolescents and young adults with phenylketonuria. *Eur J Pediatr*. 1996;155(Suppl 1):S145–S147.
107. Aung TT, Klied A, McGinn J, McGinn T. Vitamin B12 deficiency in an adult phenylketonuric patient. *J Inherit Metab Dis*. 1997;20:603–604.
108. Robinson M, White FJ, Cleary MA, Wraith E, Lam WK, Walter JH. Increased risk of vitamin B12 deficiency in patients with phenylketonuria on an unrestricted or relaxed diet. *J Pediatr*. 2000;136:545–547.
109. Hvas AM, Nexo E, Nielsen JB. Vitamin B12 and vitamin B6 supplementation is needed among adults with phenylketonuria (PKU). *J Inherit Metab Dis*. 2006;29: 47–53.
110. Lipinska L, Laskowska-Klita T, Cabalska B. Riboflavin status in phenylketonuric patients in the course of dietary treatment. *J Inherit Metab Dis*. 1994;17:242.
111. Matern D, Seydewitz HH, Lehnert W, Niederhoff H, Leititis JU, Brandis M. Primary treatment of propionic acidemia complicated by acute thiamine deficiency. *J Pediatr*. 1996;129:758–760.
112. Spraker MK, Helminski M, Elsas LJ. Peri-orificial dermatitis secondary to diet deficiency of isoleucine in treated infants with maple syrup urine disease. *J Invest Dermatol*. 1986;56:508A.

113. De Raeve L, De Meirleir L, Ramet J, Vandenplas Y, Gerlo E. Acrodermatitis enteropathica-like cutaneous lesions in organic aciduria. *J Pediatr*. 1994;124: 416–420.
114. Tain YL, Huang SC, Hung FC, Wang HS, Sun PC. Acrodermatitis enteropathica-like eruption during treatment of maple syrup urine disease: report of one case. *Zhonghua Min Guo Xiao Er Ke Yi Xue Hui Za Zhi*. 1996;37:357–360.
115. Sasaki M, Aikoh H, Sugai K, Yoshida H, Tunnessen WW Jr. Picture of the month. Cutaneous lesions associated with isoleucine deficiency. *Arch Pediatr Adolesc Med*. 1998;152:707–708.
116. Jensen GL, Binkley J. Clinical manifestations of nutrient deficiency. *JPEN J Parenter Enteral Nutr*. 2002;26:S29–S33.
117. Heimburger DC, McLaren DS, Shils ME. Clinical manifestations of nutrient deficiencies and toxicities. In: Shils ME, Shike M, Olson J, Ross AC, eds. *Modern Nutrition in Health and Disease*. Philadelphia, PA: Lippincott Williams & Wilkins; 2005:595–612.
118. Hubbard VA, Hubbard LR. Clinical assessment of nutritional status. In: Walker WA, Watkins JB, eds. *Nutrition in Pediatrics, Basic Science and Clinical Applications*. 2nd ed. Hamilton, ON, Canada: BC Decker; 1997:7–28.

Chapter 4

Rationales for and Practical Aspects of Nutrition Management

Phyllis B. Acosta

INTRODUCTION

The objectives of nutrition management of patients with inherited metabolic disorders are normal growth and development, and as an adult, to be a normal functioning member of society. Nutrition management of patients with a genetic disorder requires accurate diagnosis, early and continuous therapy, and knowledge of the pathogenesis of the disorder.[1] Without such knowledge, the nutrition prescription may not be appropriate to the patient's needs and may result in mental retardation, metabolic crises, neurologic crises, growth failure, and, with some inherited metabolic disorders, death.[2]

Rationales for Nutrition Management

Altered genes may result in non-functioning or partially functioning enzymes, which in turn may lead to defects in transport proteins, lack of essential body compound(s), accumulation of toxic compounds, and synthesis of normal substances in excess amounts, of abnormal substances, which in turn may cause excretion of essential nutrients, deficiencies of metabolites essential for de novo synthesis of required products, and failure to release nutrients in order that they may be reused.[1] Because of the results that may occur from the enzyme defect, from possible organ damage, and from loss of specific chemicals, a number of compounds may become conditionally essential. These include the amino acids arginine (ARG), cystine (CYS), and tyrosine (TYR), and other chemicals such as L-carnitine, coenzyme Q_{10}, lipoic acid, and tetrahydrobiopterin (BH_4).[3]

This text discusses 10 approaches to nutrition management of patients with an inherited metabolic disorder (IMD). The correct approach to each IMD depends on the biochemistry and pathophysiology of the disease expression. Several approaches may be used simultaneously for some disorders and may include one or more of the following[2-5]: enhance anabolism and depress catabolism, correct the primary imbalance in metabolic relationships, depress absorption of nutrients that are toxic when ingested in excess of tolerance, provide alternative metabolic pathways to decrease accumulated toxic precursors in blocked reaction sequences, supply necessary products of blocked reactions, supplement nutrients that are bound and excreted with toxic compounds, stabilize altered enzyme production, enhance coenzyme production, induce normal enzyme production, and supplement nutrients that are inadequately absorbed or not released from their apoenzyme. Examples of these various approaches are described in Chapters 5 through 11.

Practical Aspects of Nutrition Management

Evolution of Nutrition Management

Nutrition management of patients with inherited disorders of essential amino acids, carbohydrates, or essential fatty acids was difficult prior to the development of special medical foods low in or devoid of specific amino acid(s) or other poorly metabolized or absorbed nutrients. Subsequent to the demonstrations that a phenylalanine (PHE)-restricted diet would benefit development of patients with phenylpyruvic oligophrenia (little brains due to phenylpyruvic acid), now called phenylketonuria (PKU; OMIM 261600),[6] Mead Johnson Nutritionals (Evansville, Indiana) began to develop a low-PHE formula using the enzymatic casein hydrolysate prepared for Nutramigen®. Much of the PHE, tryptophan (TRP), and TYR were removed by treatment of the hydrolysate with activated charcoal. The TRP and TYR, along with corn oil, carbohydrate, and some minerals and vitamins, were added.[7] The Food and Drug Administration (FDA) ruled in the mid-1950s that special foods to treat these patients would be considered drugs and required an Investigational New Drug Application for study.[7] Clinical studies indicated safety and efficacy of Lofenalac® (Mead Johnson Nutritionals, Evansville, Indiana), and from 1958 to 1972 it was marketed in the United States as a prescription product.[7] Lofenalac initially had no added vitamin K, choline, copper, iodine, magnesium, or manganese.[8]

Several other companies also began manufacturing formulas (medical foods) for patients with PKU from casein hydrolysate, beef serum albumin, or free amino acids in the 1950s. Minafen®, a casein hydrolysate formula made by Trufoods, Ltd. (United Kingdom), contained no methionine (MET), TRP, vitamins A, D, B_{12}, and choline but had DL-MET, DL-TRP, and peanut oil (free of essential fatty acids) added. Cymogran®, also a casein hydrolysate, manufactured by Allen and Hanbury, Ltd. (United Kingdom), was free of added essential fatty acids, vitamins A, C, D, B_2, niacin, B_6, pantothenic acid, folate, biotin, E, K, and B_{12}. Albumaid XP, made from hydrolyzed beef serum albumin, was manufactured by Milner Scientific and Medical Research Co., Ltd. (Liverpool, United Kingdom) (later, Scientific Hospital Supplies, Ltd.) and was fat free and low in or devoid of minerals and vitamins.[8] The protein hydrolysates all contained some PHE and TYR. Ketonil, made from DL-amino acids by Merck, Sharpe, and Dohme (Rahway, New Jersey), had no added minerals or vitamins and required the addition of minerals, vitamins, sugar, oil, milk, and water.[9] Other approaches to simplifying nutrition management for patients with PKU included development of food lists for patients giving PHE, TYR, protein, and energy for specific portion sizes[10] and development of computer software that was used for calculating nutrient intakes from 3-day diet diaries.[11]

Branched-chain ketoaciduria (maple syrup urine disease, MSUD; OMIM 248600)[6] was first reported in 1954,[12] and several physicians used mixtures of gelatin (low in branched-chain amino acids) with added free L-amino acids, carbohydrate, fat, minerals, and vitamins for nutrition management.[13-16] By 1965, Scientific Hospital Supplies, Ltd. (Liverpool, United Kingdom) provided amino acid mixtures that could be used for nutrition management of patients with MSUD.[17] Both an amino acid mixture to add to Product 80056 (carbohydrate, fat, minerals, vitamins) (Mead Johnson Nutritionals) and a gelatin-amino acid mixture were suggested by Snyderman at a symposium held in San Diego in March, 1977.[18] By 1978, Snyderman[19] had developed a formula consisting of free amino acids and Protein-Free Diet Powder (Product 80056) and made available by Mead Johnson Nutritionals as MSUD Diet Powder®. As amino acid analyses of foods became available, "equivalency lists" of foods that contained leucine (LEU) were introduced in 1971,[20] and later extended by Bell et al.[21] Reports of isoleucine (ILE) or valine (VAL) deficiency (see Chapter 6) led to further extensions of equivalency lists by the addition of ILE, VAL, protein, and energy to the food list.[22]

Few studies have evaluated growth and nutrition status of infants and children with MSUD undergoing nutrition management. In the early report by Dent and Westall[14] therapy was begun in a severely retarded female who was < 10th centile in length and weight and who was begun on a diet containing 1500 kcal (~200 kcal/kg/day) and 40 g protein (~5.5 g/kg/day). During the following 4 months of study, diet remained the same and at 12 months, the patient had increased to the 50th centile in length and slightly less than the

50th centile in weight, at which time energy intake was ~65 kcal/kg/day and protein intake was ~1.7 g/kg/day. In 1984, Leonard et al.[23] reported height Z-scores of 3 patients with MSUD, one of whom started the diet at 1 year of age (patient A), while patients B and C started nutrition management very early in the neonatal period. Total protein intake (as intact protein and free amino acids) declined from 3.75 to 4.00 g/kg/day in early infancy to about 1.5 g/kg/day at 13 years of age. Energy intake was not given. The length Z-score of patient A declined from < –1.0 to about –3.0 at 2 years of age and gradually increased to 0.0 at 12 years. Patient B initially declined from about –0.5 to about –3.0 but by 13 years of age had a height Z-score of +1.0, while patient C declined from ~–0.33 to ~–1.0 at 6 years. Henstenburg et al.[24] reported 12 children 2.8 to 11 years of age with MSUD who were compared to 12 age- and gender-matched healthy children and found that the patients with MSUD were significantly lower in height and weight than normal children. Children with MSUD had an energy intake of 86% and a protein intake of 78% of 1989 Recommended Dietary Allowances (RDAs). Gropper et al.[25] found that 15 infants and children with MSUD had an average energy intake ~89% of 1989 RDAs and a protein intake of ~143% 1989 RDAs. No growth data were reported.

More recent data on growth of 5 patients 14 to 27 years of age with MSUD were reported as part of a study to determine branched-chain amino acid (BCAA) requirements. While energy and protein intakes during previous years of nutrition management were not reported, three patients were < 3rd centile in height, one was < 10th centile, and one was < 25th centile. Weights varied from < 3rd centile to < 50th centile.[26] Clearly, further research is needed that provides data on age at diagnosis, plasma BCAA concentrations, and intakes of BCAAs, protein, and energy, as well as growth with height and weight of parents and non-affected siblings.

In the early 1960s, tyrosinemia (hepatorenal; OMIM 276700)[6] was reported in a number of infants in the Chicoutimi region of Canada.[27] The casein hydrolysate, which was not totally free of either PHE or TYR, was used with a mixture of carbohydrate, fat, minerals, and vitamins to try nutrition management of these patients. Later, Mead Johnson Nutritionals made this product available as 3200 AB.[7]

Homocystinuria (OMIM 236200),[6] resulting from a deficiency of cystathionine-β-synthase, was first reported in Ireland in 1962[28] and in the United States in 1964.[29] Treatment with a low-methionine diet made with soy protein isolate (low in methionine) was first reported in 1966 by Brenton et al.[30] in the United Kingdom and in the United States in 1967.[31] Food lists containing MET, CYS, protein, and energy contents for specific low-protein foods were published in 1976.[22] Over the next few years, as other disorders of amino acid metabolism were reported, some physicians treated patients with very low-protein intakes that resulted in severe protein malnutrition and failure to thrive,[32] while others compounded amino acid mixes locally. The latter mixtures had no quality control. As patients with other IMDs were diagnosed and treated, commercial medical foods consisting of free amino acids, carbohydrate, fat, minerals, and vitamins became available. Lists of low-protein foods with the specific amino acids requiring restriction, protein, and energy for each portion size were published.[22]

Between 1958 and 1978, many problems attributed to non-milk-based and elemental diets were reported. These included failure to thrive,[33-37] megaloblastic anemia,[37] severe skin rashes,[38] hypoglycemia,[39] peculiar roentgenographic bone changes,[40] and seven deaths, as well as mental retardation.[41]

In 1963, the Committee on Nutrition, American Academy of Pediatrics (AAP/CON) reported nutrition problems in infants fed milk substitute formulas made with soya flour as the protein source.[42] Subsequently, the AAP/CON proposed changes in FDA regulations relevant to formula products for infants.[43] The FDA then undertook extensive review of regulations governing composition and labeling of foods for special dietary uses and in 1971 published regulations for manufacturing and marketing of infant formulas.[44] These regulations were for minimum nutrients per 100 kcal and were largely those recommended by AAP/CON.[43] However, no minimum amounts were given for copper, manganese, potassium, sodium, zinc, biotin, choline, inositol, or vitamin K.

In 1972, due to the time and cost of developing formulas labeled as drugs, AAP/CON requested the FDA to rename the special formulas "Foods for Special Dietary Uses" to be used under medical supervision. Their supervision was relegated to the Bureau of Foods.[45] The AAP was contracted to monitor the use of these products.[46] An amendment (PL 96:359) to the Food, Drug, and Cosmetic Act, named the Infant Formula Act,[47] gave the FDA authority to establish quality-control procedures for infant formula manufacturing; establish recall procedures; establish nutrient content, with revisions as necessary; and regulate labels. An AAP task force submitted revised nutrient content recommendations for infant formulas to the FDA in 1983.[48] The final rule was published by the FDA in 1985.[49] Minimum and maximum requirements per 100 kcal were specified for 9 nutrients and minimum concentrations per 100 kcal for 20 nutrients. In Subpart C, exempt infant formulas were described and were to meet all nutrient requirements described for other infant formulas unless a written medical justification was submitted and accepted by the FDA. Exempt infant formulas are described as those "represented and labeled for use by an infant who has an inborn error of metabolism or low birth weight or who otherwise has an unusual medical or dietary problem, if such formulas comply with regulations prescribed by the Secretary."[49] Manufacturers are required to analyze each lot of formula before marketing to ensure that nutrients met specifications, test samples over the shelf life of the product, code containers to identify the lot and expiration date, and make all records available to FDA investigators.

Other regulations published by the FDA in 1985 require that nutrients be given on the label in a specific order and in specific units per 100 kcal as the minimum below which no nutrient would fall at the end of its shelf life, the list of ingredients and the order in which they were to be given, directions for storing and mixing, and the specific disorder(s) for which the product was to be used. Even label print size is regulated. Other requirements included ingredients that can be used, laboratory testing to be done before release, and notification of the FDA if any major reformulation, site, or method of manufacturing occurred.[49] In 1987, proposed rules for infant formula recall were first published.[50] Later, these exempt infant formulas were defined as Special Infant Formulas by Women's Infant and Children (WIC).[51] Orphan drugs are those products required by fewer than 200,000 people in the United States (1983),[52] and in 1988 this definition was applied to medical foods.[53] In 1992, Jess Thoene[54] defined exempt infant formulas and the products for over 1 year of age as Orphan Medical Foods. A medical food is defined as "a food which is formulated to be consumed or administered enterally under the supervision of a physician and which is intended for the specific dietary management of a disease or condition for which distinctive nutritional requirements based on recognized scientific principles are established by medical evaluation."[55] Medical foods are exempt from the labeling requirements for health claims in the Nutrition Labeling and Education Act of 1990, nor do medical foods for patients over 1 year of age have to undergo premarket review, approval, or registration with the FDA.[55]

In addition to medical foods that supply protein equivalent (nitrogen, g × 6.25 = protein equivalent), minerals, and vitamins, intact food sources of protein are required that provide amino acids in prescribed amounts, as well as carbohydrate, fat, and energy. Acosta and Centerwall[10] published "serving lists" of breads/cereals, fats, fruits, and vegetables that provide PHE, protein, and energy content per serving. Later, Acosta and Elsas[22] provided "serving lists" for nutrition management of patients with PHE- and TYR-restricted diets; MET-restricted diets; and ILE-, LEU-, and VAL-restricted diets. Lists of food for patients with propionic acidemia or methylmalonic acidemia were subsequently published[56] that reported ILE, MET, threonine (THR), VAL, protein, and energy content per serving.

Recipe books to help parents and patients prepare interesting meals were published early beginning with books of recipes low in PHE.[57,58] A recipe book used to prepare foods for patients with any of the inherited disorders of amino acid metabolism was subsequently published in 1977,[59] has been revised several times, and is still available. All of these recipe books supply PHE, protein, and energy content per serving.

Hand calculation of nutrient intakes of patients, essential to determine the range of requirements for amino acids and adequacy of intake for other nutrients, was a laborious process requiring the use of several references[60-62] before the development of a computer program to conduct the task. Dietitians working with the U.S. PKU Collaborative Study met in 1969 in Los Angeles, California, with representatives of the U.S. Department of Agriculture (USDA) to request that more foods be analyzed for amino acid content. Prior to the initiation of the PKU Collaborative Study that began in 1968, a program was developed that calculated 13 nutrients for each patient based on 3-day diet diaries obtained at numerous times throughout the study.[11] In the 1980s, Kennedy and Anderson[63] developed computer software with no missing nutrient data designed to calculate nutrient intakes of patients with inherited metabolic disorders of amino acid metabolism. Foods in this software database contain information on all essential amino acids, ARG, CYS, and TYR, carbohydrate, fat, energy, seven minerals, and nine vitamins. If any nutrient was not present in the USDA database, it was obtained from manufacturers when available or calculated from very similar foods with the same kind of protein present in the USDA database. The work of Holt and Snyderman[64] in describing essential amino acid requirements of infants and of Rose and coworkers[65] for adults was essential to the development of nutrition management.

Osmolality of Medical Food Mixtures

Nutrition management to correct imbalances in metabolic relationships in patients with disorders of amino acid metabolism requires the use of elemental medical foods. Other metabolic disorders may require the use of carbohydrate, mineral, and vitamin mixtures in large amounts.[4] These medical foods, called elemental medical foods, consisting of free amino acids, carbohydrates, minerals, and vitamins in chemical form, are comprised of many small molecules that if inadequately diluted with water often provide an osmolality that exceeds the physiologic tolerance of the patient. Osmotic pressure of a diet, reported as osmolality, is a measure of the pressure the diet will exert when it contacts the semipermeable membrane of the intestinal tract. The number of particles of solute miscible in water determines osmolality and includes amino acids, protein, carbohydrate, minerals, and vitamins. Fat, not water soluble, has no effect on osmolality other than by displacement of water that may be used to prepare a specific volume.[66] Elemental medical foods, if inadequately diluted with water, often provide an osmolality that exceeds the physiologic tolerance of the patient. Abdominal cramping, diarrhea, distention, nausea, and vomiting may result from hyperosmolar feeds. Aside from gastrointestinal distress, more serious consequences can occur, such as hypertonic dehydration, hypovolemia, hypernatremia, and death. Osmolalities of selected medical foods intended for inherited disorders of amino acid metabolism have been published.[4] Whenever a medical food mixture contains greater than 24 kcal/fl oz (81 kcal/100 mL), osmolality should be determined before feeding to the very young patient. If osmolality is greater than 450 mOsm/L for the neonate, greater than 750 mOsm/L for the child, greater than 1000 mOsm/L for the adult, or greater than tolerated by the patient, the water content should be increased and the osmolality again determined.[67]

Potential Renal Solute Load

Protein, sodium, potassium chloride, and phosphorus contribute to the renal solute load of a medical food mixture. Nitrogen (as urea), sodium, chloride, potassium, and phosphorus not retained for growth or maintenance contribute most of the renal solute load that is excreted with water by the kidneys. The upper limit of renal solute load for neonates is approximately 1100 mOsm/L.[68] Protein per gram yields 5.7 mOsm, while sodium, potassium, and chloride each yield 1 mOsm/mEq. Each milligram of phosphorus yields 0.0323 mOsm (P divided by 31). The milliosmoles (mOsm) in a medical food mixture are estimated as follows:

$$\text{mOsm Potential Renal Solute Load (PRSL)} = (\text{mg dietary protein} / 175) + \text{mOsm}(\text{Na}^+ + \text{K}^+ + \text{Cl}^- + \text{P})$$

Both insensible and fecal water losses must be considered when calculating the effect of renal solute load on urine concentration. A very high environmental temperature without air conditioning, fever, diarrhea, or vomiting may increase these water losses that are normally about 10 mL/kg/day in feces and about 60 mL/kg/day of insensible loss. Urinary concentration may be estimated by dividing the PRSL contributed to the diet by the water available for urine formation using the following mathematical formula:[69]

$$\text{mOsm RSL/L} = \frac{\text{mOsm in medical food mixture} \times 1000}{\text{mL medical food mixture} - (\text{mL insensible + fecal water losses})}$$

Prescribing Nutrition Management

The nutrient prescription, when based on unit of body weight, will differ significantly for patients of similar age, height, and similar genetic potential for

Table 4.1 *Nutrient and Weight Percentiles*

	Weight percentiles	
Nutrient	**3rd**	**50th**
Protein (g)	6.4	7.9
Energy (kcal)	840	1040

growth if based on different weights. For example, a 1-year-old male at the 3rd centile weighs 8.4 kg and at the 50th centile, 10.4 kg. A prescription of 0.87 g protein/kg and 100 kcal/kg will result in the data given in Table 4.1.

If the prescription based on 3rd centile weight is inadequate to support normal growth, the patient will become farther and farther behind in both height and weight, possibly resulting in failure to thrive (see Chapter 3, Assessment of Growth). Neither the energy nor protein prescribed above is likely to be adequate for growth of the patient ingesting an elemental medical food (see Chapter 3).

Feeding for Catch-Up Growth

Many children with inherited metabolic disorders have ingested diets inadequate to maintain normal growth in length/height and weight (see Chapter 5, Table 5.7). For catch-up growth to occur, both energy and protein intakes must be increased concomitantly and maintained at the higher intakes until the patient has achieved appropriate height and weight centiles. Catch-up growth in height may lag several months behind that in weight.[70]

Estimation of energy and protein needs for catch-up growth may be achieved as follows:

1. Determine the 50th centile for the child's weight and height for age based on the National Center for Health Statistics (NCHS) growth chart.[71]
2. Determine whether the percent weight and height are greater than the present weight and height of the child. For example, the 1-year-old-male child who weighs 8.4 kg and is 70 cm in length would, at the 50th centile, weigh 10.4 kg and be 124% heavier, and at the 50th centile in length would be 75 cm or 107% taller than at 70 cm.
3. Multiply the midpoint of the energy intake recommended in Chapter 3, Table 3.1 by 1.24 to obtain the energy intake to prescribe. For example, 1350 kcal × 1.24 = 1674 kcal/day.
4. Multiply the protein in grams in Chapter 3, Table 3.1 by 1.07 to obtain the recommended protein to prescribe. For example, 35 g × 1.07 = 37.5 g/day.

Few children can increase intake rapidly to the amount recommended above. Consequently, 5 to 8% increases in energy and protein from the present usual intake every 3 to 4 days as tolerated is recommended until full prescription is achieved. Slow introduction of the recommended intake is important to prevent the refeeding syndrome, which consists of hypokalemia, hypophosphatemia, and hypomagnesemia. The hypokalemia may result from depleted body stores, hyperinsulinemia, or anabolism. Phosphorus utilization by cells is enhanced by glucose and insulin-stimulated glycolysis.[72] Patients undergoing refeeding for catch-up growth should be evaluated early and often for the refeeding syndrome, which can result in death. According to Fomon et al.,[73] daily gains in normal infants and children in height by age should decline from 1.03 mm at 0 to 3 months of age to 0.15 mm at 7 to 10 years, while daily gains in weight should vary from 20–30 g at 0 to 3 months to 5–11 g at 7 to 10 years. However, children with failure to thrive, if fed adequately, should gain greater amounts daily than normal children.

Tube Feeding and Total Parenteral Nutrition

Infants and children who routinely fail to ingest less than 75 to 80% of their prescription should be considered for tube (enteral) or parenteral feeding, particularly if falling below their appropriate length/height and weight centiles for age. Failure to ingest adequate nutrients by patients with inherited metabolic disorders leads to difficulty in controlling the disorder and failure to thrive. Other factors to consider before making a decision about tube feeding or total parenteral nutrition include amount of time required for each feeding, inability to prevent loss of liquids from the mouth, oral aversion to foods, or mechanical problems.[74] In this author's experience, patients with an organic acidemia or urea cycle enzyme defect are often very poor eaters, sometimes requiring several hours per feeding. However, many parents do not understand the need for adequate nutrient intake to control the symptoms of the disorder and may fail to consent to the placement of an enteral feeding tube or a line for venous access. Medical foods available for nutrition management of patients with inherited metabolic disorders may be tube fed when appropriately mixed with water and any other required fluids.

Different routes have been used for tube feeding and commonly include nasogastric, nasoduodenal, nasojejunal, gastrostomy, and jejunostomy and may include continuous or intermittent feeds. If not continuously fed, frequent intermittent feeds should be considered for the patient on an elemental medical food in order for its most efficient use of nutrients (see Chapter 3).

A number of complications may be associated with tube feedings, including gastrointestinal, mechanical, metabolic, and psychologic.[74] Because few of the orphan medical foods are ready to feed when purchased, most require reconstitution, and all require additives—and because patients are managed long term at home—patients or caregivers will need careful education on mixing, storing, and administering. Preparation of the mixture should be done in a container or mixer washed in a dishwasher with very hot water. If the mixture is not used immediately after preparation, it should be refrigerated and warmed to room temperature prior to use. Caregivers' hands should be carefully washed prior to transfer of the mixture from the storage container to the feeding bag, and frequent changing of the feeding bag and tube and limiting the hang time of the mixture should be practiced. Feeding bags should not be reused.[74]

Criteria suggested before home tube feeding are given.[75] Those applicable to the patient with an inherited metabolic disorder include the following:

1. A nutrition management plan is designed that is easily changed based on growth, routine biochemical monitoring of the metabolic disorder, and infectious illness or trauma.
2. The patient is medically stable and demonstrates tolerance to the nutrition management.
3. The parent or caregiver is willing and capable of mixing and administering the feeding.
4. The parent or caregiver has been educated in appropriate care in weighing or measuring the various components of the feeding, how to mix and store in a sanitary fashion as needed to prevent microorganism growth, how to connect the feeding bag and tube, how long to hang the feed, rapidity of feed, record keeping of any problem with the feeding, and has demonstrated the ability to do so.
5. The home has electricity, safe running water, refrigeration, and adequate storage space.
6. Funding for and availability of all of the components of the feeding are accessible.
7. A healthcare team consisting of a metabolic dietitian and nurse is available to provide service to the patient out of the hospital, as needed.
8. A metabolic physician with access to a laboratory that can evaluate required analytes is available to follow the patient.

For the patient who cannot tolerate enteral feeds, total parenteral nutrition is essential. In many patients with inherited metabolic disorders, metabolic decompensation can be triggered by catabolism (accompanied by the accumulation of toxic metabolites) associated with fasting, infection, trauma, immunization, or immobilization. Fasting beyond 4 hours in early infancy, 6 hours in children, and 8 hours in adults with an inherited metabolic disorder may lead to catabolism. Guttler et al.[76] reported a 900 μmol/L average increase of plasma PHE concentration during a 12-hour period overnight without eating by a child with PKU. The suggestion was made that this increase in plasma PHE concentration corresponded to the catabolism of a minimum of 2.0 g of body protein. This author observed that in patients with PKU, the longer the fast was extended, the greater was the plasma PHE concentration, suggesting continuing catabolism of body protein.

The same members of the healthcare team utilized for enteral nutrition care should be available for parenteral nutrition care of the patient with an inherited metabolic disorder. Team members who are knowledgeable in all aspects of parenteral nutrition should be consulted about vascular access, solution concentration, administration, patient monitoring for problems with parenteral nutrition, and problem management. Parenteral amino acid solutions appropriate to the metabolic disorder are available (Coram Health Care Specialty Infusion Services) and should be used. Other criteria and resources required for home parenteral nutrition are described by Cox and Melbardes.[77]

Other Practical Aspects

All measures for medical foods that are dry powders should be in metric weights or U.S. standard, level household measures. Cups and spoons intended for measuring liquids should not be used to measure powders. Many measuring cups and spoons sold in food markets are grossly inaccurate. If scales that read in grams are not available, U.S. standard measuring equipment for dry materials, calibrated by the U.S. Bureau of Standards, should be obtained. Healthcare professionals, parents, and patients should be aware that density of medical foods varies because of settling during shipping and differences in packing. Because of this variability, medical foods should be weighed on a scale that reads in grams. Weighing will take the guesswork out of determining whether the amount of medical food ingested was the same as that prescribed. Weighing of the medical food and its ingredients before mixing also helps the clinician understand why a patient may be having difficulty in tolerating the medical food mixture. To ensure accuracy, measurement of liquids used in the medical food mixture should be in a calibrated syringe or flask.[4]

For infants younger than 4 months of age, restricted amino acids are normally supplied by iron-fortified proprietary infant formulas. Use of iron-fortified products enhances the iron status of infants who may absorb less than normal amounts of iron from elemental medical foods.[78] Most proprietary infant formulas are available in ready-to-feed, concentrated liquid, and powder forms. Directions for carefully measuring the proprietary infant formula should be based on the form prescribed. Parents, caregivers, or whoever mixes the medical food should be very clear as to the form of the proprietary infant formula to be used. Nutrition management problems with excess blood concentration of the poorly metabolized amino acid(s) were observed by this author when parents failed to observe that the form of the proprietary infant formula added to the medical food was not the same as prescribed (concentrated vs ready to feed).

Baby foods (beikost) should be added slowly to the diet as the infant becomes developmentally ready and tongue-thrust disappears, sometime between 3 and 4 months of age for the developmentally normal. Prescribed amounts of selected beikost, and, later, low-protein table foods gradually displace infant formula with iron as the source of restricted amino acid(s).[4]

The Maillard reaction occurs in some foods, resulting in amino acids, peptides, and proteins condensing with sugars, forming bonds for which no digestive enzymes are available and decreasing the nutritional quality of foods.[79] The Maillard reaction is accelerated by heat although it also occurs in the container during storage at room temperature. It is characterized in its initial stage by a light-brown color, followed by buff yellow and then dark brown in the intermediate and final stages. Caramel-like and roasted aromas develop.[4] Dietitians need to be able to recognize the Maillard reaction because it causes loss of some sugars and amino acids (see Chapter 3).[4,80] For this reason, medical food mixtures should not be heated beyond 100°F because Maillard reaction products cause gastrointestinal disturbances, which can be severe. For babies in the newborn nursery and at home, the aseptic technique of mixing medical foods should be used.

Successful management of inherited metabolic disorders requires frequent monitoring of appropriate analytes. Plasma analyte concentrations should be as close to the normal range as possible because patient outcomes are the best. In the past, normal concentrations were difficult to achieve because of inadequate knowledge of requirements and food composition, infrequent monitoring, and failure to recognize the effects of fasting, infection, trauma, and catabolism on plasma amino acid concentrations.[4] Frequent monitoring of plasma amino acid concentrations and other analytes gives the physician and nutritionist data that verify the adequacy of the nutrition management prescription, if it is closely followed. These data are also useful in motivating patient/parent compliance with the prescription.[4]

Some centers may wish to draw blood to monitor plasma amino acid concentrations while the patient is fasting. If blood cannot be drawn 2 to 4 or 5 hours after feeding, local normal standards should be developed for plasma amino acid concentrations. However, prolonged fasting may cause spurious elevations of plasma amino acid concentrations that could lead to unwarranted diet changes, and blood drawn 15 minutes to one hour after a meal may also yield spuriously high concentrations.[81]

Adjusting the Prescription

Beikost should be introduced into the diet when infants are between 3 and 4 months of age or when the patient is developmentally ready. Delay in introduction of beikost or table foods beyond this "critical period" often leads to great difficulty in getting the infant to accept them at a later age.[4] Amino acid intakes recommended in this book are ranges within which requirements for many patients fall; however, the requirement of each patient will differ, with some patients tolerating the lower end of the range and others requiring the upper end.[4] The specific requirement for each patient must be determined by frequent evaluation of plasma amino acid and other biochemical evaluations of nutrition status, growth, and the clinical appearance of skin and hair (see Chapter 3). Patients who are growing well due to adequate protein intake can normally tolerate more of the restricted amino acid(s) than can poorly growing infants and children.[82-84]

When an analyte concentration that is indicative of nutrition management is elevated or below the reference range, careful questioning is required to determine the reason(s) for the abnormality. Some areas that should be explored are given below:[4]

- Whether the patient fails to ingest all of the prescribed medical food, beikost, or table food
- Whether measuring equipment is accurate and foods carefully weighed or measured
- Whether the appropriate form of proprietary infant formula (concentrated liquid, powder, ready to feed) is mixed with the medical food
- Whether siblings, relatives, neighbors, babysitters, or friends feed the patient. If "yes," whether they give foods not prescribed, or prescribed foods in greater or lesser than prescribed amounts
- If the patient is in day care or school, whether peers, teachers, or classmates give the patient food, or whether the patient is "trading" foods
- Whether the patient has eaten any excluded foods
- Whether the patient is stealing or discarding food
- Whether the patient is ill
- Whether the medical food mixture is fed at least three times daily to children after infancy

Appropriate monitoring and disciplining of the child on a special diet from an early age are essential to diet compliance.[85]

Medical foods called exempt infant formulas are designed to supply the nutrient needs of infants when they are supplemented with enough iron-fortified infant formula or low-protein foods to provide the restricted amino acid(s) and other nutrients in amounts necessary for normal growth and development. When an infant's appetite is small, infant medical food should be replaced by child/adult medical food because it usually supplies more protein equivalent than the infant medical food. This change may be immediate only if the medical food is promptly accepted by the child. Many infants and children, however, are slow to accept new flavors.[4] As infants grow into children, they become more sensitive to changes in flavors of foods,[86] a phenomenon that often complicates ingestion of medical foods. Because nutrient requirements change gradually over time, the medical food does not need to be changed abruptly. If acceptance is slow, the amount of new medical food is gradually increased as the infant medical food is gradually decreased. The change from infant to child/adult medical food may require a few days or several months. The older child or adult who has discontinued diet will have great difficulty in returning to nutrition management although it may prevent serious health problems.[87] For the pregnant woman, hyperemesis gravida may make returning to a restricted diet even more difficult than if she were not pregnant.

Foods with free amino acids containing sulfur, such as essential MET and those with acidic or basic groups, have a sulfurous, bitter, unpleasant taste that may make diet compliance difficult. Products containing free amino acids taste best when they are served very cold.[4] Patients will accept these products containing free amino acids more easily if they are served as "slushes"; that is, chilled almost to freezing. Various forms and flavors of medical foods have been developed to help alleviate the taste and odor of amino acids. However, the best approach is for the patient never to discontinue diet.

CONCLUSION

Various approaches to nutrition management of patients are often required to prevent death, mental retardation, metabolic crises, neurologic crises, or growth failure. Some of these approaches may be used singly or simultaneously. Prior to the introduction of nutrition management, special medical foods had to be developed that deleted most or all of the nutrient(s) that were toxic in excess of tolerance and those medical foods for aminoacidopathies required the manufacture of free amino acids. Development of food lists, recipe books, and computer software for calculating nutrient intake made nutrition management easier to achieve than prior to their availability. With the use of medical foods composed of free amino acids, carbohydrate, minerals, and vitamins, care is required to provide adequate fluid to prevent concentrated solutions.

As data became available that more energy and protein equivalent were required by patients ingesting free amino acids than by normal infants and children to prevent poor growth, failure to thrive in the United States became less common than in many other countries. Organic acidemias and urea cycle enzyme disorders often lead to poor appetites, and suggestions were given to prevent poor appetite as well as reasons for enteral or parenteral feeding.

REFERENCES

1. Treacy EP, Valle D, Scriver CR. Treatment of genetic disease. In: Scriver CR, Beaudet AL, Sly WS, Valle D, eds. *The Metabolic and Molecular Bases of Inherited Disease*. New York, NY: McGraw-Hill; 2001:175–191.
2. Acosta PB. Nutrition support for inborn errors. In: Samour PQ, King K, eds. *Handbook of Pediatric Nutrition*. 3rd ed. Sudbury, MA: Jones & Bartlett; 2005:239–286.
3. Elsas LJ, Acosta PB. Inherited metabolic disease: amino acids, organic acids, and galactose. In: Shils ME, Shike M, Olson J, Ross AC, Caballero B, Cousins RJ, eds. *Modern Nutrition in Health and Disease*. 10th ed. Philadelphia, PA: Lippincott Williams & Wilkins; 2005:909–959.
4. Acosta PB, Yannicelli S. *Nutrition Support Protocols*. 4th ed. Columbus, OH: Ross Products Division, Abbott Laboratories; 2001.
5. Matalon R, Michals-Matalon K, Bhatia G, et al. Double blind placebo control trial of large neutral amino acids in treatment of PKU: effect on blood phenylalanine. *J Inherit Metab Dis*. 2007;30:153–158.
6. National Center for Biotechnology Information. OMIM™—Online Mendelian Inheritance in Man™ (database). Available at: http://www.ncbi.nlm.nih.gov/sites/entrez?db=omim. Accessed February 2, 2008.
7. Sarrett H, Knauff K. Development of special formulas for the dietary management of inborn errors of metabolism. In: Wapnir RA, ed. *Congenital Metabolic Diseases*. New York, NY: Marcel Dekker; 1985.
8. Report to the Medical Research Council of a Conference on Phenylketonuria. Treatment of Phenylketonuria. *Br Med J*. 1963;1:1691–1697.
9. Armstrong MD, Tyler FH. Studies on phenylketonuria. I. Restricted phenylalanine intake in phenylketonuria. *J Clin Invest*. 1955;34:565–580.
10. Acosta PB, Centerwall WR. Phenylketonuria dietary management. *J Am Diet Assoc*. 1960;36:206–211.
11. Williamson M, Azen C, Acosta P. A computerized procedure for estimating nutrient intake. *J Toxicol Environ Health*. 1976;2:481–487.
12. Menkes JH, Hurst PL, Craig JM. A new syndrome: progressive familial infantile cerebral dysfunction associated with an unusual urinary substance. *Pediatrics*. 1954;14:462–467.
13. Holt LE Jr, Snyderman SE, Dancis J, Norton P. Treatment of a case of maple syrup urine disease. *Fed Proc*. 1960;19:10.
14. Dent CE, Westall RG. Studies in maple syrup urine disease. *Arch Dis Child*. 1961;36:259–268.
15. Westall RG. Dietary treatment of a child with maple syrup urine disease (branched-chain ketoaciduria). *Arch Dis Child*. 1963;38:485–491.
16. Snyderman SE, Norton PM, Roitman E, Holt LE Jr. Maple syrup urine disease, with particular reference to dietotherapy. *Pediatrics*. 1964;34:454–472.

17. Dickinson JP, Holton JB, Lewis GM, Littlewood JM, Steel AE. Maple syrup urine disease: four years' experience with dietary treatment of a case. *Acta Paediatr Scand*. 1969;58:341–351.
18. Snyderman SE. Medical and nutritional aspects of maple syrup urine disease. No (HSA). 79-5294. In: Koch R, Shaw KNF, Durkin F, eds. *Maple Syrup Urine Disease*. Rockville, MD: U.S. Department of Health, Education, and Welfare; 1979:18–33.
19. Snyderman SE. Diet therapy for MSUD and organic acidurias. American Academy of Pediatrics Nutrition Committee. Amino Acid Sub-Committee. Evanston, IL: American Academy of Pediatrics; 1978:1–7.
20. Smith BA, Waisman HA. Leucine equivalency system in managing branched chain ketoaciduria. *J Am Diet Assoc*. 1971;59:342–346.
21. Bell L, Chao E, Milne J. Dietary management of maple-sirup-urine disease: extension of equivalency systems. *J Am Diet Assoc*. 1979;74:357–361.
22. Acosta PB, Elsas LJ. *Dietary Management of Inherited Metabolic Disease: Phenylketonuria, Galactosemia, Tyrosinemia, Homocystinuria, Maple Syrup Urine Disease*. Atlanta, GA: ACELMU; 1976.
23. Leonard JV, Daish P, Naughten ER, Bartlett K. The management and long-term outcome of organic acidaemias. *J Inherit Metab Dis*. 1984;7(Suppl 1):13–17.
24. Henstenburg JD, Mazur AT, Kaplan PB, Stallings VA. Nutritional assessment and body composition in children with maple syrup urine disease. *J Am Diet Assoc*. 1990;90:32A.
25. Gropper SS, Naglak MC, Nardella M, Plyler A, Rarback S, Yannicelli S. Nutrient intakes of adolescents with phenylketonuria and infants and children with maple syrup urine disease on semisynthetic diets. *J Am Coll Nutr*. 1993;12:108–114.
26. Riazi R, Rafii M, Clarke JT, Wykes LJ, Ball RO, Pencharz PB. Total branched-chain amino acids requirement in patients with maple syrup urine disease by use of indicator amino acid oxidation with L-(1-13C)phenylalanine. *Am J Physiol Endocrinol Metab*. 2004;287:E142–E149.
27. Scriver CR, Larochelle J, Silverberg M. Hereditary tyrosinemia and tyrosyluria in a French Canadian geographic isolate. *Am J Dis Child*. 1967;113:41–46.
28. Carson NA, Neill DW. Metabolic abnormalities detected in a survey of mentally backward individuals in Northern Ireland. *Arch Dis Child*. 1962;37:505–513.
29. Mudd SH, Finkelstein F, Irreverre F, Lester L. Homocystinuria: an enzymatic defect. *Science*. 1964;143:1443–1445.
30. Brenton DP, Cusworth DC, Dent CE, Jones EE. Homocystinuria: clinical and dietary studies. *Q J Med*. 1966;35:325–346.
31. Chase HP, Goodman SI, O'Brien D. Treatment of homocystinuria. *Arch Dis Child*. 1967;42:514–520.
32. Nyhan WL, Fawcett N, Ando T, Rennert OM, Julius RL. Response to dietary therapy in B12 unresponsive methylmalonic acidemia. *Pediatrics*. 1973;51:539–548.
33. Coursin DB. Convulsive seizures in infants with pyridoxine-deficient diet. *J Am Med Assoc*. 1954;154:406–408.
34. Davis RA. Infantile beriberi associated with Wernicke's encephalopathy. *Pediatrics*. 1958;21:409–420.
35. Wolf IJ. Vitamin A deficiency in an infant. *J Am Med Assoc*. 1958;166:1859–1860.
36. Cochrane WA, Collins-Williams C, Donohue WL. Superior hemorrhagic polioencephalitis (Wernicke's disease) occurring in an infant—probably due to thiamine deficiency from use of a soya bean product. *Pediatrics*. 1961;28:771–777.
37. Royston NJW, Parry TE. Megaloblastic anaemia complicating dietary treatment of phenylketonuria in infancy. *Arch Dis Child*. 1962;37:430–435.

38. Mann TP, Wilson KM, Clayton BE. A deficiency state arising in infants on synthetic foods. *Arch Dis Child*. 1965;40:364–375.
39. Dodge PR, Mancall EL, Crawford JD, Knapp J, Paine RS. Hypoglycemia complicating treatment of phenylketonuria with a phenylalanine-deficient diet; report of two cases. *N Engl J Med*. 1959;260:1104–1111.
40. Feinberg SB, Fisch RO. Roentgenologic findings in growing long bones in phenylketonuria. Preliminary study. *Radiology*. 1962;78:394–398.
41. Hanley WB, Linsao L, Davidson W, Moes CA. Malnutrition with early treatment of phenylketonuria. *Pediatr Res*. 1970;4:318–327.
42. American Academy of Pediatrics Committee on Nutrition. Report of the Committee on Nutrition: appraisal of nutritional adequacy of infant formulas used as cow's milk substitutes. *Pediatrics*. 1963;31:329–338.
43. American Academy of Pediatrics Committee on Nutrition. Proposed changes in Food and Drug Administration regulations concerning formula products and vitamin-mineral dietary supplements for infants. *Pediatrics*. 1967;40:916–922.
44. Food and Drug Administration Rules and Regulations: Label statements concerning dietary properties of food purporting to be or represented for special dietary uses. *Fed Regist*. 1971;36:23553(Part 125).
45. Food and Drug Administration. Foods for special dietary uses. *Fed Regist*. 1972;37:18229.
46. Academy signs federal contract to monitor amino acid products and renew nutrition survey data. *AAP Newsletter*. 1972;23:1,4.
47. Food and Drug Administration. Infant formulas; interim guidelines for nutrient composition; notice to manufacturers, packers, and distributors. Notice. *Fed Regist*. 1980;45:17206–17207.
48. Forbes GB, Woodruff CW. *Pediatric Nutrition Handbook*. Elk Grove Village, IL: AAP; 1985.
49. Food and Drug Administration Rules and Regulations. Nutrient requirements for infant formulas (21 CFR Part 107). *Fed Regist*. 1985;50:45106–45108.
50. Food and Drug Administration Proposed Rules. Infant formula recall requirements (21 CFR Part 7). *Fed Regist*. 1987;52:30171–30174.
51. Ohio Administrative Code. Department of Health. Chapter 3701-42 WIC Program. 3701-42-01 Definitions. Available at http://codes.ohio.gov/oac/3701-42-01.gov/3701-42-01. Accessed July 31, 2007.
52. U.S. Food and Drug Administration. Orphan Drugs. Available at: http://www.fda.gov/cder/handbook/orphan.htm. Accessed September 25, 2007.
53. U.S. Food and Drug Administration. The Orphan Drug Act (as amended). Available at: http://www.fda.gov/orphan/oda.htm. Accessed March 27, 2008.
54. Thoene J. *Physicians' Guide to Rare Diseases*. Montvale, NJ: Dowden; 1992.
55. United States Food and Drug Administration Center for Food Safety and Applied Nutrition. Guidance for industry. Frequently asked questions about medical foods. Available at: http://www.cfsan.fda.gov/~dms/medquid.html. Accessed March 24, 2008.
56. Acosta PB. Serving lists for propionic acidemia and methylmalonic acidemia. *Ross Metabolic Formula System Nutrition Support Protocols*. Columbus, OH: Ross Laboratories, Division of Abbott Laboratories; 1989.
57. Acosta PB, Beckner A. *The Phenylalanine Restricted Diet Recipe Book*. Berkeley, CA: California State Department of Public Health; 1966.
58. Read E, Wenz E, Duffy RA, Wellman NS, Acosta A, Acosta PB. *The PKU Cookbook*. Albuquerque, NM: The University of New Mexico Printing Press; 1976.

59. Schuett V. *Low Protein Cookery for Phenylketonuria.* Madison, WI: University of Wisconsin Press; 1977.
60. Block RJ, Bolling D. *The Amino Acid Composition of Proteins and Foods.* 2nd ed. Springfield, IL: Charles C Thomas; 1951.
61. Orr ML, Watt BK. *Amino Acid Content of Foods.* Washington, DC: U.S. Government Printing Office; 1957.
62. Watt BK, Merrill AL. *Composition of Foods.* Washington, DC: U.S. Government Printing Office; 1963.
63. Kennedy B, Anderson K. *Amino Acid Analyzer Software.* Tallahassee, FL: Nutrition Management Systems; 1989.
64. Holt LE Jr, Snyderman SE. Protein and amino acid requirements of infants and children. *Nutr Abstr Rev.* 1965;35:1–13.
65. Rose WC. The amino acid requirements of adult man. *Nutr Abstr Rev Ser Hum Exp.* 1957;27:631–647.
66. MacLean WC Jr, Graham G. Principles of nutrition. *Pediatric Nutrition in Clinical Practice.* Menlo Park, CA: Addison-Wesley; 1982.
67. Smith JL, Heymsfield SB. Enteral nutrition support: formula preparation from modular ingredients. *JPEN J Parenter Enteral Nutr.* 1983;7:280–288.
68. Smith CA, Nelson NM. *The Physiology of the Newborn Infant.* 4th ed. Springfield, IL: Charles C Thomas; 1976.
69. Ziegler EE, Fomon SJ. Potential renal solute load of infant formulas. *J Nutr.* 1989;119(12 Suppl):1785–1788.
70. Frank DA, Zeisel SH. Failure to thrive. *Pediatr Clin North Am.* 1988;35: 1187–1206.
71. National Center for Health Statistics. 2000 CDC Growth Charts: United States. Available at: http://www.cdc.gov/growthcharts/. Accessed January 4, 2008.
72. Udall JN. Malnutrition and refeeding. In: Baker SB, Baker RD Jr, Davis A, eds. *Pediatric Enteral Nutrition.* New York, NY: Chapman & Hall; 1994:205–216.
73. Fomon SJ, Haschke F, Ziegler EE, Nelson SE. Body composition of reference children from birth to age 10 years. *Am J Clin Nutr.* 1982;35:1169–1175.
74. Nevin-Folino N, Miller M. Enteral nutrition. In: Samour PQ, King K, eds. *Handbook of Pediatric Nutrition.* 3rd ed. Sudbury, MA: Jones & Bartlett; 2005:499–524.
75. Vanderhoof JA, Young RJ. Overview of considerations for the pediatric patient receiving home parenteral and enteral nutrition. *Nutr Clin Pract.* 2003;18:221–226.
76. Guttler F, Olesen ES, Wamberg E. Diurnal variations of serum phenylalanine in phenylketonuric children on low phenylalanine diet. *Am J Clin Nutr.* 1969;22: 1568–1570.
77. Cox JH, Melbardis IM. Parenteral nutrition. In: Samour PQ, King K, eds. *Handbook of Pediatric Nutrition.* 3rd ed. Sudbury, MA: Jones & Bartlett; 2005:525–557.
78. Alexander JW, Clayton BE, Delves HT. Mineral and trace-metal balances in children receiving normal and synthetic diets. *Q J Med.* 1974;169:80–111.
79. Erbersdobler HF, Somoza V. Forty years of furosine—forty years of using Maillard reaction products as indicators of the nutritional quality of foods. *Mol Nutr Food Res.* 2007;51:423–430.
80. Rerat A, Calmes R, Vaissade P, Finot PA. Nutritional and metabolic consequences of the early Maillard reaction of heat treated milk in the pig: significance for man. *Eur J Nutr.* 2002;41:1–11.
81. Gropper SS, Acosta PB. Effect of simultaneous ingestion of L-amino acids and whole protein on plasma amino acid and urea nitrogen concentrations in humans. *JPEN J Parenter Enteral Nutr.* 1991;15:48–53.

82. Kindt E, Motzfeldt K, Halvorsen S, Lie SO. Is phenylalanine requirement in infants and children related to protein intake? *Br J Nutr.* 1984;51:435–442.
83. Acosta PB, Yannicelli S. Protein intake affects phenylalanine requirements and growth of infants with phenylketonuria. *Acta Paediatr Suppl.* 1994;407:66–67.
84. MacDonald A, Chakrapani A, Hendriksz C, et al. Protein substitute dosage in PKU: how much do young patients need? *Arch Dis Child.* 2006;91:588–593.
85. Taylor JF, Latta RS. *Why Can't I Eat That?* Saratoga, CA: R&E; 1993.
86. Schiffman SS, Hornack K, Reilly D. Increased taste thresholds of amino acids with age. *Am J Clin Nutr.* 1979;32:1622–1627.
87. Schuett VE, Brown ES, Michals K. Reinstitution of diet therapy in PKU patients from twenty-two U.S. clinics. *Am J Public Health.* 1985;75:39–42.

Chapter 5

Nutrition Management of Patients with Inherited Disorders of Aromatic Amino Acid Metabolism

Phyllis B. Acosta
Kimberlee Michals Matalon

Phenylketonuria

Introduction

Phenylketonuria (PKU), (OMIM 261600)[1] reported in 1933 by Folling[2] and named imbecillitis phenylpyruvica or phenylpyruvica oligophrenia (little brains because of phenylpyruvic acid) due to the mental retardation and excretion of phenylpyruvic acid in the urine, was found to respond to a phenylalanine (PHE)-restricted diet. Horst Bickel et al.,[3] working in the Birmingham Children's Hospital in the United Kingdom, first reported the effects of a casein hydrolysate, treated with activated charcoal to remove the PHE, on a 2-year-old female with PKU. The charcoal also removed tryptophan (TRP) and tyrosine (TYR) that were added back to the hydrolysate. Initially, the musty odor of the patient disappeared and plasma and urine PHE concentrations returned to normal while the urinary excretion of phenylpyruvic acid (PPA) ceased. Shortly thereafter, due to catabolism resulting from inadequate PHE intake, the biochemical abnormalities reappeared and small amounts of whole milk were added to the hydrolysate to provide the essential intake of PHE. While on the PHE-restricted diet with the added milk, the child learned to stand and climb on chairs; her hair grew darker and she stopped banging her head. When L-PHE (4 g) was added back to her diet daily, she regressed to her pre-treatment condition. Woolf et al.,[4] Armstrong and Tyler,[5] and Blainey and Gulliford,[6] among others, demonstrated the beneficial effects of a PHE-restricted diet on the development of children with PKU. Jervis[7] was the first to report a deficiency in the liver of the PHE-oxidizing system.

Biochemistry

The essential amino acid, PHE, with a molecular weight of 165.19, has two main functions in the body. These are tissue protein synthesis and hydroxylation to form TYR.[8] Phenylalanine hydroxylase (PAH; E.C.1.14.16.1), which catalyzes the conversion of PHE to TYR, requires the coenzyme tetrahydrobiopterin (BH_4), dihyropteridine reductase (DHPR; E.C.1.5.1.34), and NADH+H^+ (see Figure 5.1).[9] At physiological concentrations of plasma, free PHE in the person without PAH deficiency, about three-fourths of PHE

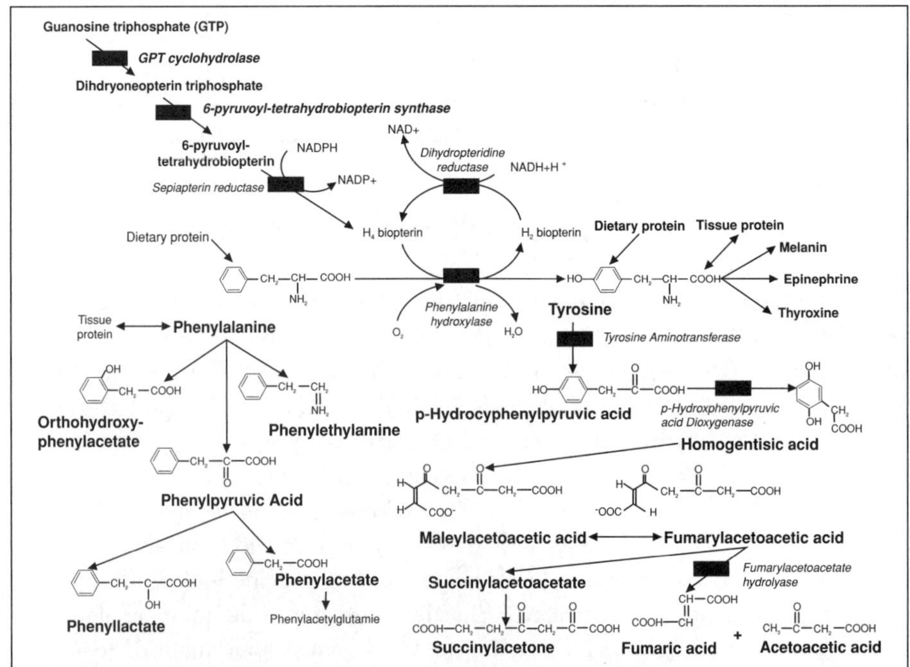

Figure 5.1 *Synthesis of Tetrahydrobiopterin and Metabolism of Aromatic Amino Acids*

Source: Modified by permission of Elsas LJ, Acosta PB. Inherited metabolic disease: amino acids, organic acids, and galactose. In: Shils ME, Shike M, Olson J, Ross AC, Caballero B, Cousins RJ, eds. *Modern Nutrition in Health and Disease*. 10th ed. Philadelphia, PA: Lippincott Williams & Wilkins; 2005:909–959. Courtesy of Wolters Kluwer Health.

Note: Black bars represent impaired enzymes in biopterin biosynthesis, phenylketonuria, and tyrosinemia.

is catalyzed to TYR and about one-fourth is used for protein synthesis.[10] While conversion of PHE to TYR is the major metabolic pathway of PHE, conversion of PHE to orthohydroxyphenylactic acid (OHPAA), PPA, and phenylethylamine occurs when PAH is nonfunctional. Phenylpyruvic acid is further catabolized to phenyllactate, and phenylacetate and phenyllactate are converted to phenylacetylglutamine[11] (see Figure 5.1).

Normal human milk-fed infants at 12 weeks of age had a mean (± SEM) plasma free PHE concentration of 30 ± 3.0 μmol/L, and infants of the same age fed formula with 15 g protein/L had a plasma PHE concentration of 46 ± 4.0 μmol.[12] Plasma TYR concentration of the human milk-fed infants was 58 ± 6.0 μmol and the formula-fed was 87 ± 9 μmol/L at the same age. Normal concentrations of plasma free PHE (mean ± SD) in children, adolescents, and adults are 68 ± 18, 60 ± 13, and 58 ± 15 μmol/L, respectively, with adolescent males having somewhat higher concentrations.[13,14] TYR, derived from either the hydrolysis of food or tissue protein or from dietary or tissue PHE, is used for synthesis of protein, catecholamines, melanin pigment, and thyroid hormones.

Hyperphenylalaninemias

Hyperphenylalaninemias (HPAs), a group of inherited disorders of PHE metabolism, result from a defect in the function of PAH. Patients with < 2% activity, if untreated by 2 weeks of age, may demonstrate PHE, PPA, and other PHE metabolites in the urine, especially if the plasma PHE concentration reaches > 900 μmol/L. By 3 to 6 months of age, developmental delay, microcephaly, and abnormal electroencephalogram often associated with seizures, eczema, musty odor, and hyperactivity occur.[15] Scriver et al.[16] classified patients with HPA at the time of diagnosis as follows:

Classical PKU = blood/plasma PHE concentration > 1200 μmol/L (> 20 mg/dL)
Mild PKU = blood/plasma PHE concentration 600–1200 μmol/L (10–20 mg/dL)
Non-PKU HPA = blood/plasma PHE concentration 120–599 μmol/L (2 <10 mg/dL)

See Appendix A for mathematical formulas for changing micromoles of amino acids to mg/dL and vice versa. Throughout this chapter, patients classified as classic or mild will be referred to as PKU while those with plasma PHE concentrations < 599 μmol/L will be referred to as non-PKU HPA.

Molecular Biology

The PAH gene is expressed primarily in liver, although significant activity is found in human kidney.[17] The human PAH gene is located on chromosome

12, band region q22–q24.1, and has 100 kilobases (kb) with 13 exons and 12 introns. Over 500 mutations[18,19] involving deletions in coding frames, missense mutations, and intron splice site mutations have been identified and cause their pathogenic effect on the PAH enzyme in at least four ways: by producing no activity, reduced activity, altered affinity for substrate or coenzyme, or increased turnover and loss.[9] The various mutations in the PAH gene result in no activity to nearly normal activity of the PAH enzyme. Ethnic variation occurs in the type and frequency of PAH mutations.[9] Defects in the synthesis of coenzyme BH_4 may also cause problems with elevated plasma PHE concentrations.

DHPR, an enzyme normally present in many tissues, reduces the quininoid form of dihydropbiopterin to BH_4 (see Figure 5.1). The gene for DHPR is located on chromosome 4p15.1–p16.1. Several other types of HPA result from defects in the synthesis of BH_4 (see Figure 5.1).[20] In addition to functioning as coenzyme for PAH, BH_4 is also required by TYR hydroxylase and TRP hydroxylase.

Newborn Screening

Because of the observation by Folling[2] that PPA reacts with ferric chloride to produce a green color, Centerwall in 1957 used the chemical principle to develop the "diaper test."[21] This test was the first step toward mass screening for PKU. Subsequently, phenistix test strips[22] were developed based on the same principle. However, PPA fails to appear in the urine until plasma PHE concentration reaches 720 to 900 μmol/L, and this concentration is not usually obtained until the untreated infant is about 6 weeks of age. Further, PPA is unstable and fresh urine is required for best results.[23,24]

Screening for PKU by a bacterial inhibition assay of blood obtained from a newborn infant and placed on a filter paper to dry was developed by Guthrie in 1962.[25] In this assay, when the blood spot from an affected infant is placed on an agar media, the bacteria in the media grow in direct relationship to the amount of PHE in the blood.

In the early 1990s, tandem mass spectrometry (see Chapter 2) was suggested as a method of screening for PKU.[26] Tandem mass spectrometry is now used in most of the United States, as well as in other countries, to screen for PKU and many other inherited metabolic disorders.

Diagnosis

Newborn screening identifies infants with plasma PHE concentrations elevated above the normal range. The cause of the elevated plasma PHE concentration must then be ascertained to determine what treatment is necessary. Diagnosis may be achieved by both biochemical and molecular means. Quantitative analysis of plasma amino acids, in particular PHE and TYR concentrations and their relationship to each other when a patient is ingesting a known quantity of protein, assay of DHPR activity and of urinary biopterin, are required. Mutational analysis of the PAH gene is recommended and may also be helpful in determining if or how the patient should be treated.[27] An estimate of the number of infants in the United States born with PKU yearly is 1 in 13,500 live births, while the estimated number born with non-PKU HPA is 1 in 19,000 live births.[28]

Outcomes if Untreated or Treatment Discontinued

Folling[2] described the two most common features of children with PKU in institutions to be mental retardation and excretion of PPA in the urine, while others[29] reported that of 55 patients identified between 1 and 6 years of age, all but two presented with mental retardation. Other clinical signs in these patients included hyperactive or bizarre behavior, signs of pigment dilution, delayed speech, skin rash, and seizures. Of 46 never-treated patients with classical or mild PKU, ranging in age from 28.8 to 71.8 years, mean plasma PHE concentration was 1180 μmol/L with a range from 784 to 1950 μmol/L. Twenty-one of the patients had an intelligence quotient (IQ) < 35, 22 an IQ of 36 to 67, and 3 with an IQ > 68. Seizures were present in 12 patients, spasticity in 4; eczema and psoriasis were common. Few of the abilities required for self-care or independent living were reported in patients with an IQ < 35.[30] Behavioral aberrations in untreated adults with PKU include hyperactivity, aggressiveness, negative mood swings, motor and attention disturbances, and self-inflicted injury.[31]

Some clinicians suggested in the past that the diet might be discontinued at 4, 6, or 12 years of age with no adverse effects.[32-34] However, studies have shown significant differences in performance and intelligence in children[35,36] and neurologic function in adults who discontinued the PHE-restricted diet compared with those who remained on the diet.[36,37] Vitamin B_{12} deficiency resulting in hematologic changes and neurologic disease occurs in off-diet patients who refuse foods of animal origin and fail to ingest PHE-free medical foods containing added B_{12}.[38,39]

In neurological studies in which the older, treated patient with PKU was his or her own control, elevated plasma PHE concentrations prolonged the performance time on neuropsychological tests of higher integrative function, reduced the mean power frequency of the electroencephalogram (EEG), and decreased urinary dopamine excretion and plasma L-DOPA in older treated patients with PKU.[40] A negative correlation was found between high plasma PHE concentrations, prolonged performance time on neuropsychological tests, and urinary dopamine in 10 patients. In eight additional patients, statistical decreases were found in the mean power frequency of the EEG and in plasma L-DOPA concentrations when plasma PHE concentrations increased.[41] When 25 patients 18 to 35 years of age still on the PHE-restricted diet were compared with 25 off-diet patients of the same age, the groups differed significantly in accuracy and speed of performance of tasks.[42] Similar results were found in 35 German patients 13 to 21 years of age compared with 35 patients with diabetes matched for age, gender, and socioeconomic status.[43] Mean ± SD of plasma PHE concentrations at the time of testing follow up was 822 ± 277 μmol/L. Performance speed of tasks was significantly reduced in patients with PKU.[43] EEG slowing occurred in PKU heterozygotes at concentration changes of plasma PHE that are induced by aspartame ingestion (150 μmol).[44] These effects were reversible and correlated in the reverse direction when plasma PHE concentration was reduced. Severe neurologic deterioration occurred in several off-diet patients with PKU.[36,37] Reversal of most of the symptoms occurred in a patient who returned to a PHE-restricted, medical food-containing diet.[37]

When the PHE-restricted diet was discontinued between 6 and 6.5 years of age in 72 patients with PKU, most of whom had been on diet since early infancy, IQ scores and school performance declined while increases occurred in mood/behavior changes, EEG abnormalities, hyperactivity, and eczema. A few patients had excessive weight gain and developed body odor, tremors, seizures, or hallucinations.[45] Neurological deterioration often occurs in young adults with PKU who have been off the PHE-restricted diet a number of years, and symptoms include ataxia, dystonia, hyperreflexia, paraparesis, seizures, tremor, inability to walk, and agoraphobia.[36,37,46] Among the agoraphobic women, 5 had plasma PHE concentrations on normal diet ranging from 1515 to 2000 μmol/L. The women with PKU appeared to be more prone to social withdrawal and fear of leaving home, while those still on the PHE-restricted diet and those with non-PKU HPA had less avoidant behavior.[46]

Although the precise pathogenesis of mental retardation in PKU is unknown, several hypotheses have been proposed.[27] Among these are accumulation of PHE or its catabolic products, deficiency of TYR or its products, or all four conditions may produce central nervous system damage if PHE in the brain accumulates above normal concentrations during critical periods of brain development. The pathologic consequences vary with the time in brain development at which the chemical insult occurs.[27] Deficient myelination and abnormalities in brain proteolysis and protein occur in the fetus of the untreated woman with HPA during late gestation and during the first 6 to 9 months of life of the child with PKU.[47] During this period, oligodendroglia migrations may also be impaired, resulting in irreversible brain damage later in childhood. The depressed protein synthesis in the brain results from competitive inhibition by high plasma PHE concentrations on blood-brain barrier transport with a resulting imbalance in intraneuronal amino acid concentrations.[48] In the mature brain, neurodegeneration, behavioral difficulties, and prolonged performance times may result from depressed neurotransmitter synthesis. Impairment of these neuropsychological functions in the mature brain may be reversible when plasma PHE returns toward normal concentrations.[44,49] However, the effect of prolonged elevated plasma PHE concentrations on function of the mature brain is unknown.

Opinions differ as to whether patients with non-PKU HPA require treatment with a PHE-restricted diet. Some investigators have failed to find deficits in cognitive (executive) functions, academic skills, behavior, or changes in cerebral white matter in these untreated patients.[50-52] Others suggest that executive function is impaired in untreated patients with non-PKU HPA as compared to the normal population.[53]

Nutrition Management

Management of plasma PHE concentrations of patients with PKU is more effective with an experienced team of healthcare professionals.[54] Differences of opinion exist among researchers in different countries and in the same country as to which patients with HPA should be treated and at what concentration plasma PHE should be maintained.[27] The United Kingdom Medical Research Council Working Party on Phenylketonuria[55] suggested that all infants whose plasma PHE concentration exceeds 400 μmol/L in the presence of normal or low plasma TYR concentration should be placed on a PHE-restricted diet. The Working Party recommended that plasma PHE concentrations remain between 120 and 360 μmol/L until 10 years of age, at which time they might be allowed to increase to 480 μmol/L until age 20, when they could be increased to 700 μmol/L.

A group of German investigators[56] suggested that patients with plasma PHE concentrations > 600 μmol/L should be treated and that plasma PHE concentrations should be maintained between 40 and 240 μmol/L. After 10 years of age, plasma PHE concentrations could be increased to < 600 μmol/L and at 20 years to < 1200 μmol/L.

The National Institutes of Health in the United States published recommendations for whom should be treated and the concentrations at which plasma PHE should be maintained throughout life.[28] The recommendations are that any newborn infant with a plasma PHE concentration > 600 μmol/L should be started on treatment as soon as possible, ideally by 7 to 10 days of age, and that plasma PHE concentrations should be maintained between 120 and 360 μmol/L through 12 years of age, and between 120 and 900 μmol/L after 12 years. However, due to the lack of data concerning brain development during adolescence, even lower plasma PHE concentrations of 120 to 600 μmol/L are recommended. Some investigators in the United States differ in whom they think should be treated and at what plasma PHE concentration they should be maintained.[27] Elsas and Acosta recommend that newborn infants with plasma PHE concentrations > 250 μmol/L or plasma TYR concentrations < 50 μmol/L with normal BH_4 should be treated at no later than 2 weeks of age with a PHE-restricted, TYR-supplemented diet.

The French have proposed that all neonates who have a plasma PHE concentration > 600 μmol/L should be placed on a diet that maintains plasma PHE concentrations between 120 and 360 μmol/L until 10 years of age. During adolescence, the plasma PHE concentration should be < 900 μmol/L and < 1200 to 1500 μmol/L in adulthood.[57] The objective of nutrition management of the patient with PKU is to maintain plasma PHE concentrations that support optimal growth, development, and mental functioning while supplying adequate PHE, TYR, protein, energy, and other nutrients to support normal biochemical indices of nutrition status.

Nutrient Requirements

PHE and TYR

Table 5.1 outlines the PHE and TYR to offer daily to a patient with PKU. A prescription must be written that is specific for age, gender, genotype,[58] growth rate,[59,60] protein intake,[61-64] and health status of each patient. According to a number of reports, protein intake affects the amount of PHE that may be ingested daily by infants, children, and pregnant women with PKU.[61-64] Twice-weekly adjustments in the diet prescription may be necessary during the first 3 to 6 months of life based on growth, hunger, and laboratory analyses of plasma PHE and TYR concentrations. The PHE ingested should maintain the 2- to 4-hour postprandial plasma PHE concentration within treatment range. PHE, an essential amino acid that cannot be synthesized in the body,[65,66] cannot be deleted from the diet without resulting in death, while excess restriction produces growth failure, including weight loss or poor weight gain, skin rashes, aminoaciduria, decreased serum proteins, anemia, bone changes, and mental retardation.[67] The full-term infant with PKU requires 20 to 70 mg PHE per kg of body weight (BW) for growth, with the younger infants and those with mild PKU requiring the larger amount.[59] The PHE requirement on a body weight basis declines rapidly between 3 and 6 months of age as growth rate decelerates, but there is considerable variation in requirement. Because amino acids are required for protein synthesis, fat mass of the patient should not be considered in determining PHE requirement. Thus, PHE prescription for overweight or obese patients should be based on ideal body weight for height for age, if not prescribed as total per day for patients. The premature infant with PKU requires greater PHE, protein, and energy to maintain in utero weight gain than full-term infants with PKU. One premature infant had daily requirements per kg BW of

Table 5.1 ***Ranges of Recommended Daily Phenylalanine and Tyrosine Intakes for Beginning Therapy of Patients With Classic Phenylketonuria or Tyrosinemia***[a]

	Phenylketonuria		***Tyrosinemia***			
			Type I		***Types II, III***	
Age	***PHE***[a] ***(mg)***	***TYR***[b] ***(mg)***	***PHE***[a] ***(mg)***	***TYR***[b] ***(mg)***	***PHE***[a] ***(mg)***	***TYR***[b] ***(mg)***
0 < 3 mos	130–430	1100–1300	185–550	95–275	340–580	170–290
3 < 6 mos	135–400	1400–2100	225–730	115–365	500–860	250–430
6 < 9 mos	145–370	2500–3000	235–775	120–390	670–1030	335–515
9 < 12 mos	135–330	2500–3000	210–825	105–415	700–1180	350–590
1 < 4 yrs	200–320	2800–3500	300–700	150–350	400–500	520–450
4 < 7 yrs	200–400	3200–4000	400–750	200–375	450–550	360–500
7 < 11 yrs	220–500	4000–5000	450–800	225–400	500–800	450–640
11 < 19 yrs	220–1000	5200–6500	500–1050	250–525	550–800	400–640
Adult	220–1100	5600–7000	600–1050	300–525	270–750	260–600
Pregnant						
Trimester 1	265–770[c]	6000–7600	ND	ND	400–700	350–600
Trimester 2	400–1650[c]	6000–7600	ND	ND	500–800	400–640
Trimester 3	700–2275[c]	6000–7600	ND	ND	1200–1500	800–1200

Sources:

Acosta PB, Centerwall WR. Phenylketonuria dietary management. *J Am Diet Assoc*. 1960;36:206–211.

Acosta PB, Matalon K, Castiglioni L, et al. Intake of major nutrients by women in the Maternal Phenylketonuria (MPKU) Study and effects on plasma phenylalanine concentrations. *Am J Clin Nutr*. 2001;73:792–796.

Acosta PB, Michals-Matalon K, Austin V, et al. Nutrition findings and requirements in pregnant women with phenylketonuria. In: Platt LD, Koch R, de la Cruz F, eds. *Genetic Disorders and Pregnancy Outcome*. New York, NY: Parthenon; 1997:21–32.

Acosta PB, Trahms C, Wellman NS, Williamson M. Phenylalanine intakes of 1- to 6-year-old children with phenylketonuria undergoing therapy. *Am J Clin Nutr*. 1983;38:694–700.

Acosta PB, Wenz E, Williamson M. Nutrient intake of treated infants with phenylketonuria. *Am J Clin Nutr*. 1977;30:198–208.

Acosta PB, Yannicelli S. Protein intake affects phenylalanine requirements and growth of infants with phenylketonuria. *Acta Paediatr Suppl*. 1994;407:66–67.

Acosta PB, Yannicelli S, Marriage B, et al. Nutrient intake and growth of infants with phenylketonuria undergoing therapy. *J Pediatr Gastroenterol Nutr*. 1998;27:287–291.

Acosta PB, Yannicelli S, Singh R, et al. Nutrient intakes and physical growth of children with phenylketonuria undergoing nutrition therapy. *J Am Diet Assoc*. 2003;103:1167–1173.

Ellaway CJ, Holme E, Standing S, et al. Outcome of tyrosinaemia type III. *J Inherit Metab Dis*. 2001;24:824–832.

Kindt E, Motzfeldt K, Halvorsen S, Lie SO. Is phenylalanine requirement in infants and children related to protein intake? *Br J Nutr*. 1984;51:435–442.

(continues)

Table 5.1 *Ranges of Recommended Daily Phenylalanine and Tyrosine Intakes for Beginning Therapy of Patients With Classic Phenylketonuria or Tyrosinemia*[a], *Continued*

MacDonald A, Chakrapani A, Hendriksz C, et al. Protein substitute dosage in PKU: how much do young patients need? *Arch Dis Child.* 2006;91:588–593

Matalon K, Acosta PB, Castiglioni L, et al. *Protocol for Nutrition Support of Maternal PKU.* Bethesda, MD: The National Institute of Child Health and Human Development. 1998;1–51.

Note: ND, no data.

[a]The requirements of any one patient usually depend on protein intake, gender, growth rate, and state of health and usually fall between the ranges for age. After 1 to 2 days of deleting PHE and TYR from the diet, introduce those amino acids at the minimum for age. Monitor plasma concentrations of amino acids frequently and modify the diet prescriptions for PHE and TYR as required to maintain their concentrations in the treatment range.

[b]L-TYR is very insoluble in water. Consequently, any supplemental L-TYR should be mixed with fruit purees, mashed potatoes, or soup, or taken as tablets. Medical food mix should be shaken often while feeding to maintain L-TYR in suspension.

[c]Recommended range of PHE intake covered about 80% of MPKUCS women studied. Initiate diet with the lowest amount recommended for trimester and age. Frequent monitoring of plasma PHE is essential to prevent deficiency or excess. Modify prescription based on frequent plasma and TYR concentrations; intakes of PHE, TYR, protein and energy; and maternal weight gain.

about 90 mg PHE, 270 to 290 mg TYR, and 5 g protein to achieve 20 g/kg daily weight gain.[68]

Frequent monitoring of plasma PHE and TYR concentrations and intakes is required to prevent excess intake when growth rate declines and to prevent inadequate intake when growth rate is at its peak, as in early infancy and during the prepubertal and pubertal growth spurts. Without adequate monitoring and adjustment of nutrient intakes, growth rate may be stunted.

TYR is an essential amino acid for the patient with PKU who is unable to normally hydroxylate PHE to TYR. For this reason, plasma TYR concentrations must be monitored, and if they are below reference range, more medical food may need to be prescribed or TYR supplements given. To supply adequate TYR to patients, about 8 to 10% of protein prescribed should be as TYR. L-TYR supplements alone will not prevent mental retardation in patients with PKU.[69] L-TYR is only very slightly soluble in water.[70] Consequently, caregivers and patients with PKU must shake the medical food mixture often during feeding to ensure that the L-TYR is in suspension.

Protein

Amino acids are rapidly oxidized to keto acids when a day's supply is given in one feed and protein synthesis cannot keep pace with its absorption.[71,72] Thus, the older patient should be fed medical food at least three times daily. Also, protein requirements are increased above recommended intakes[73] for age when a free amino acid mix rather than intact protein is the primary protein source (see Chapter 3, Table 3.1). The Medical Research Council Working Party on Phenylketonuria[55] recommend a total amino acid intake of at least 3 g/kg BW/day for children under 2 years of age and 2 g/kg BW/day for children over 2 years of age. Intact protein to supply required PHE adds additional protein to the diet.

Fat and Essential Fatty Acids

Dietary Reference Intakes (DRIs) for fat for infants are given in Chapter 3, Table 3.1, and also include DRIs for essential fatty acids, linoleic, and α-linolenic acids throughout life for normal infants, children, and adults.[73] Whether the essential fatty acids are adequate for patients with PKU to synthesize required docosahexaenoic acid is not known.

Energy and Fluid

Recommendations for energy and fluid intakes (see Chapter 3, Table 3.1) are somewhat greater than those for normal infants due to the use of free amino acids as the primary source of protein equivalent;[66,74] however, the energy should not be prescribed in amounts that could cause overweight or obesity because clinical practice has shown that weight loss elevates plasma PHE concentrations. The resting energy expenditure in children with PKU is reported to not differ from that of normal children.[75] Except when there are large fluid losses from the body, fluid intake should be about 1.5 mL for each kilocalorie ingested during early infancy and about 1.0 mL/kcal ingested by children and adults.[76] For infants, the osmolality of a medical food mixture should be < 450 mOsm/L; for children, < 750 mOsm/L; and for adults, < 1000 mOsm/L to prevent gastrointestinal upset.

Minerals and Vitamins

Mineral and vitamin intakes often must be greater than recommended intakes for age to prevent deficiency in patients on diets that are mostly elemental (see Chapter 3, Table 3.1). Alexander et al.[77] reported that a number of minerals were poorly absorbed by patients ingesting an elemental diet. Lewis et al.[78] found that metabolism of TRP to niacin was depressed in patients with PKU. Table 3.1 in Chapter 3 suggests intakes of minerals and vitamins that should prevent deficiencies if adequate medical food is prescribed and ingested.

Phenylalanine-Free Medical Foods

Intact protein cannot be ingested in adequate amounts to supply protein and amino acid requirements for growth without providing excess PHE. Intact proteins contain some 2 to 9% PHE by weight.[27] Thus, PHE-free special elemental medical foods consisting of free amino acids, carbohydrate, fat, minerals, and vitamins are used to supply a high percentage of the protein prescribed. Names and sources of medical foods that contain minerals and vitamins are given in Table 5.2. Some companies manufacture and market medical foods

Table 5.2 ***Formulation, Selected Nutrient Composition, and Sources of Medical Foods for Patients With Disorders of Aromatic Amino Acids***

Disorder/ medical foods	***Modified nutrient(s)***	***Protein equiv***[a]	***Fat***	***Carbohydrate***	***Energy***	***Linoleic acid/ α-linolenic acid***
	(mg/100 g)	(g/100 g, source)	(g/100 g, source)	(g/100 g, source)	(kcal/ 100 g/ kj/100 g)	(mg/100 g)
Phenylketonuria						
			Abbott Nutrition[b]			
Phenex-1	PHE 0 TYR 1500, L-carnitine 20 Taurine 40	15.0 Amino acids[c]	21.7 High oleic safflower, coconut, soy oils	53 Corn syrup solids	480 / 2006	3500 / 350
Phenex-2 unflavored	PHE 0 TYR 3000, L-carnitine 40 Taurine 50	30.0 Amino acids[c]	14.0 High oleic safflower, coconut, soy oils	35 Corn syrup solids	410 / 1714	2200 / 225
Phenex-2 vanilla	PHE 0 TYR 3000, L-carnitine 40 Taurine 50	30.0 Amino acids[c]	13.5 High oleic safflower, coconut, soy oils	36 Corn syrup solids	410 / 1714	2200 / 225
			Applied Nutrition Corp[d]			
PhenylAde amino acid bars	PHE 20 TYR1960, L-carnitine 20 Taurine 60	20.0 Amino acids[c]	34	38	540 / 2257	0 / 0
PhenylAde amino acid blend	PHE 0, TYR 7500, L-carnitine 100, Taurine 120	80.0 Amino acids[c]	0	0	323 / 1350	0 / 0
PhenylAde drink mix	PHE 0 TYR 2400, L-carnitine 30 Taurine 100	25.0 Amino acids[c]	13 Partially hydrogenated coconut oil	47 Sucrose, corn syrup solids, modified food starch	400 / 1672	ND / ND

(continues)

Table 5.2 ***Formulation, Selected Nutrient Composition, and Sources of Medical Foods for Patients With Disorders of Aromatic Amino Acids**, Continued*

Disorder/ medical foods	***Modified nutrient(s)***	***Protein equiv***[a]	***Fat***	***Carbohydrate***	***Energy***	***Linoleic acid/ α-linolenic acid***
PhenylAde drink mix essential	PHE 0 TYR 3000, L-carnitine 20 Taurine 80	25.0 Amino acids[c]	13 Safflower, canola, soybean, coconut, flaxseed oils	45 Modified food starch, dextrin, corn syrup solids	390 / 1630	2025 / 525
PhenylAde 40 drink mix	PHE 0 TYR 3744, L-carnitine 30 Taurine 120	40.0 Amino acids[c]	2 Partially hydrogenated coconut oil	40 Sucrose, corn syrup solids, modified food starch	336 / 1404	ND / ND
			Cambrooke Foods[e]			
PKU Drink (per 100 mL)	PHE 0 TYR 1190, L-carnitine 10 Taurine 45	10.7 Amino acids[c]	0	18.6 Sugar	106 / 443	0 / 0
			Mead Johnson Nutritionals[f]			
Phenyl-Free-1	PHE 0 TYR 1600, L-carnitine 51 Taurine 30	16.2 Amino acids[c]	26 Palm olein, soy, coconut, high oleic sunflower oils	51 Corn syrup solids, sugar, modified corn starch, maltodextrin	500 / 2090	4500 / 380
Phenyl-Free-2	PHE 0 TYR 2200, L-carnitine 49 Taurine 49	22.0 Amino acids[c]	8.6 Soy oil	60 Sugar, corn syrup solids, modified corn starch	410 / 1714	4600 / 651
Phenyl-Free-2HP	PHE 0 TYR 4000, L-carnitine 36 Taurine 63	40.0 Amino acids[c]	6.3 Soy oil	44 Sugar, corn syrup solids, modified corn starch	390 / 1630	3200 / 453
			Nutricia[g]			
LoPhlex	PHE 0 TYR 1120, L-carnitine 70 Taurine 140	69.9 Amino acids[c]	< 0.21	<0.98	287 / 1200	0 / 0

(continues)

Table 5.2 *Formulation, Selected Nutrient Composition, and Sources of Medical Foods for Patients With Disorders of Aromatic Amino Acids, Continued*

Disorder/ medical foods	*Modified nutrient(s)*	*Protein equiv*[a]	*Fat*	*Carbohydrate*	*Energy*	*Linoleic acid/ α-linolenic acid*
Periflex infant	PHE 0 TYR 1440, L-carnitine 10 Taurine 20	13.0 Amino acids[c]	19.1 Soy, coconut, high oleic safflower, M. alpine, C. cohena (Cohnii) oils	49.3 Corn syrup solids	421 / 1760	3368 / 2850
XPHE maxamaid	PHE 0 TYR 2650, L-carnitine 20 Taurine 140	25.0 Amino acids[c]	<1.0 None added	56 Corn syrup solids, sugar	324 / 1354	None / None
XPHE maxamum	PHE 0, TYR 4000, L-carnitine 39 Taurine 140	40.0 Amino acids[c]	<1.0 None added	34 Sugar	305 / 1275	None / None
PKU 3	PHE 0 TYR 6000, L-carnitine 0 Taurine 0	68.0 Amino acids[c]	0 None added	1.7 Sugar	280 / 1170	None / None
			Vitaflo US LLC[h]			
PKU cooler (per 100 mL)	PHE 0 TYR 1370, L-carnitine 12.5 Taurine 25.7	11.5 Amino acids[c]	Trace	5.9 Sugar, maltodextrin	71 / 297	0 / 0
PKU express	PHE 0 TYR 6590, L-carnitine 65.1 Taurine 129.6	60.0 Amino acids[c]	<0.5	15 Sugar, dried glucose syrup	302 / 1260	0 / 0
PKU gel	PHE 0 TYR 4630, L-carnitine 45.8 Taurine 91.1	42.0 Amino acids[c]	<0.5	43 Sugar, dried glucose syrup	342 / 1428	0 / 0

(continues)

Table 5.2 ***Formulation, Selected Nutrient Composition, and Sources of Medical Foods for Patients With Disorders of Aromatic Amino Acids***, *Continued*

Disorder/ medical foods	***Modified nutrient(s)***	***Protein equiv***[a]	***Fat***	***Carbohydrate***	***Energy***	***Linoleic acid/ α-linolenic acid***
Tyrosinemia Types I, II, III						
			Abbott Nutrition[b]			
Tyrex-1	PHE 0 TYR 0, L-carnitine 20 Taurine 40	15.0 Amino acids[c]	21.7 High oleic safflower, coconut, soy oils	53 Corn syrup solids	480 / 2006	3500 / 350
Tyrex-2	PHE 0 TYR 0, L-carnitine 40 Taurine 50	30.0 Amino acids[c]	14.0 High oleic safflower, coconut, soy oils	35 Corn syrup solids	410 / 1714	2200 / 225
			Mead Johnson Nutritionals[f]			
Tyros 1	PHE 0 TYR 0, L-carnitine 50 Taurine 30	16.7 Amino acids[c]	26 Palm olein, soy, coconut, high oleic safflower oils	51 Corn syrup solids, modified corn starch, sugar, maltodextrin	500 / 2090	4500 / 380
Tyros 2	PHE 0 TYR 0, L-carnitine 49 Taurine 49	22.0 Amino acids[c]	8.5 Soy oil	60 Corn syrup solids, sugar, modified corn starch	410 / 1714	4600 / 651
			Nutricia[g]			
XPHE, TYR analog	PHE 0 TYR 0, L-carnitine 10 Taurine 20	13.0 Amino acids[c]	20.9 High oleic safflower, soy, coconut oils	59 Corn syrup solids	475 / 1985	3025 / 428
XPHE, TYR maxamaid	PHE 0 TYR 0, L-carnitine 20 Taurine 140	25.0 Amino acids[c]	<1.0 None added	56 Sugar, corn syrup solids	324 / 1754	None / None

(continues)

Table 5.2 ***Formulation, Selected Nutrient Composition, and Sources of Medical Foods for Patients With Disorders of Aromatic Amino Acids,*** *Continued*

Disorder/ medical foods	***Modified nutrient(s)***	***Protein equiv***[a]	***Fat***	***Carbohydrate***	***Energy***	***Linoleic acid/ α-linolenic acid***
			VitaFlo USA LLC[h]			
TYR cooler	PHE 0 TYR 0 L-carnitine 13 Taurine 25	11.5 Amino acids[c]	Trace	5.9 Sugar, maltodextrin	71 / 297	ND / ND
TYR express	PHE 0 TYR 0 L-carnitine 143, Taurine 256	60.0 Amino acids[c]	<0.5	15 Sugar, modified corn starch, dried glucose syrup	302 / 1260	0 / 0
TYR gel	PHE 0 TYR 0 L-carnitine 46 Taurine 90	42.0 Amino acids[c]	<0.5	43 Sugar, modified corn starch, dried glucose syrup	342 / 1428	ND / ND

Source: Data supplied by each company.

Notes: Values listed, although accurate at time of publication, are subject to change. The most current information may be obtained by referring to product labels.

ND, no data.

[a]g protein equivalent = g nitrogen × 6.25.

[b]Abbott Nutrition, 625 Cleveland Avenue, Columbus, OH 43215; 800-551-5838.

[c]All except glycine are in the L- form.

[d]Applied Nutrition Corp., 10 Saddle Road, Cedar Knolls, NJ 07927; 800-605-0410.

[e]Cambrooke Foods, 2 Central St, Framingham, MA 01701; 866-456-9776.

[f]Mead Johnson Nutritionals, 2400 West Lloyd Expressway, Evansville, IN 47721; 800-457-3550.

[g]Nutricia North America, PO Box 117, Gaithersburg, MD 20884; 800-365-7354.

[h]Vitaflo US LLC, 123 East Neck Road, Huntington, NY 11743; 888-848-2356.

free of minerals and vitamins that could cause serious nutrient deficiencies if ingested for prolonged periods of time (see Chapter 3, Biochemical Assessment: Minerals, and Vitamins). These medical foods are not recommended, especially for infants, children, adolescents, and pregnant women.

Intact Proteins

Human milk or proprietary infant formula containing iron should be used to supply required PHE to the young infant (see Appendix B). For the infant who does not tolerate infant formulas with casein or whey, soya protein isolate formulas may be used. When the infant reaches 3 to 4 months of age and tongue thrust disappears, low-protein baby foods (beikost) gradually displace the human milk or proprietary infant formula with iron as a source of PHE. Various lists of foods have been provided to parents and patients to help simplify the PHE-restricted diet for families. One of the first, called a serving list, was based on the Diabetic Exchange List, in that foods of similar PHE content were grouped together and could be exchanged for one another within a list to vary the diet (see Table 5.3).[79] Portion sizes of foods in each

Table 5.3 ***Average Nutrient Content of Serving Lists for PHE- and/or TYR-Restricted Diets, Per Serving***

Food List	***PHE (mg)***	***TYR (mg)***	***Protein (g)***	***Fat (g)***	***Energy (kcal/ kj)***	***Linoleic acid (mg)***
Breads/cereals	30	20	0.6	0.0	30 / 125	—
Fats	5	4	0.1	5.0	60 / 250	?
Fruits	15	10	0.5	0.0	60 / 250	—
Vegetables	15	10	0.5	0.0	10 / 42	—
Free foods A[a]	5	4	0.1	0.0	65 / 272	—
Free foods B[a]	0	0	0.0	Varies	55 / 230	—
Infant formula powders, 100 g						
Enfamil® Lipil®[b]	420	490	10.9	27.1	513 / 2144	4047
Enfamil ProSobee® Lipil[b]	660	490	12.3	26.2	495 / 2069	5250
Similac® Advance®[c]	465	450	10.8	28.2	526 / 2199	5260
Similac Isomil® Advance[c]	675	465	12.6	28.0	516 / 2157	4438

Sources:

Acosta PB, Centerwall WR. Phenylketonuria dietary management. *J Am Diet Assoc.* 1960;36:206–211.

Acosta PB, Yannicelli S. Phenylketonuria (PKU). *Nutrition Support Protocols.* 4th ed. Columbus, OH: Ross Products Division, Abbott Laboratories; 2001:1–32.

Elsas LJ, Acosta PB. Inherited metabolic disease: amino acids, organic acids, and galactose. In: Shils ME, Shike M, Olson J, Ross AC, Caballero B, Cousins RJ, eds. *Modern Nutrition in Health and Disease.* 10th ed. Philadelphia, PA: Lippincott Williams and Wilkins; 2005:909–959.

Matalon K, Acosta PB, Castiglioni L, et al. *Protocol for Nutrition Support of Maternal PKU.* Bethesda, MD: The National Institute of Child Health and Human Development. 1998;1–51.

[a]Modified very-low protein cookies, pastas, and breads not included.

[b]Mead Johnson Nutritionals, 2400 West Lloyd Expressway, Evansville, IN 47721; 800-457-3550.

[c]Abbott Nutrition, 625 Cleveland Avenue, Columbus, OH 43215; 800-551-5838.

list may be found in reference 80. Many dietitians working with patients with PKU have their own special list of foods with PHE content given while others refer caregivers and patients to the U.S. Department of Agriculture website[81] for information on PHE, TYR, protein, energy, and other nutrients in food. A PKU "exchange" list, based on 15 mg PHE per "exchange," is also available.[82] Parents who are unable to read in any language will require diet instructions in pictograms.

Initiation of Nutrition Management and During Illness or Following Trauma

Plasma PHE concentration at the time of diagnosis may be rapidly lowered to treatment range by feeding the infant a 20 kcal/fl oz (67 kcal/100 mL) PHE-free formula.[83] A minimum of 120 kcal/kg BW and 3.50 g protein/kg is used to enhance a rapid decline in plasma PHE concentration. Within a mean of 4 ± 3 days (mean ± SD), plasma PHE concentration should drop to treatment range on a PHE-free formula. Treatment should be initiated in hospitalized infants, if at all possible, to enable education of parents or caregivers and to monitor plasma amino acid concentrations daily. In order to prevent PHE deficiency when using a PHE-free formula, and to enable rapid changes in diet prescription, laboratory results must be available daily. A hospitalized 3.5 kg full-term infant with a diagnostic plasma PHE concentration of 1500 μmol/L, low plasma TYR concentration, and normal tetrahydrobiopterin (BH_4) might be fed a PHE-free medical food mixture daily for 48 hours (see Table 5.4), after which a maintenance medical food mixture containing PHE should be prescribed.

Table 5.4 ***Diet Plan for a 3.5-kg Hospitalized Neonate With PKU During the First 24 to 48 Hours***

Food	***Amount***	***PHE (mg)***	***TYR (mg)***	***Protein (g)***	***Energy (kcal)***
Phenex™-1 powder	82 g	0	1230	12.3	394
Polycose® powder	7 g	0	0	0	27
Total		0	1230	12.3	421
Per kg body weight		0	351	3.5	120

- Add water to yield 620 mL (21 fl oz)
- Feed every 2.5 to 3 hours

If the patient cannot be hospitalized for initial control of plasma PHE concentration and education of parents, the diet plan in Table 5.5 may be administered. Plasma PHE concentrations should be evaluated twice weekly while feeding the PHE-containing medical food mixture to determine adequacy or excess. With this diet, plasma PHE concentrations usually decrease to treatment range within a mean (± SD) of 10 ± 5 days.[83]

Hypercatabolism is induced in patients during infectious disease or following trauma that results in protein catabolism and negative nitrogen balance, paralleling the extent of infection or injury,[84] resulting in elevated plasma PHE concentrations in patients with PKU or non-PKU HPA. Infection requires immediate diagnosis and treatment to prevent prolonged, elevated plasma PHE concentrations. Therapies to depress catabolism, maintain treatment plasma PHE concentrations, and support hydration and electrolyte balance are essential. Catabolism may be lessened and electrolyte balance maintained in the presence of vomiting or diarrhea in the infant or young child by adding Polycose® powder to Pedialyte® (Abbott Nutrition, Columbus, Ohio) (see Appendix C) and feeding often as ice chips in small amounts. One-third cup of Polycose® powder added to Pedialyte® to make 240 mL (~8 fl oz) provides energy and electrolytes when fed as tolerated. For the patient who cannot tolerate oral feeds and a rapid return to the usual prescribed PHE-restricted, TYR-supplemented diet, parenteral nutrition to supply adequate amino acids, energy, and other nutrients may be required. The pharmacy manager at a regional Coram Health Care (see Appendix D) facility should be able to provide a PHE-free parenteral amino acid solution.

Table 5.5 *Diet Plan for a Non-Hospitalized 3.5 kg Infant With PKU*

Food	*Amount*	*PHE (mg)*	*TYR (mg)*	*Protein (g)*	*Energy (kcal)*
Phenex™-1 powder	65 g	0	975	9.8	312
Similac® Advance® Infant Formula with iron powder	23 g	107	104	2.5	121
Total		107	1079	12.3	433
Per kg body weight		31	308	3.5	124

- Add water to yield 620 mL (21 fl oz)
- Feed every 2.5 to 3 hours

Long-Term Nutrition Management

Diet for life for the patient with PKU has been proposed due to the problems encountered by off-diet patients.[85] The previously described infant, now 5 months of age and weighing 5.5 kg, might receive the diet given in Table 5.6 in which the PHE is supplied by Similac® Advance® Infant Formula with Iron powder (see Appendix B) and a vegetable (see Table 5.3). The infant should be fed often to achieve the best growth and plasma PHE concentrations.[62,64]

As the infant develops hand-to-mouth movements, finger foods that will not cause choking should be added to the diet and their PHE, TYR, protein, and energy content included in the daily prescription. This is an age when a cup should be introduced to begin weaning the infant from a bottle to a cup. Because of the odor of most medical foods, a covered cup may be continued longer than it is by children without PKU. However, the introduction of a child-size cup or glass by 8 months of age should aid in discontinuing the bottle. Low-protein table foods (see Table 5.3) or cow's milk (if tolerated) should be used to displace all proprietary infant formula by about 18 months of age. However, some children have small appetites and whole, 2%, or skim cow's milk may be prescribed, as needed, to supply PHE requirements (see Appendix B).

New Approaches to Therapy

New approaches to therapy have recently been introduced and include administration of large neutral amino acids (LNAAs) and BH_4. LNAAs that share common transporters across the intestinal cell membrane and blood-brain

Table 5.6 *Diet for a 5.5 kg Infant With PKU*

Food	*Amount*	*PHE (mg)*	*TYR (mg)*	*Protein (g)*	*Energy (kcal)*
Similac Advance Infant Formula with iron powder	50 g	233	225	5.4	263
Carrots, pureed	75 g	15	10	0.7	26
Phenex-1 powder	71 g	0	1065	10.6	341
Total		248	1300	16.7	630
Per kg body weight		45	236	3.0	115

- Add water to Similac Advance and Phenex-1 powder to yield 828 mL (28 fl oz)
- Feed 4 to 6 times daily

barrier include arginine, histidine, isoleucine, leucine, lysine, methionine, phenylalanine, threonine, tryptophan, tyrosine, and valine and depend on the affinity of each amino acid for the carrier protein.[86-88] In patients with PKU, plasma PHE concentrations are much higher than that of other LNAAs; thus, PHE readily crosses the intestinal cell membrane and blood-brain barrier. Administration of LNAAs free of PHE to 8 untreated patients with PKU at 0.5 g/kg BW per day in 3 divided doses for 3 weeks and to 3 patients for 1 week at 1.0 g/kg BW daily in adults were shown to decrease elevated plasma PHE concentrations by 52 and 55%, respectively.[89] In a double-blind, placebo control trial in 20 untreated patients administered 0.5 g/kg BW per day of LNAAs for 1 week, mean plasma PHE concentration declined from 933 μmol/L to 568 μmol/L.[90] In neither of these trials was actual nutrient intake reported; thus, the change in intake of PHE or protein, if any, was considered unlikely.

Measurement of brain PHE concentration has been suggested as useful in the management of patients with PKU[91] by investigators who found a positive correlation between plasma and brain PHE concentrations when the plasma PHE concentration was < 1200 μmol/L. However, other investigators were unable to demonstrate a positive correlation between plasma and brain PHE concentrations. One report indicated anxiety levels were higher when patients were ingesting the LNAAs than when not ingesting them.[92] Long-term studies of the use of LNAAs on growth and nutrition status in patients with PKU is needed.

Tetrahydrobiopterin has been used in therapy of BH_4 deficiencies for many years. Several investigators have recently reported a decline in plasma PHE concentrations when 5 to 10 mg/kg BW/day of BH_4 was administered to patients with mutations in the PAH gene that resulted in non-PKU HPA.[93-97] In 1999, BH_4 was used for the first time in therapy of one patient with non-PKU HPA and four with mild PKU. At 24 hours after initiation of PHE intake at 80 to 90 mg/kg BW/day and BH_4 at 5 to 10 mg/kg BW/day, all except one patient had a significant decline in plasma PHE concentration. The patient who failed to respond to BH_4 administration with a decline in plasma PHE concentration had two mutant alleles for PAH: P407S and RIIIX.[93] Subsequently, investigators in Germany, The Netherlands, Spain, and the United States, among other countries, tried BH_4 for all forms of HPA while other researchers evaluated mechanisms of its actions.[94-96] Four mechanisms have been proposed for the effects of BH_4 on PAH activity. These include (1) improved binding of the mutant PAH, (2) stabilization of the active tetramer/dimer forms of the mutant PAH and protection from proteolytic cleavage, (3) BH_4-induced change in BH_4 biosynthesis, and (4) PAH messenger ribonucleic acid (mRNA) stabilization.

In a recent study, 33 children 4 to 12 years of age with non-PKU HPA or mild PKU were treated for 10 weeks with BH_4 as PHE intake was increased with non-fat dry milk or egg-white powder added to their usual PHE-restricted diet. At baseline, PHE tolerance was 17 ± 7 mg/kg BW/day, while at study end, PHE tolerance was 44 ± 25 mg/kg BW/day and plasma PHE concentration was < 360 μmol/L.[97] Unfortunately, the significant increase in intakes of protein and energy was not reported. Consequently, it is not possible to determine whether some of these 33 patients might have responded to the increase in intakes of PHE and protein alone with a decline to normal plasma PHE concentration as reported by Blaskovics[98] without the administration of BH_4. Some few patients classified with classic PKU have responded to 20 mg/kg BW/day of BH_4 with a substantial increase in PHE tolerance.[99]

For those patients who fail to have a substantial increase in PHE tolerance on administration of BH_4, there are differences of opinion as to whether they should be given a PHE-restricted diet containing medical food, as well as BH_4. One group of investigators suggested that the combination of BH_4 and the PHE-restricted diet with medical food would worsen the quality of life, increase the cost of therapy, and decrease nutrition status.[100] A group of U.S. dietitians recently suggested a protocol for nutrition management of patients who failed to respond to BH_4, with a decline in plasma PHE concentrations to < 360 μmol/L that included both BH_4 and a PHE-restricted diet containing medical food.[101] Many of the patients reported to be BH_4 responsive have mild PKU or non-PKU HPA with residual PAH activity, and in many countries would not be treated at all.[102]

Patients with biopterin-deficient forms of HPA require therapy with BH_4 and products manufactured by enzymes that require BH_4 as a coenzyme. Tyrosine hydroxylase, which is involved in synthesis of L-DOPA, and TRP hydroxylase, necessary for synthesis of serotonin, require BH_4 to function.[103] A PHE-restricted, TYR-supplemented diet used in combination with L-DOPA, carbidopa, and serotonin may improve outcome in these patients.[103-105] Age of onset of treatment appears to be a major factor in determining outcome.[106,107]

Assessment of Nutrition Management

Plasma PHE concentrations both above and below treatment range should be dealt with promptly. Excess PHE intake is the most common cause of elevated plasma PHE concentration, but it may also result from overprescription; misunderstanding of the diet; dietary noncompliance and deficient intakes of PHE, protein, and/or energy; and illness or trauma. Frequent analysis of plasma PHE and TYR concentrations with accompanying prior 3-day diet diary for calculation of intake that indicates health status is essential for determining management of the patient. Excess PHE intake, above that prescribed, requires additional education of parents, grandparents, siblings, any caregivers, school personnel, and the patient who is old enough to understand. If the PHE prescription is in excess, it should be gradually decreased with frequent analysis of plasma PHE concentration until concentration is in the treatment range.

Plasma PHE concentrations <25 μmol/L may lead to depressed appetite,[27] decreased growth, and, if prolonged, mental retardation.[67] Below treatment range plasma PHE concentrations may result from inadequate prescription of PHE, poor appetite, or misunderstanding of the diet. An inadequate prescription or poor appetite can be rectified by gradually increasing the amount of PHE prescribed and frequently evaluating plasma PHE and TYR concentrations. Analytes other than low concentrations of plasma PHE may also aid in determining whether PHE intake is inadequate. Decreased urine PHE accompanied by increased plasma alanine, β-hydroxybutyric acid, and acetoacetic acid concentrations result from muscle alanine production and β-lipolysis. The first stage of PHE deficiency, if untreated, may progress and result in an elevated plasma PHE concentration as a result of muscle protein degradation. Plasma TYR and other amino acids may be depressed. Aminoaciduria may appear because of renal tubular malabsorption. Body protein stores are catabolized, energy sources are depleted, and active membrane transport functions are impaired.[27] In the last stage of PHE deficiency before death occurs, if the deficiency is not treated immediately with PHE in the form of good quality intact protein such milk or eggs, plasma PHE concentration is significantly below normal as are the other amino acids. Clinical manifestations at this stage include growth failure, osteopenia, anemia, and loss of hair.[27] Unless the plasma PHE concentration is very low or zero, or much above treatment range, small changes in prescribed PHE intake are recommended to prevent wide swings in its concentration.

Insufficient protein intake results in an inadequate supply of essential amino acids and nitrogen for growth. When protein synthesis is decreased, PHE is no longer used for growth and accumulates in the blood. If catabolism occurs because of prolonged lack of nitrogen or amino acid intake, plasma PHE concentration increases because tissue protein contains about 5.5% PHE. In instances of protein insufficiency with adequate PHE intake, medical food intake should be increased to supply the required nitrogen or essential amino acids.[27]

Energy, the first requirement of the body, is necessary for growth. When energy is provided as carbohydrate and fat and if adequate nitrogen is available, nonessential amino acids are synthesized from their ketoacid precursors. Carbohydrate ingestion leads to insulin secretion, and insulin promotes amino acid transport into the cell and subsequent protein synthesis.[27] When energy intake is inadequate and liver glycogen stores are depleted, catabolism of muscle and fat occurs to meet energy needs. Catabolism releases PHE, leading to elevated plasma PHE concentration. Sufficient energy must be provided through the use of very-low-protein foods (see Appendix E) and adequate PHE-free medical foods to ensure normal growth rate, but very-low-protein foods and protein-free beverages should be avoided if overweight or obesity occurs. Loss of weight in the patient with PKU results in elevated plasma PHE concentration.

The first year of life is the period of most rapid growth followed by the prepubertal and pubertal growth spurt. During the first 6 months to 1 year of life, twice-weekly tests for monitoring plasma PHE and TYR concentrations and weekly measurements of length, head circumference, and weight are obtained. After 1 year of age, every-other-week blood tests may be adequate until the child reaches the prepubertal growth spurt when at least weekly tests are required. The growth of the prepubertal and pubertal child with PKU may be stunted unless very frequent plasma PHE and TYR concentrations are analyzed and diet adjusted as required. If plasma PHE concentrations are below or above treatment range, the diet prescription for PHE is modified and frequent blood tests are obtained until plasma PHE concentration is acceptable.

For blood tests to be of use in adjusting the prescription, laboratory analyses must be both accurate and prompt. Quantitative methods are preferred for monitoring PHE and TYR concentrations. If properly instructed, parents may be given responsibility for obtaining the specimens on filter paper or in microcapillary tubes and mailing them to a central laboratory.[27] A 3-day diet diary of food ingested immediately before obtaining blood for PHE and TYR analysis is essential. The correlation between the patient's intake of PHE, TYR, protein, and energy, growth, health status, and the plasma PHE and TYR concentrations must be considered before changing the diet prescription.

Results of Nutrition Management

Neurologic Outcome

Early diagnosis and treatment of infants with PKU before 2 weeks of age with a nutritionally adequate, PHE-restricted, TYR-supplemented diet promote normal growth and development. Ninety-five patients with PKU in the Phenylketonuria Collaborative Study (PKUCS) in whom the PHE-restricted diet was initiated in infancy had IQ scores evaluated at 12 years of age. The group whose mean ± SD plasma PHE concentration increased to 576 ± 150 μmol/L before 6 years of age had a full-scale IQ score of 87 ± 14, the patients who maintained plasma PHE concentration in treatment range until 10 years of age had a mean score of 96 ± 14, while those whose plasma PHE concentration remained within treatment range until 12 years of age had a mean IQ of 101 ± 11.[108]

Twenty-four adults who had participated in the PKUCS but discontinued diet at 6 years of age had a mean ± SD IQ score of 105 ± 3 with a range from 75 to 126.[109] Trefz et al.[110] reported that when plasma PHE concentration was maintained below 360 μmol/L, there was a difference in IQ by genotype in 9-year-old children. Early treated adolescent and adult patients with PKU in Germany had poorer scores on IQ, information processing, and selective and sustained attention than patients with diabetes matched for gender, age, and socioeconomic status.[43] Waisbren et al.[111] reported that for each 100 μmol increase in plasma PHE concentration between 394 and 750 μmol/L from diagnosis in the neonatal period to 18 years of age, there was a 1.3 to 3.9 point decline in IQ score.

Clinical and Biochemical Status

The semi-synthetic nature of the diet for patients with PKU, as well as the reports of nutrition problems during the first 10 to 15 years of treatment, led to questions concerning diet adequacy. Some of the early problems included hypoglycemia,[112] peculiar bone changes in a number of patients,[113] skin rash in the perineum,[114] megaloblastic anemia,[115] bone marrow vacuolizations,[116] mental retardation, and death.[67]

Although the early reports of malnutrition were followed by improvement of medical foods, nutrition problems have still occurred. However, mean serum carnitine concentrations of treated patients were in the reference range when patients were fed medical foods containing L-carnitine. Medical foods containing increased amounts of L-TYR have alleviated the problem of low plasma TYR concentrations.[117] Plasma glycine concentrations were elevated in one group of treated patients.[118] Treated patients with PKU often have below reference range concentrations of transthyretin when fed Recommended Dietary Allowances (RDAs) for protein.[119] Arnold et al.[120] and Acosta et al.[121] reported a positive correlation between height and transthyretin with concentrations < 200 mg/L associated with poor linear growth.

Growth

Physical growth during infancy and childhood is influenced by genetic and environmental factors, including nutrition. In 1970, a Canadian group[67] and in 1971, a U.S. group[122] reported poor growth in many treated patients with PKU. Linear growth, in particular, was diminished in relation to that found in children without PKU. Prior to the initiation of the PKUCS in 1967, a protocol was prepared that addressed the nutrition management of patients to be entered in the study and recommended the protein and energy to be ingested by differing ages. Growth of the patients ingesting Lofenalac® (Mead Johnson Nutritionals, Evansville, Indiana) as their primary protein source did not differ from growth of normal children (see Table 5.7).[59,60,123] Height of these

Table 5.7 ***Daily Protein and Energy Intakes, Plasma Phenylalanine Concentrations, and Linear Growth of Treated Children With PKU in Different Countries***

Country (Number)	*Age*	*Protein intake (g)*	*(g/kg)*	*Energy intake (kcal)*	*Plasma PHE concentration (µmol/L)*	*Length/height (Z-Score or percentile)*
United States (88)	Diagnosis–6 mos	20.4[a]	3.6 ± 0.8[a]	621[a]	400[a]	F +0.38, M +0.96
	7–12 mos	23.0[a]	2.6 ± 0.5[a]	788[a]	440[a]	F +0.18, M +0.42
United States (12)	Diagnosis–6 mos	16.0 ± 0.8[b]	NA	630 ± 33[b]	272 ± 44[b]	↑ from 38 ± 6 to 55 ± 8%[b]
(13)	Diagnosis–6 mos	14.2 ± 0.7[b]	NA	650 ± 32[b]	268 ± 61[b]	↓ from 60 ± 8 to 29 ± 7%[b]
United States (35)	Diagnosis–< 3 mos	15.0 ± 0.6[b]	2.8 ± 0.1[b]	596 ± 14[b]	297 ± 41[b]	59.1 ± 4.3% at 6 mos
	3 < 6 mos	19.2 ± 0.1[b]	2.5 ± 0.1[b]	658 ± 25[b]	—	
The Netherlands (174)	0 < 6 mos	NA	2.7 ± 0.5[c]	NA	NA	Mean < 0.00 with greater variability < 0.00 than > 0.00
	6 < 12 mos	NA	2.4 ± 0.5[c]			
	12 < 24 mos	NA	2.2 ± 0.6[c]			
	24 < 36 mos	NA	2.2 ± 0.6[c]			
United States (129)	1 < 4 yrs	34.0[a]	2.4 ± 0.1[a]	1235[a]	495[a]	Height of neither F nor M differed from national standards
	4 < 7 yrs	39.0[a]	1.9 ± 0.1[a]	1500[a]	625[a]	
Germany (82)	6 yrs	21.0 1st 3 yrs[d]	2.2 ± 0.5[d,e]	NA	315 ± 103	F –0.54 ± 1.24[d] with gradual increase to 6 yrs
		34.2 2nd 3 yrs[d]	2.0 ± 0.2[d,e] mean ± SD	NA	418 ± 151 mean ± SD	M –0.78 ± 0.97[d] with no catch-up
France (20)	8 mos – 7 yrs	NA	1.7 ± 0.2 mean ± SD	NA	Mean 457	–0.49, range –2.12 to +1.61 9 < –0.5, 2 = –2.0 Wt –0.71
The Netherlands (112)	6 mos – 10 yrs	NA	NA	NA	NA	–0.23 ± 0.17 mean ± SD

(continues)

Table 5.7 ***Daily Protein and Energy Intakes, Plasma Phenylalanine Concentrations, and Linear Growth of Treated Children With PKU in Different Countries**, Continued*

Country (Number)	***Age***	***Protein intake (g)***	***(g/kg)***	***Energy intake (kcal)***	***Plasma PHE concentration (µmol/L)***	***Length/ height (Z-Score or percentile)***
Austria (34)	8.7 ± 3.9 yrs 2 mos – 15 yrs	33.7 ± 10.3 mean ± SD	1.2 ± 0.3 mean ± SD	NA	456 ± 432 mean ± SD	–0.11 ± 1.10 mean ± SD
United States (58)	2.0 – 12.3 yrs	124 ± 5% RDI[b,e]	NA	83 ± 4%[b,e]	519 ± 70[b,e]	+0.06 ± 0.18[b,e]

Sources:

Acosta PB, Trahms C, Wellman NS, Williamson M. Phenylalanine intakes of 1- to 6-year-old children with phenylketonuria undergoing therapy. *Am J Clin Nutr*. 1983;38:694–700.

Acosta PB, Wenz E, Williamson M. Nutrient intake of treated infants with phenylketonuria. *Am J Clin Nutr*. 1977;30:198–208.

Acosta PB, Yannicelli S. Protein intake affects phenylalanine requirements and growth of infants with phenylketonuria. *Acta Paediatr Suppl*. 1994;407:66–67.

Acosta PB, Yannicelli S, Marriage B, et al. Nutrient intake and growth of infants with phenylketonuria undergoing therapy. *J Pediatr Gastroenterol Nutr*. 1998;27:287–291.

Acosta PB, Yannicelli S, Singh R, et al. Nutrient intakes and physical growth of children with phenylketonuria undergoing nutrition therapy. *J Am Diet Assoc*. 2003;103:1167–1173.

Dobbelaere D, Michaud L, Debrabander A, et al. Evaluation of nutritional status and pathophysiology of growth retardation in patients with phenylketonuria. *J Inherit Metab Dis*. 2003;26:1–11.

Hoeksma M, Van Rijn M, Verkerk PH, et al. The intake of total protein, natural protein and protein substitute and growth of height and head circumference in Dutch infants with phenylketonuria. *J Inherit Metab Dis*. 2005;28:845–854.

Holm VA, Kronmal RA, Williamson M, Roche AF. Physical growth in phenylketonuria: II. Growth of treated children in the PKU collaborative study from birth to 4 years of age. *Pediatrics*. 1979;63:700–707.

Schaefer F, Burgard P, Batzler U, et al. Growth and skeletal maturation in children with phenylketonuria. *Acta Paediatr*. 1994;83:534–541.

Verkerk PH, van Spronsen FJ, Smit GPA, Sengers RC. Impaired prenatal and postnatal growth in Dutch patients with phenylketonuria. *Arch Dis Child*. 1994;71:114–118.

Note: NA = not available.

[a]Food and beverage intakes recorded 3 days monthly by caregiver and mean ± SD calculated for entire period.

[b]Food and beverage intakes recorded 3 days monthly by caregiver and mean ± SEM calculated for entire period.

[c]Prescribed mean ± SD recorded but actual intakes not given.

[d]From diet plans recorded at the end of each 6-month interval. Actual intake not given.

[e]RDI for age:	Protein (g/d)	Energy (kcal/d)
2 < 4 yrs	30	1300
4 < 6 yrs	35	1700
7 < 11 yrs	40	2400
11 < 13 yrs		
F	50	2200
M	55	2700

children when assessed at 10 years of age did not differ from national standards, while the weight of females and males from 4 and 5 years of age onward, respectively, exceeded national standards.[124] Length/height, weight, and mean of median intakes of infants and children in the PKUCS, based on 3-day diet diaries recorded monthly by the caregiver prior to blood draw for plasma PHE analysis and calculated from U.S. Department of Agriculture (USDA) data, are given in Table 5.7.[59,60,125-127] Other studies of U.S. infants and children with PKU fed medical foods containing free amino acids as the protein equivalent reported excellent growth in length/height, head circumference, and weight. See Table 5.7 for length/height and intakes of protein and energy.

Mean length/height, head circumference, and weight of Dutch, German, and French infants and children undergoing nutrition management for PKU have often been reported to fall below zero Z-score for length/height and weight during much of infancy and childhood (see Table 5.7).[128-132] A 2007 report of growth during 1 year of study in treated Austrian children with PKU indicated no significant differences in growth and body composition between patients with PKU and healthy children at birth or during a 1-year study. A significant correlation was found between intact protein intake and muscle mass (see Chapter 3). A positive statistically significant correlation between head circumference, growth, and intact and total protein intake was found.[133]

Reasons for poor linear growth in patients undergoing nutrition management for PKU have been suggested and include inadequate intakes of PHE, protein, iodine, iron, and zinc.[61,62,119,120,132,134] Many of the studies of growth of children with PKU have reported neither parental heights nor actual protein and energy intakes; consequently, neither the genetic nor environmental effects on growth can be reported for many of the children in Europe or the United States undergoing nutrition management.

Cholesterol and Essential Fatty Acids

In 1955, Goldstein[135] at McGill University proposed in his doctoral dissertation that the low serum cholesterol concentrations in untreated patients with PKU might reflect a deficiency of coenzyme A necessary for its synthesis or decreased activity of enzymes needed for cholesterol production. Woolf[136] reported that untreated patients with PKU utilize large amounts of acetyl-CoA in the synthesis of phenylacetylglutamine. Acosta et al.[137] demonstrated that mean total serum cholesterol concentrations were significantly lower in both untreated and treated patients with PKU than in normal children while Galluzzo et al.[138] demonstrated a highly significant difference between treated children with PKU and normal children. Serum cholesterol concentrations were also found to be significantly lower in pregnant women with PKU than in normal control pregnant women.[63] Castillo et al. reported inhibition of brain and liver 3-hydroxy-3-methylglutaryl-CoA reductase and mevalonate-5-pyrophosphate decarboxylase in experimental HPA.[139] Colomé and coworkers[140] found an inverse correlation between plasma PHE concentrations and serum concentrations of cholesterol in patients undergoing treatment for PKU.

Fatty acids were also analyzed in four serum lipid fractions of the three groups of patients for whom total cholesterol concentrations, using a gas liquid chromatograph, were analyzed.[137] With the technology available, fatty acids longer than arachidonic acid (ARA; C20:4n-6) could not be analyzed. Treated patients were ingesting Lofenalac® (Mead Johnson Nutritionals, Evansville, Indiana) that contained corn oil as its fat. Linoleic acid (C18:2n-6) was significantly greater in serum triglycerides, phospholipids, and sterol esters, but not in free fatty acids in treated patients than in untreated patients and normal children. Alpha-linolenic acid (C18:3n-3) did not differ in any lipid fraction among the three groups.

Since the early 1970s, many publications have appeared on the topic of plasma and erythrocyte docosahexaenoic acid (DHA; C22:6n-3) concentrations in patients undergoing therapy for PKU. The suggestion has been made that the lower long-chain n-3 fatty acids were responsible for visual perception problems and other neuropathology in treated patients with PKU.[141,142] However, Acosta et al.[143] reported that 2- to 13-year-old patients undergoing management with Phenex™-1/2 (Abbott Nutrition, Columbus, Ohio), Phenyl-Free® (Mead Johnson Nutritionals, Evansville, Indiana), or XPHE Maxamaid®/Maxamum® (Nutricia, North America, Gaithersburg, Maryland) had similar percentages of fatty acids as n-3 fatty acids as their normal siblings on a normal diet with only DHA (C22:6n-3) being significantly lower in the erythrocytes of the XPHE Maxamaid®/Maxamum®-fed patients than in their normal siblings. XPHE Maxamaid® and XPHE Maxamum® are fat-free medical foods.

Whether the addition of DHA to medical foods for patients with PKU does anything more than increase plasma and erythrocyte concentrations, shorten shelf life of medical foods, and inhibit DHA synthesis[144] is not known. Campistol et al.[145] in Spain recently indicated that the n-3 fatty acids were not correlated with visual function of patients with PKU undergoing nutrition management. If fatty acids were reported as μmol/L rather than as a percentage of fatty acids, results might not differ from those found in normal individuals.

The report by the group in Spain[145] is even more important in view of the references that the liver of the human neonate desaturates the two essential fatty acids, linoleate (C18:2n-6) and α-linolenic (C18:3n-3),[146] that neonates with PKU can synthesize ARA (C20:4n-6)[147] from linoleate and other normal neonates can synthesize DHA (C22:6n-3) from α-linolenic acid,[148,149] and that astrocytes[150] and human skin fibroblasts[151] synthesize DHA by peroxisomal retroconversion of tetracosahexaenoic acid. No studies to date have demonstrated inhibition of enzymes that desaturate and elongate linoleic and α-linolenic acids by PHE and its metabolites, while studies have shown that the long-chain polyunsaturated fatty acids do inhibit their synthesis.[144] However, the possibility exists that the use of acetyl-CoA for the synthesis of phenylacetate and phenylacetylglutamine from elevated plasma PHE concentrations[136] could interfere with elongation of essential fatty acids, rather than from the lower concentrations being diet related.

Osteopenia

Despite early reports on changes in bones of patients undergoing nutrition management for PKU, no studies on bone density were published until the 1980s. Since that time many publications on this subject have appeared. Amino acid imbalances; inadequate protein, calcium, phosphorus, and vitamin D intakes; poor diet compliance with decreased medical food intake; and elevated plasma PHE concentrations have all been suggested as possible reasons for poor bone density. However, a number of reports have indicated that mean intakes of protein, calcium, phosphorus, and vitamin D met or exceeded recommended intakes.[59,126,127] Later, studies by Acosta et al.[121] evaluated bone collagen (the matrix in which minerals are deposited) loss by measurement of morning urinary deoxypyridinoline (DPYD) five times during 1 year in 2- to 13-year old children undergoing nutrition management for PKU. Intakes of PHE, protein, calcium, phosphorus, copper, zinc, and vitamin D were assessed, and concentrations of plasma PHE, plasma/serum concentrations of albumin, retinol binding protein, transthyretin, 25-hydroxycholecalciferol, calcium, phosphorus, and alkaline phosphatase activity were analyzed. Plasma/serum concentrations of all analytes except PHE were within reference ranges and the PHE concentrations increased with age. After 8 years of age, DPYD urinary excretion positively correlated with plasma PHE concentrations and was significantly greater than found in normal children of the same age. Preschool children with plasma PHE concentrations in treatment range had normal bone mineralization.[152-155] Greeves et al.[156] reported that 25% of patients with PKU, most of whom were over 8 years of age, had a history of fractures compared with 18% of normal siblings. Untreated PKU mice (PAH^{enu-2}) had reduced mean femur weight compared with treated and control mice, and shorter mean femur length than control mice.[157] These and other reports resulted in the hypothesis that osteopenia in patients with PKU may result from the following series of events: poorly controlled plasma PHE concentrations result in elevated serum prolactin concentrations[158] that result in a high prevalence of menstrual irregularities, and inhibition of cholesterol synthesis required for estrogen synthesis[135,137,140] that is necessary to enhance bone mineralization,[159-161] and hyperprolactinemia results in bone mineral loss that is reversed by therapy of hyperprolactinemia.[162,163]

Iron

In the late 1960s, Acosta and Koch found little stainable bone marrow iron; some low concentrations of hemoglobin, serum iron, and transferrin saturations; and elevated total iron binding capacity in children 9.8 to 44 months of age who were ingesting Lofenalac®.[119] Iron intake as ferrous sulfate, a usually well-absorbed source of iron, met or exceeded recommended intakes in all patients. Since that time, several references from different countries have been published concerning patients with PKU who were ingesting recommended iron intakes but had iron deficiency based on plasma ferritin concentrations.[164,165] Relatively recent publications on over 70 infants and children with PKU undergoing nutrition management reported continuing problems with iron deficiency.[166,167] Alexander and Clayton[77] reported that patients with PKU undergoing nutrition management retained significantly less iron and other minerals than normal children. Gropper et al.[168] indicated that untreated PKU mice ($PAH^{enu\text{-}2}$) on a low-protein diet had much higher iron stores in the liver than the mice on a normal protein intake. This was also found in the PKU mice on a PHE-restricted diet ingesting a low protein intake, suggesting possible excessive liver iron storage when protein intakes are low and plasma PHE concentrations are elevated.

Selenium

Selenium deficiency resulting in low plasma concentrations and low activity of selenium-dependent erythrocyte glutathione peroxidase, inadequate thyroid function, poor immune status, and life-threatening cardiac dysrythmia[169-172] was ended by the addition of selenium in adequate amounts to the medical food,[121,173] when appropriate amounts of the medical food are ingested.[166]

Zinc

Plasma/serum zinc concentrations below reference ranges have been reported in patients with PKU meeting or exceeding recommended zinc intakes.[174] However, the addition of adequate zinc to the medical foods prevents low plasma zinc concentrations.[121,166]

Vitamins

Intakes of vitamins A, D, and E by children with PKU in the United States undergoing nutrition management have all been adequate to result in concentrations of plasma/serum retinol, 25-hydroxycholecalciferol, and α-tocopherol in the reference ranges.[119,166] Intakes of thiamin, riboflavin, niacin, vitamins B_6, B_{12}, C, and folic acid met or exceeded recommended intakes when adequate medical food was ingested.[126,127] However, Lewis et al.[78]

suggested that a problem occurred in niacin metabolism in children with PKU, and La Du and Zannoni[175] reported decreased urinary excretion of niacin metabolites by children with PKU. Schulpis et al.[176] reported that patients with well-controlled plasma PHE concentrations had higher serum biotin concentrations and biotinidase activity than patients with poorly controlled plasma PHE concentrations. Twenty of 26 patients with poorly controlled plasma PHE concentrations had seborrheic dermatitis that healed after 15 days on a strict PHE-restricted diet. Further, the in vitro effects of PHE inhibited biotinidase activity. Whether the high plasma PHE concentrations or the low biotin concentrations were responsible for the dermatitis is unclear.

Maternal Phenylketonuria

Introduction

The first suggestion that untreated women with PKU would give birth to offspring with mental retardation was reported by Dent in 1957.[177] Later, 2 untreated women with PKU gave birth to 14 mentally retarded children and the suggestion was made that if maternal plasma PHE concentration was lowered by the administration of a PHE-restricted diet during pregnancy, mental retardation in their offspring could be prevented.[178] Offspring of women with PKU untreated during gestation also had intrauterine growth retardation, microcephaly, congenital anomalies, and heart disease often incompatible with life.[179] Because PHE is actively transported across the placenta to the fetus and is 1.5- to 2.0-times greater than the concentration in maternal blood, the pathogenesis of the fetal damage is believed to be related to the elevated PHE concentration in maternal blood.[179-181] The fetal plasma PHE concentration is then concentrated two to four times by the fetal blood-brain barrier to a concentration that interferes with brain development by several different mechanisms.[182,183]

Plasma PHE concentrations of women with PKU who are of childbearing age must remain < 360 µmol/L prior to and during gestation for the best fetal outcome. In fact, Smith et al.[184] has suggested plasma concentrations of 60 to 180 µmol/L in the pregnant woman with PKU. Surviving offspring of untreated or inadequately treated women fail to grow and develop normally. Five-year-old offspring of women in the International Maternal PKU Collaborative Study (MPKUCS) who had plasma PHE concentrations > 360 µmol/L throughout gestation were small at birth and failed to have catch-up growth in height or head circumference. In fact, mean head circumference Z-score of children whose mothers had plasma PHE concentrations between

360 and 600 μmol/L had a decline from –0.65 ± 0.87 at birth to –0.97 ± 1.49 at 5 years, while offspring of women with plasma PHE concentrations > 600 μmol/L had a mean head circumference Z-score at birth of –1.46 ± 1.08 that declined to –2.09 ± 1.57 at 5 years of age.[185] Results from the International MPKUCS support the premise that a PHE-restricted diet that maintains plasma concentrations < 360 μmol/L, if started prior to pregnancy, improves reproductive outcome.[186]

Untreated pregnant women with non-PKU HPA had offspring with a birth head circumference Z-score of –0.63 that negatively correlated with maternal plasma PHE concentrations. Mean IQ score of offspring of these untreated women was 96 ± 14 and was 109 ± 21 in the offspring of control women.[187]

The suggestion has been made that BH_4 may be useful in controlling plasma PHE concentrations during pregnancy in non-PKU HPA.[188] One pregnant patient whose PAH mutation was R408/F39L was treated with both a PHE-restricted diet and BH_4 under an Investigational New Drug Application that was approved by the Food and Drug Administration (FDA), and gave birth to a normal infant.[189] More information is needed to determine whether diet, BH_4, or both resulted in the normal offspring outcome.

Nutrition Management

The PHE-restricted diet should be initiated at least 3 months before a planned pregnancy by women with PKU or non-PKU HPA if they have previously discontinued diet. Protein and fat storage by the mother during early pregnancy is essential to support last trimester fetal growth. Intakes recommended after stabilization of plasma PHE concentration in treatment range are given in Table 5.1. Plasma PHE concentrations must be monitored twice weekly to maintain the targeted treatment range. Plasma TYR concentrations with recommended TYR intakes were (mean ± SD) 0.90 ± 0.40 mg/dL first trimester, 1.04 ± 0.44 mg/dL second trimester, and 0.99 ± 0.49 mg/dL third trimester.[63] Two- to 4-hour postprandial plasma PHE concentrations found in normal pregnant women in the MPKUCS are given in Chapter 3, Table 3.8.[190]

After stabilization of plasma PHE and TYR concentrations in the treatment range, frequent changes in the diet prescription are required as pregnancy progresses, based on concentrations of plasma amino acids and weight gain. The PHE and TYR requirements of each pregnant woman with PKU depend on genotype,[191] age, state of health, total amount of protein ingested[63] and trimester of pregnancy.[63,191] About mid-pregnancy, PHE tolerance increases considerably (see Table 5.1).

The amount of protein prescribed for the pregnant woman with PKU exceeds recommended intakes for normal women because of the use of free amino acids as the primary source of protein equivalent (see Chapter 3, Table 3.1). PHE-free medical foods (see Table 5.2) are used to supply most of the protein prescribed and low-protein, modified very-low-protein, and nitrogen-free foods and fats are used to provide the remaining energy needs. Supplying required energy needs during pregnancy is a challenge and requires creativity in planning by the dietitian. Sources of modified very-low-protein foods are given in Appendix E. A protocol is available that suggests how to plan and evaluate nutrition management of the pregnant woman with PKU.[190]

Linoleic acid (C18:2n-6) and α-linolenic acid (C18:3n-3) are essential for human nutrition. Intakes recommended daily are 13 g and 1.4 g, respectively, during pregnancy.[73] Women in the MPKUCS who had a good reproductive outcome had greater fat intake throughout pregnancy than women with a poorer outcome.[63] Whether the poor outcome was partly due to inadequate essential fatty acids is unclear, as these were not calculated for women in the MPKUCS. Because some of the medical foods are devoid of, or contain very little, fat and essential fatty acids (see Table 5.2), unhydrogenated canola oil or soybean oil, which contains both linoleic and α-linolenic acids, should be the fats of choice to use for cooking and salad dressings (see Appendix F).[192] Butter containing 260 mg cholesterol per 10 g may be beneficial as a fat source in the diet that contains little or none and for the pregnant woman with PKU who appears to synthesize less cholesterol than the normal pregnant woman.[63]

PHE-free medical foods that provide prescribed protein equivalent (nitrogen in grams × 6.25) for the pregnant woman with PKU also provide the required amounts of minerals and vitamins (see Chapter 3, Table 3.1). Thus, a prenatal vitamin capsule containing vitamins A and D should not be prescribed for pregnant women with PKU who are ingesting all prescribed medical food. Supplementation may, in fact, supply vitamins A and D in amounts approaching those that are teratogenic.[73,193] The critical period for fetal susceptibility to vitamin A teratogenicity is the first trimester of pregnancy and intakes > 7800 μg/day often result in craniofacial malformations and abnormalities of the central nervous system (except neural tube defects), thymus, and heart.[73] Those women who fail to ingest adequate medical food prior to and during gestation should be given supplements of folic acid and vitamin B_{12} from very early in pregnancy to help decrease the incidence of congenital heart disease in offspring.[194]

Assessment of Nutrition Management

Ongoing monitoring of pregnant women with PKU or non-PKU HPA involves analyzing plasma concentrations of PHE, TYR, and other amino acids, and assessing maternal weight gain and plasma/serum concentrations of transthyretin, ferritin, and zinc. Because pregnant women with PKU often deliver prematurely, they should be treated as high-risk patients, even if their plasma PHE concentration is in the targeted treatment range. Multiple ultrasound studies, beginning at 16 to 20 weeks gestation, should be completed to monitor fetal head size and intrauterine growth patterns. Level II ultrasound to scan for heart defects and other malformations may also be ordered.[27]

Reproductive Outcomes

Birth measurements of newborn infants of women with PKU are negatively correlated with maternal plasma PHE concentrations, and positively correlated with maternal energy and protein intakes and maternal weight gain during pregnancy.[63] Appropriate maternal weight gain is related to height and prepregnancy weight and is greater for underweight women than for women of normal weight.[195] Women who are underweight for height at conception should gain the greatest weight, both during the first trimester and throughout pregnancy.

Neurologic outcome of offspring of women with PKU was significantly improved in women with tight control of plasma PHE concentrations prior to and throughout pregnancy.[186] Reported factors that interfere with control of plasma PHE concentrations prior to and during pregnancy include young maternal age, belief that management costs complicate the diet, proof of pregnancy for eligibility to state-based assistance programs for medical food, private insurers unwilling to pay for medical foods, and few obstetricians who are knowledgeable about the PHE-restricted diet.[196]

The Australian,[197] English,[198] French,[199] and Irish[200] have reported reproductive outcomes in over 450 pregnancies in women with PKU. As found in the International MPKUCS,[186] poor metabolic control of the mother during pregnancy was associated with poor cognitive and behavioral outcomes of offspring. All of these studies clearly suggest the need for plasma PHE concentrations near the normal range, both in women with PKU and in women with non-PKU HPA during pregnancy.

Tyrosinemias

Introduction

Tyrosine is obtained from food, phenylalanine hydroxylation, and body protein catabolism (see Figure 5.1) and has several important functions in the body including use in synthesis of proteins, catecholamines, thyroid hormones, melanin pigments, and energy. Only L-TYR is metabolically active in humans and has a molecular weight of 181.19. This amino acid is only very slightly soluble in water and forms characteristic crystals at high concentrations.[70,201]

Biochemistry

Three enzymes have been identified as having little or no function in the inherited metabolic disorders discussed herein (see Figure 5.1). Tyrosine aminotransferase (TAT; E.C.2.6.1.5) is the first enzyme in TYR catabolism and requires pyridoxine as coenzyme. Its action results in the synthesis of p-hydroxyphenylpyruvic acid (p-HPPA). TAT is found only in the cytoplasm of hepatocytes. Its activity is low in the neonatal period and is the rate-limiting enzyme of TYR metabolism.[201] A deficiency in activity of TAT results in the autosomal recessively inherited tyrosinemia type II (OMIM 276600),[1] previously called Richner-Hanhart's syndrome or oculocutaneous tyrosinemia. P-hydroxyphenylpyruvic acid dioxygenase (p-HPPAD; E.C.1.13.11.27) is found in the cytoplasm of hepatocytes and renal tubular cells. Ascorbic acid is the coenzyme for p-HPPAD, and ferrous iron bound to the enzyme is catalytically important. This enzyme acts on p-HPPA to synthesize homogetisic acid. A deficiency in activity of p-HPPAD results in autosomal recessively inherited tyrosinemia type IIIa (OMIM 767710)[1] and dominantly inherited IIIb (hawkinsinuria; OMIM 140350),[1] and its late maturation in the newborn is believed to cause transient tyrosinemia. P-HPPAD is also found to be deficient in scurvy, liver disease, and in a disorder called Medes tyrosinosis.[201] Homogentisic acid oxidase (E.C.1.13.11.5), not associated with any tyrosinemias, is found in the cytoplasm of liver and kidney and catalyzes the cleavage of the aromatic ring of TYR to form maleylacetoacetic acid that is further catabolized to succinylacetoacetic acid and fumarylacetoacetic acid by maleylacetoacetate isomerase (E.C.5.2.1.2). Fumarylacetoacetic acid is catabolized to fumaric acid and acetoacetic acid by fumarylacetoacetic acid hydrolase (FAH; E.C.3.7.1.2), which is deficient in autosomal recessively inherited tyrosinemia type I (OMIM 276700),[1] also named hepatorenal tyrosinemia. FAH is found in the cytosol of liver, renal tubules, and most other tissues.[201]

Normal fasting plasma TYR concentrations range from 25 to 103 μmol/L in the newborn, from 30 to 90 μmol/L in the child, and from 35 to 90 μmol/L in the adult.[201] Picone et al.[12] reported that 2- to 4-hour postprandial plasma TYR concentrations in normal human milk-fed and in proprietary formula-fed infants with 15 g protein/L at 12 weeks of age were 58 ± 6.0 μmol/L and 87 ± 9.0 μmol/L (mean ± SEM), respectively.

Molecular Biology

The TAT gene is located on chromosome 16q22.1–22.3, has 12 exons, and is 10.9 kb in length. Over 15 mutations have been reported with no association between genotype and phenotype of the disease.[201-203] Deletions, missense, nonsense, and splice-site mutations have been reported. TAT gene mutations have been reported in patients in France, Israel, Italy, Japan, Scotland, and Tunisia,[203] and many of the patients have been of Italian descent.[204]

The gene for p-HPPAD is located on chromosome 12q24-qter, is about 21 kb in size, and contains 14 exons. Few patients have been reported with either tyrosinemia type III or hawkinsinuria, and no association has been found between genotype and phenotype.[201,205]

Tyrosinemia type I results from a defect of the enzyme FAH for which the gene is located on chromosome 15q23–q25. The human gene spans 30 to 35 kb and contains 14 exons.[201] More than 34 gene mutations have been reported,[27] resulting in patients with heterogeneous phenotypic patterns ranging from acute to chronic forms.[206] Patients have been reported from many ethnic groups and are relatively common in Quebec and Finland.[201]

Newborn Screening

Newborn screening for the tyrosinemias is by analyzing the TYR concentration in blood spots found on filter paper. Patients with blood TYR concentrations greater than the state-determined maximum concentration are referred to a metabolic center for diagnostic work-up. High-protein, proprietary infant formulas may result in elevated concentrations of both PHE and TYR on newborn screening.[207] Plasma TYR concentrations in the neonate with tyrosinemia type I may not be adequately elevated to detect on newborn screening. Thus, a number of researchers have developed other methods to analyze succinylacetone in dried blood spots.[208,209]

Diagnosis

Accurate biochemical diagnosis is important because disorders such as liver disease, scurvy, and prematurity may produce increases in plasma TYR concentrations that are not due to enzyme defects in TYR metabolism. Further, therapy differs depending on the enzyme defect present. Tyrosinemia type II (TAT deficiency) is characterized by greatly elevated concentrations of blood and urine TYR, with plasma TYR ranging from 370 to 3300 μmol/L, and increases in urinary phenolic acids, N-acetyltyrosine, and tyramine[27,201] (see Figure 5.1).

Tyrosinemia type III results from malfunctioning p-OPPAD (see Figure 5.1). Plasma TYR concentrations may range from 350 to 640 μmol/L with increased urinary excretion of p-HPPA and p-hydroxyphenylacetic acid.[201] Hawkinsinuria is named for the 2-L-cysteinyl 5-1,4-dihydroxycyclohexenyl-acetic acid that is formed from an intermediate of the impaired p-OHPPAD reaction.[27] Hawkinsin is measured using ion-exchange chromatography.[27] Neonatal tyrosinemia is associated with increased plasma and urinary concentrations of TYR and its metabolites. It may occur in up to 10% of neonates.[201]

Tyrosinemia type I (FAH deficiency) may be diagnosed by finding succinylacetone in the urine (with or without a previously elevated plasma TYR concentration), by enzyme assay, or by assessing patient tissue for gene mutations.[201,204] As liver disease progresses in FAH deficiency, plasma methionine concentration increases because the liver is its primary site of metabolism.

Outcomes if Untreated

Tyrosinemia type I is characterized by generalized renal tubular impairment with hypophosphatemic rickets, progressive liver failure resulting in cirrhosis and hepatic cancer, hypertension, acute porphyric episodes, and peripheral nerve deficiencies. Elevated concentrations of plasma PHE, TYR and succinylacetone, and δ-aminolevulinic acid (δ-ALA) excretion are found in the urine in tyrosinemia type I.[27,201] Death usually occurs around 2 years of age without treatment. Characteristic physical findings of tyrosinemia type II include corneal erosions and plaques and lesions of the soles and palms. Keratitis and hyperkeratosis occur on the fingers and palms of the hands and soles of the feet and are probably due to intracellular crystallization of TYR causing inflammatory responses. Mental retardation may occur.[27] Neurologic abnormalities including seizures, ataxia, and mental retardation have been reported in untreated patients with tyrosinemia type III.[27,201] Persistence of hypertyrosinemia in neonatal tyrosinemia may lead to impaired mental function.[210]

Nutrition Management

The objective of nutrition management of inherited tyrosinemias is to provide a biochemical environment that supports normal growth and development of intellectual potential. Nutrition management alone will prevent pathophysiologic changes only in types II and III, for which prognosis is excellent.[27] Plasma PHE concentration should be maintained between 50 and 100 μmol/L and plasma TYR concentration between 50 and 150 μmol/L.

Short-term protein restriction in the patient with neonatal tyrosinemia to 1.5 to 2.0 g/kg BW/day has lowered plasma TYR concentrations in most patients. Whether added ascorbate of 50 to 200 mg per day for a few weeks will stabilize and increase the activity of p-OHPPAD in this disorder is not clear.[201]

A relatively new drug, 2-(2-nitro-4-trifluoromethyl-benzyol)-1,3-cyclohexanedione (NTBC; ORFADIN®, RDT Rare Disease Therapeutics, Inc., Nashville, Tennessee) was first tested in the early 1990s as therapy for tyrosinemia type I. NTBC inhibits the activity of p-HPPAD, blocking its catabolic activity and preventing synthesis of fumarylacetoacetate and succinylacetone.[204] NTBC therapy in tyrosinemia type I with concomitant nutrition management to maintain plasma TYR concentration at < 500 µmol/L[211] has prevented acute porphyria episodes, decreased rates of progression of cirrhosis and Fanconi syndrome, greatly improved the survival of patients, reduced the need for liver transplantation during early childhood, and prevented deposits of TYR crystals in the eye or palms of the hands and soles of the feet. The effects of NTBC in decreasing succinylacetone production do not totally eliminate the risk for hepatocarcinoma.[212]

If NTBC is unavailable and renal impairment is present, it must also be treated in tyrosinemia type I. Generalized renal tubular failure may result in metabolic acidosis, hypophosphatemia, rickets, and hypokalemia unless treatment with bicarbonate, phosphate, 1,25-dihydroyxcholecalciferol, and potassium is instituted. Rapid treatment of infections is required to prevent an overwhelming catabolic state with excess production of succinylacetone.[27]

Many of the porphyric symptoms result from overproduction of δ-ALA due to the inhibitory effect of succinylacetone on δ-ALA dehydratase and/or decreased heme biosynthesis. Parenteral nutrition with 20 to 25% dextrose solutions has been found to control these acute porphyric attacks in some patients.[27] Loss of energy-requiring functions that involve loosely bound heme to heme-protein (plasma membrane transporters, cytochrome P-450) may be due to rapid turnover and insufficient heme biosynthesis. Infusions of hematin have produced transient decreases in δ-ALA and have improved acute attacks of intermittent porphyria, but this therapy is not recommended unless NTBC is unavailable.[213] Nutrition management, in conjunction with NTBC therapy, is essential in the treatment of patients with tyrosinemia type I.

Nutrient Requirements

A written prescription for daily amounts of PHE, TYR, protein, energy, and fluid is necessary. The prescription for PHE and TYR is based on plasma analyses correlated with intake that indicate the patient's tolerance for each amino acid (see Table 5.1). Because about 75% of PHE is normally hydroxylated to form TYR,[11] PHE is also restricted in the diet of patients with tyrosinemia. PHE requirements are greater for children with tyrosinemia than for children with PKU. Generally, the more distal the block in the catabolic pathway, the higher the amino acid requirement. TYR needs of children with tyrosinemia have been inadequately described and vary with the metabolic state of the child, plasma PHE and TYR concentrations, and the accumulation of succinylacetone in tyrosinemia type I. If plasma TYR is inadequately controlled in NTBC-treated patients, symptoms of tyrosinemia type II will occur.[211]

A 9-year-old child with TAT deficiency was noted to have plasma PHE concentrations that were very low on occasion.[214] On three consecutive days, this patient was given 20, 30, and 40 mg/kg BW of L-PHE, respectively, with the medical food mixture. Even at baseline, prior to administration of L-PHE, plasma TYR concentration was greater than 500 μmol/L. Five patients ranging in age from 1.3 to 7 years of age with FAH deficiency who also had very low plasma PHE concentrations on occasion were supplemented with 20, 30, and 40 mg/kg BW, respectively, over 3 consecutive days. Of the total of 48 blood draws on 4 patients and 8 on 1 patient (56 blood draws at 7:00, 11:00, 16:00, and 20:00 hours), 34 analyses indicated that plasma TYR concentrations were > 500 μmol/L and 40 plasma PHE concentrations were < 50 μmol/L. Whether less L-PHE or L-PHE administered in a slow-release capsule or as intact protein would have the same effect was not tried, nor was the effect of long-term L-PHE administration available. See Table 5.1 for recommended beginning intakes of dietary PHE and TYR by age. Cohn et al.[215] reported deficiency of both PHE and TYR in patients treated by diet restriction only.

Recommended protein intakes for patients with hereditary tyrosinemias are given in Chapter 3, Table 3.1. Because the primary protein equivalent (nitrogen, g × 6.25) source is free amino acids, recommended intake is greater than for normal people.[73] However, if severe liver disease is present in tyrosinemia type I, protein intake may require restriction to prevent hyperammonemia.[216]

Energy needs must be adequate to support normal growth and to prevent catabolism,[73] and fluid needs are 1.5 mL/kcal ingested by infants (see Chapter 3, Table 3.1).[76] Children and adults require about 1.0 mL/kcal ingested. Excess energy intake results in obesity while excess fluid intake may result in hyponatremia.[73]

Recommended mineral and vitamin intakes are described in Chapter 3, Table 3.1. Recommended intakes of minerals are greater in patients with any of the tyrosinemias than in normal patients due to their decreased absorption from elemental medical foods.[77] Administration of phosphorus, potassium, and 1,25-dihydroxycholecalciferol are essential for the patient with tyrosinemia type I not receiving NTBC, but will not be necessary for the patient with normal liver and renal functions.

Phenylalanine- and Tyrosine-Free Medical Foods

Intact protein cannot be used to supply all protein requirements without providing excess PHE and TYR (intact proteins contain by weight 2 to 9% PHE and 1.4 to 5.8% TYR). Thus, special medical foods that contain no PHE or TYR are used. Several medical foods free of PHE and TYR are available to provide protein equivalent. Formulations, composition of major nutrients, and sources of medical foods containing minerals and vitamins are given in Table 5.2.

Intact Proteins

Intact proteins in recommended amounts are usually used to supply PHE and TYR prescribed in the diet. Proprietary infant formula with iron is used in early infancy as the primary source of PHE and TYR. Intact low protein beikost and, later, table foods are used to supply the majority of PHE and TYR in the diet. However, if plasma PHE concentrations are below reference range or inadequate to support normal linear growth, administration of L-PHE in small amounts may be required.[214] Serving lists (see Table 5.3) used in the PHE-restricted diet have portion sizes of individual foods in each list (given in reference 80) and are helpful in diet planning. The USDA website[217] also provides information on the amino acid, protein, energy, and other nutrients in foods.

Initiation of Nutrition Management and During Illness or Following Trauma

As with PKU, the most rapid decline of plasma TYR concentration at the time of diagnosis may be obtained by feeding a 20 kcal/oz (67 kcal/dL) PHE- and TYR-free formula with no added sources of PHE and TYR for up to 48 hours. Energy intake above 120 kcal/kg/day and protein of 3.5 g/kg BW are required to prevent the early catabolic phase in the neonate. Laboratory results of plasma concentrations of PHE and TYR should be rapidly available or deficiency of PHE and TYR[214,215] could be precipitated. Catabolism due to inadequate intake of energy, PHE, TYR, or protein is particularly undesirable in treating tyrosinemia type I because a catabolic phase with overproduction of succinylacetone will worsen the clinical state. Intact protein sources containing adequate PHE and TYR to maintain treatment concentrations are usually required after 2 days of total restriction following the diagnostic period in the patient with tyrosinemia type II or III. Patients with tyrosinemia type I may tolerate more dietary PHE and TYR when managed with NTBC than in patients not receiving NTBC (see Table 5.1).[27] The protein catabolism and increased energy expenditure that result from infection or following trauma[84] require therapy to depress catabolism and maintain electrolyte homeostasis if vomiting or diarrhea is present. As in PKU, rapid diagnosis and treatment to prevent prolonged elevated plasma PHE and TYR concentrations and support hydration and electrolyte balance are essential. (See this chapter: Phenylketonuria: Initiation of Nutrition Management and During Illness or Following Trauma.)

Assessment of Nutrition Management

Frequency of assessment depends on the type of tyrosinemia and clinical course of the patient. In patients with tyrosinemias, vital signs, height, weight, head circumference, neurologic examination, and development are documented weekly for the first 3 months, biweekly for the second 3 months, and monthly from 6 months of life and onward. Plasma amino acids, succinylacetone, and p-hydroxyphenyl organic acids are assessed routinely in patients with tyrosinemia type I. Laboratory studies in tyrosinemia type I include urinary δ-ALA, blood and urine assessment of renal losses (HCO_3, K+, Na+), and liver status (1,25-dihydroxycholecalciferol, α-fetoprotein, and liver function tests). Clinical status, dietary intake, and laboratory data for assessment of biochemical status (see Chapter 3) should be monitored and correlated in managing tyrosinemia at intervals indicated if required by the clinical course.[27] Application for eventual liver transplant should be initiated early in life for patients with tyrosinemia type I. Patients with tyrosinemia type II will require routine assessment of eyes and skin, particularly if plasma TYR concentrations are not well controlled.

Results of Nutrition Management

With early diagnosis and control of plasma TYR concentrations in treatment range, ocular and cutaneous lesions as well as mental retardation may be prevented in patients with tyrosinemia type II, although mental retardation is variable and occurs in less than half the patients.[201,218,219] Of 12 patients with tyrosinemia type III, 5 of whom were diagnosed and treated from the newborn period, 3 were developmentally normal. Of the seven late-diagnosed patients, two were lost to follow up, and five were intellectually impaired. From this report,[220] it is unclear whether a PHE- and TYR-restricted diet alters the outcome of patients with tyrosinemia type III, but did appear to be beneficial in three of the patients in whom it was begun in infancy. Few children have been symptomatic with hawkinsinuria, although symptoms have occurred in some infants following weaning from human milk.[201]

Hawkinsinuria has not been reported to occur after infancy, despite progressive discontinuation of diet.

Tyrosinemia type I due to FAH deficiency, when untreated by a PHE- and TYR-restricted diet and NTBC, results in death of most patients in early childhood. Infants treated before the age of 2 months with diet and NTBC had a 4-year survival rate of 88% vs 29% of those treated with diet alone, while children treated by diet and NTBC after 6 months of age had a 10-year survival rate of 85% vs 60% of those treated by diet only. Early NTBC treatment with diet also reduced the incidence of liver transplantation.[212]

Maternal Tyrosinemia

Introduction

Since TYR, like PHE, is actively transported across the placenta, concentrations in maternal amniotic and fetal fluids are increased during pregnancy of untreated women with tyrosinemia type II. Whether these elevated concentrations affect fetal development is unclear. Although offspring of some untreated mothers have developed normally,[201,221] others have presented with mental retardation, seizures, and malformations.[201,222]

Nutrition Management

Careful control of plasma TYR concentrations during pregnancy resulted in a normal infant.[221] Consequently, in order to avoid risk to the fetus, maternal plasma TYR concentrations during pregnancy should be maintained between 75 and 150 µmol/L.[221] Recommendations for beginning therapy are given in Table 5.1. Both PHE and TYR intakes require modification if plasma concentration of either is not in treatment range. By mid-gestation, requirements for both PHE and TYR will have usually doubled. Protein intake, when free amino acids are used as the major source of protein equivalent (nitrogen, g × 6.25), should be greater than recommended intakes (see Chapter 3, Table 3.1).[73] Energy intake should provide for appropriate weight gain, and should be greater for the underweight woman than for the normal or overweight (see Chapter 3, Table 3.1). Modified very-low-protein foods (see Appendix E), along with fats that contain adequate linoleic and α-linolenic acids (see Appendix F), should be provided to supply energy and essential fatty acids. Recommended fluid intake is about 1 mL/kcal. Mineral and vitamin intakes recommended for the pregnant woman ingesting elemental medical foods are given in Chapter 3, Table 3.1, and are greater than recommended by RDA[73] due to poor absorption.[77]

Assessment of Nutrition Management

Twice-weekly assessment of nutrient intake from a prior 3-day diet diary maintained by the pregnant woman just prior to obtaining blood for analysis of plasma PHE and TYR concentrations is essential to quality care. See Chapter 3, Table 3.8 for 2- to 5-hour postprandial selected plasma amino acid concentrations in normal pregnant women. Routine assessment of other biochemical indices of nutrition status are required (see Chapter 3, Table 3.7), and assessment of fetal growth during pregnancy is useful.[27]

CONCLUSION

Nutrition management of patients with PKU or tyrosinemia type II can result in normal growth and development if started early in the neonatal period, plasma concentrations of specific analytes are maintained in appropriate ranges, and nutrient intakes are adequate. For offspring of women with an inherited metabolic disorder to grow and develop normally, nutrition management, if previously discontinued, should be initiated prior to conception and plasma concentrations of specific analytes controlled throughout pregnancy. For best functioning as an adult, nutrition management should be lifelong.

REFERENCES

1. National Center for Biotechnology Information. OMIM™-Online Mendelian Inheritance in Man™ (database). Available at: http://www.ncbi.nlm.nih.gov/sites/entrez?db=omim. Accessed February 2, 2008.
2. Folling A. The original detection of phenylketonuria. In: Bickel H, Hudson FP, Woolf LI, eds. *Phenylketonuria and Some Other Inborn Errors of Amino Acid Metabolism*. Stuttgart, Germany: Georg Thieme Verlag; 1971:1–3.
3. Bickel H, Gerrard E, Hickmans M. Influence of phenylalanine intake on phenylketonuria. *Lancet*. 1953;265:812–813.
4. Woolf LI, Griffiths R, Moncrieff A. Treatment of phenylketonuria with a diet low in phenylalanine. *Br Med J*. 1955;1:57–64.
5. Armstrong MD, Tyler FH. Studies on phenylketonuria. I. Restricted phenylalanine intake in phenylketonuria. *J Clin Invest*. 1955;34:565–580.
6. Blainey JR, Gulliford R. Phenylalanine-restricted diets in the treatment of phenylketonuria. *Arch Dis Child*. 1956;31:452–466.
7. Jervis GA. Phenylpyruvic oligophrenia deficiency of phenylalanine-oxidizing system. *Proc Soc Exp Biol Med*. 1953;82:514–515.
8. Matthews DM. Protein and amino acids. In: Shils ME, Shike M, Olson J, Ross AC, Caballero B, Coursins RJ, eds. *Modern Nutrition in Health and Disease*. 10th ed. Philadelphia, PA: Lippincott Williams & Wilkins; 2005:23–51.
9. Scriver CR, Kaufman S. The hyperphenylalaninemias. In: Scriver CR, Beaudet AL, Sly WS, Valle D, eds. *The Metabolic and Molecular Bases of Inherited Disease*. 8th ed. New York, NY: McGraw-Hill; 2001:1667–1724.

10. Salter M, Knowles RG, Pogson CI. Quantification of the importance of individual steps in the control of aromatic amino acid metabolism. *Biochem J.* 1986;234: 635–647.
11. Rampini S, Vollmin JA, Bosshard HR, Muller M, Curtius HC. Aromatic acids in urine of healthy infants, persistent hyperphenylalaninemia, and phenylketonuria, before and after phenylalanine load. *Pediatr Res.* 1974;8:704–709.
12. Picone TA, Benson JD, Moro G, et al. Growth, serum biochemistries, and amino acids of term infants fed formulas with amino acid and protein concentrations similar to human milk. *J Pediatr Gastroenterol Nutr.* 1989;9:351–360.
13. Gregory DM, Sovetts D, Clow CL, Scriver CR. Plasma-free amino acid values in normal children and adolescents. *Metabolism.* 1986;35:967–969.
14. Scriver CR, Gregory DM, Sovetts D, Tissenbaum G. Normal plasma-free amino acid values in adults: the influence of some common physiological variables. *Metabolism.* 1985;34:868–873.
15. Centerwall WR, Centerwall SA, Armon V, Mann LB. Phenylketonuria. II. Results of treatment of infants and young children. A report of 10 cases. *J Pediatr.* 1961; 59:102–118.
16. Scriver CR, Waters PJ, Sarkissian C, et al. PAHdb: a locus-specific knowledgebase. *Hum Mutat.* 2000;15:99–104.
17. Lichter-Konecki U, Hipke CM, Konecki DS. Human phenylalanine hydroxylase gene expression in kidney and other nonhepatic tissues. *Mol Genet Metab.* 1999;67:308–316.
18. Scriver CR. The PAH gene, phenylketonuria, and a paradigm shift. *Hum Mutat.* 2007;28:831–845.
19. PAHdb. Phenylalanine hydroxylase locus knowledgebase. Available at: http://www.pahdb.mcgill.ca. Accessed January 5, 2008.
20. Thony B, Blau N. Mutations in the BH_4-metabolizing genes GTP cyclohydrolase I, 6-pyruvoyl-tetrahydropterin synthase, sepiapterin reductase, carbinolamine-4α-dehydratase, and dihydropteridine reductase. *Hum Mutat.* 2006;27:870–878.
21. Koch JH. *Robert Guthrie: The PKU Story.* Pasadena, CA: Hope Publishing House; 1997:24.
22. Nellhaus G. Clinical use of phenistix reagent strip method of testing urine samples. *J Am Med Assoc.* 1959; 170:1052–1053.
23. Bickel H. Inborn errors of metabolism associated with brain damage. Recent advances in early detection and prevention of their manifestations. In: Holt LS, Coffey VP, eds. *Some Recent Advances in Inborn Errors of Metabolism.* London, England: E&S Livingstone; 1968:39–60.
24. Shaw KNF. Biochemical aspects of phenylketonuria. In: Shaw KNF, Koch R, Schild MSW, Ragsdale N, Fishler K, Acosta PB, eds. *The Clinical Team Looks at Phenylketonuria.* Washington, DC: U.S. Government Printing Office; 1961:1–7.
25. Guthrie R, Susi R. A simple phenylalanine method for detecting phenylketonuria in large populations of newborn infants. *Pediatrics.* 1963;32:338–343.
26. Chace DH, Millington DS, Terada N, Kahler SG, Roe CR, Hofman LF. Rapid diagnosis of phenylketonuria by quantitative analysis for phenylalanine and tyrosine in neonatal blood spots by tandem mass spectrometry. *Clin Chem.* 1993;39:66–71.
27. Elsas LJ, Acosta PB. Inherited metabolic disease: amino acids, organic acids, and galactose. In: Shils ME, Shike M, Olson J, Ross AC, Caballero B, Cousins RJ, eds. *Modern Nutrition in Health and Disease.* 10th ed. Philadelphia, PA: Lippincott Williams & Wilkins; 2005:909–959.

28. National Institutes of Health Consensus Statement. *Phenylketonuria (PKU): Screening and Management*. Bethesda, MD: National Institutes of Health; 2000; 1–31.
29. Koch R, Acosta PB, Shaw KNF, et al. Clinical aspects of phenylketonuria. In: Bickel H, Hudson FP, Woolf LI, eds. *Phenylketonuria and Some Other Inborn Errors of Amino Acid Metabolism*. Stuttgart, Germany: Georg Thieme Verlag; 1971:20–25.
30. Pitt DB, Danks DM. The natural history of untreated phenylketonuria over 20 years. *J Paediatr Child Health*. 1991;27:189–190.
31. Brunner RL, Brown EH, Berry HK. Phenylketonuria revisited: treatment of adults with behavioural manifestations. *J Inherit Metab Dis*. 1987;10:171–173.
32. Horner FA, Streamer CW, Alejandrino LL, Reed LH, Ibbott F. Termination of dietary treatment of phenylketonuria. *N Engl J Med*. 1962;266:79–81.
33. Hudson FP. Termination of dietary treatment of phenylketonuria. *Arch Dis Child*. 1967;42:198–200.
34. Holtzman NA, Kronmal RA, van Doorninck W, Azen C, Koch R. Effect of age at loss of dietary control on intellectual performance and behavior of children with phenylketonuria. *N Engl J Med*. 1986;314:593–598.
35. Seashore MR, Friedman E, Novelly RA, Bapat V. Loss of intellectual function in children with phenylketonuria after relaxation of dietary phenylalanine restriction. *Pediatrics*. 1985;75:226–232.
36. Thompson AJ, Smith I, Brenton D, et al. Neurological deterioration in young adults with phenylketonuria. *Lancet*. 1990;336:602–605.
37. Villasana D, Butler IJ, Williams JC, Roongta SM. Neurological deterioration in adult phenylketonuria. *J Inherit Metab Dis*. 1989;12:451–457.
38. Aung TT, Klied A, McGinn J, McGinn T. Vitamin B_{12} deficiency in an adult phenylketonuric patient. *J Inherit Metab Dis*. 1997;20:603–604.
39. Hanley WB, Feigenbaum A, Clarke JT, Schoonheyt W, Austin V. Vitamin B_{12} deficiency in adolescents and young adults with phenylketonuria. *Lancet*. 1993;342: 997.
40. Krause W, Epstein C, Averbook A, Dembure P, Elsas L. Phenylalanine alters the mean power frequency of electroencephalograms and plasma L-dopa in treated patients with phenylketonuria. *Pediatr Res*. 1986;20:1112–1116.
41. Elsas LJ, Trotter JF. Changes in physiological concentrations in blood phenylalanine produce changes in sensitive parameters of human brain function. *Dietary Phenylalanine and Brain Function*. Boston, MA: Birkhauser; 1987:187–195.
42. Channon S, Goodman G, Zlotowitz S, Mockler C, Lee PJ. Effects of dietary management of phenylketonuria on long-term cognitive outcome. *Arch Dis Child*. 2007;92:213–218.
43. Feldmann R, Denecke J, Grenzebach M, Weglage J. Frontal lobe-dependent functions in treated phenylketonuria: blood phenylalanine concentrations and long-term deficits in adolescents and young adults. *J Inherit Metab Dis*. 2005;28: 445–455.
44. Krause W, Halminski M, McDonald L, et al. Biochemical and neuropsychological effects of elevated plasma phenylalanine in patients with treated phenylketonuria. A model for the study of phenylalanine and brain function in man. *J Clin Invest*. 1985;75:40–48.
45. Schuett VE, Brown ES, Michals K. Reinstitution of diet therapy in PKU patients from twenty-two U.S. clinics. *Am J Public Health*. 1985;75:39–42.
46. Waisbren SE, Levy HL. Agoraphobia in phenylketonuria. *J Inherit Metab Dis*. 1991;14:755–764.

47. Dobbing J. The later development of the brain and its vulnerability. In: Davis JA, Dobbing J, eds. *Scientific Foundations of Paediatrics*. London, England: Heinemann; 1981:2073–2078.
48. Pardridge WM, Choi TB. Neutral amino acid transport at the human blood-brain barrier. *Fed Proc*. 1986;45:2073–2078.
49. Epstein CM, Trotter JF, Averbook A, Freeman S, Kutner MH, Elsas LJ. EEG mean frequencies are sensitive indices of phenylalanine effects on normal brain. *Electroencephalogr Clin Neurophysiol*. 1989;72:133–139.
50. Weglage J, Ullrich K, Pietsch M, Funders B, Guttler F, Harms E. Intellectual, neurologic, and neuropsychologic outcome in untreated subjects with nonphenylketonuria hyperphenylalaninemia. German Collaborative Study on Phenylketonuria. *Pediatr Res*. 1997;42:378–384.
51. Smith ML, Saltzman J, Klim P, Hanley WB, Feigenbaum A, Clarke JT. Neuropsychological function in mild hyperphenylalaninemia. *Am J Ment Retard*. 2000;105:69–80.
52. Weglage J, Pietsch M, Feldmann R, et al. Normal clinical outcome in untreated subjects with mild hyperphenylalaninemia. *Pediatr Res*. 2001;49:532–536.
53. Gassio R, Artuch R, Vilaseca MA, et al. Cognitive functions in classic phenylketonuria and mild hyperphenylalaninaemia: experience in a paediatric population. *Dev Med Child Neurol*. 2005;47:443–448.
54. Camfield CS, Joseph M, Hurley T, Campbell K, Sanderson S, Camfield PR. Optimal management of phenylketonuria: a centralized expert team is more successful than a decentralized model of care. *J Pediatr*. 2004;145:53–57.
55. Report of Medical Research Council Working Party on Phenylketonuria. Recommendations on the dietary management of phenylketonuria. *Arch Dis Child*. 1993;68:426–427.
56. Burgard P, Bremer HJ, Buhrdel P, et al. Rationale for the German recommendations for phenylalanine level control in phenylketonuria 1997. *Eur J Pediatr*. 1999;158: 46–54.
57. Abadie V, Berthelot J, Feillet F, et al. Management of phenylketonuria and hyperphenylalaninemia: the French guidelines (French). *Arch Pediatr*. 2005;12: 594–601.
58. Guldberg P, Mikkelsen I, Henriksen KF, Lou HC, Guttler F. In vivo assessment of mutations in the phenylalanine hydroxylase gene by phenylalanine loading: characterization of seven common mutations. *Eur J Pediatr*. 1995;154:551–556.
59. Acosta PB, Wenz E, Williamson M. Nutrient intake of treated infants with phenylketonuria. *Am J Clin Nutr*. 1977;30:198–208.
60. Acosta PB, Trahms C, Wellman NS, Williamson M. Phenylalanine intakes of 1- to 6-year-old children with phenylketonuria undergoing therapy. *Am J Clin Nutr*. 1983;38:694–700.
61. Kindt E, Motzfeldt K, Halvorsen S, Lie SO. Is phenylalanine requirement in infants and children related to protein intake? *Br J Nutr*. 1984;51:435–442.
62. Acosta PB, Yannicelli S. Protein intake affects phenylalanine requirements and growth of infants with phenylketonuria. *Acta Paediatr Suppl*. 1994;407:66–67.
63. Acosta PB, Michals-Matalon K, Austin V, et al. Nutrition findings and requirements in pregnant women with phenylketonuria. In: Platt LD, Koch R, de la Cruz F, eds. *Genetic Disorders and Pregnancy Outcome*. New York, NY: Parthenon; 1997: 21–32.
64. MacDonald A, Chakrapani A, Hendriksz C, et al. Protein substitute dosage in PKU: how much do young patients need? *Arch Dis Child*. 2006;91:588–593.

65. Snyderman SE, Pratt EL, Cheung MW, et al. The phenylalanine requirement of the normal infant. *J Nutr*. 1955;56:253–263.
66. Rose WC. Amino acid requirements of man. *Fed Proc*. 1949;8:546–552.
67. Hanley WB, Linsao L, Davidson W, Moes CA. Malnutrition with early treatment of phenylketonuria. *Pediatr Res*. 1970;4:318–327.
68. Shortland D, Smith I, Francis DEM, Ersser R, Wolff OH. Amino acid and protein requirements in a preterm infant with classic phenylketonuria. *Arch Dis Child*. 1985;60:263–265.
69. Batshaw ML, Valle D, Bessman SP. Unsuccessful treatment of phenylketonuria with tyrosine. *J Pediatr*. 1981;99:159–160.
70. Ajinomoto. *Amino Acids*. 8th ed. Teaneck, NJ: Ajinomoto, USA; 1997:132–133.
71. Herrmann ME, Brosicke HG, Keller M, Monch E, Helge H. Dependence of the utilization of a phenylalanine-free amino acid mixture on different amounts of single dose ingested. A case report. *Eur J Pediatr*. 1994;153:501–503.
72. Schoeffer A, Herrmann ME, Brosicke HG, Moench E. Effect of dosage and timing of amino acid mixtures on nitrogen retention in patients with phenylketonuria. *J Nutr Med*. 1994;4:415–418.
73. Otten JJ, Hellwig JP, Meyers LD. *Dietary Reference Intakes: The Essential Guide to Nutrient Requirements*. Washington, DC: National Academies Press; 2006.
74. Pratt EL, Snyderman SE, Cheung MW, et al. The threonine requirement of the normal infant. *J Nutr*. 1955;56:231–251.
75. Allen JR, McCauley JC, Waters DL, O'Connor J, Roberts DC, Gaskin KJ. Resting energy expenditure in children with phenylketonuria. *Am J Clin Nutr*. 1995;62: 797–801.
76. MacLean W, Graham G. *Pediatric Nutrition in Clinical Practice*. Menlo Park, CA: Addison-Wesley; 1982.
77. Alexander JW, Clayton BE, Delves HT. Mineral and trace-metal balances in children receiving normal and synthetic diets. *Q J Med*. 1974;169:80–111.
78. Lewis JS, Loskill S, Bunker ML, Acosta PB, Kim R. N-methylnicotinamide excretion of phenylketonuric children and a child with Hartnup disease before and after phenylalanine and tryptophan load. *Fed Proc*. 1974;33:666A.
79. Acosta PB, Centerwall WR. Phenylketonuria dietary management. *J Am Diet Assoc*. 1960;36:206–211.
80. Acosta PB, Yannicelli S. Phenylketonuria (PKU). *Nutrition Support Protocols*. 4th ed. Columbus, OH: Ross Products Division, Abbott Laboratories; 2001:1–32.
81. USDA Agricultural Research Service. *Nutrient Data Laboratory*. Available at: http://www.nal.usda.gov/fnic/foodcomp/search/. Accessed January 5, 2008.
82. Singh RH, Lesperance E, Crawford K. *PKUfoodlist*. Atlanta, GA: Division of Medical Genetics, Department Human Genetics, Emory University School of Medicine; 2006.
83. Acosta PB, Wenz E, Williamson M. Methods of dietary inception in infants with PKU. *J Am Diet Assoc*. 1978;72:164–169.
84. Lowry SF, Perez JM. The hypercatabolic state. In: Shils ME, Shike M, Olson J, Ross AC, Caballero B, Cousins RJ, eds. *Modern Nutrition in Health and Disease*. 10th ed. Philadelphia, PA: Lippincott Williams & Wilkins; 2005: 1381–1400.
85. Merrick J, Aspler S, Schwarz G. Phenylalanine-restricted diet should be life long. A case report on long-term follow-up of an adolescent with untreated phenylketonuria. *Int J Adolesc Med Health*. 2003;15:165–168.

86. Pardridge WM. Kinetics of competitive inhibition of neutral amino acid transport across the blood-brain barrier. *J Neurochem*. 1977;28:103–108.
87. Pardridge WM. Blood-brain barrier amino acid transport: clinical implications. In: Cockburn F, Gitzelmann R, eds. *Inborn Errors of Metabolism in Humans*. Lancaster, United Kingdom: MTP Press; 1982:87–99.
88. Hidalgo IJ, Borchardt RT. Transport of a large neutral amino acid (phenylalanine) in a human intestinal epithelial cell line: Caco-2. *Biochim Biophys Acta*. 1990; 1028:25–30.
89. Matalon R, Michals-Matalon K, Bhatia G, et al. Large neutral amino acids in the treatment of phenylketonuria (PKU). *J Inherit Metab Dis*. 2006;29:732–738.
90. Matalon R, Michals-Matalon K, Bhatia G, et al. Double-blind placebo control trial of large neutral amino acids in treatment of PKU: effect on blood phenylalanine. *J Inherit Metab Dis*. 2007;30:153–158.
91. Moats RA, Koch R, Moseley K, et al. Brain phenylalanine concentration in the management of adults with phenylketonuria. *J Inherit Metab Dis*. 2000;23:7–14.
92. Schindeler S, Ghosh-Jerath S, Thompson S, et al. The effects of large neutral amino acid supplements in PKU: an MRS and neuropsychological study. *Mol Genet Metab*. 2007;91:48–54.
93. Kure S, Hou DC, Ohura T, et al. Tetrahydrobiopterin-responsive phenylalanine hydroxylase deficiency. *J Pediatr*. 1999;135:375–378.
94. Blau N, Koch R, Matalon R, Stevens RC. Five years of synergistic scientific effort on phenylketonuria therapeutic development and molecular understanding. *Mol Genet Metab*. 2005;86:S1.
95. Perez B, Desviat LR, Gomez-Puertas P, Martinez A, Stevens RC, Ugarte M. Kinetic and stability analysis of PKU mutations identified in BH_4-responsive patients. *Mol Genet Metab*. 2005;86(Suppl 1):S11–S16.
96. Pey AL, Martinez A. The activity of wild-type and mutant phenylalanine hydroxylase and its regulation by phenylalanine and tetrahydrobiopterin at physiological and pathological concentrations: an isothermal titration calorimetry study. *Mol Genet Metab*. 2005;86(Suppl 1):S43–S53.
97. Trefz F, Burton B, Longo N, et al. PKU 006: the effect of sapropterin dihydrochloride (tetrahydrobiopterin 6R- BH_4) treatment on phenylalanine (PHE) tolerance in children with phenylketonuria controlled on a PHE-restricted diet. *J Inherit Metab Dis*. 2007;30(Suppl 1):17A.
98. Blaskovics ME. Hyperphenylalaninaemic variants. In: Seakins JWT, Saunders RA, Toothill C, eds. *Treatment of Inborn Errors of Metabolism*. Edinburgh, Scotland: Churchill Livingstone; 1973:23–29.
99. Hennermann JB, Buhrer C, Blau N, Vetter B, Monch E. Long-term treatment with tetrahydrobiopterin increases phenylalanine tolerance in children with severe phenotype of phenylketonuria. *Mol Genet Metab*. 2005;86(Suppl 1):S86–S90.
100. Lambruschini N, Perez-Duenas B, Vilaseca MA, et al. Clinical and nutritional evaluation of phenylketonuric patients on tetrahydrobiopterin monotherapy. *Mol Genet Metab*. 2005;86(Suppl 1):S54–S60.
101. Singh RH, Jurecki E, Rohr F. Recommendations for personalized dietary adjustments based on patient response to tetrahydrobiopterin (BH_4) in phenylketonuria. *TICN*. 2008;22:149–157.
102. Gramer G, Burgard P, Garbade SF, Lindner M. Effects and clinical significance of tetrahydrobiopterin supplementation in phenylalanine hydroxylase-deficient hyperphenylalaninaemia. *J Inherit Metab Dis*. 2007;30:556–562.

103. Blau N, Thony B, Cotton RGH, Hyland K. Disorders of tetrahydrobiopterin and related biogenic amines. In: Scriver CR, Beaudet AL, Sly WS, Valle D, eds. *The Metabolic and Molecular Bases of Inherited Disease*. New York, NY: McGraw-Hill; 2001:1725–1776.
104. Shintaku H. Disorders of tetrahydrobiopterin metabolism and their treatment. *Curr Drug Metab*. 2002;3:123–131.
105. Tanaka Y, Kato M, Muramatsu T, et al. Early initiation of L-dopa therapy enables stable development of executive function in tetrahydrobiopterin (BH_4) deficiency. *Dev Med Child Neurol*. 2007;49:372–376.
106. Wang L, Yu WM, He C, et al. Long-term outcome and neuroradiological findings of 31 patients with 6-pyruvoyltetrahydropterin synthase deficiency. *J Inherit Metab Dis*. 2006;29:127–134.
107. Jaggi L, Zurfluh MR, Schuler A, et al. Outcome and long-term follow-up of 36 patients with tetrahydrobiopterin deficiency. *Mol Genet Metab*. 2008;93:295–305.
108. Azen CG, Koch R, Friedman EG, et al. Intellectual development in 12-year-old children treated for phenylketonuria. *Am J Dis Child*. 1991;145:35–39.
109. Brumm VL, Azen C, Moats RA, et al. Neuropsychological outcome of subjects participating in the PKU adult collaborative study: a preliminary review. *J Inherit Metab Dis*. 2004;27:549–566.
110. Trefz FK, Burgard P, Konig T, et al. Genotype-phenotype correlations in phenylketonuria. *Clin Chim Acta*. 1993;217:15–21.
111. Waisbren SE, Noel K, Fahrbach K, et al. Phenylalanine blood levels and clinical outcomes in phenylketonuria: a systematic literature review and meta-analysis. *Mol Genet Metab*. 2007;92:63–70.
112. Dodge PR, Mancall EL, Crawford JD, Knapp J, Paine RS. Hypoglycemia-complicating treatment of phenylketonuria with a phenylalanine-deficient diet; report of two cases. *N Engl J Med*. 1959;260:1104–1111.
113. Fisch RO, Gravem HJ, Feinberg SB. Growth and bone characteristics of phenylketonurics. Comparative analysis of treated and untreated phenylketonuric children. *Am J Dis Child*. 1966;112:3–10.
114. Wilson KM, Clayton BE. Importance of choline during growth, with particular reference to synthetic diets in phenylketonuria. *Arch Dis Child*. 1962;37:565–577.
115. Royston NJW, Parry TE. Megaloblastic anaemia complicating dietary treatment of phenylketonuria in infancy. *Arch Dis Child*. 1962;37:430–435.
116. Sherman JD, Greenfield JB, Ingall D. Reversible bone-marrow vacuolizations in phenylketonuria. *N Engl J Med*. 1964;270:810–814.
117. Acosta PB, Yannicelli S, Marriage B, et al. Protein status of infants with phenylketonuria undergoing nutrition management. *J Am Coll Nutr*. 1999;18:102–107.
118. Buist NR, Prince AP, Huntington KL, Tuerck JM, Waggoner DD. A new amino acid mixture permits new approaches to the treatment of phenylketonuria. *Acta Paediatr Suppl*. 1994;407:75–77.
119. Acosta PB, Greene C, Yannicelli S. Nutrition studies in treated infants with phenylketonuria. *Int Pediatr*. 1993;8:6–16.
120. Arnold GL, Vladutiu CJ, Kirby RS, Blakely EM, Deluca JM. Protein insufficiency and linear growth restriction in phenylketonuria. *J Pediatr*. 2002;141:243–246.
121. Acosta PB, Yannicelli S. Nutrient intake and biochemical status of children with phenylketonuria undergoing nturition management. Unpublished data. Columbus, OH: Ross Products Division, Abbott Laboratories; 2003.

122. Sibinga MS, Friedman CJ, Steisel IM, Baker EC. The depressing effect of diet on physical growth in phenylketonuria. *Dev Med Child Neurol*. 1971;13:63–70.
123. Holm VA, Kronmal RA, Williamson M, Roche AF. Physical growth in phenylketonuria: II. Growth of treated children in the PKU collaborative study from birth to 4 years of age. *Pediatrics*. 1979;63:700–707.
124. McBurnie MA, Kronmal RA, Schuett VE, Koch R, Azen CG. Physical growth of children treated for phenylketonuria. *Ann Hum Biol*. 1991;18:357–368.
125. Williamson M, Azen C, Acosta P. A computerized procedure for estimating nutrient intake. *J Toxicol Environ Health*. 1976;2:481–487.
126. Acosta PB, Yannicelli S, Marriage B, et al. Nutrient intake and growth of infants with phenylketonuria undergoing therapy. *J Pediatr Gastroenterol Nutr*. 1998;27: 287–291.
127. Acosta PB, Yannicelli S, Singh R, et al. Nutrient intakes and physical growth of children with phenylketonuria undergoing nutrition therapy. *J Am Diet Assoc*. 2003; 103:1167–1173.
128. Verkerk PH, van Spronsen FJ, Smit GPA, Sengers RC. Impaired prenatal and postnatal growth in Dutch patients with phenylketonuria. *Arch Dis Child*. 1994;71: 114–118.
129. Hoeksma M, Van Rijn M, Verkerk PH, et al. The intake of total protein, natural protein and protein substitute and growth of height and head circumference in Dutch infants with phenylketonuria. *J Inherit Metab Dis*. 2005;28:845–854.
130. Schaefer F, Burgard P, Batzler U, et al. Growth and skeletal maturation in children with phenylketonuria. *Acta Paediatr*. 1994;83:534–541.
131. Dhondt JL, Largilliere C, Moreno L, Farriaux JP. Physical growth in patients with phenylketonuria. *J Inherit Metab Dis*. 1995;18:135–137.
132. Dobbelaere D, Michaud L, Debrabander A, et al. Evaluation of nutritional status and pathophysiology of growth retardation in patients with phenylketonuria. *J Inherit Metab Dis*. 2003;26:1–11.
133. Huemer M, Huemer C, Moslinger D, Huter D, Stockler-Ipsiroglu S. Growth and body composition in children with classical phenylketonuria: results in 34 patients and review of the literature. *J Inherit Metab Dis*. 2007;30:694–699.
134. van Spronsen FJ, Verkerk PH, van Houten M, et al. Does impaired growth of PKU patients correlate with the strictness of dietary treatment? National Dutch PKU Steering Committee. *Acta Paediatr*. 1997;86:816–818.
135. Goldstein FB. Phenylpyruvic oligophrenia. PhD thesis. McGill University. 1955.
136. Woolf LI. Excretion of conjugated phenylacetic acid in phenylketonuria. *Biochem J*. 1951;49:ix–x.
137. Acosta PB, Alfin-Slater RB, Koch R. Serum lipids in children with phenylketonuria (PKU). *J Am Diet Assoc*. 1973;63:631–635.
138. Galluzzo CR, Ortisi MT, Castelli L, Agostoni C, Longhi R. Plasma lipid concentrations in 42 treated phenylketonuric children. *J Inherit Metab Dis*. 1985;8(Suppl 2): 129.
139. Castillo M, Zafra MF, Garcia-Peregrin E. Inhibition of brain and liver 3-hydroxy-3-methylglutaryl-CoA reductase and mevalonate-5-pyrophosphate decarboxylase in experimental hyperphenylalaninemia. *Neurochem Res*. 1988;13:551–555.
140. Colomé C, Artuch R, Lambruschini N, Cambra FJ, Campistol J, Vilaseca M. Is there a relationship between plasma phenylalanine and cholesterol in phenylketonuric patients under dietary treatment? *Clin Biochem*. 2001;34:373–376.

141. Galli C, Agostoni C, Mosconi C, Riva E, Salari PC, Giovannini M. Reduced plasma C-20 and C-22 polyunsaturated fatty acids in children with phenylketonuria during dietary intervention. *J Pediatr*. 1991;119:562–567.
142. Sanjurjo P, Perteagudo L, Rodriguez-Soriano J, Vilaseca A, Campistol J. Polyunsaturated fatty acid status in patients with phenylketonuria. *J Inherit Metab Dis*. 1994;17:704–709.
143. Acosta PB, Yannicelli S, Singh R, et al. Intake and blood levels of fatty acids in treated patients with phenylketonuria. *J Pediatr Gastroenterol Nutr*. 2001;33: 253–259.
144. Carnielli VP, Simonato M, Verlato G, et al. Synthesis of long-chain polyunsaturated fatty acids in preterm newborns fed formula with long-chain polyunsaturated fatty acids. *Am J Clin Nutr*. 2007;86:1323–1330.
145. Campistol J, Fons C, Vilaseca MA, et al. Visual function abnormalities in PKU patients: lack of correlation with deficient plasma docosahexaenoic acid. *J Inherit Metab Dis*. 2007;30:12A.
146. Poisson JP, Dupuy RP, Sarda P, et al. Evidence that liver microsomes of human neonates desaturate essential fatty acids. *Biochim Biophys Acta*. 1993;1167: 109–113.
147. Demmelmair H, von Schenck U, Behrendt E, Sauerwald T, Koletzko B. Estimation of arachidonic acid synthesis in full term neonates using natural variation of 13C content. *J Pediatr Gastroenterol Nutr*. 1995;21:31–36.
148. Carnielli VP, Wattimena DJ, Luijendijk IH, Boerlage A, Degenhart HJ, Sauer PJ. The very low birth weight premature infant is capable of synthesizing arachidonic and docosahexaenoic acids from linoleic and linolenic acids. *Pediatr Res*. 1996;40: 169–174.
149. Salem N Jr, Wegher B, Mena P, Uauy R. Arachidonic and docosahexaenoic acids are biosynthesized from their 18-carbon precursors in human infants. *Proc Natl Acad Sci USA*. 1996;93:49–54.
150. Moore SA, Yoder E, Murphy S, Dutton GR, Spector AA. Astrocytes, not neurons, produce docosahexaenoic acid (22:6 omega-3) and arachidonic acid (20:4 omega-6). *J Neurochem*. 1991;56:518–524.
151. Moore SA, Hurt E, Yoder E, Sprecher H, Spector AA. Docosahexaenoic acid synthesis in human skin fibroblasts involves peroxisomal retroconversion of tetracosahexaenoic acid. *J Lipid Res*. 1995;36:2433–2443.
152. Al Qadreh A, Schulpis KH, Athanasopoulou H, Mengreli C, Skarpalezou A, Voskaki I. Bone mineral status in children with phenylketonuria under treatment. *Acta Paediatr*. 1998;87:1162–1166.
153. Carson DJ, Greeves LG, Sweeney LE, Crone MD. Osteopenia and phenylketonuria. *Pediatr Radiol*. 1990;20:598–599.
154. Hillman L, Schlotzhauer C, Lee D, et al. Decreased bone mineralization in children with phenylketonuria under treatment. *Eur J Pediatr*. 1996;155(Suppl 1): S148–S152.
155. McMurry MP, Chan GM, Leonard CO, Ernst SL. Bone mineral status in children with phenylketonuria—relationship to nutritional intake and phenylalanine control. *Am J Clin Nutr*. 1992;55:997–1004.
156. Greeves LG, Carson DJ, Magee A, Patterson CC. Fractures and phenylketonuria. *Acta Paediatr*. 1997;86:242–244.
157. Yannicelli S, Medeiros DM. Elevated plasma phenylalanine concentrations may adversely affect bone status of phenylketonuric mice. *J Inherit Metab Dis*. 2002;25:347–361.

158. Schulpis KH, Papakonstantinou E, Michelakakis H, Theodoridis T, Papandreou U, Constantopoulos A. Elevated serum prolactin concentrations in phenylketonuric patients on a "loose diet." *Clin Endocrinol (Oxf)*. 1998;48:99–101.
159. Tanko LB, Bagger YZ, Nielsen SB, Christiansen C. Does serum cholesterol contribute to vertebral bone loss in postmenopausal women? *Bone*. 2003;32:8–14.
160. Boivin G, Vedi S, Purdie DW, Compston JE, Meunier PJ. Influence of estrogen therapy at conventional and high doses on the degree of mineralization of iliac bone tissue: a quantitative microradiographic analysis in postmenopausal women. *Bone*. 2005;36:562–567.
161. Suganuma N, Furuhashi M, Hirooka T, et al. Bone mineral density in adult patients with Turner's syndrome: analyses of the effectiveness of GH and ovarian steroid hormone replacement therapies. *Endocr J*. 2003;50:263–269.
162. Hillman L, Sateesha S, Haussler M, Wiest W, Slatopolsky E, Haddad J. Control of mineral homeostasis during lactation: interrelationships of 25-hydroxyvitamin D, 24,25-dihydroxyvitamin D, 1,25-dihydroxyvitamin D, parathyroid hormone, calcitonin, prolactin, and estradiol. *Am J Obstet Gynecol*. 1981;139: 471–476.
163. Klibanski A, Greenspan SL. Increase in bone mass after treatment of hyperprolactinemic amenorrhea. *N Engl J Med*. 1986;315:542–546.
164. Bodley JL, Austin VJ, Hanley WB, Clarke JT, Zlotkin S. Low iron stores in infants and children with treated phenylketonuria: a population at risk for iron-deficiency anaemia and associated cognitive deficits. *Eur J Pediatr*. 1993;152: 140–143.
165. Gropper SS, Trahms C, Cloud HH, Isaacs JS, Malinauskas B. Iron deficiency without anemia in children with phenylketonuria. *Int Pediatr*. 1994;9:237–243.
166. Acosta PB, Yannicelli S. Plasma micronutrient concentrations in infants undergoing therapy for phenylketonuria. *Biol Trace Elem Res*. 1999;67:75–84.
167. Acosta PB, Yannicelli S, Singh RH, Elsas LJ, Mofidi S, Steiner RD. Iron status of children with phenylketonuria undergoing nutrition therapy assessed by transferrin receptors. *Genet Med*. 2004;6:96–101.
168. Gropper SS, Yannicelli S, White BD, Medeiros DM. Plasma phenylalanine concentrations are associated with hepatic iron content in a murine model for phenylketonuria. *Mol Genet Metab*. 2004;82:76–82.
169. Lombeck I, Kasperek K, Feinendegen LE, Bremer HJ. Serum-selenium concentrations in patients with maple-syrup-urine disease and phenylketonuria under dietotherapy. *Clin Chim Acta*. 1975;64:57–61.
170. Darling G, Mathias P, O'Regan M, Naughten E. Serum selenium levels in individuals on PKU diets. *J Inherit Metab Dis*. 1992;15:769–773.
171. Collins RJ, Boyle PJ, Clague AE, Barr AE, Latham SC. In vitro OKT3-induced mitogenesis in selenium-deficient patients on a diet for phenylketonuria. *Biol Trace Elem Res*. 1991;30:233–244.
172. Greeves LG, Carson DJ, Craig BG, McMaster D. Potentially life-threatening cardiac dysrhythmia in a child with selenium deficiency and phenylketonuria. *Acta Paediatr Scand*. 1990;79:1259–1262.
173. Calomme M, Vanderpas J, Francois B, et al. Effects of selenium supplementation on thyroid hormone metabolism in phenylketonuria subjects on a phenylalanine restricted diet. *Biol Trace Elem Res*. 1995;47:349–353.
174. Acosta PB, Fernhoff PM, Warshaw HS, et al. Zinc status and growth of children undergoing treatment for phenylketonuria. *J Inherit Metab Dis*. 1982;5: 107–110.

175. La Du BN, Zannoni VG. Basic biochemical disturbances in aromatic amino acid metabolism in phenylketonuria. In: Bickel H, Hudson FP, Woolf LI, eds. *Phenylketonuria and Some Other Inborn Errors of Amino Acid Metabolism.* Stuttgart, Germany: Georg Thieme Verlag; 1971:6–13.
176. Schulpis KH, Nyalala JO, Papakonstantinou ED, et al. Biotin recycling impairment in phenylketonuric children with seborrheic dermatitis. *Int J Dermatol.* 1998;37:918–921.
177. Dent CE. The relation of biochemical abnormality to the development of the mental defect in phenylketonuria. Report of the Twenty-Third Ross Pediatric Research Conference. Columbus, OH: Ross Laboratories; 1957:28–33.
178. Mabry CC, Denniston JC, Nelson TL, Son CD. Maternal phenylketonuria. A cause of mental retardation in children without the metabolic defect. *N Engl J Med.* 1963;269:1404–1408.
179. Lenke RR, Levy HL. Maternal phenylketonuria and hyperphenylalaninemia. An international survey of the outcome of untreated and treated pregnancies. *N Engl J Med.* 1980;303:1202–1208.
180. Kudo Y, Boyd CA. Transport of amino acids by the human placenta: predicted effects thereon of maternal hyperphenylalaninaemia. *J Inherit Metab Dis.* 1990;13:617–626.
181. Hanley WB, Clarke JTR, Schoonheyt W. Maternal phenylketonuria (PKU)—a review. *Clin Biochem.* 1987;20:149–156.
182. Kirby ML, Miyagawa ST. The effects of high phenylalanine concentration on chick embryonic development. *J Inherit Metab Dis.* 1990;13:634–640.
183. Okano Y, Chow IZ, Isshiki G, Inoue A, Oura T. Effects of phenylalanine loading on protein synthesis in the fetal heart and brain of rat: an experimental approach to maternal phenylketonuria. *J Inherit Metab Dis.* 1986;9:15–24.
184. Smith I, Glossop J, Beasley M. Fetal damage due to maternal phenylketonuria: effects of dietary treatment and maternal phenylalanine concentrations around the time of conception. *J Inherit Metab Dis.* 1990;13:651–657.
185. Michals-Matalon K, Acosta PB, Azen C. Five-year postnatal growth of offspring of women with phenylketonuria in the Maternal PKU Collaborative Study. *J Inherit Metab Dis.* 2007;30:19A.
186. Koch R, Hanley W, Levy H, et al. The Maternal Phenylketonuria International Study: 1984–2002. *Pediatrics.* 2003;112:1523–1529.
187. Levy HL, Waisbren SE, Guttler F, et al. Pregnancy experiences in the woman with mild hyperphenylalaninemia. *Pediatrics.* 2003;112:1548–1552.
188. Trefz FK, Blau N. Potential role of tetrahydrobiopterin in the treatment of maternal phenylketonuria. *Pediatrics.* 2003;112:1566–1569.
189. Koch R, Moseley K, Guttler F. Tetrahydrobiopterin and maternal PKU. *Mol Genet Metab.* 2005;86(Suppl 1):S139–S141.
190. Matalon K, Acosta PB, Castiglioni L, et al. Protocol for nutrition support of maternal PKU. Bethesda, MD: The National Institute of Child Health and Human Development. 1998;1–51.
191. Acosta PB, Matalon K, Castiglioni L, et al. Intake of major nutrients by women in the Maternal Phenylketonuria (MPKU) Study and effects on plasma phenylalanine concentrations. *Am J Clin Nutr.* 2001;73:792–796.
192. Hunter JE. n-3 fatty acids from vegetable oils. *Am J Clin Nutr.* 1990;51:809–814.
193. Rothman KJ, Moore LL, Singer MR, Nguyen US, Mannino S, Milunsky A. Teratogenicity of high vitamin A intake. *N Engl J Med.* 1995;333:1369–1373.

194. Matalon KM, Acosta PB, Azen C. Role of nutrition in pregnancy with phenylketonuria and birth defects. *Pediatrics*. 2003;112:1534–1536.
195. Subcommittee on Nutritional Status and Weight Gain During Pregnancy. *Nutrition and Pregnancy*. Washington, DC: National Academy Press; 1990:1–233.
196. Brown AS, Fernhoff PM, Waisbren SE, et al. Barriers to successful dietary control among pregnant women with phenylketonuria. *Genet Med*. 2002;4:84–89.
197. Ng TW, Rae A, Wright H, Gurry D, Wray J. Maternal phenylketonuria in Western Australia: pregnancy outcomes and developmental outcomes in offspring. *J Paediatr Child Health*. 2003;39:358–363.
198. Lee PJ, Ridout D, Walter JH, Cockburn F. Maternal phenylketonuria: report from the United Kingdom Registry 1978–97. *Arch Dis Child*. 2005;90:143–146.
199. Feillet F, Abadie V, Berthelot J, et al. Maternal phenylketonuria: the French survey. *Eur J Pediatr*. 2004;163:540–546.
200. Magee AC, Ryan K, Moore A, Trimble ER. Follow up of fetal outcome in cases of maternal phenylketonuria in Northern Ireland. *Arch Dis Child Fetal Neonatal Ed*. 2002;87:F141–F143.
201. Mitchell GA, Grompe M, Lambert M, Tanguay RM. Hypertyrosinemia. In: Scriver CR, Beaudet AL, Sly WS, Valle D, eds. *The Metabolic and Molecular Bases of Inherited Disease*. 8th ed. New York, NY: McGraw-Hill; 2001:1777–1805.
202. Charfeddine C, Monastiri K, Mokni M, et al. Clinical and mutational investigations of tyrosinemia type II in Northern Tunisia: identification and structural characterization of two novel TAT mutations. *Mol Genet Metab*. 2006;88:184–191.
203. Maydan G, Andresen BS, Madsen PP, et al. TAT gene mutation analysis in three Palestinian kindreds with oculocutaneous tyrosinaemia type II; characterization of a silent exonic transversion that causes complete missplicing by exon 11 skipping. *J Inherit Metab Dis*. 2006;29:620–626.
204. Held PK. Disorders of tyrosine catabolism. *Mol Genet Metab*. 2006;88:103–106.
205. Ruetschi U, Cerone R, Perez-Cerda C, et al. Mutations in the 4-hydroxyphenylpyruvate dioxygenase gene (HPD) in patients with tyrosinemia type III. *Hum Genet*. 2000;106:654–662.
206. Arranz JA, Pinol F, Kozak L, et al. Splicing mutations, mainly IVS6-1(G>T), account for 70% of fumarylacetoacetate hydrolase (FAH) gene alterations, including 7 novel mutations, in a survey of 29 tyrosinemia type I patients. *Hum Mutat*. 2002;20:180–188.
207. Techakittiroj C, Cummingham A, Hopper PF, Andersson HC, Thoene J. High protein diet mimics hypertyrosinemia in newborn infants. *J Pediatr*. 2005;146: 281–282.
208. Allard P, Grenier A, Korson MS, Zytkovicz TH. Newborn screening for hepatorenal tyrosinemia by tandem mass spectrometry: analysis of succinylacetone extracted from dried blood spots. *Clin Biochem*. 2004;37:1010–1015.
209. Matern D, Tortorelli S, Oglesbee D, Gavrilov D, Rinaldo P. Reduction of the false-positive rate in newborn screening by implementation of MS/MS-based second-tier tests: the Mayo Clinic experience (2004–2007). *J Inherit Metab Dis*. 2007;30: 585–592.
210. Rice DN, Houston IB, Lyon IC, et al. Transient neonatal tyrosinaemia. *J Inherit Metab Dis*. 1989;12:13–22.
211. Holme E, Lindstedt S. Nontransplant treatment of tyrosinemia. *Clin Liver Dis*. 2000; 4:805–814.
212. Nitisinone: new drug. Type 1 tyrosinemia: an effective drug. *Prescrire Int*. 2007; 16:56–58.

213. Rank JM, Pascual-Leone A, Payne W, et al. Hematin therapy for the neurologic crisis of tyrosinemia. *J Pediatr*. 1991;118:136–139.
214. Wilson CJ, Van Wyk KG, Leonard JV, Clayton PT. Phenylalanine supplementation improves the phenylalanine profile in tyrosinaemia. *J Inherit Metab Dis*. 2000; 23:677–683.
215. Cohn RM, Yudkoff M, Yost B, Segal S. Phenylalanine-tyrosine deficiency syndrome as a complication of the management of hereditary tyrosinemia. *Am J Clin Nutr*. 1977;30:209–214.
216. Lieber CS. Nutrition in liver disorders. In: Shils ME, Shike M, Olson J, Ross AC, Caballero B, Cousins RJ, eds. *Modern Nutrition in Health and Disease*. 10th ed. Philadelphia, PA: Lippincott Williams & Wilkins; 2005:1235–1259.
217. United States Department of Agriculture Agricultural Research Service. Nutrient Data Laboratory. Available at: http://www.nal.usda.gov/fnic/foodcomp/search/. Accessed January 5, 2008.
218. Macsai MS, Schwartz TL, Hinkle D, Hummel MB, Mulhern MG, Rootman D. Tyrosinemia type II: nine cases of ocular signs and symptoms. *Am J Ophthalmol*. 2001;132:522–527.
219. Madan V, Gupta U. Tyrosinaemia type II with diffuse plantar keratoderma and self-mutilation. *Clin Exp Dermatol*. 2006;31:54–56.
220. Ellaway CJ, Holme E, Standing S, et al. Outcome of tyrosinaemia type III. *J Inherit Metab Dis*. 2001;24:824–832.
221. Francis DE, Kirby DM, Thompson GN. Maternal tyrosinaemia II: management and successful outcome. *Eur J Pediatr*. 1992;151:196–199.
222. Cerone R, Fantasia AR, Castellano E, Moresco L, Schiaffino MC, Gatti R. Pregnancy and tyrosinaemia type II. *J Inherit Metab Dis*. 2002;25:317–318.

Chapter 6

Nutrition Management of Patients with Inherited Disorders of Branched-Chain Amino Acid Metabolism

Barbara Marriage

INTRODUCTION

The branched-chain amino acids (BCAAs), leucine (LEU), valine (VAL), and isoleucine (ILE), are essential amino acids and cannot be deleted from the diet. The initial step in metabolism is transamination to the corresponding branched-chained organic acids and decarboxylation to form branched-chain acyl coenzyme A (CoA) products.[1] Maple syrup urine disease (MSUD) is caused by a deficiency of branched-chain α-ketoacid dehydrogenase (BCKD). Different pathways are utilized to metabolize each CoA product from LEU (isovaleryl–CoA), ILE (α-methylbutyryl-CoA), and VAL (isobutyryl-CoA). Defects in these pathways cause additional disorders referred to as branched-chain organic acidurias. The disorders for which nutrition management are outlined in this chapter are MSUD, isovaleric acidemia (IVA), β-methylcrotonyl-CoA carboxylase deficiency (βMCC), β-hydroxy-β-methylglutaryl-CoA (HMGCOA) lyase deficiency, and mitochondrial acetoacetyl-CoA thiolase deficiency, commonly known as β-ketothiolase (βKT) deficiency. A brief description of β-methylglutaconyl-CoA hydratase deficiency and β-hydroxy-α-methylbutyryl-CoA dehydrogenase deficiency is also included.

Maple Syrup Urine Disease

Introduction

MSUD (OMIM 24860)[2], or branched-chain α-ketoaciduria,[3] is an autosomal recessive disorder first described by Menkes, Hurst, and Craig in 1954. They observed four cases of familial cerebral degenerative disease in the first week of life resulting in death within three months. The urine of these infants smelled like maple syrup. The compounds accumulating in the plasma and urine were identified as BCAAs and their corresponding α-ketoacids (BCKAs).[4,5] In 1960, Dancis et al. demonstrated that the pathway was blocked at the decarboxylation of the respective BCKAs and the transamination of the BCAAs was not affected.[6] Pettit et al. confirmed that a single mitochondrial branched-chain α-ketoacid dehydrogenase complex was responsible for the decarboxylation of the three BCKAs.[7] In 1964, Snyderman at al. reported their experience with a restricted BCAA diet in seven patients with MSUD[8] and it was demonstrated that neurological manifestations could be prevented if nutrition management is instituted early.[8] This established the basis for long-term nutrition management of patients with MSUD.

Biochemistry

The BCAAs, LEU, ILE, and VAL, are neutral aliphatic amino acids, with a branched methyl group in the side chain. BCAAs account for approximately 35% of the essential amino acids in muscle and 40% of the essential amino acids required by humans.[1,9] Ingested BCAAs provide a major source for protein synthesis, but are also metabolized by skeletal muscle as an alternative energy source.[10] In humans, skeletal muscle is the major site of both transamination and oxidation of the BCAAs, followed by the liver, brain, kidney, and gastrointestinal tract.[11] The initial step in catabolism of LEU, ILE, and VAL is reversible transamination to form the respective BCKAs: α-ketoisocaproic acid, α-keto-β-methylvaleric acid, and α-ketoisovaleric acid (see Figure 6.1). The second step is the irreversible oxidative decarboxylation by the mitochondrial BCKD complex. The coenzymes thiamine pyrophosphate, lipoic acid, CoA, and nicotinamide adenine dinucleotide (NAD^+) are required for the reaction.[12] The defect in MSUD is the impairment of the BCKD complex (see Figure 6.1).

Molecular Biology

The BCKD complex (EC 1.2.4.4) is comprised of three enzymes: branched-chain α-ketoacid decarboxylase (E1), dihydrolipoamide acyltransferase (E2), and dihydrolipoyl dehydrogenase (E3; EC 1.8.1.4).[11] The mammalian BCKD

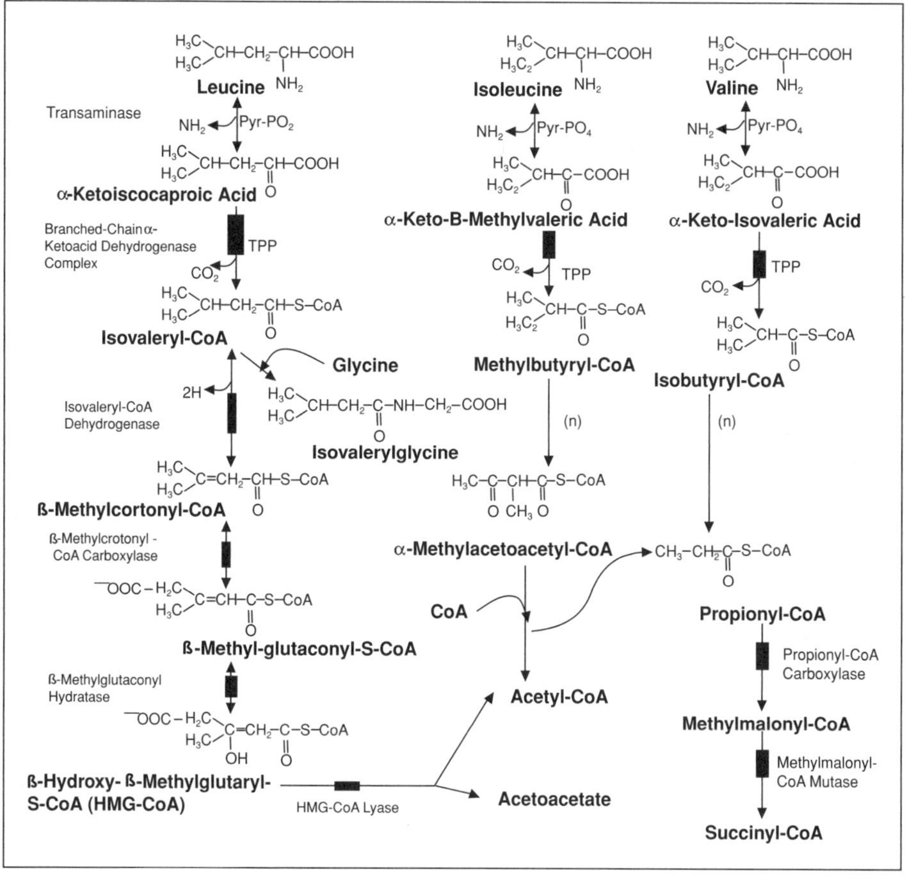

Figure 6.1 *Metabolism of Branched-Chain Amino Acids*

Source: Modified by permission of Elsas LJ, Acosta PB. Inherited metabolic disease: amino acids, organic acids, and galactose. In: Shils ME, Shike M, Olson J, Ross AC, Caballero B, Cousins RJ, eds. *Modern Nutrition in Health and Disease*. 10th ed. Philadelphia, PA: Lippincott Williams & Wilkins; 2005: 909–959. Courtesy of Wolters Kluwer Health.

Notes: Black bars indicate sites of enzyme defects.

(n) indicates several steps.

TPP = Thiamine pyrophosphate.

complex also contains a specific kinase and phosphatase that regulates activity through phosphorylation (inactivation) and dephosphorylation (activation).[1] The human E1 component contains two α and two β subunits: E1α is mapped to chromosome 19q13.1-q13.2, and E1β is localized to chromosome 6q14. The E2 gene is mapped to chromosome 1p31 and E3 is localized to chromosome 7q31-q32.[1] E3 is a component of the pyruvate dehydrogenase complex and α-ketoglutarate dehydrogenase complex, in addition to the BCKD complex. More than 60 mutations in the E1α, E1β, E2, and E3 subunits have been identified with the majority affecting the E1 gene. Evaluation of 63 cell lines from clinically diagnosed patients with MSUD indicated the following frequencies for the mutations: 33% for E1α, 38% for E1β, 19% for E2, and 10% unknown.[13] A similar distribution of mutations was found in a study of 15 patients with variant forms of MSUD: 37% of mutations in the E1α loci, 46% in the E1β, and 13% in the E2 domain[14] (see Chapter 1).

Newborn Screening

Newborn screening for MSUD has been performed since 1964 by the Guthrie bacterial inhibition assay on dried blood spots.[15] Since the early 1990s, tandem mass spectrometry (MS/MS) (see Chapter 2) has been the most common method for screening MSUD.[16] A blood LEU concentration greater than 153 μmol/L (2 mg/dL) or greater than 305 μmol/L (4 mg/dL) is used to identify newborns at risk for MSUD. There is not general agreement in the United States or other countries as to the concentration of LEU to be utilized in identifying possible cases of MSUD. Patients with the intermittent form of MSUD may not be detected by newborn screening, as blood concentrations of BCAAs are normal when the person is asymptomatic.[1]

Diagnosis

Newborn screening will identify patients with blood LEU concentrations above normal ranges. Amino acid and organic acid analyses are performed to confirm diagnosis, or when a patient presents with clinical symptoms. The BCAAs are markedly increased in blood, urine, and cerebrospinal fluid. The impaired ILE metabolism leads to the formation of alloisoleucine, a specific and sensitive diagnostic marker for MSUD.[17] The measurement of BCKD activity in cultured skin fibroblasts and lymphoblasts may be used to establish the deficiency of the complex, but it is not required for routine diagnosis. Compared to other single-gene disorders such as phenylketonuria, few MSUD mutations have been identified and the mutation analyses have not established a genotype/phenotype correlation. The most prevalent MSUD mutation is the Y393N mutation in the E1α subunit, found in the Mennonite population with MSUD.[18] The incidence of patients with MSUD varies with the population studied, from 1 in 560,000 live births in Japan to 1 in 176 live births in the Mennonite population of the eastern United States.[18,19] The worldwide incidence has been estimated at 1 in 185,000 live births.[1]

Clinical Phenotypes

Patients with MSUD can be divided into five clinical phenotypes—classic, intermediate, intermittent, thiamine-responsive, and dihydrolipoyl dehydrogenase (E3)-deficient MSUD.[1]

Classic

Approximately 80% of patients diagnosed with MSUD have the severe classic type with 0 to 2% of normal enzyme activity.[1,20] More than 50% of the BCKAs are derived from LEU; thus, tolerance for LEU is low. Infants may present within the first 2 weeks of life with poor feeding, lethargy, hypertonia, hypotonia, dystonia, ketoacidosis, and encephalopathic crisis.

Intermediate

The intermediate form of MSUD has residual BCKD enzyme activity ranging from 3 to 40% of normal and a clinical phenotype ranging from asymptomatic to severe developmental delay.[1,20,21] Patients with the intermediate form have higher tolerance for BCAAs than do patients with classic MSUD, and do not usually present with severe metabolic decompensation in the first weeks of life. Caution is advised, however, because these patients are at risk for metabolic decompensation in catabolic situations. Two patients have demonstrated a larger excretion of α-keto-β-methylvaleric acid (ILE derivative) compared to the amount of α-ketoisocaproic acid (LEU derivative) excretion typically seen in patients with classic MSUD.[21,22]

Intermittent

Patients with the intermittent form of MSUD usually show normal early growth and development. Plasma BCAA concentrations are normal when the patient is asymptomatic and residual enzyme activity ranges from 5 to 20% of normal.[1] During catabolic stress such as fasting, illness, infections, or surgery, clinical symptoms may present and plasma BCAA concentrations are markedly elevated. Although the initial symptoms generally appear between 5 months and 2 years, a case of a 46-year-old female has been reported, who was identified upon diagnosis of the disorder in her 2-year-old daughter.[23] Residual BCKD activity in fibroblasts was 12 to 16% of normal.[23]

Thiamine-Responsive

Patients with thiamine-responsive MSUD have been described with a clinical course similar to that found in patients with intermediate MSUD. The initial patient described was placed on 10 mg of thiamine per day with a resulting decrease in plasma BCAA concentrations.[24,25] Additional patients have been reported who have responded to thiamine dosages ranging from 10 to 1000 mg per day.[26-28] All treated patients have been on combined therapy of thiamine administration and BCAA restriction. The mechanism proposed is that ingested thiamine increases thiamine pyrophosphate and saturates the binding sites on the BCKD complex, inducing a conformational change making it more resistant to degradation and thereby increasing its activity.[27]

Dihydrolipoyl Dehydrogenase (E3)-Deficient MSUD

Dihydrolipoyl dehydrogenase deficiency is a rare disorder (fewer than 20 reported cases), and patients present with severe lactic acidosis in addition to elevated plasma concentrations of BCAAs.[1] These patients have a deficiency of three dehydrogenase complexes: BCKD, pyruvate dehydrogenase, and α-ketoglutarate dehydrogenase.

Outcomes if Untreated

Patients with untreated classic MSUD have severe mental and physical disabilities, and death may occur within a few weeks or months of life due to metabolic decompensation. The outcome of patients with MSUD has improved with early diagnosis and effective nutrition management, but complications may still arise due to catabolic stress and dietary noncompliance. Ophthalmic complications in untreated or late-diagnosed patients include optic atrophy, grey optic papilla, nystagmus, bilateral ptosis, strabismus, and cortical blindness.[29,30] A 6-month-old infant diagnosed with intermittent MSUD had cortical visual impairment and absent visual evoked potentials, which reversed over a period of 3 months with nutrition management.[30]

Cerebral edema with increased intracranial pressure has been described in neonates and in older patients during intercurrent illness. The pathogenesis of cerebral edema in MSUD is unknown, but altered amino acid metabolism affecting the blood–brain barrier, dehydration with increased osmolality, and rapid overhydration may contribute.[31]

Pancreatitis has been reported in patients with MSUD, generally preceded or accompanied by metabolic decompensation.[32,33] Pancreatitis with retinopathy was reported in a 7-year-old child with MSUD during an episode of gastroenteritis.[33] Recurrent infections are a common feature in patients with MSUD and it is postulated that elevated concentrations of the BCAAs and the corresponding ketoacids may act as immunosuppressants.[34]

Computerized tomography (CT) and magnetic resonance imaging (MRI) reveal dysmyelinating changes in patients with classic MSUD, which is related to chronic exposure to elevated BCAA concentrations.[35,36] In 14 patients (11 to 28 years old), the patients with good metabolic control (BCAAs below twice the normal concentration) showed near normal radiological examinations, whereas chronic elevations of BCAAs (BCAAs more than 4 times the normal concentration) were associated with severe radiological changes.[36] Although the pathogenesis of the neurological damage is poorly understood, LEU and the corresponding α-ketoisocaproic acid are thought to be the main contributors to the chronic brain dysfunction.[35,37]

The most important factor in determining intellectual outcome in patients with MSUD is the duration of time that the plasma BCAAs and metabolites are elevated in the neonatal period.[38-42] In addition, long-term metabolic control and acute decompensations have a major impact on the cognitive outcome of patients with MSUD.[39-41,43] Early diagnosis plus careful nutrition and medical management of patients with MSUD can result in normal intellectual outcome.[41,44]

Nutrition Management

The management of patients with MSUD consists of limiting the intake of BCAAs while maintaining normal growth and development. Early studies indicated that the optimal intake of BCAAs may be one-half to two-thirds of recommended requirements and must be individualized for each patient.[45] The goal of long-term therapy is to maintain postprandial (2 to 4 hours after a meal) plasma concentrations of the BCAAs in the following ranges: LEU, 80 to 200 μmol/L; ILE, 40 to 90 μmol/L; and VAL, 200 to 425 μmol/L.[44] To achieve optimal intellectual outcome, the target range for plasma LEU concentrations in infants and children is less than 200 μmol/L,[43] while adults may be able to tolerate plasma LEU concentrations up to 500 μmol/L without detrimental effects.[46]

Nutrient Requirements

BCAAs

The requirements for essential LEU, ILE, and VAL are outlined in Table 6.1. The requirements vary widely depending on the patient's age, growth rate, energy and protein intakes, health status, and amount of BCKD activity. The goal is to provide sufficient intake for normal growth without toxicity. The BCAA requirements for patients with MSUD appear to be 50 to 65% of the recommended intakes for healthy individuals.[44,45,47,48] The requirement for BCAAs declines rapidly during the first year of life; thus, it is recommended that plasma BCAA concentrations be monitored weekly during the first year of life.[48] Stabilization of the LEU requirement in classic MSUD occurs at 2 or 3 years of life and remains fairly constant until puberty.[49] A consistent daily intake of intact protein minimizes the occurrence of BCAA toxicity and possible negative nitrogen balance.

The content of ILE and VAL in intact protein is lower than LEU, which may necessitate the supplementation of these amino acids to maintain normal plasma concentrations. This can be achieved by use of LEU-free medical food or supplementation of L-ILE and L-VAL. Sources of purified free amino acids are given in Appendix G.

Table 6.1 ***Recommended Daily Nutrient Intakes for Infants, Children, and Adults with MSUD***

	Nutrient					
Age	*LEU (mg per kg)*	*ILE (mg per kg)*	*VAL (mg per kg)*	*Protein (g per kg)*	*Energy (kcal per kg)*	*Fluid (mL per kg)*
Infants, mo						
0 to 6	40–100	30–90	40–95	2.5–3.5	95–145	125–160
7 to 12	40–75	30–70	30–80	2.5–3.0	80–135	125–145
Children, yr						
1 to 3	40–70	20–70	30–70	1.5–2.5	80–130	115–135
4 to 8	35–65	20–30	30–50	1.3–2.0	50–120	90–115
9 to 13	30–60	20–30	25–40	1.2–1.8	40–90	70–90
14 to 18	15–50	10–30	15–30	1.2–1.8	35–70	40–60
Adults, yr						
Over 19	15–50	10–30	15–30	1.1–1.7	35–45	40–50

Sources:

Acosta PB, Yannicelli S. Protocol 5. Maple syrup urine disease (MSUD). *Nutrition Support Protocols.* Columbus, OH: Ross Products Division, Abbott Laboratories; 2001.

De Raeve L, De Meirleir L, Ramet J, Vandenplas Y, Gerlo E. Acrodermatitis enteropathica-like cutaneous lesions in organic aciduria. *J Pediatr.* 1994;124:416–420.

Elsas LJ, Acosta PB. Inherited metabolic disease: amino acids, organic acids and galactose. In: Shils ME, Shike M, Ross AC, Cabellero B, Cousins RJ, eds. *Modern Nutrition in Health and Disease.* 10th ed. Philadelphia, PA: Lippincott Williams & Wilkins; 2005:909–959.

Institute of Medicine of the National Academies. *Dietary Reference Intakes for Energy, Carbohydrate, Fiber, Fat, Fatty Acids, Cholesterol, Protein, and Amino Acids.* Washington, DC: National Academies Press; 2005.

Kindt E, Halvorsen S. The need of essential amino acids in children: an evaluation based on the intake of phenylalanine, tyrosine, leucine, isoleucine, and valine in children with phenylketonuria, tyrosine amino transferase defect, and maple syrup urine disease. *Am J Clin Nutr.* 1980;33:279–286.

Parsons HG, Carter RJ, Unrath M, Snyder FF. Evaluation of branched-chain amino acid intake in children with maple syrup urine disease and methylmalonic aciduria. *J Inherit Metab Dis.* 1990;13:125–136.

Note: Amino acid intake based on plasma amino acid concentrations. If protein is inadequate to support normal linear growth, see Chapter 3, Table 3.1, for recommended intake. Increase fluid intake during illness to enhance urinary ketoacid excretion.

Deficiencies or imbalances in BCAAs, particularly ILE deficiency, can result in dermatologic complications.[50-55] In 1973, Diliberti et al. reported a case of acrodermatitis enteropathica-like rash that they suggested was caused by an elevated LEU to ILE ratio.[51] Several cases of similar skin lesions in MSUD have been reported since that time.[52-54] The rash resolves within 24 to 48 hours after treatment with the deficient BCAAs. An isolated ILE deficiency has been reported that caused an acrodermatits enteropathica-like syndrome, emphasizing the importance of ILE in keratinocyte and enterocyte growth and differentiation.[55] In addition to skin lesions, corneal ulceration caused by an acute ILE deficiency has been reported in a newly diagnosed newborn with MSUD, emphasizing the importance of careful monitoring of BCAA concentrations during initiation of nutrition management.[56]

Protein and BCAA-Free Medical Foods

Because the primary source of protein equivalent (nitrogen, g × 6.25) is free amino acids, the recommended protein intake for patients with MSUD is higher (see Chapter 3) than the amounts specified by the Recommended Dietary Allowances (RDAs). Suggested protein intakes for patients with MSUD are outlined in Table 6.1, but should be individualized for each patient, if necessary to achieve normal linear growth. Table 6.2 gives sources and selected nutrient composition of BCAA-free medical foods.

A more rapid and elevated increase in plasma amino acid concentrations, followed by a rapid decline, has been noted after ingestion of free amino acids compared to an equivalent amount of amino acids provided as intact protein.[57] BCAA-free medical food should be consumed with other foods or beverages to try to slow the absorption rate. Frequent consumption of the medical food throughout the day is recommended.

In the first few months of life, proprietary infant formula or human milk is used to supply the BCAAs (see Appendix B). At 4 to 6 months of age, low-protein food choices gradually replace human milk or proprietary infant formula as a source of BCAAs. Several food lists are available to assist parents, caregivers, and patients with MSUD plan their BCAA-restricted diets.[58,59] In addition, the U.S. Department of Agriculture (USDA) website contains a nutrient database that is a reliable source of information for the nutrient composition of foods and includes amino acid data for most foods.[60] The amount of BCAAs allowed from intact protein is generally based on the LEU content, as LEU is more abundant than VAL and ILE in foods. The average LEU content of intact protein is approximately 8%, with a range of 3.5 to 10%.[44] Table 6.3 illustrates how to estimate the LEU content of foods when specific LEU information is not available.

Amino acid-based medical foods free of BCAAs (nitrogen, g × 6.25 = g protein equivalent) are utilized to supply the majority of the protein required in the diet. Most medical foods for MSUD contain fat, carbohydrate, vitamins, and minerals. Medical foods containing vitamins and minerals for the nutrition management of patients with MSUD are included in Table 6.2. If medical foods that do not contain vitamins and minerals are prescribed, they must be supplemented with multivitamin, multimineral sources to avoid nutrient deficiencies.

Table 6.2 *Nutrient Composition and Sources of Branched-Chain Amino Acid-Free Medical Foods*

Medical Foods	***Modified[a] Nutrient(s) (mg/100 g)***	***Protein Equiv[b] (g/100 g, source)***	***Fat (g/100 g, source)***	***Carbohydrate (g/100 g, source)***	***Energy (kcal/100 g/ kJ/100 g)***	***Linoleic Acid/ α-Linolenic Acid (mg/100 g)***
			Abbott Nutrition[c]			
Ketonex®-1	L-carnitine 100 Taurine 40	15 Amino acids[d]	21.7 High-oleic safflower, coconut, and soy oils	53 Corn syrup solids	480/2006	3500/350
Ketonex®-2	L-carnitine 200 Taurine 50	30 Amino acids[d]	14 High-oleic safflower, coconut, and soy oils	35 Corn syrup solids	410/1714	2200/230
			Applied Nutrition[e]			
Complex® MSUD Drink Mix	L-carnitine 30 Taurine 100	25 Amino acids[d]	14 Partially hydrogenated coconut oil	45 Sucrose, corn syrup solids, modified food starch	410/1714	380/60
Complex® Essential MSD	L-carnitine 550 Taurine NA	25 Amino acids[d]	13 Safflower, canola, soybean, coconut oils	45 Sugar, modified cornstarch, corn syrup solids	400/1672	2025/525
			Cambrooke Foods[f]			
Camino pro™ MSUD Drink	L-carnitine 30 Taurine NA	15 Amino acids[d]	0	26 Sugar	149/623	NA
Camino pro™ MSUD Bar	LEU 14, ILE 8, VAL 10, L-carnitine 9.57, Taurine NA	10 Amino acids[d]	3.6	39 Sugar	165/690	NA
Camino pro™ MSUD Sorbet Stix	L-carnitine 20.1 Taurine NA	10 Amino acids[d]	0	10.9 Sugar	70/293	NA

Table 6.2 *Nutrient Composition and Sources of Branched-Chain Amino Acid-Free Medical Foods, Continued*

Medical Foods	Modified[a] Nutrient(s) (mg/100 g)	Protein Equiv[b] (g/100 g, source)	Fat (g/100 g, source)	Carbohydrate (g/100 g, source)	Energy (kcal/100 g/ kJ/100 g)	Linoleic Acid/ α-Linolenic Acid (mg/100 g)
Mead Johnson[g]						
BCAD 1	L-carnitine 50 Taurine added	16.2 Amino acids[d]	26 Palm olein, soy, coconut, high oleic sunflower oils	51 Corn syrup solids, sugar, modified cornstarch, maltodextrin	500/2090	4500/380
BCAD 2	L-carnitine 49 Taurine added	24 Amino acids[d]	8.5 Soy oil	57 Corn syrup solids, sugar, modified cornstarch	410/1714	4600/610
Nutricia[h]						
Acerflex™	L-carnitine 20 Taurine 140	20 Amino acids[d]	17 Canola, high oleic safflower oils	40.5 Corn syrup solids	395/1651	2689/NA
MSUD Analog™	L-carnitine 10 Taurine 20	13 Amino acids[d]	20.9 High oleic safflower, coconut, soy oils	59 Corn syrup solids	475/1985	3025/NA
Milupa MSUD 2	L-carnitine 0 Taurine 0	54 Amino acids[d]	0	21 Sugar	300/1254	0
MSUD Maxamaid®	L-carnitine 20 Taurine 140	25 Amino acids[d]	<0.1	56 Sugar, corn syrup solids	324/1354	0

(continues)

Table 6.2 *Nutrient Composition and Sources of Branched-Chain Amino Acid-Free Medical Foods, Continued*

Medical Foods	*Modified[a] Nutrient(s) (mg/100 g)*	*Protein Equiv[b] (g/100 g, source)*	*Fat (g/100 g, source)*	*Carbohydrate (g/100 g, source)*	*Energy (kcal/100 g/ kJ/100 g)*	*Linoleic Acid/ α-Linolenic Acid (mg/100 g)*
MSUD Maxamum®	L-carnitine 39 Taurine 140	40 Amino acids[d]	<1	34 Sugar, corn syrup solids	305/1275	0
			Vitaflo[i]			
MSUD gel™	L-carnitine 12 Taurine 91.1	42 Amino acids[d]	<0.5	43 Sugar, starch, modified cornstarch	342/1428	NA
MSUD express™	L-carnitine 165.6 Taurine 129.6	60 Amino acids[d]	<0.5	15 Dried glucose syrup	302/1260	NA
MSUD express cooler	L-carnitine 0 Taurine NA	15 Amino acids[d]	<0.1	7.8 Sugar	92/385	NA

Notes:
NA = not available.
Values listed, although accurate at time of publication, are subject to change. The most current information may be obtained by referring to product labels.
[a]LEU-, ILE-, VAL-free unless specified.
[b]Nitrogen, g $\times$ 6.25 = g protein.
[c]Abbott Nutrition, 3300 Stelzer Road, Columbus, Ohio, 43219. 800-551-5838.
[d]All except glycine are in the L-form.
[e]Applied Nutrition Corp, 10 Saddle Road, Cedar Knolls, New Jersey 07927. 800-605-0410.
[f]Cambrooke Foods, Two Central Street, Framingham, Massachusetts 01701. 866-456-9776.
[g]Mead Johnson Nutritionals, 2400 West Lloyd Expressway, Evansville, Indiana 47721. 800-457- 3550.
[h]Nutricia North America, PO Box 117, Gaithersburg, Maryland 20884. 800-365-7354.
[i]Vitaflo US LLC, 123 East Neck Road, Huntington, New York 11743. 888-848-2356.

Table 6.3 *Estimation of the LEU Content of Foods*

Food	*Approx LEU (mg/g protein)*	*Example*
Fruits	40	1 cup raspberries = 1.5 g protein 1.48 × 40 = **60 mg LEU**
Vegetables	50	½ cup sweet pepper = 0.8 g protein 0.8 × 50 = **40 mg LEU**
Bread, crackers, and other starches	70	2 sq graham crackers = 1.0 g protein 1 × 70 = **70 mg LEU** 1 slice white bread = 2.3 g protein 2.3 × 70 = **161 mg LEU**
Meat, poultry, and fish	80	1 oz ham = 5.0 g protein 5 × 80 = **400 mg LEU**
Dairy products	100	½ cup milk = 4.0 g protein 4 × 100 = **400 mg LEU**

Source: USDA Agricultural Research Service. Nutrient Data Laboratory. Available at: http://www.nal.usda.gov/fnic/foodcomp/search/. Accessed July 8, 2008.

Note: The quick calculation method in Table 6.3 may be used to estimate the LEU content of food when specific LEU information is not available; this provides an estimate only.

Fat and Essential Fatty Acids

Because medical foods provide less fat than proprietary infant formulas and intact protein, sources of essential fatty acids to meet recommended intakes may need to be supplied (see Appendix F). See Chapter 3, Table 3.1 for recommended intakes of fat and essential fatty acids.

Energy and Fluid

Suggested energy and fluid requirements are listed in Table 6.1. Carbohydrate and fat in the diet decrease the rate of amino acid oxidation and facilitate protein synthesis. Carbohydrate intake, with its use mediated by insulin, decreases both LEU release from protein breakdown and LEU oxidation, lowering the plasma concentration.[61] A high carbohydrate and energy intake during metabolic decompensation is necessary to decrease plasma LEU concentration and correct the ketoacidosis. Protein-free energy sources are available in Appendix C and very-low-protein food sources are found in Appendix E.

Fluid requirements, especially during infancy, are higher for children with MSUD than in normal infants due to the use of amino acids as the protein source, and the additional fluid required to excrete toxic metabolites.[62] Amino acid-based medical foods have a higher osmolality than intact protein formulas. Recommendations for infant medical food mixtures are an osmolality of less than 460 mOsm per kg water.[63] In children and adults, additional water may need to be added if formula osmolality is greater than 1000 mOsm per kg water.

Minerals and Vitamins

Intake of minerals and vitamins may need to be higher than RDAs for age, due to ingestion of elemental medical foods resulting in less than normal absorption (see Chapter 3, Table 3.1). Medical foods supply the majority of vitamins and minerals needed for growth and development. Selenium deficiency and a decrease in glutathione peroxidase has been reported when patients with MSUD were consuming a medical food that did not contain selenium.[64,65]

Initiation of Nutrition Management and During Critical Illness or Following Trauma

Emergency treatment of an infant with MSUD requires rapid removal of the toxic metabolites, elimination of catabolism, and promotion of anabolism. A delay in diagnosis may cause extremely high blood and tissue concentrations of BCAAs and their corresponding ketoacids, necessitating the use of hemodialysis, exchange transfusions, or peritoneal dialysis.[66,67] These invasive measures are rarely needed when screening and diagnosis occur very early in life, but if required, they must be combined with prompt nutrition support. Even with plasma LEU concentrations 10 to 20 times above normal, nutrition therapy, which promotes anabolism and thereby avoids accumulation of toxic metabolites, is the preferred treatment.[67-69] A combination of parenteral and enteral nutrition is more effective than dialysis or hemoperfusion in lowering plasma LEU concentrations.[69] In comatose or neurologically compromised patients who cannot tolerate oral feeds, parenteral nutrition of BCAA-free amino acids, glucose, and lipid may be required. Parenteral amino acid solutions free of BCAAs have been developed for this purpose (see Appendix D).

The goal of hyperalimentation is to provide 120 to 140 kcal per kg per day for infants, 80 to 100 kcal per kg per day for children, and 40 to 45 kcal per kg per day for adults.[44,68] The BCAA-free solution for the neonate should provide 2.5 to 3.0 g of protein per kg per day.[44,68] Plasma concentrations of ILE and VAL decrease more rapidly than LEU and must be added to the intravenous solution when plasma concentrations reach the upper limit of treatment range to promote protein synthesis.[37,44] ILE and VAL supplementation should be initiated at the lower limit of recommended intake for age (see Table 6.1). Plasma concentration of LEU will not decrease if ILE or VAL is deficient. Monitor plasma amino acids closely and add LEU when the plasma LEU concentration reaches 200 μmol/L. Normalization of all 3 plasma BCAAs usually occurs within 48 to 72 hours.[68,69] Insulin may be administered if hyperglycemia occurs due to the large infusions of glucose that are needed to promote anabolism.[37,68,70]

Enteral feeding should be initiated as soon as possible. Start a BCAA-free medical food when the patient is able to tolerate nasogastric or gastrostomy feeds (see Table 6.2) and maintain energy and fluid intake by intravenous infusions of glucose and lipid.

Monitor plasma amino acid concentrations and add ILE and VAL to the medical food mixture when plasma concentrations reach the upper limit of the treatment range. When the BCAA concentrations have reached the treatment range, an intact protein source such as proprietary infant formula, expressed human milk, or cow's milk (for children or adults; see Appendix B) must be added to meet essential LEU requirements. A sample prescription for initiation of nutrition support for a newly diagnosed infant with MSUD is illustrated in Table 6.4.

Acute metabolic decompensation is a medical emergency, and the patient should be managed in a hospital setting with a medical team that is familiar with the acute management of patients with an inherited metabolic disorder. Intercurrent illness, surgery, injury, diet indiscretions, and the initial neonatal episode also require emergency management. Several authors have reported their experiences and provided practical treatment protocols for an acute crisis.[66-76] Each episode raises the risk for cerebral edema, necessitating careful monitoring of hydration status, electrolyte balance, and clinical symptoms. An emergency protocol for managing patients with an acute illness in MSUD has been developed by the New England Consortium of Metabolic Physicians. It is available online at http://www.childrenshospital.org/newenglandconsortium/NBS/MSUD.html.[77] Nutrition management is critical in patients with MSUD and prompt attention to control of catabolism during illness is essential to prevent a neurological crisis.

Long-Term Nutrition Management

The goal of long-term nutrition management of patients with MSUD is to achieve near normal plasma concentrations of BCAAs while supplying adequate nutrients necessary for growth and development. To achieve this goal, the use of medical foods free of BCAAs (see Table 6.2) in combination with an intact protein source is required. It may be necessary to supplement the diet with L-ILE and L-VAL to maintain plasma concentrations in the treatment range. In patients with residual BCKD activity, a trial of thiamine (100 to 500 mg per day) should be prescribed for a period of up to 3 months.[27] Evaluation of plasma concentrations of BCAAs before and after supplementation are recommended to assess responsiveness. Branched-chain amino

Table 6.4 ***Initiation of Nutrition Management for a Patient with MSUD***

A 7-day-old 3.5 kg neonate newly diagnosed with MSUD with clinical history of poor feeding. The plasma LEU concentration is 1005 μmol/L.

1. Provide energy needed for anabolism (125 to 145 kcal/kg).
2. Provide extra fluid and adequate sodium to treat dehydration, maintain urine output, and avoid hyponatremia.
3. Provide protein equivalent source free of BCAAs[a] (2.5 to 3.5 g/kg).

A. Initial Prescription

	Amount	*LEU (mg)*	*ILE (mg)*	*VAL (mg)*	*Sodium (mEq)*	*Protein (g)*	*Energy (kcal)*	*Fluid (mL)*
Ketonex®-1 powder	70 g	—	—	—	5.8	10.5	336	—
Polycose® powder	35 g	—	—	—	2.0	—	133	—
Water to make*								~640
Total per day					7.8	10.5	469	640
Total per kg					2.2	3.0	134	183

*Water to make final volume of 640 mL (~22 fl oz).

4. Monitor plasma amino acid and serum sodium concentrations. May need to adjust sodium intake to 4 mEq/kg.
5. Add ILE (~45 mg/kg) and VAL (~50 mg/kg) when plasma concentrations reach the upper limits of treatment range. These may be added as L-ILE and L-VAL or by using a LEU-free medical food.
6. When plasma LEU concentration reaches ~200 μmol/L, add an intact protein source to provide LEU (85 mg/kg).

	Amount	*LEU (mg)*	*ILE (mg)*	*VAL (mg)*	*Sodium (mEq)*	*Protein (g)*	*Energy (kcal)*	*Fluid (mL)*
Ketonex®-1 powder	50 g	—	—	—	4.2	7.5	240	—
Similac® Advance® RTF[a]	200 mL	294	149	163	1.4	2.8	135	200
Polycose® powder	20 g	—	—	—	1.1	—	76	—
Water to make[b]								~600
Total per day		294	149	163	6.7	10.3	451	600
Total per kg		84	43	47	2.0	2.9	129	170

Notes:

[a]RTF = Ready to feed.

[b]Water to make final volume of 600 mL (~20 fl oz).

Estimated osmolarity 370 mOsm per L. Caloric density 22 kcal per fl oz.

7. Monitor plasma amino acids closely and adjust medical food mixture to maintain BCAA concentrations within treatment range.
8. If patient's linear growth is below normal, see recommended protein intake in Chapter 3, Table 3.1.

acid content of small portion sizes of foods is given in references 58 and 59 and for 100 g portions in reference 60.

Assessment of Nutrition Management

Plasma BCAA concentrations should be maintained as close as possible to the normal range. In the initial stages, plasma amino acids may need to be monitored daily. The frequency of assessment is determined by the age of the patient, clinical course of the disease, and diet adherence. Generally, plasma amino acid concentrations are monitored weekly in the first year of life and every 2 weeks or monthly during childhood. Elevated plasma LEU concentrations may be a result of diet non-adherence, over prescription, inadequate intake of protein and energy, infections, or illness. Inadequate protein and energy intakes result in catabolism of the body protein and an increase in plasma concentrations of BCAAs. Adequate energy and protein intakes are required for protein synthesis, growth, and normal body processes. Deficiency of VAL or ILE will also cause LEU concentrations to rise due to decreased protein synthesis or muscle catabolism. Elevated plasma concentrations of LEU and the corresponding ketoacid, α-ketoisocaproic, may also contribute to immune suppression.[34] Plasma concentrations of amino acids in addition to anthropometrics, nutrient intakes, clinical evaluation for nutrient deficiencies, and laboratory assessment of protein, vitamin, and mineral status indices should be monitored at regular intervals as determined by age and clinical course (see Chapter 3).

The urine should be free of ketoacids at all times. Home monitoring using 2,4-dinitrophenylhydrazine (DNPH) is a method of detecting the presence of α-ketoacids in urine. The DNPH combined with hydrochloric acid reacts with the α-ketoacids in urine to form hydrazones that precipitate. A yellow precipitate indicates the presence of α-ketoacids. DNPH is available from companies that produce and distribute laboratory-grade chemicals. Although not as specific as the DNPH test, Ketostix® Reagent Strips or Keto-Diastix® (Bayer Healthcare, Morristown, New Jersey) may be used as a simple means of detecting the presence of ketones in urine. A positive result from either method requires further analysis of plasma BCAA concentrations and consultation with the metabolic healthcare team. Although there is a correlation between plasma LEU concentration and the corresponding ketoacid, the appearance of clinical symptoms is most closely related to the degree of elevation of plasma LEU concentration.[78]

The aroma of maple syrup in the urine of patients with MSUD is due to a substance called sotolone, derived from accumulating ILE or alloisoleucine.[79] Fenugreek is an herb ingested by mothers to induce labor or enhance milk production, and is sometimes given to infants and children to treat illness, which is a common practice in Indian, Mediterranean, and Middle East cultures.[80] Fenugreek exposure may be a cause of the characteristic maple syrup-like odor and may lead to a false suspicion of metabolic imbalance in a previously diagnosed patient with MSUD.

Results of Nutrition Management

Early diagnosis and attentive medical and nutrition management in MSUD can result in normal growth and development. Intellectual outcome is negatively correlated with long-term plasma LEU concentrations and duration of elevated plasma LEU concentrations during the neonatal period.[43]

The effect of BCAA-restricted diets on nutrition status was evaluated in 12 children with MSUD. Lean body mass and percent body fat were not different from controls, but height for age was significantly less than in controls, indicating possible chronic malnutrition.[81] The energy and protein intakes were, respectively, 86% and 78% of the RDA.[81] Normal growth can be achieved when adequate energy, protein, and BCAAs are consumed.

Alternative Approaches to Therapy

Although advances in newborn screening, diagnosis, and nutrition management have improved the prognosis of patients with MSUD, the risk of acute metabolic decompensation with resulting brain injury is always present. Liver transplantation was initially performed in two patients with liver failure due to hepatitis A infection, and in one patient with hypervitaminosis A.[82,83] The transplantation significantly decreased plasma BCAA concentrations, but alloisoleucine was detected at low concentrations in both patients. In the third patient, alloisoleucine was detectable only during catabolic stress. Elective liver transplantation for MSUD has been reported in 10 additional children with stabilization of plasma BCAA concentrations despite an increase in LEU intake from 15 to 37 mg per kg per day to 145 to 350 mg per kg per day.[83] Alloisoleucine remained detectable in plasma at low concentrations. Branched-chain amino acid oxidation occurs in skeletal muscle, kidney, and other organs in addition to the liver; thus it is evident that transplantation does not completely cure the disease. The amount of enzyme activity appeared similar to that observed in patients with the mild variant form of MSUD. The liver of a 25-year-old man with MSUD was used as a domino graft for a man with hepatocellular carcinoma.[84] Both patients tolerate a normal protein intake although mild impairment of BCAA metabolism is evident.[84] Although the risk of surgery and immunosuppression must be considered, liver transplantation is a treatment option that reduces plasma

BCAA concentrations, relaxes BCAA restrictions, and eliminates the risk of metabolic decompensation during catabolic events.

Maternal Maple Syrup Urine Disease

Introduction

Successful pregnancy outcomes in women with MSUD have been reported. Unlike phenylketonuria, nothing is known concerning the potential harmful effects of elevated plasma BCAAs and the corresponding ketoacid concentrations on the developing fetus. Data do not exist for women with classic MSUD who have discontinued or relaxed nutrition management. Five normal pregnancy outcomes have been reported in two women with intermittent MSUD.[23,85] The women were undiagnosed at the time of their pregnancies and did not receive nutrition therapy. The female reported by Lie et al. had 50% residual enzyme activity in leukocytes and 12 to 16% activity in cultured fibroblasts.[23] Residual enzyme activity of 12% was reported in the woman whom Zaleski et al. presented.[85]

Nutrition Management

Metabolic decompensation due to the stress of the pregnancy is a major concern for women with MSUD. Marked increase in LEU tolerance during pregnancy is also reported.[86,87] Van Calcar et al. outlined a pregnancy in a woman treated for MSUD since 11 days of age.[86] When she presented to the clinic at 2 months gestation, the plasma BCAA concentrations were within normal range. In the first trimester, the diet consisted of 0.6 g per kg per day of intact protein and 0.6 g per kg per day protein equivalents from the BCAA-free medical food. The diet was similar to prepregnancy intake with the exception of a 0.2 g per kg per day increase in protein from the BCAA-free medical food. Intact protein intake was increased to 0.8 g per kg per day to maintain normal plasma BCAA concentrations in the second trimester. L-carnitine supplementation of 50 mg per kg per day was prescribed to maintain normal blood concentrations. At 28 weeks gestation, a low plasma-free carnitine concentration was found as a result of noncompliance with the L-carnitine supplement for a 1-month period. The plasma carnitine profile in nonpregnant women is significantly higher than in pregnant women.[88,89] Urinary excretion of carnitine increases during the first and second trimester of pregnancy and decreases in the third trimester.[89] Since plasma carnitine concentrations decrease during situations of high energy needs such as pregnancy, it is important to monitor and supplement as necessary to maintain normal concentrations. At week 37 of gestation, the woman was hospitalized due to a low concentration of plasma L-carnitine and slow fetal growth. Intact protein intake was increased to 1.5 g per kg per day and carnitine was supplemented at 150 mg per kg per day.

A healthy 2600 g girl was delivered at 40 weeks gestation with intravenous glucose administered for 12 hours postdelivery. Intact protein was limited to 1.0 g per kg per day and L-carnitine supplementation was decreased to 50 mg per kg per day following delivery. At 9 days postpartum, clinical symptoms of lethargy and dizziness were noted in the mother with an accompanying plasma LEU concentration of 1015 μmol/L. Frequent carbohydrate feedings were initiated and plasma LEU concentrations returned to normal within 5 days. The combination of high intake of intact protein and nitrogenous products from the involutional changes of the uterus may have contributed to the elevation of plasma concentrations of BCAAs.[1] Grünewald et al.[87] presented a favorable pregnancy outcome in a woman with MSUD who maintained plasma LEU concentrations between 100 and 300 μmol/L. Leucine tolerance increased progressively from 350 mg per day starting at week 22 of gestation to 2100 mg per day at the end of gestation. Requirements for BCAAs increase during the course of the pregnancy, but modifications to intake should be based on plasma concentrations.

Subsequent pregnancies in women with MSUD have been followed with two requiring supplementation of L-ILE and L-VAL. In some cases the increase in intact protein appears to maintain the plasma concentrations of ILE and VAL in the normal ranges (S. van Calcar, personal communication, March 21, 2008).

Recommended energy, protein, essential fatty acids, vitamin, and mineral intakes for pregnancy are outlined in Chapter 3, Table 3.1. Essential plasma amino acid concentrations during pregnancy in normal women are included in Chapter 3, Table 3.8.

Assessment of Nutrition Management

Weekly assessment of BCAA concentrations during pregnancy is ideal. More frequent monitoring of BCAA may be required during illness or if the pregnant woman experiences loss of appetite. Nutrient intake 3 days prior to blood collection should be included as part of the assessment. Routine biochemical measurements of nutrition status are required (see Chapter 3, Table 3.7), in addition to assessment of fetal growth. Monitoring during the entire pregnancy, labor, delivery, and postpartum period is essential to decrease the risk of metabolic decompensation.

Isovaleric Acidemia

Introduction

Isovaleric acidemia (IVA; OMIM 243500)[2] or isovaleryl-CoA dehydrogenase deficiency is an autosomal recessive disorder first described by several investigators in the mid-1960s.[90,91] The two phenotypes described were an acute neonatal presentation and a chronic intermittent type. The initial patient was a neonate who presented with metabolic acidosis due to accumulation of isovaleric acid and a characteristic odor of "sweaty feet."[90] The infant had severe neurological impairment and died following a pulmonary hemorrhage. The subsequent cases, siblings of 2 and 4 years of age, experienced recurrent episodes of vomiting, lethargy, and metabolic acidosis associated with intercurrent infections or excess LEU ingestion as intact protein.[91] The characteristic odor and elevations in the concentrations of isovaleric acid in serum and urine were noted. Oral L-LEU loading resulted in neurological symptoms and marked increases in serum isovaleric acid concentrations.[91] A deficiency of isovaleryl-CoA dehydrogenase (IVD) was later identified in mitochondria isolated from fibroblasts derived from patients with IVA.[92]

Recent advances in newborn screening have identified a third group of patients who can be asymptomatic, but have mild biochemical abnormalities.[93] Unlike the two phenotypes initially described, there is a spectrum of disease with severity of the symptoms and the timing of the presentation dependent on the amount of residual enzyme activity, modifying effects on the enzyme, and environmental factors.[93]

Biochemistry

IVA is a disorder of LEU catabolism caused by a deficiency of IVD (EC 1.3.99.10), which catalyzes the oxidation of isovaleryl-CoA to β-methylcrotonyl-CoA (see Figure 6.1). IVD, a member of the acyl-CoA dehydrogenase family, is a mitochondrial flavoenzyme transferring electrons to electron transfer flavoprotein (ETF).[94]

The major metabolite that accumulates is isovalerylglycine, produced by conjugation with glycine. Normal excretion of isovalerylglycine is less than 15 μmol per day, but amounts of 2000 to 15,000 μmol per day are detected in the urine of patients with IVA.[94] Concentrations of this nontoxic metabolite are highest during an acute episode, but remain elevated during periods of remission. During catabolic stress, the capacity of the alternative pathway through glycine-N-acylase (EC 2.31.13) to produce isovalerylglycine is exceeded and the toxic metabolite isovaleric acid becomes elevated in plasma. The phenotype results from an accumulation of isovaleric acid. Additional metabolites of isovaleryl-CoA including β-hydroxyisovaleric acid, 4-hydroxyisovaleric acid, and isovalerylglucuronide are detected in the urine of patients with IVA during acute illness.[94]

Molecular Biology

The human IVD gene consists of 12 exons and is located on chromosome 15q13-q15.[95] Five classes of mutations have been identified that produce proteins of different molecular size (see Chapter 1). These variants are caused by point mutations, splice-site mutations, or premature terminations, resulting in residual IVD activity from 0 to 3% of normal, and no correlation has been found between genotype and phenotype in these mutations.[96,97] The clinical heterogeneity may be caused by nongenetic factors, as both the acute neonatal presentation and the chronic intermittent type can occur in the same family.[94] Recently, a mild or asymptomatic phenotype with partial IVD activity has been recognized due to MS/MS newborn screening. A missense mutation, 932C-T (A282V) was identified in 18 (47%) of 38 mutant alleles.[93] The need for nutrition therapy and the long-term clinical outcome in patients with this mutation are not known.

Newborn Screening

Previously, diagnosis of IVA was based on the large urinary excretion of isovaleryl-CoA metabolites in symptomatic patients. MS/MS analysis of acylcarnitines is now the most commonly used method to identify patients with possible IVA (see Chapter 2).

Isovalerylcarnitine (C5) is elevated in blood in both IVA and α-methylbutyrylglycinuria (also called short-chain-branched acyl-CoA dehydrogenase). Additional analysis of plasma acylcarnitines and urine organic acids is required to determine the diagnosis. An elevated plasma C5 concentration in combination with an elevated urinary C5 leads to the diagnosis of IVA. Although there is variation in detection limits among newborn screening laboratories, a dried blood spot containing 0.8 to 6 μmol/L of C5 may indicate a milder phenotype of IVA, whereas a blood concentration of C5 up to 21.7 μmol/L may represent a more severe phenotype.[98] A false-positive result has been reported in a human milk-fed infant whose mother was ingesting a pivalic acid-containing antibiotic, as pivaloylcarnitine has the same molecular mass as C5.[99] Newborns treated with antibiotics have also demonstrated elevated C5 concentrations.[100] The medication history of the mother and infant or a second-tier analysis examining isovalerylglycine in the dried blood spot may eliminate false-positive results.

Diagnosis

Increases in amounts of isovalerylglycine in urine and C5 in plasma are hallmarks of IVA. These metabolites are elevated in patients with IVA irrespective of the metabolic condition.[98] Isovalerylglycine is detected in the urine of patients with IVA (1000 to 3000 mmol/mol of creatinine) during remission, while during an acute crisis, isovalerylglycine amounts of 2000 to 9000 mmol/mol creatinine, plus elevations of urinary β-hydroxyisovaleric acid have been reported.[94] Analysis of IVD activity in fibroblasts or lymphocytes is used to confirm the diagnosis but correlation with clinical phenotype is poor.[96] Molecular genetic evaluation has revealed a common mutation, 932C-T(A282V), in patients with mild elevations in blood isovaleryl-CoA metabolites.[93] Based on newborn screening results, the incidence of IVA is reported as 1 in 62,500 live births in Germany, 1 in 250,000 live births in the United States, and 1 in 365,000 live births in Taiwan.[93,101]

Outcomes if Untreated

The clinical presentations of patients with IVA include an acute neonatal form, a chronic intermittent type, and more recently, a mild or asymptomatic presentation. Infants with acute IVA appear normal at birth but develop poor feeding, vomiting, diarrhea, and lethargy within the first few weeks of life. Hypothermia, severe acidosis, hyperammonemia, seizures, pancytopenia, neutropenia, thrombocytopenia, and death due to cerebral edema, hemorrhage, severe metabolic acidosis, or infection have been reported.[94,96] Advances in diagnosis and improvements in acute therapy have markedly improved outcomes. The subsequent course for infants who survive the neonatal period is that of the chronic intermittent form, which is characterized by episodes of vomiting, lethargy, and acidosis. The symptoms are more frequent in the first few years of life and are precipitated by illness, infections, or increased LEU intake. The characteristic odor of "sweaty feet" and clinical progression similar to the neonatal course will occur if not treated promptly.

Nutrition Management

The management of patients with IVA consists of restriction of LEU, supplementation with single or combined glycine, and L-carnitine therapy, plus prevention of metabolic crisis. The goal of nutrition therapy is to avoid the presence of isovaleric acid and β-hydroxyisovaleric acid in the urine. It is not known whether nutrition therapy is necessary for patients diagnosed to be carrying the 932C-T mutation.[98]

Nutrient Requirements

Leucine

The requirements for LEU are outlined in Table 6.5 and are dependent on age, growth rate, energy and protein intake, health status, and the avoidance of isovaleric acid in plasma and urine. The amount of LEU required per unit of body weight declines with age and must be individually determined. Patients with IVA who are supplemented with glycine and/or L-carnitine appear to have a higher LEU tolerance than those who are not supplemented.

Table 6.5 ***Recommended Daily Nutrient Intakes for Infants, Children, and Adults with LEU Catabolism Disorders***

	Nutrient			
Age	*LEU*[a] *(mg/kg)*	*Protein*[b] *(g/kg)*	*Energy*[c] *(kcal/kg)*	*Fluid*[d] *(mL/kg)*
Infants, mo				
0 to 6	65–120	2.5–3.5	95–145	125–160
7 to 12	50–90	2.5–3.0	80–135	125–145
Children, yr				
1 to 3	40–90	1.5–2.5	80–130	115–135
4 to 8	40–60	1.3–2.0	50–120	90–115
9 to 13	40–60	1.2–1.8	40–90	70–90
14 to 18	30–60	1.2–1.8	35–70	40–60
Adults, yr				
Over 19	30–60	1.1–1.7	35–45	40–50

Sources:

Acosta PB, Yannicelli S. Protocol 5. Maple syrup urine disease (MSUD). *Nutrition Support Protocols.* Columbus, OH: Ross Products Division, Abbott Laboratories; 2001.

De Raeve L, De Meirleir L, Ramet J, Vandenplas Y, Gerlo E. Acrodermatitis enteropathica-like cutaneous lesions in organic aciduria. *J Pediatr.* 1994;124:416–420.

Elsas LJ, Acosta PB. Inherited metabolic disease: amino acids, organic acids and galactose. In: Shils ME, Shike M, Ross AC, Cabellero B, Cousins RJ, eds. *Modern Nutrition in Health and Disease.* 10th ed. Philadelphia, PA: Lippincott Williams & Wilkins; 2005:909–959.

Institute of Medicine of the National Academies. *Dietary Reference Intakes for Energy, Carbohydrate, Fiber, Fat, Fatty Acids, Cholesterol, Protein, and Amino Acids.* Washington, DC: National Academies Press; 2005.

Kindt E, Halvorsen S. The need of essential amino acids in children: an evaluation based on the intake of phenylalanine, tyrosine, leucine, isoleucine, and valine in children with phenylketonuria, tyrosine amino transferase defect, and maple syrup urine disease. *Am J Clin Nutr.* 1980;33:279–286.

Parsons HG, Carter RJ, Unrath M, Snyder FF. Evaluation of branched-chain amino acid intake in children with maple syrup urine disease and methylmalonic aciduria. *J Inherit Metab Dis.* 1990;13:125–136.

Note: Adjust amino acid intake based on plasma amino acid concentrations. If protein is inadequate to support normal linear growth, see Chapter 3, Table 3.1. Increase fluid intake during illness to enhance urinary ketoacid excretion.

Glycine

Glycine supplementation in combination with or without a LEU-restricted diet has been utilized in long-term maintenance to enhance isovalerylglycine excretion.[102-104] Under stable conditions, glycine supplementation of 60 to 150 mg per kg per day has been recommended.[102,103] The advantages of combined glycine and L-carnitine supplementation in long-term management warrant further investigation. The combination of glycine and L-carnitine therapy may maximize excretion of isovaleryl-CoA metabolites and lessen the severity of metabolic crisis.[105] The L-carnitine and glycine contributed by the LEU-free medical food (see Table 6.6) should be calculated before prescribing additional supplementation.

Protein and Leucine-Free Medical Foods

A moderate protein restriction of 1.5 to 2.0 g per kg per day has been used to manage patients with IVA. The value of protein restriction is questioned in light of the finding that protein catabolism due to inadequate intake contributes significantly to production of isovaleric acid.[94,106] Additionally, in the investigation of urinary metabolites in 6 patients with IVA, 19 isovaleryl- and acetyl-amino acid conjugates were identified.[107] The abnormal amino acid conjugation and protein restriction caused a depletion of free amino acids in these patients when compared to healthy controls.[108] The authors suggested that the toxic metabolites and amino acid depletion may help explain some of the clinical symptoms of IVA. Importantly, this research discourages the use of protein restriction and supports the use of LEU restriction with addition of LEU-free medical foods to meet protein requirements.[108] Protein should be higher than RDAs for age when the major source of protein is free amino acids (see Chapter 3, Table 3.1). Selected nutrient composition and sources of LEU-free medical foods are reported in Table 6.6. Proprietary infant formula or human milk is used to supply LEU in the first months of life (see Appendix B). Food lists and the USDA nutrient database containing the LEU content of foods can help individuals and families plan the LEU-restricted diet.[58-60] A rough guideline to estimate the LEU content of foods is outlined in Table 6.4. Most medical foods for IVA contain fat, carbohydrate, vitamins, and minerals. Some of the medical foods contain additional glycine and L-carnitine.

Fat and Essential Fatty Acids

Because medical foods provide less fat than proprietary infant formulas or intact protein, sources of essential fatty acids to meet recommended intakes may need to be supplied (see Appendix F). See Chapter 3, Table 3.1 for recommended intakes of fat and essential fatty acids.

Table 6.6 *Nutrient Composition and Sources of LEU-Free Medical Foods*

Medical Foods	Modified[a] Nutrient(s) (mg/100 g)	Protein Equiv[b] (g/100 g, source)	Fat (g/100 g, source)	Carbohydrate (g/100 g, source)	Energy (kcal/100 g/kJ/100 g)	Linoleic Acid/ α-Linolenic Acid (mg/100 g)
Abbott Nutrition[c]						
I-Valex®-1	Glycine 1000 L-carnitine 900 Taurine 40	15 Amino acids[d]	21.7 High-oleic safflower, coconut, and soy oils	53 Corn syrup solids	480/2006	3500/350
I-Valex®-2	Glycine 2000 L-carnitine 1800 Taurine 50	30 Amino acids[d]	14.0 High-oleic safflower, coconut, and soy oils	35 Corn syrup solids	410/1714	2200/230
Mead Johnson[e]						
LMD	Glycine 1100 L-carnitine 50 Taurine added	16.2 Amino acids[d]	26 Palm olein, soy, coconut, and high-oleic sunflower oils	51 Corn syrup solids, sugar, modified cornstarch, maltodextrin	500/2090	4500/380

(continues)

Table 6.6 ***Nutrient Composition and Sources of LEU-Free Medical Foods**, Continued*

Medical Foods	**Modified[a] Nutrient(s) (mg/100 g)**	**Protein Equiv[b] (g/100 g, source)**	**Fat (g/100 g, source)**	**Carbohydrate (g/100 g, source)**	**Energy (kcal/100 g/kJ/100 g)**	**Linoleic Acid/ α-Linolenic Acid (mg/100 g)**
			Nutricia[f]			
XLeu Analog™	Glycine 2050 L-carnitine 10 Taurine 20	13 Amino acids[c]	20.9 High oleic safflower, coconut, and soy oils	59 Corn syrup solids, galactose	475/1985	3025/NA
XLeu Maxamaid®	Glycine 3990 L-carnitine 20 Taurine 140	25 Amino acids[c]	<0.1	56 Sugar, corn syrup solids	324/1754	0
XLeu Maxamum®	Glycine 6300 L-carnitine 39 Taurine 140	40 Amino acids[c]	<1	34 Sugar, corn syrup solids	305/1275	0

Notes:
NA = not available.
Values listed, although accurate at time of publication, are subject to change. For current information, refer to product labels.
[a]LEU-free.
[b]Nitrogen, g × 6.25 = g protein.
[c]Abbott Nutrition, 3300 Stelzer Road, Columbus, Ohio, 43219. 800-551-5838.
[d]All except glycine are in the L-form.
[e]Mead Johnson Nutritionals, 2400 West Lloyd Expressway, Evansville, Indiana 47721. 800-457-3550.
[f]Nutricia North America, PO Box 117, Gaithersburg, Maryland 20884. 800-365-7354.

Energy and Fluid

Energy intake must be adequate to support normal growth for infants and children, appropriate weight for height for adults, and prevent protein catabolism. Adequate carbohydrate and fat intakes will facilitate the decrease in protein use for energy purposes, decrease catabolism, and enhance protein synthesis.[61] An increased intake of energy during catabolic stress is recommended to help decrease catabolism and accumulation of toxic metabolites. Fluid and energy recommendations are included in Table 6.5.

Minerals and Vitamins

Recommendations for minerals and vitamins are higher than RDAs for age due to ingestion of elemental diets as the major protein source (see Chapter 3, Table 3.1). If a patient with IVA is consuming a restricted protein diet without medical foods as a source of protein equivalent, mineral and vitamin intakes should be carefully evaluated.

Initiation of Nutrition Management and During Critical Illness or Following Trauma

Acute episodes of metabolic illness require a LEU-free protein intake, high-energy intake, appropriate fluid therapy, and correction of the metabolic acidosis. During periods of illness, endogenous LEU from protein catabolism is the main source of isovaleryl-CoA metabolites.[94] Increased energy intake in addition to a reduction in LEU intake is necessary to promote anabolism during illness. An adequate intake of a LEU-free medical food (see Table 6.6) will help decrease the amount of body protein breakdown with release of LEU. After approximately 24 to 48 hours, an intact source of protein is required to provide LEU to prevent further protein catabolism. During acute episodes additional glycine and L-carnitine may be required to promote excretion of isovalerylglycine and isovalerylcarnitine. Glycine is required for the synthesis of isovalerylglycine and concentrations of plasma glycine decrease during acute episodes.[94]

Glycine supplementation up to 600 mg per kg per day has been utilized during acute episodes.[102] Monitoring of plasma glycine concentrations, urinary isovalerylglycine excretion, and clinical status is necessary when utilizing doses over 300 mg per kg per day.[102,109] Lethargy and ataxia have been reported with elevated plasma glycine concentrations,[109] and the increase in glycine from 300 to 600 mg per kg per day may actually decrease urinary excretion of isovalerylglycine.[102] This effect could be due to inhibition of glycine-N-acylase by high concentrations of glycine or depletion of isovaleryl-CoA.[102] L-Carnitine supplementation of 100 to 200 mg per kg per day in combination with glycine resulted in an increase in both isovalerylcarnitine and isovalerylglycine excretion during illness and in response to an L-LEU load.[110,111] Combined glycine and L-carnitine therapy may be important during periods of metabolic stress to enhance isovaleryl-CoA metabolite excretion.[110-112] A sample emergency protocol for IVA is available online at http://www.childrenshospital.org/newenglandconsortium/NBS/IVA/IVA_protocol.htm.[77] Newborn screening has enabled identification, diagnosis, and treatment of patients with IVA before clinical symptoms develop. A sample prescription for an asymptomatic newborn with IVA is illustrated in Table 6.7.

Long-Term Nutrition Management

The goal of nutrition management of patients with IVA is to avoid elevations of isovaleric acid in plasma and urine while supplying LEU, energy, protein, essential fatty acids, vitamins, and minerals needed for normal growth and development. A LEU-free medical food (see Table 6.6) with the addition of intact protein to supply essential LEU is recommended. The clinical benefit of combined glycine and L-carnitine therapy in long-term management of patients with IVA remains controversial.

Decreased concentrations of total carnitine with elevations of acylcarnitine have been detected in the plasma of patients with IVA, suggesting an increased excretion of carnitine as a possible cause.[110,113,114] Several investigators have presented case reports of patients supplemented with L-carnitine alone at 100 mg per kg per day. The patients maintained normal plasma carnitine concentrations and achieved effective urinary excretion of isovaleryl-CoA metabolites.[113-115] A 12-year-old girl with IVA treated with 100 mg per kg per day of L-carnitine for a month demonstrated improved exercise tolerance.[116]

Table 6.7 ***Nutrition Management for a Patient with IVA***

A 10-day-old asymptomatic 3.2 kg neonate diagnosed with IVA.

	Amount	*LEU (mg)*	*GLY (mg)*	*Carnitine (mg)*	*Protein (g)*	*Energy (kcal)*	*Fluid (mL)*
I-Valex®-1 powder	55 g	—	550	495	8.3	264	—
Similac® Advance® RTF[a]	200 mL	294	56	2	2.8	135	200
Water to make[b]							~530
Total per day		294	606	497	11.1	399	530
Total per kg		92	189	155	3.5	125	165

Note: Estimated osmolarity of 395 mOsm per L. Caloric density of 22 kcal per fl oz.
[a]RTF = ready-to-feed.
[b]Water to make final volume of 530 mL (18 fl oz).

Assessment of Nutrition Management

The goal of therapy is to avoid accumulation of toxic isovaleryl-CoA metabolites. Vockley and Ensenauer suggest that urinary isovalerylglycine amounts of 15 to 195 mmol/mol creatinine are associated with a mild or intermediate phenotype while urine isovalerylglyine concentrations up to 3300 mmol/mol creatinine indicate a metabolically severe phenotype.[98] Acute episodes cause a marked increase in urinary isovalerylglycine plus the appearance of urinary isovaleric acid and β-hydroxyisovaleric acid. The goal of therapy is to maintain the urine free of isovaleric acid and β-hydroxyisovaleric acid. Monitoring of urinary organic acids to assess presence of toxic metabolites should be performed weekly to monthly as determined by the clinical course of the disease. Evaluation of plasma concentrations of amino acids, carnitine, anthropometrics, nutrient intake, and laboratory indices of mineral and vitamin status should be conducted regularly (see Chapter 3, Tables 3.1 through 3.7).

Results of Nutrition Management

Early diagnosis, proper nutrition management, and prompt medical treatment of metabolic decompensation can result in normal outcomes. The neurological impairment reported is generally the result of overwhelming illness in the initial presentation.[94] Advances in newborn screening and improved nutrition management have resulted in lower morbidity than previously reported in patients with IVA.

Maternal Isovaleric Acidemia

Two cases of successful pregnancy outcomes in patients with IVA have been reported. The first report was a woman who was diagnosed at 5 years of age and had nutrition treatment up until 21 years of age and during pregnancy ingested a self-limited low-protein intake.[117] The second woman received L-carnitine and glycine in addition to a low-protein diet throughout the pregnancy.[118] These reports confirm that patients with uncomplicated maternal IVA can have apparently normal outcome.

β-Methylcrotonyl-CoA Carboxylase Deficiency

Introduction

β-Methylcrotonyl-CoA carboxylase (βMCC) deficiency (OMIM 210200)[2] is an autosomal recessive disorder of LEU catabolism. The disorder is often referred to as β-methylcrotonylglycinuria or isolated βMCC deficiency to distinguish it from the biotin-responsive multiple carboxylase deficiencies: biotinidase deficiency and holocarboxylase synthetase deficiency (see Chapter 8). The disorder was first described in the 1970s with a clinical phenotype of feeding problems, failure to thrive, neurological dysfunction, and severe metabolic acidosis.[119] Subsequent reports have revealed a broad spectrum of clinical presentations ranging from asymptomatic to early onset necrotizing encephalopathy, severe hypoglycemia, metabolic stroke, status epilepticus, cardiomyopathy, developmental delay, and adult-onset muscle pain and disability.[120-126] Markedly different clinical presentations have been reported within an individual family.[124] The recent introduction of expanded newborn screening for βMCC deficiency has revealed that less than 10% of persons with the deficiency may develop symptoms.[127] The outcome measures are difficult to validate as the affected newborns were treated with mild protein restriction, L-carnitine supplementation, and counseling to prevent catabolic episode.[127] Guidelines for nutrition management are lacking and long-term outcomes of patients who are diagnosed presymptomatically are not known.

Biochemistry

βMCC deficiency is caused by an isolated deficiency of the biotin-dependent enzyme β-methylcrotonyl-CoA carboxylase (EC 6.4.1.4). βCC carboxylates β-methylcrotonyl-CoA to form β-methylglutaconyl-CoA (see Figure 6.1). Increased concentrations of 3-hydroxyisovaleric acid and β-methylcrotonylglycine are found in urine with the absence of methylcitrate, and α-methyl-β-hydroxybutyrate is found in combined carboxylase deficiency.[128] The presence of β-hydroxyisovalerylcarnitine (C5OH) in plasma and urine is characteristic of the disorder.[129] A secondary carnitine deficiency with an elevated ratio of acylcarnitine to free carnitine in plasma is a common feature.[130]

Molecular Biology

βMCC is comprised of two subunits: MCCα (OMIM 609010)[2] that covalently binds biotin, and a MCCβ subunit (OMIM 609014)[2] that contains a binding site for the acyl-CoA substrate[127] (see Chapter 1). The MCCα or MCCA gene is located on chromosome 3q26-28 and consists of 19 exons, and the MCCβ or MCCB gene is localized to chromosome 5q13 and contains 17 exons.[127] Mutations have been identified in both subunits with no prevalent mutation identified and poor phenotype/genotype correlation.[131] Other factors such as modifying genes or environmental factors may have a major influence on the phenotype of βMCC deficiency. An unusual mutation has been reported (MCCA-R385S) that is a dominant negative allele and results in clinical symptoms in patients who are heterozygous.[132] The term "dominant negative" is applied to mutations that lead to the production of a mutant protein that interferes with the protein of the normal allele in these patients.[133] Two patients have been described: one patient with clinical symptoms of seizures and psychomotor delay; and the second with biochemical abnormalities of βMCC deficiency, despite partial enzyme deficiency.[132] Clinical symptoms improved and biochemical abnormalities resolved with biotin therapy.[132-134] A biotin-responsive form had not previously been reported.

Newborn Screening

Expanded newborn screening by MS/MS (see Chapter 2) demonstrated that βMCC deficiency is one of the most common organic acidemias detected. An incidence of 1 in 36,000 live births was reported in an 8-year review of neonatal screening in North Carolina.[135] The overall frequency, combining data from Europe, Australia, and North America is estimated at 1 in 50,000 live births.[131] The inclusion of βMCC deficiency in newborn screening protocols varies among countries due to the large percentage of asymptomatic patients who have been identified.[127] Stadler et al. presented data to support the exclusion of βMCC deficiency from newborn screening in Germany, stating that the individual preventive benefits did not outweigh the possible stigmatization of patients and unnecessary intervention and financial burden for the healthcare system.[127] Clinical symptoms in women who were diagnosed with βMCC deficiency upon detection of elevated blood C5OH concentrations in their newborns suggest that exclusion of βMCC deficiency from the newborn screening panel requires further study.[136] An elevated blood concentration of C5OH is the first step in identification of possible βMCC deficiency. An initial blood C5OH concentration of 1.36 μmol/L was established as a cutoff value in the North Carolina newborn screening program.[135] A concentration of 2.6 μmol/L on the initial blood sample or on a repeat sample was shown to have a positive predictive value of 80% in the North Carolina screening program.[130]

Diagnosis

A panel of 15 experts in inherited metabolic disorders was organized to develop consensus-based guidelines for the diagnosis and management of βMCC-deficient screen-positive infants and their mothers.[137] They recommended that all screen-positive infants have analysis of urine organic acids and plasma acylcarnitine concentrations for further diagnosis of βMCC deficiency.[137] A biotinidase assay should be performed if this was not done on the newborn screen.[137]

For asymptomatic infants, determination of plasma carnitine concentration is recommended due to significant carnitine deficiency detected in affected patients. The addition of a complete blood count with differential, plasma concentrations of electrolytes, glucose, ammonia, blood gases, liver function tests, and urinalysis is suggested for the infant with clinical symptoms.[137]

The identification of abnormal metabolites of maternal origin emphasizes the importance of analyzing urine organic acids and plasma acylcarnitine concentrations in mothers of suspected infants.[130,136-138] βMCC deficiency has been diagnosed in mothers from detection of abnormal acylcarnitine profiles in their infants.[130,136,138] Clinical symptoms and biochemical abnormalities in the affected mothers included myopathy, weakness, increased liver enzyme activities and plasma uric acid concentrations, fatty livers, and carnitine deficiency.[127,138] In asymptomatic infants with affected mothers, the metabolites in the formula-fed infant should be reevaluated in approximately one month to confirm that the concentrations in the infant are normalizing. In the human milk-fed infant of affected mothers testing should be done after weaning.[137]

The initial blood C5OH concentrations may not differentiate between affected and unaffected infants.[130] Transient elevations of urinary β-hydroxyisovaleric acid have been found in infants with normal βMCC activity in lymphocytes,[130] and absent or trace amounts of urinary β-methylcrotonylglycine have been reported in two patients in whom βMCC deficiency was confirmed by enzyme activity and mutation analysis.[128] The clinical course of the patients should be monitored in combination with the presence of persistent abnormal metabolites. Although plasma concentrations of metabolites twice the normal range may be diagnostic, the diagnosis should be confirmed by enzyme assay.[137] A case report of an infant with failure to thrive, gastrointestinal dysfunction, and hypertonia demonstrated βMCC activity that was 46% of normal in lymphocytes but 8 to 12% of normal activity in cultured fibroblasts.[139] Other investigators have confirmed this finding, reporting an infant with lymphocyte βMCC activity that was 63% of normal while βMCC activity in cultured fibroblasts was 3% of normal.[130] In symptomatic infants with a normal lymphocyte assay, repeating βMCC enzyme analysis in fibroblasts should be considered.

Outcomes if Untreated

The clinical presentation and outcome of undiagnosed or untreated patients are varied, ranging from asymptomatic to profound metabolic acidosis, cerebral edema, and death. Stadler et al. reviewed published data from 37 patients with clinically diagnosed βMCC deficiency and indicated that only 27% were completely asymptomatic.[127] The retrospective analysis may reflect bias of selection as overt clinical symptoms lead to the diagnosis. It is not known whether asymptomatic patients detected by newborn screening will develop clinical symptoms if untreated. Clinical symptoms have been reported in women who were diagnosed upon detection of abnormal metabolites in their newborns. Symptoms improved after 4 weeks of L-carnitine supplementation.[140] An infant diagnosed by newborn screening who discontinued the low-protein diet and L-carnitine supplementation presented at 19 months with metabolic decomposition.[141] The severe acidosis and hypoglycemia were associated with an upper respiratory infection, stressing the importance of emergency protocols and nutrition management during periods of illness.

Nutrition Management

Nutrition management of patients with βMCC deficiency involves management of intercurrent illness, correction of carnitine deficiency, if present, and possible LEU restriction.

Initiation of Nutrition Management and During Critical Illness or Following Trauma

Patients with βMCC deficiency, even if asymptomatic when well, may be more susceptible to metabolic decompensation during intercurrent illness than normal persons. Prior clinical history of a woman diagnosed following her infant's newborn positive screen included recurrent emesis requiring intravenous fluids with minor illnesses.[130] During periods of illness nonprotein energy should be increased, intact protein intake should be decreased, and adequate fluid intake must be administered. Additional L-carnitine (100 mg per kg per day) may be administered during illness to facilitate the excretion of β-hydroxyisovaleric acid.[141] Patients with βMCC deficiency can develop a deficiency of free carnitine due to increased formation and excretion of acylcarnitine.[142] Emergency protocol for acute illness includes correction of the metabolic acidosis and hypoglycemia. A sample protocol for emergency management of βMCC deficiency is available online at http://www.childrenshospital.org/newengland consortium/NBS/MMC.html.[77]

Long-Term Nutrition Management

Although controversy exists regarding the nutrition management of patients with βMCC deficiency, the potential for problems due to low plasma carnitine concentration and metabolite decompensation during illness is well documented.[130,139-142] Secondary carnitine deficiency is commonly observed in newborns, children, and adults diagnosed with βMCC deficiency. Four women diagnosed when their newborns had elevated blood C5OH concentration demonstrated L-carnitine deficiency that resolved after 4 weeks of L-carnitine supplementation at 50 mg per kg per day.[140] Symptoms of fatigue, joint and muscle pain, headaches, and short-term memory improved after L-carnitine supplementation.[140] Carnitine plays a key role in excretion of potential toxic acyl groups as acylcarnitines.[143] Secondary carnitine deficiency may cause the excretory mechanisms to fail leading to clinical consequences.[144] In symptomatic patients who may be susceptible to metabolic decompensation, supplementation of L-carnitine may be necessary regardless of plasma carnitine concentrations as they decrease during intercurrent illness and fasting.[137] Case reports of combined glycine and L-carnitine supplementation have shown reduction in both plasma concentrations of β-methylcrotonylglycine and of β-hydroxyisovaleric acid, but it is not known whether the biochemical improvements altered the clinical outcome.[145,146] Biotin-responsiveness is rare, but improvements in biochemical markers and clinical symptoms have been reported in patients with the MCCA-R385S mutation.[132,134] The efficacy of intact protein or LEU-restricted diets is difficult to determine as randomized clinical studies have not been performed and clinical symptoms range from asymptomatic to severe phenotypes.

Guidelines for nutrition management were developed at the University of North Carolina based on biochemical phenotypes and experience with previously undiagnosed patients (D. Frazier, personal communication, July 8, 2008). Infants with a newborn screening blood C5OH concentration of less than or equal to 3 to 4 μmol/L continue on human milk or proprietary infant formula and receive L-carnitine supplementation if plasma carnitine concentrations are low. L-carnitine administration of 50 mg per kg per day is recommended during illness. Protein intake after infancy is based on RDAs for age.[47] A more prudent guideline for newborns or mothers with blood C5OH concentration greater than 3 to 4 μmol/L was established due to low plasma carnitine concentration in both infants and mothers, plus clinical symptoms associated with higher protein intakes above RDA reported by mothers with previously undiagnosed βMCC deficiency. Infants are placed on a LEU-free medical food (see Table 6.6) to provide approximately 50% of the protein requirement. L-carnitine is added to provide 50 to 100 mg per kg per day if not present in sufficient quantities in the medical food. Human milk or proprietary infant formula, followed by low-protein food choices, is used to provide essential LEU at the upper limit of requirement for age and size (see Appendix B). After infancy, a LEU-free medical food and unrestricted vegan diet is recommended. Other investigators have placed patients on milk-protein-restricted diets and reported improvements in clinical symptoms,[139,141] but further study is required to determine the extent of LEU restriction that may be optimal.

Assessment of Nutrition Management

Poor correlation exists between urinary excretion of β-hydroxyisovaleric acid and β-methylcrotonylglycine and clinical symptoms.[147] These urinary metabolites may be elevated when patients are well, but β-methylcrotonylglycine may also be absent.[128,147] Most treated patients continue to have abnormal plasma C5OH concentrations, although normal results have been reported.[130] Plasma concentrations of carnitine, indices of protein status, plasma amino acids minerals, and vitamins, plus anthropometrics and nutrient intakes should be monitored (see Chapter 3). The frequency and type of monitoring is dependent on the age of the patient, extent of diet restriction, and clinical course of the disorder.

Results of Nutrition Management

Assessment of the results of nutrition management on long-term outcomes is difficult as some patients with βMCC deficiencies have remained asymptomatic without treatment. Conversely, severe neurological dysfunction, cerebral edema, and death have been reported in some untreated persons. Diagnosis in presymptomatic patients has the advantage of counseling them and their parents to prevent possible metabolic decompensation and ensure a good prognosis. Although the long-term outcome is not known, it appears that early detection and appropriate treatment of patients will reduce morbidity and mortality.

β-Hydroxy-β-Methylglutaryl-CoA Lyase Deficiency

Introduction

β-Hydroxy-β-methylglutaryl-CoA (HMG-CoA) lyase deficiency (OMIM 24640)[2] or β-hydroxy-β-methylglutaric aciduria is a disorder of LEU catabolism and ketone body production. Faull et al. reported the first patient in 1976 who presented with vomiting and diarrhea, and developed cyanosis and apnea requiring resuscitation.[148] A marked deficiency of HMG-CoA lyase activity was found in leukocytes.[149] HMG-CoA lyase deficiency may present in infancy with vomiting, lethargy, metabolic acidosis, hypoglycemia, hyperammonemia, and hepatomegaly, frequently triggered by intercurrent illness or fasting.[94,150]

Biochemistry

HMG-CoA lyase (EC 4.1.3.4) is a mitochondrial enzyme that catabolizes HMG-CoA to acetyl-CoA and acetoacetate. This reaction is the final step in LEU catabolism and ketone production[150] (see Figures 6.1 and 6.2). The enzyme deficiency results in a reduced ability to produce ketones and process LEU. Infection, high intact protein intake, and prolonged fasting lead to metabolic decompensation, resulting in hypoketotic hypoglycemia and marked increase in several organic acids. The inability to produce ketones in response to fasting can cause severe hypoglycemia, which can lead to death if untreated.[151] The disorder is characterized by urinary excretion of β-hydroxy-β-methylglutaric, β-methylglutaconic, β-methylglutaric, and β-hydroxyisovaleric acids.[94,150]

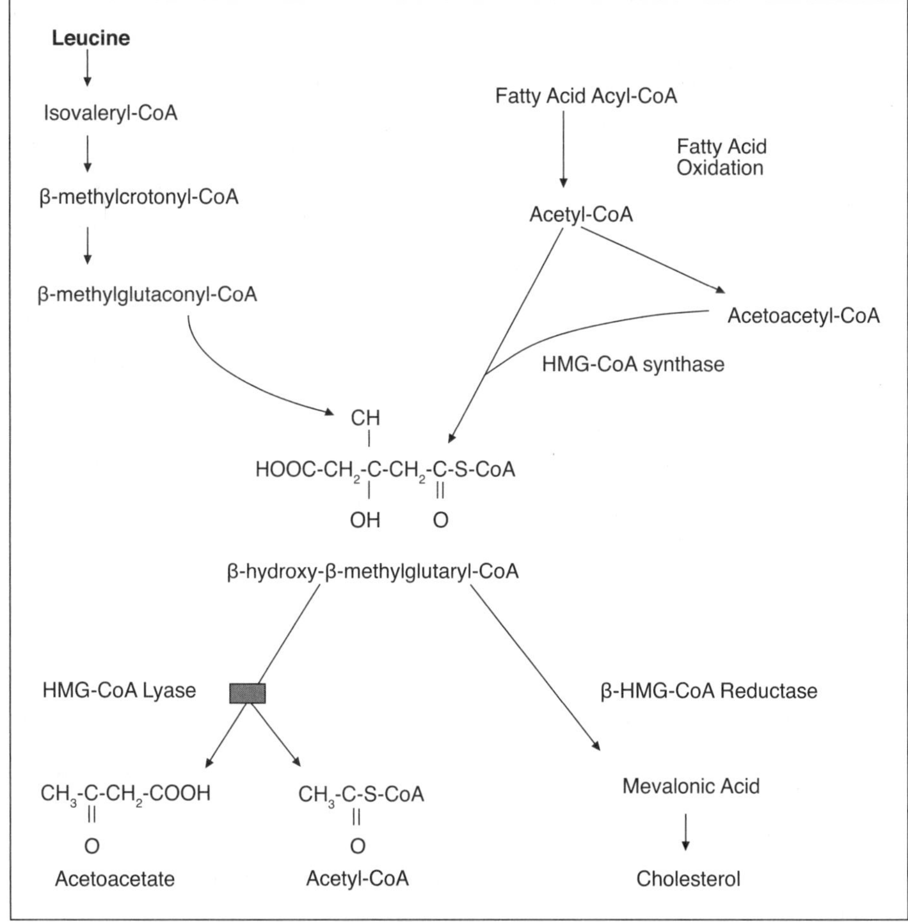

Figure 6.2 *Metabolism in HMG-CoA Lyase Deficiency*

Note: Black bar indicates site of enzyme defect.

Molecular Biology

The human gene for HMG-CoA lyase was cloned in 1993, is localized to chromosome 1pter-p33,[152] and contains 9 exons and codes for 298 peptide residues[152] (see Chapter 1). More than 90 cases of HMG-CoA lyase deficiency have been reported with 28 different mutations.[153] Two common mutations, 122G-A and 109G-A, have been found in patients in the Saudi Arabian and Iberian peninsulas (Portugal and Spain) accounting for approximately 90% of the mutations.[153] The genotype/phenotype correlation is hard to establish as the clinical phenotype is more related to the effects of hypoglycemia.[153]

Newborn Screening and Diagnosis

The incidence of this rare autosomal recessive disorder is not known. The disorder is more frequent in Saudi Arabia, Portugal, Spain, and Brazil[153,154] than reported elsewhere. An elevation of β-hydroxyisovalerylcarnitine (C5OH), included in newborn screening programs, is the first step in identifying potential cases of HMG-CoA lyase deficiency (see Chapter 2). Elevation of plasma concentrations of β-methylglutarylcarnitine, in addition to increased blood C5OH concentration, may be found. Confirmatory tests include evaluation of urinary organic acids with a characteristic elevation of β-hydroxy-β-methylglutaric acid. The urinary concentration of β-hydroxy-β-methylglutaric acid ranges from 200 to 4000 mmol/mol of creatinine when patients are well and may rise to 1500 to 19,000 mmol/mol creatinine during metabolic crisis.[94] During illness, urinary concentrations of β-hydroxyisovaleric acid, β-methylcrotonylglycine, β-methylglutaric acid, and β-methylglutaconic acid may also be increased.[94,155] To confirm the diagnosis, enzyme activity in leukocytes or fibroblasts must be performed. The diagnosis should be considered in infants and children presenting with Reye-like symptoms including neurological dysfunction, tachypnea, vomiting, nonketotic hypoglycemia, hyperammonemia, and hepatomegaly.[94]

Outcomes if Untreated

Patients who present in the neonatal period with severe nonketotic hypoglycemia, metabolic acidosis, and hyperammonemia may progress to coma and death if untreated.[94,151,156] Neonatal onset of HMG-CoA lyase deficiency is lethal in 20% of cases if untreated, although symptoms tend to be milder after childhood. Prior to newborn screening by MS/MS, approximately 30% of patients presented between 2 and 5 days of life and 70% between 3 and 11 months.[94] Acute pancreatitis, cerebral infarctions, stroke-like encephalopathy, and macrocephaly have been presenting symptoms in previously undiagnosed patients.[157-160] A clinical course of seizures, recurrent metabolic disturbances, and severe leukoencephalopathy was reported in a 36-year-old patient diagnosed after an acute episode of hypoglycemia.[161] The importance of nutrition management is illustrated in a 6-year-old girl who was identified after the diagnosis was made in a 5-day-old sibling. The child had followed a self-imposed protein and fat restriction and remained symptom free.[162] The nutrient restrictions lead to growth failure, but psychomotor development was normal.[162] Nutrition intervention results in good outcomes, although risk of decompensation exists during illness and prolonged fasting.

Nutrition Management

Nutrition management of patients with HMG-CoA lyase deficiency consists of limited intact protein (restricting intake of LEU) and fat intakes, L-carnitine supplementation, avoidance of fasting, and prompt attention to intercurrent illness.

Nutrient Requirements

Leucine, Protein, and Leucine-Free Medical Foods

Moderate intact protein restriction alone or in combination with LEU restriction has been utilized in the nutrition management of patients with HMG-CoA lyase deficiency. Protein intakes of 2.0 g per kg per day in infants and 1.5 g per kg per day in children have been reported.[150,163] Leupold et al. reported a fivefold increase in excretion of urinary metabolites when intact protein intake in a 5-month-old infant was increased from 1.8 to 2.5 g per kg per day.[160] Lower LEU intakes resulting from lower intakes of intact protein resulted in a decrease in urinary excretion of abnormal metabolites while preserving acceptable plasma LEU concentrations and normal growth.[160,163] LEU intakes in case reports of infants with HMG-CoA lyase deficiency have ranged from 50 to 120 mg per kg per day.[150,156,160,161,163-166] Suggested requirements for LEU are outlined in Table 6.5. During infancy and childhood LEU intake should be restricted by using LEU-free medical foods (see Table 6.6) in combination with an intact protein source. Growth failure was reported in a child who self-restricted protein and fat and did not consume a LEU-free medical food.[162] Proprietary infant formula, human milk, or a low-fat protein source is used to supply LEU in the first few months of life. The addition of a carbohydrate source may be necessary to maintain total fat intake to approximately 25% of energy. LEU content of foods should be considered when planning the diet as the child progresses to table foods.[58-60] Guidelines for estimating the LEU content of foods are provided in Table 6.3. Most LEU-free medical foods contain fat, carbohydrate, vitamins, and minerals. It is not known whether a moderate restriction of intact protein without the use of a LEU-free medical food is adequate after childhood, as symptoms tend to become milder.[154-156,166] Treatment recommendations for older children and adults are varied and optimal management has not been established.

Energy, Fat, and Fluid

Fluid and energy recommendations are included in Table 6.5. Due to the inability to produce ketones for energy during fasting, frequent feedings may be required during infancy and early childhood. A high carbohydrate intake with reduced fat intake is required to prevent accumulation of metabolites arising from fatty acid oxidation. Supplementation with glucose polymers or uncooked cornstarch may be required during periods of illness. Studies in patients with HMG-CoA lyase deficiency indicate that alterations in fat metabolism play a significant role in metabolic decompensation and support recommendations that restriction of dietary fat is warranted.[150,156,157,163,167] Stable isotope studies indicate that LEU oxidation, protein mobilization, and urinary excretion of LEU metabolites increase significantly during infection.[150] During fasting, despite a marked increase in urinary excretion of LEU metabolites, the LEU oxidation was unchanged and protein catabolism was slightly decreased.[150] The excretion of LEU metabolites derived from fat is accentuated during periods of fasting, accounting for approximately 70% of abnormal metabolite excretion.[150] During periods of good metabolic control, excretion of LEU metabolites increased significantly when fat intake was increased from 15 to 49 g per day in 2 children with HMG-CoA lyase deficiency.[168,169] In addition, the accumulation of CoA derivatives may further inhibit gluconeogenesis, contributing to the development of hypoglycemia.[170,171] Fat restriction to 20 to 25% of total energy is suggested and adequate intake of the essential fatty acids linoleic and α-linolenic is necessary (see Chapter 3, Table 3.1).

L-Carnitine

L-carnitine is prescribed to facilitate removal of acyl-CoA derivatives and prevent secondary carnitine deficiency.[150,163] High concentrations of urinary acylcarnitines with low concentrations of plasma-free carnitine have been reported.[144,155,161] L-carnitine doses have ranged from 50 to 100 mg per kg per day in infants and children and 1500 mg per day total in an adult.[94,155,161,163,165] Some LEU-free medical foods may contain enough L-carnitine to eliminate the need for supplemental L-carnitine. A sample prescription for an infant with HMG-CoA lyase deficiency is illustrated in Table 6.8.

Table 6.8 *Nutrition Management of a Patient with HMG-CoA Lyase Deficiency*

An 11-day-old asymptomatic 3.2 kg neonate diagnosed with HMG-CoA lyase deficiency.

	Amount	*LEU (mg)*	*Carnitine (mg)*	*Fat*[a] *(g)*	*Protein (g)*	*Energy (kcal)*	*Fluid (mL)*
I-Valex®-1 powder	30 g	—	270	6.5	4.5	144	—
ProViMin® powder	3 g	217	1.5	—	2.2	9	—
Polycose® powder	45 g	—	—	—	—	171	—
Human milk	120 mL	114	1.5	5.2	1.3	84	120
Water to make[b]							515
Total per day		331	273	11.7	8.0	408	515
Total per kg		103	85	3.6	2.5	128	161

Note: If protein is inadequate to support normal linear growth, see Chapter 3, Table 3.1.
[a]Twenty-six percent of energy provided as fat.
[b]Water to make final volume of 515 mL (~17 fl oz).

Initiation of Nutrition Management and During Critical Illness or Following Trauma

Although hypoglycemic episodes during illness are a feature in most cases of HMG-CoA lyase deficiency, the precise cause of hypoglycemia is not known. Gluconeogensis may be inhibited by the accumulation of CoA derivatives causing insufficient glucose production, while glucose consumption is increased due to absence of ketone bodies.[170,171] The importance of ketogenesis in preventing hypoglycemia was illustrated by administration of β-hydroxybutyrate to a patient that resulted in normalization of blood glucose concentration.[164] During acute illness, if the patient is unable to consume a high intake of carbohydrate orally, a 10% intravenous glucose solution at 150% of fluid requirements may be required.[165] Metabolic acidosis may require treatment with intravenous sodium bicarbonate.[165] L-carnitine (100 to 150 mg per kg per day) may be administered to promote excretion of abnormal metabolites.[144,165] Restriction of fat and LEU is recommended to minimize the acetoacetate produced and to decrease accumulation of abnormal LEU metabolites.[150,163] Hyperammonemia may occur during acute metabolic decompensation due to accumulation of β-hydroxy-β-methylglutaric acid and other metabolites, which may be toxic to the urea cycle.[150] Emergency treatment requires immediate correction of hypoglycemia and metabolic acidosis. A sample protocol for emergency management of patients with HMG-CoA lyase deficiency is available online at http://www.childrenshospital.org/newenglandconsortium/NBS/HMG.html.[77]

Long-Term Nutrition Management

The goal of long-term nutrition management is to prevent hypoglycemia, limit long periods of fasting, and minimize plasma elevations of LEU metabolites. A high-carbohydrate, low-fat diet with LEU restriction results in normal growth and development and minimizes urinary excretion of β-hydroxy-β-methylglutaric acid.[156,163,166,172]

Assessment of Nutrition Management

Elevations of urinary β-hydroxy-β-methylglutaric acid persist during periods of good metabolic control but increase significantly during periods of illness.[94,150,169] Urinary organic acid excretion is evaluated as part of clinical monitoring and needs to be assessed frequently during periods of illness. Evaluation for clinical symptoms associated with nutrient deficiencies, plasma concentrations of amino acids and carnitine, plus anthropometrics, diet intakes, and laboratory assessment of indices of protein, vitamin, and mineral status should be monitored regularly (see Chapter 3).

Results of Nutrition Management

Early diagnosis, prompt attention to illness, and adequate nutrition management can result in a clinical course free of symptoms with normal growth and development. Avoidance of fasting and immediate management of intercurrent illness will help eliminate hypoglycemia, metabolic acidosis, and the possible resulting clinical consequences.

Mitochondrial Acetoacetyl-CoA Thiolase Deficiency (β-Ketothiolase Deficiency)

Introduction

Mitochondrial acetoacetyl-CoA thiolase, mitochondrial β-ketoacyl-CoA thiolase, or β-ketothiolase (BKT) deficiency (OMIM 203750)[2] is an autosomal recessive disorder of ILE and ketone body metabolism. The disorder was initially described in 1971 in a child with intermittent metabolic acidosis and was identified as a defect in the catabolism of ILE, due to large urinary excretion of α-methyl-β-hydroxybutyric acid and α-methylacetoacetic acid during acidosis and after an ILE load.[173,174] The age of onset occurred from approximately 6 to 24 months with symptoms precipitated by an intercurrent illness in more than 50% of the cases.[175] In a review of 26 patients with BKT deficiency the median age of onset for the first ketoacidotic episode was 15 months.[176] Vomiting, dehydration, rapid respirations, diarrhea, hyperglycinemia, and severe ketoacidosis have been reported.[177,178] The onset of symptoms can be induced by high intakes of intact protein or illness causing body protein catabolism.[178] Episodes were reported to reoccur when appropriate treatment was not instituted following the initial episode.

Biochemistry

Mitochondrial acetoacetyl-CoA thiolase (EC 2.3.1.16) catalyzes two reversible mitochondrial reactions affecting ILE catabolism and ketone body metabolism. In the catabolism of ILE, the enzyme converts methylacetoacetyl-CoA into acetyl-CoA and propionyl-CoA (see Figure 6.3). In hepatic tissues during ketogenesis, βKT converts acetyl-CoA to acetoacetyl-CoA, while in non-hepatic tissues during the ketolytic process the enzyme converts acetoacetyl-CoA into acetyl-CoA (see Figure 6.3). Although βKT plays a role in both ketolysis and ketogenesis, patients with βKT deficiency generally present with ketoacidosis, illustrating that the ketolytic reaction is more dependent on the functioning of the βKT enzyme than the ketogenic reaction.[179] At least five thiolases have been identified in mammals: βKT, mitochondrial medium-chain β-ketoacyl-CoA thiolase, mitochondrial trifunctional protein, cytosolic acetoacetyl-CoA thiolase, and peroxisomal β-ketoacyl-CoA thiolase.[171] βKT is specific for methylacetoacetyl-CoA.[175,180] This specificity illustrates the key role for βKT in ILE metabolism. Deficiency of βKT results in urinary excretion of α-methyl-β-hydroxybutyric acid, α-methylacetoacetic acid, and tiglylglycine.[94,175] The urinary metabolite most characteristic of βKT deficiency is α-methyl-β-hydroxybutyric acid, as patients may have only trace amounts of α-methylacetoacetic acid and may not excrete tiglylglycine.

Molecular Biology

The human mitochondrial acetoacetyl-CoA thiolase gene was cloned in 1990 and mapped to chromosome 11q22.3-q23.1 in 1992[181,182] (see Chapter 1). The gene is approximately 1.5 kb in length and contains 12 exons and 11 introns.[182] More than 40 mutations have been identified including missense, nonsense, and splice-site mutations in addition to deletions.[176-180] A correlation between clinical severity and genotype has not been found but correlation between biochemical phenotype and genotype has been reported.[183] Patients with null mutations (severe mutations) compared with those who have residual enzyme activity (mild mutations) demonstrated differences in amounts of urinary organic acid excreted and plasma acylcarnitine profiles during stable

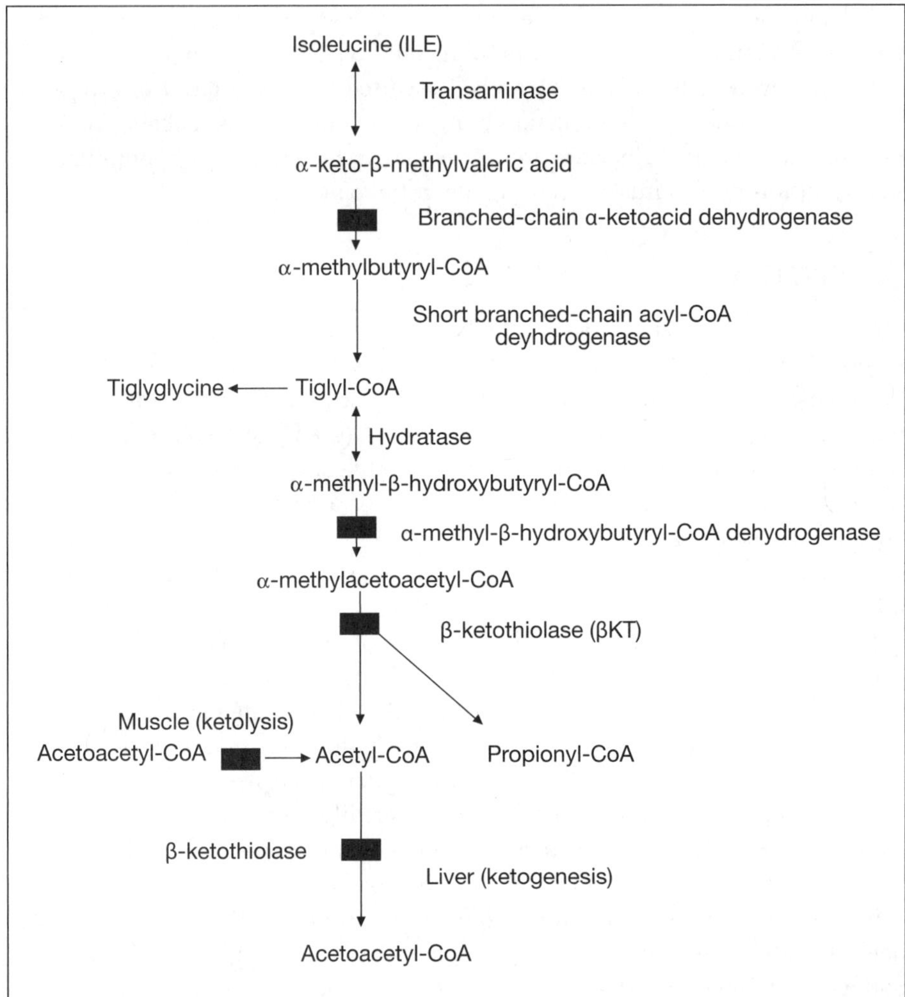

Figure 6.3 *Metabolism of Isoleucine*

Note: **Black bars indicate sites of enzyme defects.**

conditions.[183] However, patients with mild mutations did not differ from those with severe mutations with regard to prognosis or frequency and severity of ketoacidotic episodes.[183]

Newborn Screening and Diagnosis

βKT deficiency was previously suspected in infants and children who presented with intermittent ketoacidosis. This diagnosis was based on the abnormal urinary excretion of α-methyl-β-hydroxybutyric acid and possible tiglylglycine, and α-methylacetoacetic acid with ILE loading.[178] Starting in the early 2000s in the United States and many other countries, however, βKT deficiency began to be seen as part of the differential diagnosis when an elevated concentration of blood β-hydroxyisovalerylcarnitine (C5OH; see Chapter 2) or tiglylcarnitine (C5:1) was identified.[184] The next step in confirming the diagnosis is the elevation of α-methyl-β-hydroxybutyric acid and associated metabolites in urine. This abnormal pattern of urinary excretion has been detected in persons with normal thiolase activity, necessitating further investigation to confirm the diagnosis.[175]

The normal urinary excretion of α-methyl-β-hydroxybutyric acid is 1 to 9 mmol/mol of creatinine but, with any type of ketosis, excretion can increase up to 200 mmol/mol of creatinine.[94] Mildly affected patients with βKT deficiency can have α-methyl-β-hydroxybutyric acid excretion in the normal range or a slightly elevated amount when they are stable or during illness.[94] The most severely affected patients may have amounts in the range of 100 to 14,000 mmol/mol of creatinine.[94] In addition to mild urinary increases of α-methyl-β-hydroxybutyric acid in patients with residual enzyme activity, another disorder of ILE metabolism, α-methyl-β-hydroxybutyryl-CoA dehydrogenase deficiency, has similar urinary organic acid and acylcarnitine profiles.[185,186] The ambiguous urinary organic acids and acylcarnitine profiles necessitate the use of enzyme assay or DNA analysis to confirm the diagnosis. The activity of βKT is differentiated from other thiolases, as it is the only thiolase activated by potassium.[187,188] The ratio of enzyme activity in the absence and presence of potassium in combination with immunoblot analysis can identify heterozygotes and be used for prenatal diagnosis.[180,189,190] Enzyme analysis can be performed in lymphocytes, fibroblasts, aminocytes, and liver.[189,190]

More than 50 patients with βKT deficiency have been reported, but the incidence is not known. The disorder appears to be more frequent in Japan than in other countries, but patients from Tunisia (North Africa) and Arab countries have been reported.[191] It is unknown whether these patients carry more severe mutations resulting in clinical symptoms and subsequent diagnosis.

Outcome if Untreated

Untreated patients with βKT deficiency may present with a wide spectrum of clinical symptoms, ranging from normal growth and development despite recurrent ketoacidosis to severe neurological damage or death as a result of decompensation.[192] An asymptomatic course was reported in a 36-year-old father of an affected child, despite abnormal urinary metabolite excretion and absence of βKT activity in fibroblasts.[193] Coma, confusion, and lethargy have been reported in 18 patients during the initial episode of ketoacidosis, and follow-up observations on them demonstrated three patients with impaired cognitive development, one with ataxia, and one who died.[176]

Nutrition Management

Clinical consequences may be avoided with early diagnosis, avoidance of fasting, prompt management of ketoacidosis, and modest protein (ILE) restriction.

Initiation of Nutrition Management and During Critical Illness or Following Trauma

In the acute phase with ketoacidosis and dehydration, intravenous (IV) fluids with glucose, electrolytes, and bicarbonate may be required.[175,194] L-carnitine administration (200 mg per kg per day) during acute episodes has been suggested to remove tiglyl-CoA and other CoA esters, but it is not known whether it significantly improves the acute management of the patient.[175] During periods of illness such as gastroenteritis it is advisable to restrict the intake of ILE. Energy intake must be increased, especially if temperature is increased.

Long-Term Nutrition Management

Long-term nutrition management requires mild restriction of ILE and avoidance of fasting. Limited data are available on the efficacy of nutrition management and heterogeneity in the clinical presentation emphasizes the need for individualized treatment. No consensus exists whether an ILE-restricted diet with a BCAA-free medical food (see Table 6.2) is required or whether the disorder can be managed with mild intact protein restriction. During infancy and subsequent periods of rapid growth, ILE restriction along with addition of a BCAA-free medical food to provide adequate protein for normal growth and development may be required. Limited data exist regarding BCAA requirements in normal infants and children. The Dietary Reference Intakes (DRIs) for LEU, VAL, and ILE in school-age children are 52, 34, and 24 mg per kg per day, respectively, or a total BCAA intake of 110 mg per kg per day.[47] Mager et al. estimated BCAA requirements (using indicator amino acid oxidation methods) of 6 to 10-year-old children to be significantly higher at 147 mg per kg per day.[195] These requirements are based on healthy children with normal body weight. The BCAA requirements for obese or overweight persons are not known. Adequate intakes for infants from birth to

6 months are based on human milk consumption and estimated at 156, 87, and 88 mg per kg per day for LEU, VAL, and ILE, respectively.[47] Avoidance of fasting is recommended to eliminate or limit reoccurrence of ketoacidotic episodes.[175] Frequent feeding and mild restriction of both intact protein and fat have been suggested in one report.[196]

Carnitine deficiency was reported in 19-month-old male twins suspected of having βKT deficiency and in a pregnant woman with βKT deficiency.[194,197] The proposal was made that tiglyl-CoA may be trapped as tiglylcarnitine contributing to the low free plasma carnitine concentrations detected.[175,197] L-carnitine supplementation of 100 mg per kg per day was prescribed for the pregnant women with βKT deficiency.[197] A sample prescription for a neonate with βKT deficiency using a BCAA-free medical food is illustrated in Table 6.9.

Assessment and Results of Nutrition Management

The presence of α-methyl-β-hydroxybutyric acid in urine is not an indicator of metabolic control, as some patients have continued elevations when asymptomatic, while in others the metabolite is not detected.[94] Adequate total protein, energy, vitamin, and mineral intakes for growth and development should be prescribed, and plasma amino acids and carnitine concentrations monitored to avoid deficiencies (see Chapter 3). A moderate restriction of intact protein (ILE) and avoidance of fasting will prevent or limit ketoacidotic episodes and ensure a favorable long-term outcome.

Table 6.9 ***Nutrition Management of a Patient with β-Ketothiolase Deficiency***

A 12-day-old 3.5 kg neonate diagnosed with β-ketothiolase deficiency.

	Amount	*LEU (mg)*	*ILE (mg)*	*VAL (mg)*	*Protein (g)*	*Energy (kcal)*	*Fluid (mL)*
Ketonex®-1 powder	25 g	—	—	—	3.8	120	—
Human milk	500 mL	335	550	450	4.5	350	500
Water to make[a]							680
Total per day		335	550	450	8.3	470	680
Total per kg		95	157	128	2.4	134	194

Note: If protein is inadequate to support normal linear growth, see Chapter 3, Table 3.1.
[a]Water to make final volume of 680 mL (~23 fl oz).

β-Methylglutaconyl-CoA Hydratase Deficiency (β-Methylglutaconic Aciduria–Type I)

β-methylglutaconyl-CoA hydratase deficiency (OMIM 250950)[2] is one of four types of β-methylglutaconic aciduria (βMGA). βMGA Type I is a rare autosomal recessive disorder of LEU catabolism with only 14 patients reported in the literature as of 2003.[198] βMGA Type II (Barth syndrome; OMIM 302060)[2] is an X-linked disorder with dilated cardiomyopathy, growth retardation, and neutropenia. βMGA Type III (Costeff optic atrophy syndrome; OMIM 258501)[2] is associated with optic atrophy, nystagmus, cerebellar ataxia, and spastic paraparesis, while βMGA Type IV (OMIM 250951)[2] or "unclassified," has diverse clinical symptoms, and some patients are found to have abnormalities in the electron transport chain. Although all four disorders have increased urinary excretion of β-methylglutaconic acid, deficiency of β-methylglutaconyl-CoA hydratase has been demonstrated only in βMGA Type I.[94] β-methylglutaconyl-CoA hydratase (E.C.4.2.1.18) is involved in the conversion of β-methylglutaconyl-CoA to β-hydroxy-β-methylglutaryl-CoA (see Figure 6.1). The enzyme defect results in elevated urinary excretion of β-methylglutaconic acid in addition to β-methylglutaric and β-hydroxyisovaleric acid excretion.[94,199] The enzyme is identical to an RNA-binding protein (designated AUH) and molecular analysis has discovered four mutations in the AUH gene in patients with βMGA Type I.[200] Elevation of C5OH blood concentration on newborn screening with accompanying urinary excretion of β-methylglutaconic acid may identify possible cases of βMGA Type I. Clinical symptoms are variable, ranging from isolated speech retardation to psychomotor abnormalities, microcephaly, macrocephaly, seizures, neurological impairment, and progressive leukoencephalopathy in late adulthood.[198-205] An initial presentation of Reye-like symptoms including hypoglycemia, acidosis, and hyperammonemia has been reported.[202]

The goal of treatment during acute episodes is prevention of catabolism by carbohydrate administration and correction of the acidosis. The efficacy of long-term nutrition management of this rare disorder has not been established. L-carnitine supplementation has been reported to have beneficial effects in some cases.[199,206,207] LEU restriction has resulted in decreased urinary excretion of β-hydroxyisovaleric and β-methylglutaconic acids.[201,204] Neurological status remained unchanged during 1 year of follow up in a 55-year-old woman with progressive leukoencephalopathy who was placed on a low intact protein diet with a LEU-free medical food added.[203] The therapeutic benefit of a LEU-restricted diet on long-term outcome remains to be established by neonatal diagnosis and institution of long-term nutrition management.

α-Methyl-β-Hydroxybutyryl-CoA Dehydrogenase Deficiency (α-Methyl-β-Hydroxybutyric Aciduria)

First reported in 2000, α-methyl-β-hydroxybutyryl-CoA dehydrogenase (MHBD) deficiency (OMIM 300438)[2] is a new disorder of ILE and α-methyl-branched-chain fatty acid metabolism.[186] The enzyme (EC 1.1.1.178) dehydrogenates α-methyl-β-hydroxybutyryl-CoA to α-methyl-acetoacetyl-CoA (see Figure 6.3). A defect in multifunctional mitochondrial MHBD results in increased urinary excretion of α-methyl-β-hydroxybutyric acid and tiglylglycine.[208] In contrast to β-ketothiolase deficiency, α-methylacetoacetic acid is not present, and recurrent ketoacidotic episodes are not a characteristic finding.[209] The disorder is inherited as an X-linked recessive trait and mutations have been identified in the HADH2 gene.[210] The HADH2 gene has been mapped to Xp11.2 and in addition to its role in ILE metabolism, the gene may induce mitochondrial dysfunction by interaction with amyloid-β peptide-binding protein.[210,211] This interaction may play a role in the pathogenesis of Alzheimer's disease.[210]

The elevation of C5OH and C5:1 blood concentrations on newborn screening may lead to identification of possible cases of MHBD deficiency. A number of children with elevated concentrations of α-methyl-β-hydroxybutyric acid and tiglylglycine have been suspected of β-ketothiolase deficiency, although normal enzyme activity was found.[212] The importance of enzyme assay or molecular analysis is emphasized when impaired ILE metabolism is detected.

Since the initial description of a 4-month-old infant with a neurodegenerative presentation,[186] 10 additional cases have been reported that exhibit a wide array of clinical symptoms. The clinical presentations have included severe neurological regression with hypotonia, cortical blindness, myotonic seizures, and spastic diplegia.[186,209,212-215] A milder phenotype without regression has been reported in a female with developmental delay and in a 6-year-old male with normal development who experienced motor and cognitive deterioration after a febrile illness.[214,215] The disorder is generally milder in heterozygote females due to X-inactivation than in males.

ILE loading (100 mg per kg per day) resulted in a sixfold increase in urinary excretion of α-methyl-β-hydroxybutyric acid and tiglylglycine.[186,209] An ILE-restricted diet has been instituted in several patients with resulting decrease in abnormal urinary metabolite excretion and stabilization of neurological symptoms.[186,211,214,216] Sutton et al. noted minimal improvement in neurodevelopment and seizure activity in an 8-year-old male despite ILE restriction.[213] The multiple roles of the enzyme in metabolism and the present understanding of the pathophysiology of the disorder suggest that nutrition management may not significantly impact clinical symptoms in severe cases.[208] It is not known whether early diagnosis and ILE restriction before the development of clinical symptoms will alter the long-term outcome.

CONCLUSION

Nutrition management plays a key role in many inherited metabolic disorders that have been identified in the metabolism of the branched-chain amino acids. The term "organic acidemia" (or "organic aciduria") alludes to the excretion of non-amino organic acids in urine that characterize most of the disorders. The enzyme defect in MSUD involves alterations in the metabolism of all three branched-chain amino acids. Propionic and methylmalonic acidemias are disorders derived in part from the catabolism of ILE and VAL (see Chapter 8). LEU catabolism disorders include IVA, βMCC deficiency, HMG-CoA lyase deficiency, and βMGA Type I. Disorders in ILE metabolism outlined in this chapter include βKT deficiency and MHBD deficiency. Disorders affecting ILE metabolism and fatty acids including short-branched-chain acyl-CoA dehydrogenase (SBCAD) deficiency (OMIM 600301)[2] and α-methyl-CoA dehydrogenase deficiency (OMIM 61006)[2] have been recently described. SBCAD deficiency in the Hmong communities in Minnesota and Wisconsin appears to be a benign condition.[217] The clinical spectrum and effect of nutrition management in SBCAD among other ethnic groups is not known as fewer than 10 patients have been reported.[208] Disorders of VAL metabolism are extremely rare: β-hydroxyisobutyric aciduria (OMIM 236795)[2] has been identified as possibly responding to VAL restriction and L-carnitine supplementation.[94] Early diagnosis, prompt attention to intercurrent illness, and adequate nutrition management have markedly improved long-term outcomes of patients with these disorders.

REFERENCES

1. Chuang DT, Shih VE. Maple syrup urine disease (branched-chain ketoaciduria). In: Scriver CR, Beaudet AL, Sly WS, Valle D, eds. *The Metabolic and Molecular Bases of Inherited Disease*. 8th ed. New York, NY: McGraw-Hill; 2001:1971–2005.
2. National Center for Biotechnology Information. OMIM™—Online Mendelian Inheritance in Man™ (database). Available at: http://www.ncbi.nlm.nih.gov/sites/entrez?db=omim. Accessed February 2, 2008.
3. Menkes JH, Hurst PL, Craig JM. A new syndrome: progressive familial infantile cerebral dysfunction associated with an unusual urinary substance. *Pediatrics*. 1954;14:462–467.
4. Menkes JH. Maple syrup disease; isolation and identification of organic acids in the urine. *Pediatrics*. 1959;23:348–353.
5. Dancis J, Levitz M, Westall RG. Maple syrup urine disease: branched-chain ketoaciduria. *Pediatrics*. 1960;25:72–79.

6. Dancis J, Hurtzler J, Levitz M. Metabolism of the white blood cells in maple-syrup-urine disease. *Biochim Biophys Acta*. 1960;43:342–343.
7. Pettit FH, Yeaman SJ, Reed LJ. Purification and characterization of branched chain alpha-keto acid dehydrogenase complex of bovine kidney. *Proc Natl Acad Sci USA*. 1978;75:4881–4885.
8. Snyderman SE, Norton PM, Roitman E, Holt LE Jr. Maple syrup urine disease, with particular reference to dietotherapy. *Pediatrics*. 1964;34:454–472.
9. Schadewaldt P, Wendel U. Metabolism of branched-chain amino acids in maple syrup urine disease. *Eur J Pediatr*. 1997;156(Suppl 1)S62–S66.
10. Matthews DE. Observations of branched-chain amino acid administration in humans. *J Nutr*. 2005;135:1580S–1584S.
11. Suryawan A, Hawes JW, Harris RA, Shimomura Y, Jenkins AE, Hutson SM. A molecular model of human branched-chain amino acid metabolism. *Am J Clin Nutr*. 1998;68:72–81.
12. Peinemann F, Danner DJ. Maple syrup urine disease 1954 to 1993. *J Inherit Metab Dis*. 1994;17:3–15.
13. Nellis MM, Danner DJ. Gene preference in maple syrup urine disease. *Am J Hum Genet*. 2001;68:232–237.
14. Flaschker N, Feyen O, Fend S, Simon E, Schadewaldt P, Wendel U. Description of the mutations in 15 subjects with variant forms of maple syrup urine disease. *J Inherit Metab Dis*. 2007;30:903–909.
15. Naylor EW, Guthrie R. Newborn screening for maple syrup urine disease (branched-chain ketoaciduria). *Pediatrics*. 1978;61:262–266.
16. Chace DH, Hillman SL, Millington DS, Kahler SG, Roe CR, Naylor EW. Rapid diagnosis of maple syrup urine disease in blood spots from newborns by tandem mass spectrometry. *Clin Chem*. 1995;41:62–68.
17. Schadewaldt P, Bodner-Leidecker A, Hammen HW, Wendel U. Significance of L-alloisoleucine in plasma for diagnosis of maple syrup urine disease. *Clin Chem*. 1999;45:1734–1740.
18. Fisher CR, Fisher CW, Chuang DT, Cox RP. Occurrence of a Tyr393-Asn (Y393N) mutation in the E1 alpha gene of the branched-chain alpha-keto acid dehydrogenase complex in maple syrup urine disease patients from a Mennonite population. *Am J Hum Genet*. 1991;49:429–434.
19. Mitsubuchi H, Owada M, Endo F. Markers associated with inborn errors of metabolism of branched-chain amino acids and their relevance to upper levels of intake in healthy people: an implication from clinical and molecular investigations on maple syrup urine disease. *J Nutr*. 2005;135:1565S–1570S.
20. Simon E, Flaschker N, Schadewaldt P, Langenbeck U, Wendel U. Variant maple syrup urine disease (MSUD)—the entire spectrum. *J Inherit Metab Dis*. 2006;29:716–724.
21. Fischer MH, Gerritsen T. Biochemical studies on a variant of branched chain ketoaciduria in a 19-year-old female. *Pediatrics*. 1971;48:795–801.
22. Duran M, Tielens AG, Wadman SK, Stigter JC, Kleijer WJ. Effects of thiamine in a patient with a variant form of branched-chain ketoaciduria. *Acta Paediatr Scand*. 1978;67:367–372.
23. Lie IE, Haugstad S, Holm H. Tailoring of the diet for the individual in maple syrup urine disease: long-term home dietary treatment of an adult patient with MSUD by monitoring of daily intake with a personal computer. A case report. *Hum Nutr Appl Nutr*. 1985;39:130–136.

24. Scriver CR, Mackenzie S, Clow CL, Delvin E. Thiamine-responsive maple-syrup-urine disease. *Lancet*. 1971;1:310–312.
25. Scriver CR, Clow CL, George H. So-called thiamin-responsive maple syrup urine disease: 15-year follow-up of the original patient. *J Pediatr*. 1985;107:763–765.
26. Duran M, Wadman SK. Thiamine-responsive inborn errors of metabolism. *J Inherit Metab Dis*. 1985;8(Suppl 1):70–75.
27. Fernhoff PM, Lubitz D, Danner DJ, et al. Thiamine response in maple syrup urine disease. *Pediatr Res*. 1985;19:1011–1016.
28. Delis D, Michelakakis H, Katsarou E, Bartsocas CS. Thiamin-responsive maple syrup urine disease: seizures after 7 years of satisfactory metabolic control. *J Inherit Metab Dis*. 2001;24:683–684.
29. Burke JP, O'Keefe M, Bowell R, Naughten ER. Ophthalmic findings in maple syrup urine disease. *Metab Pediatr Syst Ophthalmol*. 1991;14:12–15.
30. Backhouse O, Leitch RJ, Thompson D, et al. A case of reversible blindness in maple syrup urine disease. *Br J Ophthalmol*. 1999;83:250–251.
31. Riviello JJ Jr., Rezvani I, DiGeorge AM, Foley CM. Cerebral edema causing death in children with maple syrup urine disease. *J Pediatr*. 1991;119:42–45.
32. Kahler SG, Sherwood WG, Woolf D, et al. Pancreatitis in patients with organic acidemias. *J Pediatr*. 1994;124:239–243.
33. Danias J, Raab EI, Friedman AH. Retinopathy associated with pancreatitis in a child with maple syrup urine disease. *Br J Ophthalmol*. 1998;82:841–842.
34. Wajner M, Schlottfeldt JL, Ckless K, Wannmacher CM. Immunosuppressive effects of organic acids accumulating in patients with maple syrup urine disease. *J Inherit Metab Dis*. 1995;18:165–168.
35. Treacy E, Clow CL, Reade TR, Chitayat D, Mamer OA, Scriver CR. Maple syrup urine disease: interrelations between branched-chain amino-, oxo- and hydroxy-acids; implications for treatment; associations with CNS dysmyelination. *J Inherit Metab Dis*. 1992;15:121–135.
36. Schonberger S, Schweiger B, Schwahn B, Schwarz M, Wendel U. Dysmyelination in the brain of adolescents and young adults with maple syrup urine disease. *Mol Genet Metab*. 2004;82:69–75.
37. Heldt K, Schwahn B, Marquardt I, Grotzke M, Wendel U. Diagnosis of MSUD by newborn screening allows early intervention without extraneous detoxification. *Mol Genet Metab*. 2005;84:313–316.
38. Naughten ER, Jenkins J, Francis DE, Leonard JV. Outcome of maple syrup urine disease. *Arch Dis Child*. 1982;57:918–921.
39. Nord A, van Doorninck WJ, Greene C. Developmental profile of patients with maple syrup urine disease. *J Inherit Metab Dis*. 1991;14:881–889.
40. Hilliges C, Awiszus D, Wendel U. Intellectual performance of children with maple syrup urine disease. *Eur J Pediatr*. 1993;152:144–147.
41. Kaplan P, Mazur A, Field M, et al. Intellectual outcome in children with maple syrup urine disease. *J Pediatr*. 1991;119:46–50.
42. Simon E, Fingerhut R, Baumkotter J, Konstantopoulou V, Ratschmann R, Wendel U. Maple syrup urine disease: favourable effect of early diagnosis by newborn screening on the neonatal course of the disease. *J Inherit Metab Dis*. 2006; 29:532–537.
43. Hoffmann B, Helbling C, Schadewaldt P, Wendel U. Impact of longitudinal plasma leucine levels on the intellectual outcome in patients with classic MSUD. *Pediatr Res*. 2006;59:17–20.

44. Elsas LJ, Acosta PB. Inherited metabolic disease: amino acids, organic acids and galactose. In: Shils ME, Shike M, Ross AC, Cabellero B, Cousins RJ, eds. *Modern Nutrition in Health and Disease*. 10th ed. Philadelphia, PA: Lippincott Williams & Wilkins; 2005:909–959.
45. Snyderman SE. Treatment outcome of maple syrup urine disease. *Acta Paediatr Jpn*. 1988;30:417–424.
46. le Roux C, Murphy E, Hallam P, Lilburn M, Orlowska D, Lee P. Neuropsychometric outcome predictors for adults with maple syrup urine disease. *J Inherit Metab Dis*. 2006;29:201–202.
47. Institute of Medicine of the National Academies. *Dietary Reference Intakes for Energy, Carbohydrate, Fiber, Fat, Fatty Acids, Cholesterol, Protein, and Amino Acids*. Washington, DC: National Academies Press; 2005.
48. Kindt E, Halvorsen S. The need of essential amino acids in children: an evaluation based on the intake of phenylalanine, tyrosine, leucine, isoleucine, and valine in children with phenylketonuria, tyrosine amino transferase defect, and maple syrup urine disease. *Am J Clin Nutr*. 1980;33:279–286.
49. Parsons HG, Carter RJ, Unrath M, Snyder FF. Evaluation of branched-chain amino acid intake in children with maple syrup urine disease and methylmalonic aciduria. *J Inherit Metab Dis*. 1990;13:125–136.
50. De Raeve L, De Meirleir L, Ramet J, Vandenplas Y, Gerlo E. Acrodermatitis enteropathica-like cutaneous lesions in organic aciduria. *J Pediatr*. 1994;124:416–420.
51. Diliberti JH, DiGeorge AM, Auerbach VH. Abnormal leucine/isoleucine ratio and the etiology of acrodermatitis enteropathica-like rash in maple syrup urine disease. *Pediatr Res* 1973;7:382.
52. Northrup H, Sigman ES, Hebert AA. Exfoliative erythroderma resulting from inadequate intake of branched-chain amino acids in infants with maple syrup urine disease. *Arch Dermatol*. 1993;129:384–385.
53. Giacoia GP, Berry GT. Acrodermatitis enteropathica-like syndrome secondary to isoleucine deficiency during treatment of maple syrup urine disease. *Am J Dis Child*. 1993;147:954–956.
54. Koch SE, Packman S, Koch TK, Williams ML. Dermatitis in treated maple syrup urine disease. *J Am Acad Dermatol*. 1993;28:289–292.
55. Bosch AM, Sillevis Smitt JH, van Gennip AH, et al. Iatrogenic isolated isoleucine deficiency as the cause of an acrodermatitis enteropathica-like syndrome. *Br J Dermatol*. 1998;139:488–491.
56. Tornqvist K, Tornqvist H. Corneal deepithelialization caused by acute deficiency of isoleucine during treatment of a patient with maple syrup urine disease. *Acta Ophthalmol Scand Suppl*. 1996;48–49.
57. Gropper SS, Gropper DM, Acosta PB. Plasma amino acid response to ingestion of L-amino acids and whole protein. *J Pediatr Gastroenterol Nutr*. 1993;16: 143–150.
58. Acosta PB, Yannicelli S. Protocol 5. *Maple Syrup Urine Disease (MSUD). Nutrition Support Protocols*. Columbus, OH: Ross Products Division, Abbott Laboratories; 2001.
59. Singh R, Lesperance E, Crawford K. *MSUD Food List*. Atlanta, GA: Division of Medical Genetics, Department of Human Genetics, Emory University School of Medicine; 2002.
60. USDA Agricultural Research Service. Nutrient Data Laboratory. Available at: http://www.nal.usda.gov/fnic/foodcomp/search/. Accessed July 8, 2008.

61. Krempf M, Hoerr RA, Pelletier VA, Marks LM, Gleason R, Young VR. An isotopic study of the effect of dietary carbohydrate on the metabolic fate of dietary leucine and phenylalanine. *Am J Clin Nutr.* 1993;57:161–169.
62. Curran JS, Barness LA. Nutrition. In: Behrman RE, Kliegman RM, Jenson HB, eds. *Nelson Textbook of Pediatrics.* 16th ed. Philadelphia, PA: WB Saunders; 2000:138–149.
63. Nevin-Folino N, Miller M. Enteral nutrition. In: Queen Samour P, King K, eds. *Handbook of Pediatric Nutrition.* 3rd ed. Sudbury, MA: Jones and Bartlett; 2005: 499–524.
64. Gropper SS, Naglak MC, Nardella M, Plyler A, Rarback S, Yannicelli S. Nutrient intakes of adolescents with phenylketonuria and infants and children with maple syrup urine disease on semisynthetic diets. *J Am Coll Nutr.* 1993;12:108–114.
65. Barschak AG, Sitta A, Deon M, et al. Erythrocyte glutathione peroxidase activity and plasma selenium concentration are reduced in maple syrup urine disease patients during treatment. *Int J Dev Neurosci.* 2007;25:335–338.
66. Puliyanda DP, Harmon WE, Peterschmitt MJ, Irons M, Somers MJ. Utility of hemodialysis in maple syrup urine disease. *Pediatr Nephrol.* 2002;17:239–242.
67. Jouvet P, Jugie M, Rabier D, et al. Combined nutritional support and continuous extracorporeal removal therapy in the severe acute phase of maple syrup urine disease. *Intensive Care Med.* 2001;27:1798–1806.
68. Berry GT, Heidenreich R, Kaplan P, et al. Branched-chain amino acid-free parenteral nutrition in the treatment of acute metabolic decompensation in patients with maple syrup urine disease. *N Engl J Med.* 1991;324:175–179.
69. Morton DH, Strauss KA, Robinson DL, Puffenberger EG, Kelley RI. Diagnosis and treatment of maple syrup disease: a study of 36 patients. *Pediatrics.* 2002;109: 999–1008.
70. Wendel U, Langenbeck U, Lombeck I, Bremer HJ. Maple syrup urine disease—therapeutic use of insulin in catabolic states. *Eur J Pediatr.* 1982;139:172–175.
71. Nyhan WL, Rice-Kelts M, Klein J, Barshop BA. Treatment of the acute crisis in maple syrup urine disease. *Arch Pediatr Adolesc Med.* 1998;152:593–598.
72. Parini R, Sereni LP, Bagozzi DC, et al. Nasogastric drip feeding as the only treatment of neonatal maple syrup urine disease. *Pediatrics.* 1993;92:280–283.
73. Dixon MA, Leonard JV. Intercurrent illness in inborn errors of intermediary metabolism. *Arch Dis Child.* 1992;67:1387–1391.
74. Hmiel SP, Martin RA, Landt M, Levy FH, Grange DK. Amino acid clearance during acute metabolic decompensation in maple syrup urine disease treated with continuous venovenous hemodialysis with filtration. *Pediatr Crit Care Med.* 2004;5:278–281.
75. Thompson GN, Francis DEM, Halliday D. Acute illness in maple syrup urine disease: dynamics of protein metabolism and implications for management. *J Pediatr.* 1991;119:35–41.
76. Wajner M, Coelho DM, Barschak AG, et al. Reduction of large neutral amino acid concentrations in plasma and CSF of patients with maple syrup urine disease during crises. *J Inherit Metab Dis.* 2000;23:505–512.
77. New England Consortium at Children's Hospital Boston. Acute Illness Protocols. Children's Hospital Boston. Available at: http://www.childrenshospital.org/newenglandconsortium/MSUD. Accessed July 8, 2008.

78. Snyderman SE, Goldstein F, Sansaricq C, Norton PM. The relationship between the branched chain amino acids and their alpha-ketoacids in maple syrup urine disease. *Pediatr Res*. 1984;18:851–853.
79. Monastiri K, Limame K, Kaabachi N, et al. Fenugreek odour in maple syrup urine disease. *J Inherit Metab Dis*. 1997;20:614–615.
80. Korman SH, Cohen E, Preminger A. Pseudo-maple syrup urine disease due to maternal prenatal ingestion of fenugreek. *J Paediatr Child Health*. 2001;37:403–404.
81. Henstenburg JD, Mazur AT, Kaplan PB, Stallings VA. Nutritional assessment and body composition in children with maple syrup urine disease (MSUD). *J Am Diet Assoc* 1990;90:32A.
82. Wendel U, Saudubray JM, Bodner A, Schadewaldt P. Liver transplantation in maple syrup urine disease. *Eur J Pediatr*. 1999;158(Suppl 2):S60–S64.
83. Strauss KA, Mazariegos GV, Sindhi R, et al. Elective liver transplantation for the treatment of classical maple syrup urine disease. *Am J Transplant*. 2006;6:557–564.
84. Khanna A, Hart M, Nyhan WL, Hassanein T, Panyard-Davis J, Barshop BA. Domino liver transplantation in maple syrup urine disease. *Liver Transpl*. 2006;12: 876–882.
85. Zaleski LA, Dancis J, Cox RP, Hutzler J, Zaleski WA, Hill A. Variant maple syrup urine disease in mother and daughter. *Can Med Assoc J*. 1973;109:299–300.
86. van Calcar SC, Harding CO, Davidson SR, Barness LA, Wolff JA. Case reports of successful pregnancy in women with maple syrup urine disease and propionic acidemia. *Am J Med Genet*. 1992;44:641–646.
87. Grünewald S, Hinrichs F, Wendel U. Pregnancy in a woman with maple syrup urine disease. *J Inherit Metab Dis*. 1998;21:89–94.
88. Koumantakis E, Sifakis S, Koumantaki Y, et al. Plasma carnitine levels of pregnant adolescents in labor. *J Pediatr Adolesc Gynecol*. 2001;14:65–69.
89. Cho SW, Cha YS. Pregnancy increases urinary loss of carnitine and reduces plasma carnitine in Korean women. *Br J Nutr*. 2005;93:685–691.
90. Newman CG, Wilson BD, Callaghan P, Young L. Neonatal death associated with isovalericacidaemia. *Lancet*. 1967;2:439–442.
91. Tanaka K, Budd MA, Efron ML, Isselbacher KJ. Isovaleric acidemia: a new genetic defect of leucine metabolism. *Proc Natl Acad Sci USA*. 1966;56:236–242.
92. Rhead WJ, Tanaka K. Demonstration of a specific mitochondrial isovaleryl-CoA dehydrogenase deficiency in fibroblasts from patients with isovaleric acidemia. *Proc Natl Acad Sci USA*. 1980;77:580–583.
93. Ensenauer R, Vockley J, Willard JM, et al. A common mutation is associated with a mild, potentially asymptomatic phenotype in patients with isovaleric acidemia diagnosed by newborn screening. *Am J Hum Genet*. 2004;75:1136–1142.
94. Sweetman L, Williams JC. Branched chain organic acidurias. In: Scriver CR, Beaudet AL, Sly WS, Valle D, eds. *The Metabolic and Molecular Bases of Inherited Disease*. 8th ed. New York, NY: McGraw-Hill; 2001:2125–2163.
95. Kraus JP, Matsubara Y, Barton D, et al. Isolation of cDNA clones coding for rat isovaleryl-CoA dehydrogenase and assignment of the gene to human chromosome 15. *Genomics*. 1987;1:264–269.
96. Ikeda Y, Keese SM, Tanaka K. Molecular heterogeneity of variant isovaleryl-CoA dehydrogenase from cultured isovaleric acidemia fibroblasts. *Proc Natl Acad Sci USA*. 1985;82:7081–7085.

97. Vockley J, Parimoo B, Tanaka K. Molecular characterization of four different classes of mutations in the isovaleryl-CoA dehydrogenase gene responsible for isovaleric acidemia. *Am J Hum Genet*. 1991;49:147–157.
98. Vockley J, Ensenauer R. Isovaleric acidemia: new aspects of genetic and phenotypic heterogeneity. *Am J Med Genet C Semin Med Genet*. 2006;142C:95–103.
99. Abdenur JE, Chamoles NA, Guinle AE, Schenone AB, Fuertes AN. Diagnosis of isovaleric acidaemia by tandem mass spectrometry: false positive result due to pivaloylcarnitine in a newborn screening programme. *J Inherit Metab Dis*. 1998;21: 624–630.
100. Shigematsu Y, Hata I, Tanaka Y. Stable-isotope dilution measurement of isovalerylglycine by tandem mass spectrometry in newborn screening for isovaleric acidemia. *Clin Chim Acta*. 2007;386:82–86.
101. Lin WD, Wang CH, Lee CC, Lai CC, Tsai Y, Tsai FJ. Genetic mutation profile of isovaleric acidemia patients in Taiwan. *Mol Genet Metab*. 2007;90:134–139.
102. Naglak M, Salvo R, Madsen K, Dembure P, Elsas L. The treatment of isovaleric acidemia with glycine supplement. *Pediatr Res*. 1988;24:9–13.
103. Elsas LJ, Naglak M. Acute and chronic-intermittent isovaleric acidemia: diagnosis and glycine therapy. *Acta Paediatr Jpn*. 1988;30:442–451.
104. Cohn RM, Yudkoff M, Rothman R, Segal S. Isovaleric acidemia: use of glycine therapy in neonates. *N Engl J Med*. 1978;299:996–999.
105. Berry GT, Yudkoff M, Segal S. Isovaleric acidemia: medical and neurodevelopmental effects of long-term therapy. *J Pediatr*. 1988;113:58–64.
106. Millington DS, Roe CR, Maltby DA, Inoue F. Endogenous catabolism is the major source of toxic metabolites in isovaleric acidemia. *J Pediatr*. 1987;110:56–60.
107. Loots DT, Erasmus E, Mienie LJ. Identification of 19 new metabolites induced by abnormal amino acid conjugation in isovaleric acidemia. *Clin Chem*. 2005;51: 1510–1512.
108. Loots DT, Mienie LJ, Erasmus E. Amino-acid depletion induced by abnormal amino-acid conjugation and protein restriction in isovaleric acidemia. *Eur J Clin Nutr*. 2007;61:1323–1327.
109. Chalmers RA, de Sousa C, Tracey BM, Stacey TE, Weaver C, Bradley D. L-carnitine and glycine therapy in isovaleric acidaemia. *J Inherit Metab Dis*. 1985;8(Suppl 2): 141–142.
110. de Sousa C, Chalmers RA, Stacey TE, Tracey BM, Weaver CM, Bradley D. The response to L-carnitine and glycine therapy in isovaleric acidaemia. *Eur J Pediatr*. 1986;144:451–456.
111. Fries MH, Rinaldo P, Schmidt-Sommerfeld E. Isovaleric acidemia: response to a leucine load after three weeks of supplementation with glycine, L-carnitine, and combined glycine-carnitine therapy. *J Pediatr*. 1996;129:449–452.
112. Itoh T, Ito T, Ohba S, et al. Effect of carnitine administration on glycine metabolism in patients with isovaleric acidemia; significance of acetylcarnitine determination to estimate the proper carnitine dose. *Tohoku J Exp Med*. 1996;179:101–109.
113. Roe CR, Millington DS, Maltby DA, Kahler SG, Bohan TP. L-carnitine therapy in isovaleric acidemia. *J Clin Invest*. 1984;74:2290–2295.
114. Mayatepek E, Kurczynski TW, Hoppel CL. Long-term L-carnitine treatment in isovaleric acidemia. *Pediatr Neurol*. 1991;7:137–140.
115. van Hove JLK, Kahler SG, Millington DS, et al. Intravenous L-carnitine and acetyl-L-carnitine in medium-chain acyl-coenzyme A dehydrogenase deficiency and isovaleric acidemia. *Pediatr Res*. 1994;35:96–101.

116. Lee PJ, Harrison EL, Jones MG, Chalmers RA, Leonard JV, Whipp BJ. Improvement in exercise tolerance in isovaleric acidaemia with L-carnitine therapy. *J Inherit Metab Dis*. 1998;21:136–140.
117. Shih VE, Aubry RH, DeGrande G, Gursky SF, Tanaka K. Maternal isovaleric acidemia. *J Pediatr*. 1984;105:77–78.
118. Spinty S, Rogozinski H, Lealman GT, Wraith JE. Second case of a successful pregnancy in maternal isovaleric acidaemia. *J Inherit Metab Dis*. 2002;25:697–698.
119. Finnie MD, Cottrall K, Seakins JW, Snedden W. Massive excretion of 2-oxoglutaric acid and 3-hydroxyisovaleric acid in a patient with a deficiency of 3-methylcrotonyl-CoA carboxylase. *Clin Chim Acta*. 1976;73:513–519.
120. Baykal T, Gokcay GH, Ince Z, et al. Consanguineous 3-methylcrotonyl-CoA carboxylase deficiency: early-onset necrotizing encephalopathy with lethal outcome. *J Inherit Metab Dis*. 2005;28:229–233.
121. Oude Luttikhuis HG, Touati G, Rabier D, Williams M, Jakobs C, Saudubray JM. Severe hypoglycaemia in isolated 3-methylcrotonyl-CoA carboxylase deficiency; a rare, severe clinical presentation. *J Inherit Metab Dis*. 2005;28:1136–1138.
122. Pinto L, Zen P, Rosa R, et al. Isolated 3-methylcrotonyl-coenzyme A carboxylase deficiency in a child with metabolic stroke. *J Inherit Metab Dis*. 2006;29:205–206.
123. Dirik E, Yis U, Pasaoglu G, Chambaz C, Baumgartner MR. Recurrent attacks of status epilepticus as predominant symptom in 3-methylcrotonyl-CoA carboxylase deficiency. *Brain Dev*. 2008;30:218–220.
124. Visser G, Suormala T, Smit GP, et al. 3-methylcrotonyl-CoA carboxylase deficiency in an infant with cardiomyopathy, in her brother with developmental delay and in their asymptomatic father. *Eur J Pediatr*. 2000;159:901–904.
125. Yap S, Monavari AA, Thornton P, Naughten E. Late-infantile 3-methylcrotonyl-CoA carboxylase deficiency presenting as global developmental delay. *J Inherit Metab Dis*. 1998;21:175–176.
126. Boneh A, Baumgartner M, Hayman M, Peters H. Methylcrotonyl-CoA carboxylase (MCC) deficiency associated with severe muscle pain and physical disability in an adult. *J Inherit Metab Dis*. 2005;28:1139–1140.
127. Stadler SC, Polanetz R, Maier EM, et al. Newborn screening for 3-methylcrotonyl-CoA carboxylase deficiency: population heterogeneity of MCCA and MCCB mutations and impact on risk assessment. *Hum Mutat*. 2006;27:748–759.
128. Wolfe LA, Finegold DN, Vockley J, et al. Potential misdiagnosis of 3-methylcrotonyl-coenzyme A carboxylase deficiency associated with absent or trace urinary 3-methylcrotonylglycine. *Pediatrics*. 2007;120:e1335–e1340.
129. Van Hove JL, Rutledge SL, Nada MA, Kahler SG, Millington DS. 3-hydroxyisovalerylcarnitine in 3-methylcrotonyl-CoA carboxylase deficiency. *J Inherit Metab Dis*. 1995;18:592–601.
130. Koeberl DD, Millington DS, Smith WE, et al. Evaluation of 3-methylcrotonyl-CoA carboxylase deficiency detected by tandem mass spectrometry newborn screening. *J Inherit Metab Dis*. 2003;26:25–35.
131. Baumgartner MR, Almashanu S, Suormala T, et al. The molecular basis of human 3-methylcrotonyl-CoA carboxylase deficiency. *J Clin Invest*. 2001;107:495–504.
132. Baumgartner MR, Dantas MF, Suormala T, et al. Isolated 3-methylcrotonyl-CoA carboxylase deficiency: evidence for an allele-specific dominant negative effect and responsiveness to biotin therapy. *Am J Hum Genet*. 2004;75:790–800.
133. Baumgartner MR. Molecular mechanism of dominant expression in 3-methylcrotonyl-CoA carboxylase deficiency. *J Inherit Metab Dis*. 2005;28:301–309.

134. Friebel D, von der HM, Baumgartner ER, et al. The first case of 3-methylcrotonyl-CoA carboxylase (MCC) deficiency responsive to biotin. *Neuropediatrics*. 2006;37: 72–78.
135. Frazier DM, Millington DS, McCandless SE, et al. The tandem mass spectrometry newborn screening experience in North Carolina: 1997–2005. *J Inherit Metab Dis*. 2006;29:76–85.
136. Lussky RC, Cifuentes RF. False positive newborn screens secondary to a maternal inborn error of metabolism. *Clin Pediatr (Phila)*. 2006;45:471–474.
137. Arnold GL, Koeberl DD, Matern D, et al. A Delphi-based consensus clinical practice protocol for the diagnosis and management of 3-methylcrotonyl CoA carboxylase deficiency. *Mol Genet Metab*. 2008;93:363–370.
138. Gibson KM, Bennett MJ, Naylor EW, Morton DH. 3-methylcrotonyl-coenzyme A carboxylase deficiency in Amish/Mennonite adults identified by detection of increased acylcarnitines in blood spots of their children. *J Pediatr*. 1998;132:519–523.
139. Tuchman M, Berry SA, Thuy LP, Nyhan WL. Partial methylcrotonyl-coenzyme A carboxylase deficiency in an infant with failure to thrive, gastrointestinal dysfunction, and hypertonia. *Pediatrics*. 1993;91:664–666.
140. Frazier DM, Koepke J, Wood T, Pritchett T. Maternal 3-MCC deficiency as a model for long-term outcome. *Mol Genet Metab* 2008;93:250.
141. Ficicioglu C, Payan I. 3-methylcrotonyl-CoA carboxylase deficiency: metabolic decompensation in a noncompliant child detected through newborn screening. *Pediatrics*. 2006;118:2555–2556.
142. Roschinger W, Millington DS, Gage DA, et al. 3-hydroxyisovalerylcarnitine in patients with deficiency of 3-methylcrotonyl CoA carboxylase. *Clin Chim Acta*. 1995;240:35–51.
143. Stanley CA, Berry GT, Bennett MJ, Willi SM, Treem WR, Hale DE. Renal handling of carnitine in secondary carnitine deficiency disorders. *Pediatr Res*. 1993;34:89–97.
144. Chalmers RA, Roe CR, Stacey TE, Hoppel CL. Urinary excretion of L-carnitine and acylcarnitines by patients with disorders of organic acid metabolism: evidence for secondary insufficiency of L-carnitine. *Pediatr Res*. 1984;18:1325–1328.
145. Pearson MA, Aleck KA, Heidenreich RA. Benign clinical presentation of 3-methylcrotonylglycinuria. *J Inherit Metab Dis*. 1995;18:640–641.
146. Rutledge SL, Berry GT, Stanley CA, Van Hove JL, Millington D. Glycine and L-carnitine therapy in 3-methylcrotonyl-CoA carboxylase deficiency. *J Inherit Metab Dis*. 1995;18:299–305.
147. Lehnert W, Niederhoff H, Suormala T, Baumgartner ER. Isolated biotin-resistant 3-methylcrotonyl-CoA carboxylase deficiency: long-term outcome in a case with neonatal onset. *Eur J Pediatr*. 1996;155:568–572.
148. Faull KF, Bolton PD, Halpern B, Hammond J, Danks DM. The urinary organic acid profile associated with 3-hydroxy-3-methylglutaric aciduria. *Clin Chim Acta*. 1976; 73:553–559.
149. Wysocki SJ, Hahnel R. 3-hydroxy-3-methylglutaric aciduria: 3-hydroxy-3-methylglutaryl-coenzyme A lyase levels in leucocytes. *Clin Chim Acta*. 1976; 73:373–375.
150. Thompson GN, Chalmers RA, Halliday D. The contribution of protein catabolism to metabolic decompensation in 3-hydroxy-3-methylglutaric aciduria. *Eur J Pediatr*. 1990;149:346–350.

151. Wysocki SJ, Hahnel R. 3-hydroxy-3-methylglutaryl-coenzyme a lyase deficiency: a review. *J Inherit Metab Dis*. 1986;9:225–233.
152. Mitchell GA, Robert MF, Hruz PW, et al. 3-hydroxy-3-methylglutaryl coenzyme A lyase (HL). Cloning of human and chicken liver HL cDNAs and characterization of a mutation causing human HL deficiency. *J Biol Chem*. 1993;268:4376–4381.
153. Pie J, Lopez-Vinas E, Puisac B, et al. Molecular genetics of HMG-CoA lyase deficiency. *Mol Genet Metab*. 2007;92:198–209.
154. Vargas CR, Sitta A, Schmitt G, et al. Incidence of 3-hydroxy-3-methylglutaryl-coenzyme A lyase (HL) deficiency in Brazil, South America [published online ahead of print December 17, 2007]. *J Inherit Metab Dis*. 2007.
155. Roe CR, Millington DS, Maltby DA. Identification of 3-methylglutarylcarnitine: a new diagnostic metabolite of 3-hydroxy-3-methylglutaryl-coenzyme A lyase deficiency. *J Clin Invest*. 1986;77:1391–1394.
156. Gibson KM, Breuer J, Nyhan WL. 3-hydroxy-3-methylglutaryl-coenzyme A lyase deficiency: review of 18 reported patients. *Eur J Pediatr*. 1988;148:180–186.
157. Wilson WG, Cass MB, Sovik O, Gibson KM, Sweetman L. A child with acute pancreatitis and recurrent hypoglycemia due to 3-hydroxy-3-methylglutaryl-CoA lyase deficiency. *Eur J Pediatr*. 1984;142:289–291.
158. Muroi J, Yorifuji T, Uematsu A, Nakahata T. Cerebral infarction and pancreatitis: possible complications of patients with 3-hydroxy-3-methylglutaryl-CoA lyase deficiency. *J Inherit Metab Dis*. 2000;23:636–637.
159. Huemer M, Muehl A, Wandl-Vergesslich K. Stroke-like encephalopathy in an infant with 3-hydroxy-3-methylglutaryl-coenzyme A lyase deficiency. *Eur J Pediatr*. 1998;157:743–746.
160. Leupold D, Bojasch M, Jakobs C. 3-hydroxy-3-methylglutaryl-CoA lyase deficiency in an infant with macrocephaly and mild metabolic acidosis. *Eur J Pediatr*. 1982;138:73–76.
161. Bischof F, Nagele T, Wanders RJ, Trefz FK, Melms A. 3-hydroxy-3-methylglutaryl-CoA lyase deficiency in an adult with leukoencephalopathy. *Ann Neurol*. 2004;56: 727–730.
162. Bakker HD, Wanders RJA, Schutgens RBH. 3-hydroxy-3-methylglutaryl-CoA lyase deficiency: absence of clinical symptoms due to a self-imposed dietary fat and protein restriction. *J Inherit Metab Dis*. 1993;16:1061–1062.
163. Dasouki M, Buchanan D, Mercer N, Gibson KM, Thoene J. 3-hydroxy-3-methylglutaric aciduria: response to carnitine therapy and fat and leucine restriction. *J Inherit Metab Dis*. 1987;10:142–146.
164. Francois B, Bachman C, Schutgens RBH. Glucose metabolism in a child with 3-hydroxy-3-methylglutaryl-coenzyme A lyase deficiency. *J Inherit Metab Dis*. 1981;4:163–164.
165. Urganci N, Arapoglu M, Evruke M, Aydin A. A rare cause of hepatomegaly: 3-hydroxy-3-methylglutaryl coenzyme-A lyase deficiency. *J Pediatr Gastroenterol Nutr*. 2001;33:339–341.
166. Ozand PT, al Aqeel A, Gascon G, Brismar J, Thomas E, Gleispach H. 3-hydroxy-3-methylglutaryl-coenzyme A (HMG-CoA) lyase deficiency in Saudi Arabia. *J Inherit Metab Dis*. 1991;14:174–188.
167. Holmes HC, Burns SP, Chalmers RA, Bain MS, Iles RA. Ketogenic flux from lipids and leucine, assessment in 3-hydroxy-3-methylglutaryl CoA lyase deficiency. *Biochem Soc Trans*. 1995;23:489S.

168. Norman EJ, Denton MD, Berry HK. Gas-chromatographic/mass spectrometric detection of 3-hydroxy-3-methylglutaryl-CoA lyase deficiency in double first cousins. *Clin Chem*. 1982;28:137–140.
169. Stacey TE, de Sousa C, Tracey BM, et al. Dizygotic twins with 3-hydroxy-3-methylglutaric aciduria; unusual presentation, family studies and dietary management. *Eur J Pediatr*. 1985;144:177–181.
170. Robinson BH, Oei J, Sherwood WG, Slyper AH, Heininger J, Mamer OA. Hydroxymethylglutaryl CoA lyase deficiency: features resembling Reye syndrome. *Neurology*. 1980;30:714–718.
171. Mitchell GA, Fukao T. Inborn errors of ketone body metabolism. In: Scriver CR, Beaudet AL, Sly WS, Valle D, eds. *The Metabolic and Molecular Bases of Inherited Disease*. 8th ed. New York, NY: McGraw-Hill; 2001:2327–2356.
172. Pospisilova E, Mrazova L, Hrda J, Martincova O, Zeman J. Biochemical and molecular analyses in three patients with 3-hydroxy-3-methylglutaric aciduria. *J Inherit Metab Dis*. 2003;26:433–441.
173. Daum RS, Lamm PH, Mamer OA, Scriver CR. A "new" disorder of isoleucine catabolism. *Lancet*. 1971;2:1289–1290.
174. Daum RS, Scriver CR, Mamer OA, Delvin E, Lamm P, Goldman H. An inherited disorder of isoleucine catabolism causing accumulation of alpha-methylacetoacetate and alpha-methyl-beta -hydroxybutyrate, and intermittent metabolic acidosis. *Pediatr Res*. 1973;7:149–160.
175. Sovik O. Mitochondrial 2-methylacetoacetyl-CoA thiolase deficiency: an inborn error of isoleucine and ketone body metabolism. *J Inherit Metab Dis*. 1993;16: 46–54.
176. Fukao T, Scriver CR, Kondo N. The clinical phenotype and outcome of mitochondrial acetoacetyl-CoA thiolase deficiency (beta-ketothiolase or T2 deficiency) in 26 enzymatically proved and mutation-defined patients. *Mol Genet Metab*. 2001; 72:109–114.
177. Hillman RE, Keating JP. Beta-ketothiolase deficiency as a cause of the "ketotic hyperglycinemia syndrome." *Pediatrics*. 1974;53:221–225.
178. Middleton B, Bartlett K, Romanos A, et al. 3-ketothiolase deficiency. *Eur J Pediatr*. 1986;144:586–589.
179. Kayer MA. Disorders of ketone production and utilization. *Mol Genet Metab*. 2006;87:281–283.
180. Fukao T, Yamaguchi S, Orii T, Hashimoto T. Molecular basis of beta-ketothiolase deficiency: mutations and polymorphisms in the human mitochondrial acetoacetyl-coenzyme A thiolase gene. *Hum Mutat*. 1995;5:113–120.
181. Fukao T, Yamaguchi S, Kano M, et al. Molecular cloning and sequence of the complementary DNA encoding human mitochondrial acetoacetyl-coenzyme A thiolase and study of the variant enzymes in cultured fibroblasts from patients with 3-ketothiolase deficiency. *J Clin Invest*. 1990;86:2086–2092.
182. Masuno M, Kano M, Fukao T, et al. Chromosome mapping of the human mitochondrial acetoacetyl-coenzyme A thiolase gene to 11q22.3-q23.1 by fluorescence in situ hybridization. *Cytogenet Cell Genet*. 1992;60:121–122.
183. Zhang GX, Fukao T, Rolland MO, et al. Mitochondrial acetoacetyl-CoA thiolase (T2) deficiency: T2-deficient patients with "mild" mutation(s) were previously misinterpreted as normal by the coupled assay with tiglyl-CoA. *Pediatr Res*. 2004; 56:60–64.
184. Sweetman L, Millington DS, Therrell BL, et al. Naming and counting disorders (conditions) included in newborn screening panels. *Pediatrics*. 2006;117:S308–S314.

185. Fukao T, Zhang GX, Sakura N, et al. The mitochondrial acetoacetyl-CoA thiolase (T2) deficiency in Japanese patients: urinary organic acid and blood acylcarnitine profiles under stable conditions have subtle abnormalities in T2-deficient patients with some residual T2 activity. *J Inherit Metab Dis*. 2003;26:423–431.
186. Zschocke J, Ruiter JP, Brand J, et al. Progressive infantile neurodegeneration caused by 2-methyl-3-hydroxybutyryl-CoA dehydrogenase deficiency: a novel inborn error of branched-chain fatty acid and isoleucine metabolism. *Pediatr Res*. 2000;48:852–855.
187. Middleton B, Bartlett K. The synthesis and characterisation of 2-methylacetoacetyl coenzyme A and its use in the identification of the site of the defect in 2-methylacetoacetic and 2-methyl-3-hydroxybutyric aciduria. *Clinica Chimica Acta*. 1983;128:291–305.
188. Nagasawa H, Yamaguchi S, Orii T, Schutgens RB, Sweetman L, Hashimoto T. 3-ketothiolase deficiency: heterogeneity in a defect of mitochondrial acetoacetyl-CoA thiolase biosynthesis in fibroblasts from four patients. *J Inherit Metab Dis*. 1989;12:368–372.
189. Yamaguchi S, Sakai A, Fukao T, et al. Biochemical and immunochemical study of seven families with 3-ketothiolase deficiency: diagnosis of heterozygotes using immunochemical determination of the ratio of mitochondrial acetoacetyl-CoA thiolase and 3-ketoacyl-CoA thiolase proteins. *Pediatr Res*. 1993;33:429–432.
190. Fukao T, Wakazono A, Song XQ, et al. Prenatal diagnosis in a family with mitochondrial acetoacetyl-coenzyme A thiolase deficiency with the use of the polymerase chain reaction followed by the heteroduplex detection method. *Prenat Diagn*. 1995;15:363–367.
191. Monastiri K, Amri F, Limam K, Kaabachi N, Guediche MN. Beta-ketothiolase (2-methylacetoacetyl-CoA thiolase) deficiency: a frequent disease in Tunisia? *J Inherit Metab Dis*. 1999;22:932–933.
192. Wakazono A, Fukao T, Yamaguchi S, et al. Molecular, biochemical, and clinical characterization of mitochondrial acetoacetyl-coenzyme A thiolase deficiency in two further patients. *Hum Mutat*. 1995;5:34–42.
193. Schutgens RB, Middleton B, vd Blij JF, et al. Beta-ketothiolase deficiency in a family confirmed by in vitro enzymatic assays in fibroblasts. *Eur J Pediatr*. 1982;139:39–42.
194. Aramaki S, Lehotay D, Sweetman L, Nyhan WL, Winter SC, Middleton B. Urinary excretion of 2-methylacetoacetate, 2-methyl-3-hydroxybutyrate and tiglylglycine after isoleucine loading in the diagnosis of 2-methylacetoacetyl-CoA thiolase deficiency. *J Inherit Metab Dis*. 1991;14:63–74.
195. Mager DR, Wykes LJ, Ball RO, Pencharz PB. Branched-chain amino acid requirements in school-aged children determined by indicator amino acid oxidation (IAAO). *J Nutr*. 2003;133:3540–3545.
196. Mrazova L, Fukao T, Halovd K, et al. Two novel mutations in mitochondrial acetoacetyl-CoA thiolase deficiency. *J Inherit Metab Dis*. 2005;28:235–236.
197. Sewell AC, Herwig J, Wiegratz I, et al. Mitochondrial acetoacetyl-CoA thiolase (beta-ketothiolase) deficiency and pregnancy. *J Inherit Metab Dis*. 1998;21:441–442.
198. Illsinger S, Lucke T, Zschocke J, Gibson KM, Das AM. 3-methylglutaconic aciduria type I in a boy with fever-associated seizures. *Pediatr Neurol*. 2004;30:213–215.
199. Narisawa K, Gibson KM, Sweetman L, Nyhan WL, Duran M, Wadman SK. Deficiency of 3-methylglutaconyl-coenzyme A hydratase in two siblings with 3-methylglutaconic aciduria. *J Clin Invest*. 1986;77:1148–1152.

200. Ly TB, Peters V, Gibson KM, et al. Mutations in the AUH gene cause 3-methylglutaconic aciduria type I. *Hum Mutat*. 2003;21:401–407.
201. Duran M, Beemer FA, Tibosch AS, Bruinvis L, Ketting D, Wadman SK. Inherited 3-methylglutaconic aciduria in two brothers—another defect of leucine metabolism. *J Pediatr*. 1982;101:551–554.
202. Hou JW, Wang TR. 3-methylglutaconic aciduria presenting as Reye syndrome in a Chinese boy. *J Inherit Metab Dis*. 1995;18:645–646.
203. Eriguchi M, Mizuta H, Kurohara K, et al. 3-methylglutaconic aciduria type I causes leukoencephalopathy of adult onset. *Neurology*. 2006;67:1895–1896.
204. Shoji Y, Takahashi T, Sawaishi Y, et al. 3-methylglutaconic aciduria type I: clinical heterogeneity as a neurometabolic disease. *J Inherit Metab Dis*. 1999;22:1–8.
205. Ensenauer R, Muller CB, Schwab KO, Gibson KM, Brandis M, Lehnert W. 3-methylglutaconyl-CoA hydratase deficiency: a new patient with speech retardation as the leading sign. *J Inherit Metab Dis*. 2000;23:341–344.
206. Gibson KM, Lee CF, Wappner RS. 3-methylglutaconyl-coenzyme-A hydratase deficiency: a new case. *J Inherit Metab Dis*. 1992;15:363–366.
207. Gibson KM, Wappner RS, Jooste S, et al. Variable clinical presentation in three patients with 3-methylglutaconyl-coenzyme A hydratase deficiency. *J Inherit Metab Dis*. 1998;21:631–638.
208. Korman SH. Inborn errors of isoleucine degradation: a review. *Mol Genet Metab*. 2006;89:289–299.
209. Poll-The BT, Wanders RJ, Ruiter JP, et al. Spastic diplegia and periventricular white matter abnormalities in 2-methyl-3-hydroxybutyryl-CoA dehydrogenase deficiency, a defect of isoleucine metabolism: differential diagnosis with hypoxic-ischemic brain diseases. *Mol Genet Metab*. 2004;81:295–299.
210. Ofman R, Ruiter JP, Feenstra M, et al. 2-methyl-3-hydroxybutyryl-CoA dehydrogenase deficiency is caused by mutations in the HADH2 gene. *Am J Hum Genet*. 2003;72:1300–1307.
211. Perez-Cerda C, Garcia-Villoria J, Ofman R, et al. 2-methyl-3-hydroxybutyryl-CoA dehydrogenase (MHBD) deficiency: an X-linked inborn error of isoleucine metabolism that may mimic a mitochondrial disease. *Pediatr Res*. 2005;58:488–491.
212. Sass JO, Forstner R, Sperl W. 2-methyl-3-hydroxybutyryl-CoA dehydrogenase deficiency: impaired catabolism of isoleucine presenting as neurodegenerative disease. *Brain Dev*. 2004;26:12–14.
213. Sutton VR, O'Brien WE, Clark GD, Kim J, Wanders RJ. 3-hydroxy-2-methylbutyryl-CoA dehydrogenase deficiency. *J Inherit Metab Dis*. 2003;26:69–71.
214. Ensenauer R, Niederhoff H, Ruiter JP, et al. Clinical variability in 3-hydroxy-2-methylbutyryl-CoA dehydrogenase deficiency. *Ann Neurol*. 2002;51:656–659.
215. Cazorla MR, Verdu A, Perez-Cerda C, Ribes A. Neuroimage findings in 2-methyl-3-hydroxybutyryl-CoA dehydrogenase deficiency. *Pediatr Neurol*. 2007;36:264–267.
216. Olpin SE, Pollitt RJ, McMenamin J, et al. 2-methyl-3-hydroxybutyryl-CoA dehydrogenase deficiency in a 23-year-old man. *J Inherit Metab Dis*. 2002;25:477–482.
217. Matern D, He M, Berry SA, et al. Prospective diagnosis of 2-methylbutyryl-CoA dehydrogenase deficiency in the Hmong population by newborn screening using tandem mass spectrometry. *Pediatrics*. 2003;112:74–78.

Chapter 7

Nutrition Management of Patients with Inherited Disorders of Sulfur Amino Acid Metabolism

Sandra van Calcar

INTRODUCTION

The sulfur amino acids (SAAs), methionine (MET) and cysteine/cystine (CYS), are linked by the methylation cycle (see Figure 7.1). The indispensable amino acid MET is not only required for protein synthesis, but also is converted to the intermediate S-adenosylmethionine (SAM) by methionine adenosyltransferase (MAT; EC 2.5.1.6). SAM is the primary biological methyl donor in vivo for a wide range of transmethylation reactions, including synthesis of creatine, phosphotidylcholine, and various DNA and RNA intermediates (see Figure 7.1).[1,2] With each methyl transfer, SAM is converted to S-adenosylhomocysteine (AdoHcy), which is then cleaved to homocysteine (HCY) and adenosine by S-adenosylhomocysteine hydrolase (EC 3.3.1.1). Many SAM-dependent methyltransferases are strongly inhibited by AdoHcy. The SAM to AdoHcy ratio may play an important role in regulation of methylation of various compounds.[1,2]

Transsulfuration, the irreversible conversion of HCY and serine to cystathionine and CYS, requires cystathionine-β-synthase (CβS; EC 4.2.1.22) and γ-cystathionase (EC 4.4.1.1), both pyridoxine-dependent enzymes. Cysteine is required for protein synthesis and is a precursor of taurine, sulfate, and glutathione.[3-5] Cysteine spares MET by providing an additional source of methyl groups for remethylation of HCY.[6,7] Cysteine has been considered a possible essential amino acid in neonates; however, recent studies in piglets[8] and human neonates[9] have not supported this observation.

Remethylation of HCY to MET involves methyl transfer from either 5-methyl-tetrahydrofolate (THF) or betaine. Enzymes involved in this process are 5-methyl THF-homocysteine methyltransferase (methionine synthase; EC 2.1.1.13) or betaine-homocysteine methyltransferase (BHMT; EC 2.1.1.5; see Figure 7.1).[1,2] CYS is used as an abbreviation for both cystine and cysteine since interconnection in the body is nonenzymatic.

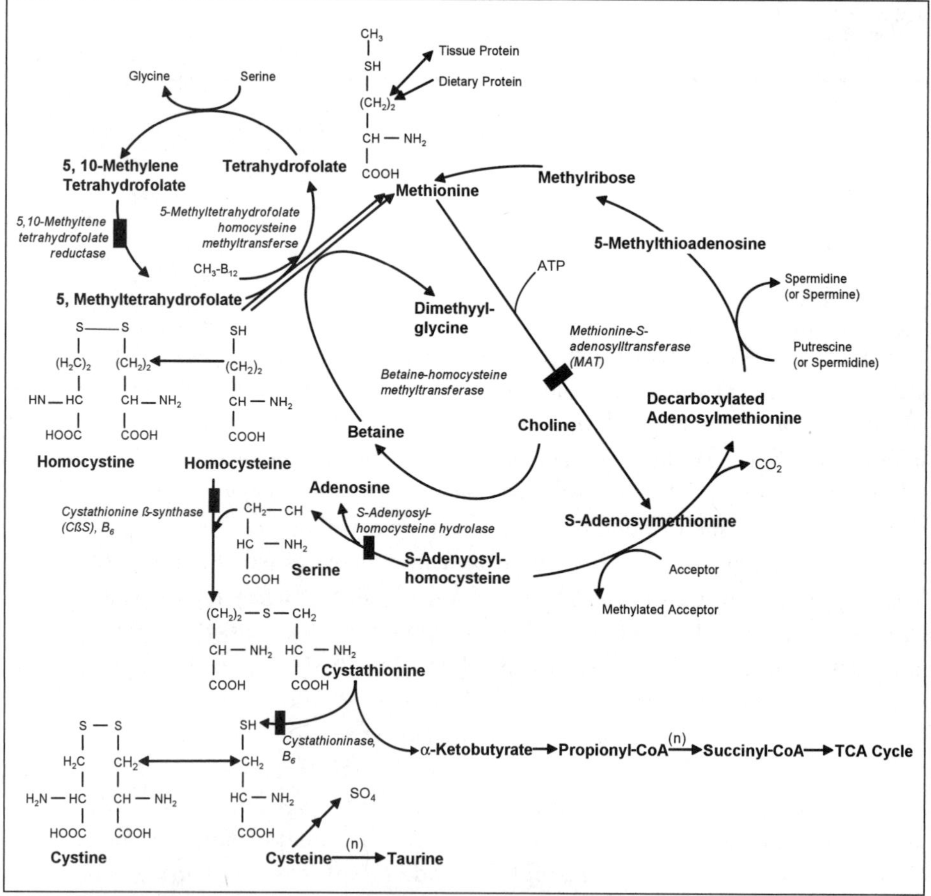

Figure 7.1 *Metabolic Pathways of Sulfur Amino Acids*

Source: Modified by permission of Elsas LJ, Acosta PB. Inherited metabolic disease: amino acids, organic acids, and galactose. In: Shils ME, Shike M, Olson J, Ross AC, Caballero B, Cousins RJ, eds. *Modern Nutrition in Health and Disease*. 10th ed. Philadelphia, PA: Lippincott Williams & Wilkins; 2005:909–959. Courtesy of Wolters Kluwer Health.

Note: The black bars represent impaired reactions in inherited metabolic disorders affecting metabolism of sulfur amino acids.

Homocystinuria

The clinical phenotypes of metabolic disorders involving SAAs vary widely from benign to a constellation including profound developmental delay, corneal dislocation, and thromboembolism. This later presentation is often called classical homocystinuria and was first described in 1962 in individuals with mental retardation in Northern Ireland.[10] Soon after, a CβS deficiency was shown to be the primary defect in this autosomal recessive disorder.[11,12] This chapter focuses on CβS deficiency, but other disorders of sulfur amino acid metabolism are addressed as well.

Biochemistry

The most common inborn error in MET metabolism is deficiency of CβS (OMIM 236200)[13] (see Figure 7.1). The accumulation of intracellular HCY, rather than elevations in MET, is believed to be the primary cause of toxicity in this disorder.[1] Since transmethylation of HCY to cystathionine is completely, or at least partially blocked, CYS becomes a conditionally essential amino acid in CβS deficiency.

CβS requires pyridoxal 5′phosphate (PLP) and heme as cofactors and is stimulated by SAM.[14,15] CβS consists of 551 base pairs and contains a heme-binding domain, a catalytic domain, and 2 regulatory domains, CβS1 and CβS2. A large number of mutations in different regions of human CβS have been found in patients with homocystinuria.[16,17] About half of these mutations result in a pyridoxine (B_6)-responsive clinical phenotype, although responsiveness is highly variable among patients.

For those responsive to vitamin B_6 supplementation, the mutant enzyme has moderately reduced affinity for PLP. In a nonresponsive phenotype, the enzyme is more likely to have little or no affinity for PLP.[17] To determine responsiveness in vivo, a trial of vitamin B_6, with measurement of various biochemical markers, is required since in vitro enzymatic response to B_6 cannot adequately predict a responsive patient from a nonresponsive one.[18] In general, B_6-responsive patients will have a less severe phenotype than nonresponsive patients.[19]

Molecular Biology

The human CβS gene, which has been mapped to chromosome 21q22.3,[20] encodes a CβS subunit of 63 kD.[21] The human cDNA for CβS was cloned and fully sequenced in 1993 and contains 18 exons and 17 introns[22] (see

Chapter 1). Many mutations have been described in the CβS gene; most are private genes or restricted to only a few pedigrees. However, some mutations are relatively common in various populations. The genomic 833T>C transition, which causes an amino acid substitution at position I278T, has been found in alleles from patients of different ethnic backgrounds and accounts for nearly 25% of all reported alleles in classical homocystinuria.[23] Homozygosity of this mutation is associated with B_6-responsiveness and a relatively mild clinical phenotype.[23-26]

Another common mutation, a 919G>A transition causing a substitution at G307S, results in a more severe nonresponsive phenotype. In Ireland, this mutation accounts for approximately 70% of the defective CβS alleles.[27] The G307S mutation has been detected primarily in patients of "Celtic" background in the United States, Australia, and various European countries.[23,28,29] The third most frequent alteration, an IVS11-2A-C splice mutation, causes skipping of exon 12 and has been detected in patients from Central and Eastern Europe.[30]

Some mutations have been associated with more centralized ethnic or racial populations. For instance, a 797G>A transition is a frequent cause of B_6-responsive homocystinuria in Norwegian patients[31] and an A114V mutation is found in the Italian population.[26] In addition, a unique 1058C>T transition resulting in a T353M mutation was found in four African Americans with B_6-nonresponsive homocystinuria.[32]

Although generalizations about B_6-responsiveness can be assigned based on gene mutation status, the mutations do not necessarily predict responsiveness in all patients. In a Dutch cohort, only 58% of those homozygous for the I278T mutation showed the expected B_6 response in vivo.[25] Further information about various mutations can be found at http://www.uchsc.edu/sm/cbs.

The estimated worldwide prevalence of CβS deficiency is 1 in 300,000 births and in Ireland, the estimated prevalence is 1 in 65,000 births.[33,34] These estimates may be falsely low because they only include those patients detected in early screening programs with a severe clinical presentation. Using molecular techniques, it appears that the incidence of CβS deficiency may be much greater. For instance, DNA sequencing to search for the 833T>C mutation in the Danish population estimated a prevalence of 1 in 20,000 births.[35] Screening for 6 mutations in the Norwegian population resulted in an estimated prevalence of 1 in 6400 births.[36]

Newborn Screening

Newborn screening for disorders causing hypermethioninemia is available and becoming more widespread as tandem mass spectrometry (MS/MS) technology is instituted[37] (see Chapter 2). Unlike many inborn errors of amino acid metabolism, there are no characteristic signs or symptoms if homocystinuria remains undiagnosed during infancy. In nonresponsive cases, the first sign of disease is often development of myopia and/or developmental delays at age 1 to 2 years.[19] In B_6-responsive cases, symptoms may not be detected for years and, for some, symptoms can be delayed into adulthood.[1,2]

Newborn screening for elevated MET concentrations from blood spots is successful in detecting syndromes causing isolated hypermethioninemia such as MET adenosyltransferase (MAT I/III) deficiency. However, because screening does not measure HCY concentrations, it is not possible to identify all neonates with homocystinuria on the basis of screening for hypermethioninemia.[34,38,39] Thus, current screening techniques do not detect all cases of CβS deficiency, particularly the vitamin B_6-responsive phenotype. In the B_6-responsive form of CβS deficiency, MET concentrations are slow to increase, particularly in human milk-fed infants who consume a lower protein intake than proprietary formula-fed infants. Also, the trend toward earlier hospital discharge may prevent sufficient increases in blood MET concentrations for detection by screening.[40]

When CβS deficiency is diagnosed based on clinical symptomology, about half of those diagnosed will have the B_6-nonresponsive form and about half will be considered B_6-responsive.[19] With screening, the B_6-responsive forms are rarely detected and some nonresponsive cases have been missed.[38,39] Reducing the screening cutoff for blood MET concentration from 2 mg/dL to 1 mg/dL improved detection of infants with nonresponsive CβS deficiency, but did not increase the detection of infants with responsive forms.[38] It has been estimated that screening misses at least one in every five infants with CβS deficiency; others estimate the false negative rate may be even higher.[35,38,39]

However, despite the inability of newborn screening to detect all infants with CβS deficiency, early detection followed by diagnosis and nutrition management has proven to reduce clinical sequelae.[33,38,39] This was clearly shown in an Irish study investigating the clinical outcome of 25 cases of CβS deficiency (age range 4.4 to 28.4 years) detected over a 25-year period (1971–1996).[33] Twenty-one of 25 were detected by screening; the remaining four cases were missed and detected clinically. All 21 screened cases were B_6-nonresponsive. Of the four missed cases, three were human milk-fed and one was B_6-responsive. For all positively screened cases, a restricted MET diet was instituted by 6 weeks of age. Of the 21 cases treated by diet, 15 had a lifetime median of plasma-free HCY concentration ≤ 11 μmol/L.[33] Three of the 21 patients were on nutrition management, but maintained a higher lifetime median of plasma-free HCY concentration and developed myopia as a first symptom of the disorder. Three of the 21 were not compliant with diet recommendations for durations of 2 to 8 years; of these, 2 developed ectopic lentis (lens dislocation), 1 developed osteoporosis, and 2 developed cognitive delays. Further, the newborn-screened compliant group had a mean full-scale intelligence quotient (IQ) of 105.8 (range 84–120) and no significant differences were found in psychomotor test scores between this group of patients and their unaffected siblings.[41] These outcomes suggest that newborn screening, diagnosis, early initiation of nutrition management, and a lifetime median of plasma-free HCY < 11 μmol/L significantly reduce the probability of developing complications when compared to those patients with untreated CβS deficiency.[33,41]

MS/MS screening (see Chapter 2) is expected to improve specificity for detection of disorders associated with elevated blood MET concentrations and reduce the probability of a false-negative result.[37] Until the development of MS/MS screening (see Chapter 2), hypermethioninemia was detected by a bacterial assay, which required separate analysis from the newborn screening card.[42-44] Because not all infants with CβS deficiency were detected, many screening programs stopped or did not include screening for blood MET concentration as part of their screening panel.[37] With MS/MS screening, one test can detect elevated blood MET concentrations while testing for more prevalent amino acid disorders such as phenylketonuria (PKU), tyrosinemia, and branched-chain ketoaciduria (maple syrup urine disease; MSUD). This improves the cost effectiveness of screening for hypermethioninemias and, now, programs that previously did not screen for homocystinuria have added it to their detection panel.[37] Use of ratios, such as MET to leucine (LEU) and isoleucine (ILE + MET:LEU + ILE), can also help reduce false detection of hypermethioninemia.[37]

However, because widespread use of MS/MS screening is relatively new, its effect on detection rates of patients with CβS deficiency remains to be determined. An additional test for screening newborns for CβS deficiency would be to measure elevated HCY in blood or urine. However, no such method for screening is available at this time[1] and affected neonates may not accumulate sufficient HCY by 24 to 48 hours of age for detection.[45]

Diagnosis

Patients with CβS deficiency are typically first ascertained by analysis of plasma amino acid and HCY concentrations (see Table 7.1). In a standard plasma amino acid panel, fasting plasma concentrations of MET can be elevated to 2000 μmol/L.[46] Normal MET concentration in plasma is less than 35 μmol/L. Total plasma CYS concentrations can be low in amino acid analysis, although low CYS without elevated MET would not be expected in CβS deficiency.[46] Elevations of HCY can also be measured in urine.

Table 7.1 ***Biochemical Findings in Plasma of Patients with Inherited Metabolic Disorders of Sulfur Amino Acid Metabolism***

Disorder[a]	***Methionine (P)***[b]	***Free Cystine (P)***	***Total Homocysteine (P)***	***Homocysteine (U)***	***Cystathionine (P)***
	(5–35 μmol/L)[c]	(100–125 μmol/L)	(5–15 μmol/L)	(< 1 mmol/mol creatinine)	(50–340 nmol/L)
MAT I/III deficiency	↑[d]	N	N–↑	0	N–↑
GNMT deficiency	↑↑	N	N–↑	N	N
S-AdoHcy hydrolase deficiency	↑↑	N	N–↑	ND	N
CβS deficiency	↑	↓	↑↑↑	↑↑↑	↓–N
γ-CTH deficiency	N	↓↓	N	0	↑↑[e]
MTHFR deficiency	↓–N	N	↑↑	↑↑	N–↑
MS/MSR deficiency, cblG, cblE defect	↓–N	N	↑	↑	N

Sources:

Andria G, Fowler B, Sebastio G. Disorders of sulfur amino acid metabolism. In: Fernandes J, Saudubray JM, van den Berghe G, Walter JH, eds. *Inborn Metabolic Disease: Diagnosis and Treatment*. 4th ed. Heidelberg, Germany: Springer Medizin Verlag; 2006:273–282.

Baric I, Fumic K, Glenn B, et al. S-adenosylhomocysteine hydrolase deficiency in a human: a genetic disorder of methionine metabolism. *Proc Natl Acad Sci USA*. 2004;101:4234–4239.

Gaull GE, Tallan HH, Lonsdale D, Przyrembel H, Schaffner F, von Bassewitz DB. Hypermethioninemia associated with methionine adenosyltransferase deficiency: clinical, morphologic, and biochemical observations on four patients. *J Pediatr*. 1981;98:734–741.

Levy HL, Mudd SH, Uhlendorf BW, Madigan PM. Cystathioninuria and homocystinuria. *Clin Chim Acta*. 1975;58:51–59.

Mudd SH, Cerone R, Schiaffino MC, et al. Glycine N-methyltransferase deficiency: a novel inborn error causing persistent isolated hypermethioninaemia. *J Inherit Metab Dis*. 2001;24:448–464.

Mudd SH, Levy HL, Kraus JP. Disorders of transsulfuration. In: Valle D, Beaudet AL, Vogelstein B, eds. *The Metabolic and Molecular Bases of Inherited Disease*. New York, NY: McGraw-Hill Medical; 2007. Available at: http://www.ommbid.com/OMMBID/the_online_metabolic_and_molecular_bases_of_inherited_diseases/b/fulltext/part8/Ch88. Accessed September 15, 2008.

(continues)

Table 7.1 ***Biochemical Findings in Plasma of Patients with Inherited Metabolic Disorders of Sulfur Amino Acid Metabolism, Continued***

Rosenblatt DS, Fenton W. Inherited disorders of folate and cobalamin transport and metabolism. In: Valle D, Beaudet AL, Vogelstein, B, eds. *The Metabolic and Molecular Bases of Inherited Disease*. New York, NY: McGraw-Hill Medical; 2007. Available at: http://www.ommbid.com/OMMBID/the_online_metabolic_and_molecular_bases_of_inherited_disease/b/abstract/part17/ch155. Accessed September 15, 2008.

Skovby F. Disorders of sulfur amino acids. In: Blau N, Duran M, Blaskovics ME, Gibson KM, eds. *Physician's Guide to the Laboratory Diagnosis of Metabolic Diseases*. 2nd ed. Berlin, Germany: Springer-Verlag; 2002:243–260.

Tada H, Takanashi J, Barkovich AJ, Yamamoto S, Kohno Y. Reversible white matter lesion in methionine adenosyltransferase I/III deficiency. *AJNR Am J Neuroradiol*. 2004;25:1843–1845.

[a]MAT I/III = Methionine adenosyltransferase, GNMT = Glycine-N-methyltransferase, S-AdoHcy hydrolase = S-adenosylhomocysteine hydrolase, CβS = Cystathionine β-synthase, γ-CTH = γ-cystathionase, MTHFR = 5,10-methylenetetrahydrofolate reductase, MS = Methionine synthase, MSR = Methionine synthase reductase.

[b]P = Plasma, U = Urine.

[c]Normal reference range.

[d]Arrows indicate direction of laboratory change in each disorder: N = Normal; 0 = None detected.

[e]Urine cystathionine is greatly increased in γ-CTH deficiency.

Homocysteine exists in plasma in several forms:[47] a thiol homocysteine (HCYH), a disulfide combining two HCY molecules labeled homocystine (HCY–HCY), and also as mixed disulfides, such as CYS–HCY and homocystine–cysteinylglycine. The disulfides, primarily, are measured in standard amino acid analysis and are labeled as "free HCY."[47]

Some HCY in blood is also bound to protein. Total HCY contains both protein-bound and free HCY fractions. This measurement requires chemical reduction and derivitization with a fluorophore before high performance liquid chromatography (HPLC) analysis and will not be reflected on a standard plasma amino acid panel.[48] The proportion of free HCY in total HCY is dependent on the total concentration of HCY present in the blood. As plasma total HCY increases, the contribution of plasma-free HCY rises disproportionately.[49-51] When total HCY is less than 60 µmol/L, the increase in free HCY is minimal. When total HCY ranges from 60 to 150 µmol/L, free HCY increases from less than 1 to 20 µmol/L, indicating that only a portion of total HCY continues to bind to protein. As total HCY increases proportionately from 150 to 250 µmol/L, free HCY increases above 20 µmol/L indicating that the protein-binding capacity for HCY has been exceeded.[52] Plasma total HCY must reach a concentration of at least 50 µmol/L, or about 4 times the upper limit of normal, before any free HCY is detectable by standard amino acid analysis.[53] When evaluating HCY concentrations, it is important to determine whether the concentrations represent free or total HCY.[47]

Processing of serum or plasma samples for amino acid analysis can affect detection of HCY. Free HCY readily undergoes disulfide exchange, binds to other proteins, and rapidly disappears as a free amino acid. This takes place even in frozen samples. Thus, deproteinization of samples is required within 30 minutes of a blood draw to accurately measure the free HCY concentration by amino acid analysis.[53] Delay in diagnosis of CβS deficiency has been reported as a result of this phenomenon.[54] In contrast, total HCY is less affected by sample storage and it is a more sensitive procedure to identify increased HCY concentrations in plasma.[53-56] Thus, measurement of total plasma HCY is the preferred method for diagnosis of homocystinuria; total HCY in a neonate with classical homocystinuria is typically >50 µmol/L (0.7 mg/dL).[53-56]

CβS deficiency is typically verified by analysis of enzyme activity in fibroblast cultures. Molecular genetic testing can be completed with targeted mutation analysis of the more common alleles (I278T; G307S) followed by sequence analysis of the entire coding region, if indicated.[47]

Once the diagnosis of CβS deficiency is strongly suspected or confirmed, a trial of vitamin B_6 is required to determine B_6-responsiveness. Although there is a strong relationship between responsiveness and presence of residual CβS activity in liver, activity of CβS in fibroblasts can vary greatly in responsive patients. Some patients demonstrate responsiveness even if CβS activity is not detected in fibroblast studies.[18] Although many mutations in the cDNA of CβS have been classified as "responsive" or "nonresponsive," the majority of patients are heterozygous for different alleles. This makes prediction of responsiveness difficult from mutation data.[1,47,57] Thus, in vivo testing of responsiveness is necessary no matter what enzyme or mutation studies suggest.

Determination of B_6-Responsiveness

Responsiveness to vitamin B_6 supplementation is not uniform in all patients. With B_6 supplementation, approximately 13% of patients display an intermediate response with continued slight elevations in plasma HCY concentrations.[19] Even those with clear B_6-responsiveness may show elevated plasma HCY concentrations and continued elevations of MET concentrations after excessive intact protein intake, although biochemical parameters will be clearly improved over the untreated state.[58] Also, responsiveness is constant within sibships.[19]

When a diagnosis of CβS deficiency is confirmed or strongly suggested, responsiveness to B_6 needs to be assessed. A decrease in free HCY concentrations in plasma below 20 μmol/L and/or a decrease of total HCY concentrations below 50 μmol/L, suggest that the patient is B_6-responsive.[59] Others suggest that the plasma concentration of free HCY needs to average < 11 μmol/L to prevent long-term complications.[33]

Methods for determining B_6-responsiveness vary widely in the literature. For instance, Yap and Naughton[33] provided oral vitamin B_6 at a dose of 50 mg 3 times a day and total plasma HCY, free HCY, and CYS concentrations were determined every 3 days. Although specific biochemical changes were not defined in this paper, rapidly falling plasma MET and clearing of free HCY concentrations suggested a responsive case. Nonresponsive cases continued to have persistently elevated or increasing plasma MET and detectable free HCY concentrations during the trial.[33] Similarly, Wilcken and Wilcken[59] provided a total vitamin B_6 dose of 100 to 200 mg/day. Others advocate higher doses. Kluijtmans et al.[25] prescribed vitamin B_6 for 3 weeks in doses of 750 mg/day to adults and 200 to 500 mg/day to children. According to Perry,[60] a patient should not be considered nonresponsive until a dose of 500 to 1000 mg/day has been given for several weeks.

More recently, Mudd and Levy suggested the following protocol:[46]

- Measure baseline plasma amino acid concentrations while the patient is ingesting his or her usual diet.
- Give 100 mg B_6 orally and remeasure plasma amino acid concentrations 24 hours later. Reductions of 30% in plasma HCY and/or MET concentrations indicate responsiveness.

- If HCY or MET concentrations do not change significantly, a 200 mg dose of B_6 is given and plasma amino acid concentrations are assessed again in 24 hours.
- If responsiveness is still not found, a maximum dose of 300 mg for infants or 500 mg for a child or adult is given and plasma amino acid concentrations are rechecked in 24 hours.
- If a 30% reduction in plasma HCY or MET concentration is still not detectable after this trial, the patient is considered nonresponsive.[46]

Once responsiveness has been determined, some advocate reducing the vitamin B_6 dose in 50 mg increments to determine the lowest dose of vitamin B_6 that still allows for a positive metabolic response.[59] Overall nutrition status can affect the results of a B_6 trial. Patients must not be folate deficient as this may prevent accurate determination of responsiveness.[61,62]

Outcomes if Untreated

The classical features of patients with untreated CβS deficiency include ectopic lentis and/or severe myopia, thromboembolisms, skeletal abnormalities, and mental retardation. Less common features include seizures, psychiatric problems, dystonia, and hypopigmentation.[1,63] The age of onset and severity of clinical manifestations vary widely among affected individuals.

A large international survey of 629 patients, published in 1985, described the natural history of CβS deficiency.[19] Among patients not diagnosed through newborn screening, vitamin B_6-responsive individuals, in general, had significantly better mental capabilities and lower incidence and reduced severity of other clinical features associated with this disorder. In this cohort, there was a continuum of B_6-responsiveness: 44% were nonresponsive, 44% were responsive, and 13% were considered intermediate in response.[19]

In untreated B_6-nonresponsive patients with CβS deficiency, mental retardation often presents as developmental delay between 1 and 2 years of age.[19] Among untreated patients with CβS deficiency, a wide range of mental capabilities was measured with mean IQ ranging from 10 to 138. However, for those who were classified as B_6-nonresponsive, the median IQ was 64 compared to a median IQ of 78 for those classified as B_6-responsive.[19] When compared to unaffected siblings, 34% of B_6-responsive patients had IQ scores comparable to their siblings, while 63% had lower scores. This contrasts to nonresponsive patients, among whom 94% had IQ scores lower than their unaffected siblings.[19]

Homocystinuria has also been implicated in development of various psychiatric manifestations in patients with CβS deficiency. Early reports suggested a high incidence of schizophrenia in untreated patients with CβS deficiency,[64,65] and led to the "transmethylation hypothesis" as a cause of schizophrenia.[66] However, using current diagnostic criteria, review of these studies did not verify this diagnosis.[66] Abbott et al.[67] completed a survey of 63 patients with late-treated CβS deficiency and found that 51% of the group showed a clinically significant psychiatric disorder from 4 primary diagnostic categories: episodic depression (10%), chronic disorders of behavior (17%), chronic obsessive-compulsive disorder (5%), and personality disorders (19%). Aggressive behavior and other disorders of conduct were particularly common among those with mental retardation and among vitamin B_6 nonresponders.[67] Seizures have also been reported in patients with late-treated CβS deficiency; the incidence of seizures was 23.4% among late-detected nonresponsive patients and 16.8% among B_6-responsive patients.[19]

The etiology of central nervous system (CNS) abnormalities in patients with CβS deficiency is unclear. It has been suggested that a chemical abnormality of the CNS might contribute to the neurological difficulties and mental retardation. Diminished cerebral concentrations of adenosine and disruptions of the ratio of SAM to AdoHcy have been implicated.[68] AdoHcy, when applied to rat sensorimotor cortex, decreases the rates of methylation of proteins and phosphotidylethanolamine derivatives.[69] Another hypothesis suggested that HCY metabolites might be potent neuronal excitotoxins causing overstimulation of various neuronal receptors.[69-71] Small but repeated cerebral vascular thromboses may be sufficient to produce abnormalities leading to development of various CNS sequelae.[60]

For untreated patients with CβS deficiency, myopia, followed by ocular dislocations, are often the first clinical sign of this disorder and can be detected at 1 to 2 years of age.[72] Mudd et al.[19] found that 82% of untreated nonresponsive patients and 50% of untreated responsive patients developed ectopic lentis by the age of 10 years, and in another study, 25% developed optic atrophy at later ages.[72] Visual prognosis deteriorates the later a diagnosis is made and treatment started; ectopic lentis can progress despite tight biochemical control in late-detected cases.[73] In addition, long-term biochemical control is necessary to maintain ocular health in patients with CβS. Early-treated patients with poor metabolic control in their teens or early twenties developed significant progression of myopia in two studies.[72,73]

The etiology of ocular deterioration in patients with CβS deficiency is not well understood, but evidence suggests that it is related to abnormally elevated plasma HCY and low CYS concentrations. Lens zonules normally have a high CYS content and deficiency of this amino acid may affect normal zonular development.[74] In addition, HCY inhibits cross-linkage in collagen, which may predispose zonule fibers to degeneration,[75] and this may cause a release of zonal tension allowing spherical deformation of the lens.[76]

Mudd et al. found that 27% of untreated B_6-nonresponsive patients developed a clinically detectable thromboembolic event by the age of 15 years. These events were the primary cause of death in 71% of reported deaths in this international survey.[19] Of the 253 recorded thromboembolic events in 181 patients, 51% affected peripheral veins with 25% of these causing pulmonary embolism, 32% were cerebrovascular accidents, 11% affected peripheral arteries, and 4% produced myocardial infarctions. The distribution of these types of thromboembolic events was only marginally related to the B_6-responsiveness of the patients.[19] Postoperative thromboembolic complications have also been reported.[19,77]

The mechanism for HCY toxicity on vascular connective tissue is not well defined. Yap[78] summarized various animal studies that demonstrated that exposure to SAAs and HCY causes myointimal hyperplasia, accumulation of extracellular matrix and fibrils, and fragmentation of elastic lamellae and internal elastic membrane. These findings are similar to those found in early atherosclerotic lesions, and endothelial dysfunction seen in patients with CβS deficiency.[79,80]

Tsai et al.[81] established in vitro that plasma HCY, at concentrations consistent with those seen in untreated patients with CβS deficiency, enhances smooth-muscle cell proliferation. Other work supported the "oxidant stress theory" of vascular dysfunction in which the sulfhydryl group of HCY undergoes auto-oxidation, generating superoxide radicals (O_2) that consume the vasodilator nitrous oxide.[82] Other studies demonstrated that plasma HCY initiates a cascade of inflammatory mediators and inflammatory transcription factors.[83-85]

Using purified plasma and fibrinogen from healthy adults, a recent study by Marchi et al.[86] found that fibrin polymerization was affected at a plasma HCY concentration greater than 52 μmol/L, and higher concentrations of HCY (> 400 μmol/L) altered fibrin formation. Another recent study suggested that abnormal HCY metabolites replace dehydroascorbic acid in connective tissue metabolism.[84] This may be pathogenic by depleting ascorbic acid required for collagen synthesis and may cause abnormal cross-linkage of collagen molecules. In addition, HCY metabolites attached to collagen molecules may render them antigenic and trigger an autoimmune response.[87]

Mudd et al.[19] found that 64% of those patients with untreated B_6-nonresponsive CβS deficiency developed radiological evidence of spinal osteoporosis by the age of 20 years and found a significantly greater progression of skeletal abnormalities in B_6-nonresponsive patients. Scoliosis, dolichostenomelia (thinning and lengthening of the long bones), and pes cavus are other common skeletal abnormalities in this population.[1]

Defective cross-linking of collagen has been suggested as a possible mechanism for the skeletal abnormalities seen in this disorder. In vitro, HCY was shown to interfere with the formation of collagen cross-links, prevent fibril insolubility, inhibit lysyl oxidase, and delay synthesis of crosslinks in mature collagen.[88] In 10 patients with elevated total plasma HCY concentrations, plasma concentrations of various indicators of bone remodeling were measured. Serum carboxy-terminal telopeptide of collagen type I, an indicator of collagen type I cross-linkage, was significantly decreased in these patients.[89]

Nutrition Management

Three primary modalities to treat CβS deficiency currently exist. For those who are B_6-responsive, vitamin B_6, often in combination with folic acid and vitamin B_{12}, is prescribed.[59] For those who do not respond to B_6 supplementation, a MET-restricted, CYS-supplemented diet is instituted.[90] For those receiving nutrition management, B_6, folic acid, and B_{12} are often included as coenzymes of MET metabolism. Finally, betaine, a methyl donor that aids in remethylation of HCY to MET, is used as an adjunct to therapy, primarily for those patients nonresponsive to B_6.[91]

Patients with B_6-Responsiveness

Based on historical clinical experience, approximately 50% of patients with CβS deficiency will respond to B_6 supplementation.[19] If a patient responds to a B_6 challenge, then long-term vitamin B_6 supplementation, usually in the form of pyridoxine hydrochloride, should be instituted. For some with classical homocystinuria, treatment with vitamin B_6 alone can completely normalize plasma HCY concentrations. For partial responders, a combination of B_6, low-protein diet, betaine, folate, and vitamin B_{12} is often necessary.[59,92,93] Some suggest that nutrition management with moderate MET restriction should be initiated even for patients with maximum vitamin B_6-responsiveness. These patients have demonstrated reduced tolerance to MET when challenged with a MET load test and showed elevated plasma MET concentrations with ingestion of high intact protein meals.[94-96]

The amount of vitamin B_6 prescribed to a B_6-responsive patient on a long-term basis varies widely. Barber and Spaeth prescribed doses of 250 to 500 mg/day,[92] Kluijtmans et al. used 750 mg/day in adults and at least 200 mg/day in children,[25] and Gaull et al. used 800 to 1200 mg/day.[96] In contrast, Wilcken and Wilcken prescribed a maximum of 200 mg/day and found that long-term free plasma HCY concentrations below 20 μmol/L and total plasma HCY below 50 μmol/L can be attained at this lower dose if sufficient folate and vitamin B_{12} status is maintained.[59] Some patients may respond to long-term doses as low as 25 mg/kg.[97]

Pyridoxine can be toxic at high intakes.[98] One study found impaired propioception, paresthesis of the feet, and/or abnormal sural nerve conduction in seven patients with nonresponsive CβS deficiency receiving doses of 900 to 1200 mg/day for periods of 4 to 22 years.[99] Sensory neuropathy induced by high B_6 consumption was suggested as a potential cause for the observed symptomology. Another study, however, did not find signs or symptoms suggestive of sensory neuropathy in 17 patients treated with 200 to 500 mg B_6 for up to 24 years; 12 of these patients received total B_6 doses exceeding 1000 mg/day.[100] The upper limit for B_6 established by the National Research Council is 100 mg/day for adults.[101] In homocystinuria, higher doses are often given without side effects, but awareness of symptomology associated with toxicity is suggested.[1] For infants, a vitamin B_6 dose above 300 mg/day is not recommended because some infants have experienced apnea or unresponsiveness requiring respiratory support at higher dosages.[102] Similar symptoms have been observed in infants given as little as 50 mg B_6 orally or 5 to 50 mg intramuscularly.[103-105]

Patients with B_6 Nonresponsiveness

Nutrient Requirements

There are several modalities to treat those patients with classical homocystinuria who are partially or completely nonresponsive to B_6 supplementation. These include a MET-restricted diet, vitamin B_6, folate, vitamin B_{12}, and/or betaine.

MET and CYS

Methionine and CYS requirements have been studied extensively over the past decade using ^{13}C-tracer balance approaches.[6,9,106-111] These studies demonstrated that the MET requirement is much lower when CYS is in sufficient supply to contribute to overall methyl-group needs. For instance, in the presence of excess dietary CYS (> 21 mg/kg), the obligatory MET requirement in adult men averaged 4.5 mg/kg/day. The minimum obligatory MET requirement is defined as the intake that cannot be replaced by CYS. From this finding, a population-safe minimum intake (+ 2 SD from mean) for MET was estimated at 10.1 mg/kg/day.[109-111] In contrast, when adult men were fed a diet devoid of CYS, MET needs were greater, with a mean of 12.6 mg/kg and a population-safe estimate of 21 mg/kg/day.[109] Similar studies have also been completed in 7 to 11-year-old children.[111]

The estimated requirements for both MET and CYS in disorders of sulfur amino acids are given in Table 7.2. The listed MET requirements encompass recent findings about minimum MET needs.[6,106-114] Because of the block in transsulfuration of HCY to CYS in CβS deficiency, CYS becomes an essential amino acid in this disorder.[1,2] The listed CYS requirements are elevated beyond minimum needs to ensure an adequate supply of CYS to spare MET as a methyl donor and allow for the lowest MET intake for protein synthesis.

Protein

Protein needs of patients with disorders of sulfur amino acid metabolism have not been individually studied. Therefore, general recommendations in Chapter 3, Table 3.1, are given. Information in references 112, 115, and 116 is useful in actual diet planning.

Fat and Essential Fatty Acids

Dietary reference intakes (DRIs) for fat for infants are given in Chapter 3, Table 3.1, and also include DRIs for essential fatty acids, linoleic, and α-linolenic acids, throughout life for normal infants, children, and adults.[113]

Energy and Fluid

Once the patient's MET prescription is supplied by intact protein and total protein needs are provided by a MET-free medical food, additional energy may still be necessary to meet the infant's energy requirement (see Chapter 3, Table 3.1). Often, a protein-free medical food may be prescribed for this purpose (see Appendix C). These medical foods vary in fat, carbohydrate, and micronutrient content. With free amino acids as the primary protein source, total energy needs for patients with inherited metabolic disorders may be somewhat greater than energy needs established for healthy persons (see Chapter 3, Table 3.1). Frequent monitoring of weight gain is necessary to ensure adequate energy intake for normal growth.

Minerals and Vitamins

An infant consuming a combination of medical food and human milk/proprietary infant formula may not require additional mineral and vitamin supplementation beyond the B-vitamins required as coenzymes in MET metabolism (described below). However, if a patient is consuming a medical food, because of the poor absorption, a mineral and vitamin supplement will likely be required to supply amounts suggested in Chapter 3, Table 3.1. Periodic assessment of micronutrient intake and status are necessary as diet changes occur over the lifespan.

MET-Free Medical Foods

Various medical foods are commercially available to manage infants with homocystinuria (see Table 7.3). These infant medical foods contain a varying

Table 7.2 ***Recommended Methionine and Cystine Intakes for Infants, Children, and Adults with Homocystinuria***

Age	*MET[a] (mg/kg)*	*L-CYS[b] (mg/kg)*
Infants, mo		
0 < 3	15–60	85–150
3 < 6	15–50	85–150
6 < 9	12–43	85–150
9 < 12	12–43	85–150
Girls and Boys, yr		
1 < 4	9–28	60–100
4 < 7	7–22	50–80
7 < 11	7–22	30–50
Women, yr		
11 < 15	7–21	30–50
15 < 19	6–19	25–40
≥ 19	5–19	20–30
Men, yr		
11 < 15	7–22	30–50
15 < 19	7–21	25–40
≥ 19	5–19	20–30

Sources:

Acosta PB, Yannicelli S. *Protocol 8. Homocystinuria. Nutrition Support Protocols*. 4th ed. Columbus, OH: Ross Products Division, Abbott Laboratories; 2001:137–165.

Ball RO, Courtney-Martin G, Pencharz PB. The in vivo sparing of methionine by cysteine in sulfur amino acid requirements in animal models and adult humans. *J Nutr*. 2006;136:1682S–1693S.

Courtney-Martin G, Chapman KP, Moore AM, Kim JH, Ball RO, Pencharz PB. Total sulfur amino acid requirement and metabolism in parenterally fed postsurgical human neonates. *Am J Clin Nutr*. 2008;88: 115–124.

Di Buono M, Wykes LJ, Ball RO, Pencharz PB. Dietary cysteine reduces the methionine requirement in men. *Am J Clin Nutr*. 2001;74:761–766.

Di Buono M, Wykes LJ, Ball RO, Pencharz PB. Total sulfur amino acid requirement in young men as determined by indicator amino acid oxidation with L-(1-13C)phenylalanine. *Am J Clin Nutr*. 2001;74:756–760.

Humayun MA, Turner JM, Elango R, et al. Minimum methionine requirement and cysteine sparing of methionine in healthy school-age children. *Am J Clin Nutr*. 2006;84:1080–1085.

Institute of Medicine. *Protein and Amino Acids. Dietary Reference Intakes*. Washington, DC: National Academies Press; 2005:589–768.

Otten JJ, Hellwig JP, Meyers LD. *Dietary Reference Intakes: The Essential Guide to Nutrient Requirements*. Washington, DC: National Academies Press; 2006.

Pencharz P. The Hospital for Sick Children. University of Toronto, Toronto, Canada. Personal Communication; 2008.

Raguso CA, Regan MM, Young VR. Cysteine kinetics and oxidation at different intakes of methionine and cystine in young adults. *Am J Clin Nutr*. 2000;71:491–499.

Turner JM, Humayun MA, Elango R, et al. Total sulfur amino acid requirement of healthy school-age children as determined by indicator amino acid oxidation technique. *Am J Clin Nutr*. 2006;83:619–623.

[a]For pyridoxine nonresponsive CβS deficiency, initiate prescription with lowest amount for patient's age. For patients with pyridoxine responsive CβS deficiency, initiate prescription in midrange for patient's age. Adjust intake based on plasma MET concentrations and clinical status.

[b]L-CYS may be prescribed above estimated requirements. Increase dose if plasma CYS concentrations are < 170 μmol/L.

Table 7.3 ***Formulation, Nutrient Composition, and Sources of Medical Foods per 100 g Powder for Patients with Disorders of Sulfur Amino Acids***

Disorder/ Medical Foods	*Modified Nutrient(s) (mg/100 g)*	*Protein Equiv*[a] *(g/100 g, source)*	*Fat (g/100 g, source)*	*Carbohydrate (g/100 g, source)*	*Energy (kcal/100 g/kJ/100 g)*	*Linoleic acid/ α-Linolenic acid (mg/100 g)*
			Abbott Nutrition[b]			
Hominex-1	L-MET 0 L-CYS 450 L-carnitine 20 Taurine 40	15 Amino acids[c]	21.7 High oleic safflower, coconut, soy oils	53 Corn syrup solids	480/2006	3500/350
Hominex-2 Unflavored	L-MET 0 L-CYS 900 L-carnitine 40 Taurine 50	30 Amino acids[c]	14.0 High oleic safflower, coconut, soy oils	35 Corn syrup solids	410/1714	2200/225
			Mead Johnson Nutritionals[d]			
HCY 1	L-MET 0 L-CYS 600 L-carnitine Added Taurine 30	16.2 Amino acids[c]	26 Palm olein, soy, coconut, high oleic sunflower oils	51 Corn syrup solids	500/2090	4500/380
HCY 2	L-MET 0 L-CYS 810 L-carnitine added Taurine 57	22 Amino acids[c]	8.5 Soy oil	61 Sucrose, corn syrup solids	410/1714	4600/610

(continues)

Table 7.3 ***Formulation, Nutrient Composition, and Sources of Medical Foods per 100 g Powder for Patients with Disorders of Sulfur Amino Acids,*** *Continued*

Disorder/ Medical Foods	Modified Nutrient(s) (mg/100 g)	Protein Equiv[a] (g/100 g, source)	Fat (g/100 g, source)	Carbohydrate (g/100 g, source)	Energy (kcal/100 g/kJ/100 g)	Linoleic acid/ α-Linolenic acid (mg/100 g)
Nutricia North America[e]						
Methionaid	L-MET 0 L-CYS 3700 L-carnitine ND Taurine ND	60 Amino acids[c]	0	3 Hydrolyzed cornstarch	250/1045	0/0
XMET Analog	L-MET 0 L-CYS 390 L-carnitine 10 Taurine 20	13 Amino acids[c]	20.9 High oleic safflower, coconut, soy oils	59 Galactose	475/1986	3025/ND
XMET Maxamaid	L-MET 0 L-CYS 750 L-carnitine 20 Taurine 140	25 Amino acids[c]	<0.1	57 Sugar, corn syrup solids	324/1354	0/0
XMET Maxamum	L-MET 0 L-CYS 1200 L-carnitine 390 Taurine 140	40 Amino acids[c]	<1.0	34 Sugar	305/1275	0/0
Milupa HOM 2	L-MET 0 L-CYS 3400 L-carnitine 0 Taurine 0	69 Amino acids[c]	0.0	3.8 Sugar	290/1212	0/0

(continues)

Table 7.3 ***Formulation, Nutrient Composition, and Sources of Medical Foods per 100 g Powder for Patients with Disorders of Sulfur Amino Acids****, Continued*

Disorder/ Medical Foods	***Modified Nutrient(s) (mg/100 g)***	***Protein Equiv[a] (g/100 g, source)***	***Fat (g/100 g, source)***	***Carbohydrate (g/100 g, source)***	***Energy (kcal/100 g/kJ/100 g)***	***Linoleic acid/ α-Linolenic acid (mg/100 g)***
			Vitaflo US LLC[f]			
HCU Cooler (per 100 mL)	L-MET 0 L-CYS 410 L-carnitine 13 Taurine 25	11.5 Amino acids[c]	Trace	5.9 Sugar, maltodextrin	71/297	0/0
HCU Express	L-MET 0 L-CYS 1920 L-carnitine 158 Taurine 238	60 Amino acids[c]	<0.5	15 Sugar, starch, dried glucose syrup	302/1260	0/0
HCU Gel	L-MET 0 L-CYS 1370 L-carnitine 50 Taurine 90	42 Amino acids[c]	<0.5	43 Sugar, starch, dried glucose syrup	342/1428	0/0

Source: Data supplied by each company.

Notes: ND = no data.

Values listed, although accurate at time of publication, are subject to change. The most current information may be obtained by referring to product labels.

[a]Protein equivalent, g = g nitrogen × 6.25.

[b]Abbott Nutrition, 625 Cleveland Avenue, Columbus, Ohio 43215. 800-551-5838.

[c]All except glycine are in the L-form.

[d]Mead Johnson Nutritionals, 2400 West Lloyd Expressway, Evansville, Indiana 47721. 800-457-3550.

[e]Nutricia North America, PO Box 117, Gaithersburg, Maryland 20884. 800-365-7354.

[f]Vitaflo US LLC, 123 East Neck Road, Huntington, New York 11743. 888-848-2356.

macronutrient profile but all contain protein equivalent (nitrogen, g × 6.25), fat, and carbohydrate. Many of the medical foods for children and adults are free of fat.

In all medical foods designed to manage patients with homocystinuria, the source of protein is free amino acids. The essential amino acid MET is removed and CYS, which is an essential amino acid in CβS deficiency, is supplemented in these medical foods (see Table 7.3). The total protein provided by both medical food and intact protein should exceed current protein recommendations[112,113] (see Chapter 3, Table 3.1).

For some patients, MET tolerance may be great enough that a medical food may not be required to meet protein needs. However, it is still highly desirable for a teenager or adult to continue ingesting a medical food. Use of a medical food allows for greater flexibility in food choices and can help improve overall metabolic control.[112]

For those patients who are not detected by newborn screening but present with clinical symptoms, initiating a MET-restricted diet and medical food at a later age may be difficult.[93] There are many medical food choices for children and adults with homocysteinuria; some are protein-dense, which may allow for a lower daily intake than do medical foods containing smaller amounts of protein equivalent (see Table 7.3).

Intact Protein

Initial MET needs can be estimated from recommendations based on age and weight of the infant (see Table 7.2). For B_6-nonresponsive infants, the initial MET prescription should be based on requirements at the lower end of the treatment range.[112] For partially responsive infants, starting with a value in the mid to upper treatment range is suggested. An infant's MET prescription can be filled with either human milk or a standard proprietary infant formula (see Appendix B).

For a mother who wishes to continue human milk-feeding, the procedure used to allow infants with PKU to breast-feed can be applied to an infant with CβS deficiency.[117] With human milk, approximately two-thirds of total protein intake will be provided from medical food and the remaining one-third from human milk.[33] However, this is only a rough guideline and frequent monitoring of plasma amino acid and total HCY concentrations needs to occur. For human milk-fed infants, adjustments are prescribed in the volume of medical food to effectively increase or decrease human milk consumption.[112] For infants consuming a proprietary infant formula as the MET source, the volume prescribed is adjusted to change MET intake.[112] Infants with early-treated CβS deficiency typically do not exhibit developmental delays that could hamper their ability to feed.[33]

Other Nutrition Therapies for Nonresponsiveness

Supplementation with L-CYS, folic acid, B_{12}, B_6, and betaine has been found beneficial in helping maintain metabolic control in patients with CβS deficiency. In patients with CβS deficiency, plasma concentrations of both total and free cyst(e)ine may be significantly reduced.[118] Cystine supplementation is often overlooked in treatment of patients with CβS deficiency, but can help improve metabolic control. In plasma samples collected from patients with classical homocystinuria, Lee et al.[118] found that when plasma CYS concentrations were below 170 μmol/L, free HCY was elevated up to 30 μmol/L. When plasma CYS concentrations were above 170 μmol/L, free HCY remained below 5 μmol/L. These results suggest that selective supplementation of CYS for patients with total CYS concentrations < 170 μmol/L may be beneficial in attaining a small, but potentially clinically significant, reduction in plasma-free HCY concentrations.[118]

Medical foods designed to treat homocystinuria are supplemented with CYS (Table 7.3). Unless medical food intake is limited, L-CYS supplementation is often not required. However, for patients consuming limited amounts of medical food, supplementation to increase plasma CYS concentrations may be necessary. L-CYS is insoluble, but cystine dihyrochloride and calcium cystinate are soluble forms of this amino acid.[119] For patients, a solution (10 mg/mL) can be used for CYS supplementation.[120] L-CYS can also be given in powder or capsule form to older patients. Periodic monitoring of plasma cyst(e)ine concentrations is recommended to determine whether L-CYS supplementation is necessary.[121]

Sulfur amino acid metabolism involves both folic acid and vitamin B_{12} enzymatic systems for remethylation of HCY to MET (see Figure 7.1). Methyl transfer from 5-methyl-tetrahydrofolate (THF) is required for MET synthase (5-methylTHF-homocystine methyltransferases) activity. In addition, the cobalamin cofactors, Cbl E and Cbl G, are necessary for MET synthase reductase and MET synthase activity, respectively.[1] Thus, patients with CβS deficiency require an adequate supply of both B-vitamins.

Folate depletion has been found in a number of patients with CβS deficiency.[61,122] The majority of patients require additional folate, irrespective of their responsiveness to B_6.[59] In patients with CβS deficiency, folate supplementation typically ranges from 1 to 5 mg/day.[1,59] Some clinicians supplement with folate only if a patient is found to be deficient,[33] while others routinely supplement.[1,59]

When supplementing with vitamin B_{12}, an oral supplement or periodic intramuscular (IM) injections of hydroxycobalamin can be prescribed. Wilcken and Wilcken[59] advocate IM injections of hydroxycobalamin every 1 to 3 months to nonresponsive patients, irrespective of their serum B_{12}

concentration. Others supplement with B_{12} only if deficiency is found.[1,33] For B_{12} injections, the hydroxycobalamin form was found to decrease both plasma HCY and urine methylmalonic acid (MMA) concentrations further than the cyanocobalamin form in patients with CblC disease.[120] If B_{12} absorption is a concern, IM injections are preferred over oral supplementation. Poor absorption of B_{12} is frequently found in the elderly.[123,124]

Even for patients found to be B_6-nonresponsive, some clinicians routinely prescribe vitamin B_6 to ensure an adequate supply as a coenzyme in SAA metabolism.[59,125] B_6 doses recommended for nonresponsive patients typically range from 100 to 200 mg daily.[59]

Betaine (Cystadane®, Accredo Health Group, Inc., Memphis, Tennessee) significantly lowers plasma HCY concentrations in patients with nonresponsive homocystinuria and can be an effective adjunct therapy to a MET-restricted diet.[91,126-131] In one study, 15 nonresponsive patients receiving 6 to 9 g/day of betaine, in addition to their standard treatment, showed a mean decrease of 74% in free plasma HCY concentration during an average treatment period of 11 years.[59] Betaine treatment may be especially effective in preventing thromboembolic events in patients with CβS deficiency.[91,126-131] Supplementation with betaine lowers plasma HCY concentrations by providing additional methyl groups to increase the rate of HCY remethylation through the activity of betaine-HCY-S-methyltransferase (BHMT; see Figure 7.1).[1,130] Betaine treatment also significantly reduces total HCY concentrations in cerebrospinal fluid (CSF).[125] With betaine treatment, plasma MET concentrations increase; however, MET contributes less to the pathophysiology of CβS deficiency than does HCY itself.[1,46] Plasma CYS concentrations also increase with betaine therapy.[49,91]

Betaine is typically prescribed at a dose of 6 to 9 g/day to adults or 200 to 250 mg/kg/day in divided doses to children.[59,125] However, a study investigating the pharmokinetics of betaine in six CβS-deficient patients, ages 6 to 17 years, showed minimal additional plasma HCY reduction when a daily betaine dose of 150 mg/kg/day was exceeded.[130,132]

Although several studies have shown that addition of betaine lowers plasma HCY concentrations in patients with nonresponsive CβS deficiency, a recent study by Singh et al.[127] investigated betaine's ability to further decrease plasma HCY concentrations in patients already on strict nutrition management for this disorder. In this study, nutrition management of five B_6-nonresponsive patients was optimized prior to starting betaine by instituting a MET-restricted diet providing < 30 mg MET/kg with a MET-free medical food, and B_6 up to 20 mg/kg to decrease plasma MET and free and total HCY concentrations. Even with strict nutrition management, 2 of 5 patients with CβS deficiency could not attain total plasma HCY concentrations below 50 μmol/L. Betaine was then initiated at 20 to 50 mg/kg and increased incrementally to 120 to 150 mg/kg until stabilization of total HCY was achieved over a 3- to 6-month period. With betaine therapy, all patients showed significant reductions in total plasma HCY (mean decrease 47.4 μmol/L, range 21 to 104 μmol/L) regardless of plasma MET concentrations. In addition, mutation analysis was completed for all patients. Betaine response was greatest among patients with mutations described as B_6-nonresponsive compared to patients heterozygous for mutant alleles classified as B_6-responsive.[127]

Adverse effects from betaine treatment appear to be rare; however, cerebral edema has been reported in two patients.[133,134] A 10-year-old female with B_6-nonresponsive CβS deficiency was noncompliant with treatment until she developed pancreatitis with splenic vein thrombosis. After surgery, she restarted betaine at 200 mg/kg, but remained noncompliant with diet resulting in plasma MET concentrations above 3000 μmol/L. She developed progressive cerebral edema over a 3-month period, which resolved once betaine was discontinued.[135] These authors suggested elevated CSF MET concentrations might have caused intracellular osmotic stress leading to edema.[135] In a later report, cerebral edema was reported in a 5-year-old boy; however, he maintained MET dietary restriction and his plasma MET concentrations remained below 1200 μmol/L. His symptoms also resolved after discontinuing betaine.[134] These authors suggested that elevated CSF betaine concentrations might have caused the edema and suggested that long-term plasma MET concentrations should remain below 1000 μmol/L in patients taking betaine.[134]

Cerebral edema was also found in a patient with MATI/III deficiency with plasma MET concentrations ≥ 1500 μmol/L who was initially treated with betaine and B_6. The edema resolved when therapy was discontinued.[135] These studies suggest that plasma MET concentrations should be included in routine monitoring of patients treated with betaine. In addition, signs of increased intracranial pressure such as headache, vomiting, change in mental status, or new neurological symptoms should be investigated.[128,133-135]

Concern has also been raised about prescribing betaine to infants who are poorly controlled on a MET-restricted diet. The infantile brain lacks BHMT activity and the effect of this lack of activity on total HCY metabolism is unclear.[125] All efforts toward dietary adherence and metabolic control should be pursued before considering the addition of betaine in the treatment of nonresponsive infants.[1]

Vitamin A status may be impaired in patients with CβS deficiency since concentrations of serum retinol were subnormal after retinol administration.[136] Oxidation of retinol by the –SH groups of HCY secreted into the gut was hypothesized as the cause of the reduction. Elevated plasma copper and ceruloplasmin concentrations were found in 15 patients with classical homocystinuria; no relationship between copper status and plasma HCY concentrations was found.[137,138] P. B. Acosta[139] found low serum retinol and elevated copper concentrations in twin boys with CβS deficiency. In addition, supplementation of selenium was required to maintain normal serum selenium concentrations in these boys.

Initiation of Nutrition Management and During Illness or Following Trauma

The concern of thromboembolism exists during both illness and surgical procedures. During all episodes of acute illness, prompt treatment of the illness with additional supportive care, including adequate hydration and aspirin or dipyridamole, is given to prevent blood stasis.[33] The danger of thromboembolism increases postoperatively in patients with CβS deficiency. This risk was lessened by increasing hydration with IV fluids pre- and postoperatively; intravenous B_6 was given during surgery in two cases.[140,141] If parenteral nutrition is required, see Chapter 4.

Table 7.4 outlines a diet plan for a 3.5-kg infant diagnosed with vitamin B_6-nonresponsive homocystinuria with plasma MET concentration at 150 µmol/L (normal 5-35 µmol/L). Subsequent testing found an elevation in total plasma HCY of 200 µmol/L (normal 5 to 15 µmol/L). After the diagnosis of CβS deficiency was confirmed, a trial of vitamin B_6 ruled out B_6-responsiveness. Thus, a MET-restricted diet was initiated at 20 mg/kg, the lower end of MET requirements for neonates.

Table 7.4 ***Diet Plan for a Neonate Who Weighs 3.5 kg Diagnosed with Vitamin B_6 Nonresponsive Homocystinuria***

Food	***Amount***	***MET (mg)***	***CYS (mg)***	***Protein (g)***	***Energy (kcal)***
Similac® Advance® infant formula with iron, powder	26 g	71	42	2.8	137
Hominex®-1 powder	63 g	0	284	9.5	302
Cystine solution (13 mg/100 mL)[a]	600 mL	0	78	0.0	0
Water to make[b]					615
Total		71	404	12.3	615
Per kg body weight		20	115	3.5	125

[a]L-CYS has a solubility of ~13 mg/100 g water at room temperature. *Source:* Ajinomoto. *Amino Acid Handbook*. Ajinomoto, Japan: 2004.

[b]Add water to yield a total 615 mL (~21 fl oz @ 20 kcal/ fl oz).

Long-Term Nutrition Management

As with most infants, beikost (baby foods) can be started at 4 to 6 months of age. Resources listing MET content of various baby foods are available.[112,115,116] As the intake of beikost increases, reduction in proprietary infant formula or human milk becomes necessary to allow for continued reduction in plasma MET concentrations.

Table 7.5 is a diet plan for a 6-month-old infant with mild developmental delay who was found to have an elevated plasma MET concentration of 60 μmol/L and elevated total HCY concentration of 80 μmol/L. The diagnosis was confirmed, and a trial of B_6 found the infant to respond to B_6 with lowered plasma HCY and MET concentrations. The infant was treated daily with 25 mg B_6 and 1 mg folate. A moderately MET-restricted diet was initiated at 42 mg/kg, the higher end of MET requirements for this age group.

As the infant grows older, beikost will be replaced by table foods. Methionine content of various foods is available but not all foods have been analyzed, especially processed products.[112,115,116] Methionine content of intact protein varies greatly, ranging from 0.3 to 5.0% of total amino acid content.[115]

Table 7.5 ***Diet Plan for a 6-Month-Old Infant Who Weighs 8 kg Diagnosed with Vitamin B_6 Responsive Homocystinuria***

Food	*Amount*	*MET (mg)*	*CYS (mg)*	*Protein (g)*	*Energy (kcal)*
Similac® Advance® infant formula with iron, powder	90 g	245	146	9.7	473
Hominex® I powder	55 g	0	248	8.3	264
Cystine solution (13 mg/ 100[a] mL)	900 mL	0	117	0.0	0
Water[b]					
Rice cereal (dry)	24 g	57	57	2.1	90
1st Foods® bananas	52 g	10	10	0.6	52
1st Foods® green beans	66 g	20	16	0.8	20
Total		332	594	21.5	899
Per kg body weight		42	74	2.7	112

Note: Vitamin B_6 (250 mg) and folate (1 mg) are also prescribed.

[a]L-CYS has a solubility of ~13 mg/100 g water at room temperature. *Source:* Ajinomoto. *Amino Acid Handbook*. Ajinomoto, Japan: 2004.

[b]Add water to yield a total of 950 mL (~34 fl oz @ 22 kcal/fl oz).

Especially for patients who are partially responsive to vitamin B_6, MET tolerance may be greater than that observed in some other amino acid disorders such as PKU or branched-chain ketoaciduria. Thus, protein rather than MET is often counted as a child with CβS deficiency grows older. Resources, such as the *Low Protein Food List for PKU*, provide a more accurate protein content of foods than that listed on product labels.[116] Use of very-low-protein bread, pasta, and other products also allows for greater flexibility in diet choices (see Appendix E).

Assessment of Specific Aspects of Nutrition Management

A monitoring schedule should be established for all patients with CβS deficiency, irrespective of their B_6-responsiveness. Monitoring includes growth parameters, various laboratory analyses specific for CβS deficiency and general nutrition status (see Chapter 3), and nutrient intake evaluation. At a minimum, biochemical laboratory analyses should include plasma concentrations of MET, CYS, and free and total HCY.[1]

Growth

Standard growth parameters need to be monitored closely. Monthly evaluation of length and weight is suggested for infants. Measurements are suggested every 3 months for children up to age 4 years and every 6 months for older children and adolescents.[112] Height and weight for age for infants and young children, and body mass index (BMI) for older children and adults need to be assessed (see Chapter 3).[129] If a patient's growth falls below his or her usual growth channels, then a more extensive work-up is recommended. Deficient intakes of MET and CYS, total protein, medical food, and/or total energy can all adversely affect growth and each should be evaluated when assessing growth problems.

Biochemical Monitoring

Biochemical goals for long-term treatment of patients with CβS deficiency include maintenance of plasma MET concentrations within or near the normal range (20 to 40 µmol/L), free plasma HCY concentrations below 20 µmol/L, and total HCY concentrations below 50 µmol/L.[59] Yap and Naughten[33] observed better long-term clinical outcomes in those patients maintaining free plasma HCY concentrations < 11 μmol/L. Walter et al.[93] also recommended plasma-free HCY concentrations < 10 μmol/L for good biochemical control.

In classical homocystinuria, the toxic compound is HCY rather than MET. However, by achieving normal, or near normal, MET concentrations, HCY concentrations will be reduced.[1,121] Methionine is a relatively benign amino acid, but very high concentrations (≥ 1200 μmol/L) have resulted in cerebral edema in two cases of CβS deficiency and one case of MAT I/III deficiency.[133-135]

Plasma Amino Acid Concentrations

In a standard plasma amino acid profile, concentrations of both MET and CYS need to be evaluated. The goal is to normalize concentrations of both amino acids, although, even with strict nutrition management, some individuals will not be able to maintain plasma MET concentrations in the reference range.[127] Initially, plasma amino acid concentrations should be measured one to two times weekly until the approximate needs of both amino acids are determined.[112,121] If plasma MET concentrations are elevated, the MET prescription should be reduced by 5 to 10% and plasma amino acids remeasured in 3 to 7 days.[112,121] If plasma CYS concentrations are low, supplementation with L-CYS needs to be considered.[121] Immediate processing of plasma samples within 30 minutes of the blood draw is necessary for accurate measurement of CYS concentrations. As with free HCY, free CYS rapidly binds to protein and falsely low CYS concentrations may be found without proper handling of the sample.[142]

Free and Total Plasma Homocysteine Concentrations

As discussed previously, only free plasma HCY is measured in a standard amino acid profile.[49] If free HCY is undetectable, this suggests that the total HCY concentration is below 50 μmol/L.[52,53] Although not as accurate as measuring total HCY concentration, maintaining free HCY concentrations below detection limits in a standard amino acid profile can be used as a guide for successful nutrition management.[121] However, periodic determination of total plasma HCY concentrations is suggested because total HCY is more stable in plasma samples and better reflects the HCY concentration in a patient with CβS deficiency than does free HCY.[53-56]

In the newborn period, patients may accumulate relatively more plasma MET and less HCY than adult patients.[143] Conversely, some untreated adult patients will show normal plasma MET concentrations in the presence of elevated HCY in plasma and urine.

Folate

Monitoring folate status is important, especially in patients who do not routinely take a folate supplement. Low-serum folate concentration (< 6 μg/dL) indicates folate deficiency; reduced RBC folate concentration (< 20 μg/dL) can be seen in both folate and/or B_{12} deficiency.[144,145] If folate above that amount in the diet is required, 500 μg/day additional is suggested with reevaluation of serum concentrations in 1 month.[112] For those taking a daily folate supplement, monitoring of B_{12} status is important because large doses of folate can mask megaloblastic anemia and accelerate the neurological complications associated with vitamin B_{12} deficiency.[146,147]

Vitamin B_{12} Status

Vitamin B_{12} status should be evaluated in patients with CβS deficiency, especially those who are not routinely supplemented with this vitamin.[148] Monitoring includes measurement of both serum B_{12} and MMA concentrations. MMA is considered a more sensitive indicator of compromised B_{12} nutriture than is serum B_{12} concentration.[145,149] The definition of B_{12} deficiency varies, but serum B_{12} concentrations < 150 pg/mL and serum MMA > 0.4 μmol/L are considered indications of poor B_{12} status.[124,144]

Betaine

To evaluate the effectiveness of betaine treatment, plasma HCY concentrations are measured. Plasma MET concentrations should be evaluated as well because betaine can increase plasma concentrations, especially if the patient is not well controlled on nutrition management.[133] The ratio of plasma MET and HCY (MET/total HCY), which increases with betaine therapy, has also been used as an indicator of the response to betaine.[127]

Various laboratory analyses should be included in the monitoring protocol for CβS deficiency. To assess protein status, albumin, transthyretin (prealbumin), and retinol-binding protein have been suggested[144,150] (see Chapter 3, Table 3.7). Iron status can be measured with ferritin, hemoglobin, and hematocrit concentrations.[145,151] Given the concerns about vitamin A, copper, and selenium status, measurement of concentrations of serum retinol and various trace minerals and vitamins may be indicated.[112,122,136-139]

Calculation of a 3-day diet diary recorded prior to each blood draw is recommended to assess MET, CYS, total protein, energy, and intakes of other nutrients.[112] Various nutrient calculation programs are available for this purpose including Amino Acid Analyzer® (Abbott Nutrition, Columbus, Ohio) and Food Processor® (ESHA Research, Inc., Salem, Oregon).

Bone Health

Given the high incidence of osteoporosis and other skeletal anomalies in untreated patients with CβS deficiency, periodic monitoring of bone status is recommended even for those treated for this disorder.[1,89] Various protocols for assessing bone status have been published.[144,152,153] A screening protocol developed at the University of Wisconsin–Madison Osteoporosis Clinic and Research Program includes yearly measurement of plasma/serum calcium, phosphorus, and 25-hydroxyvitamin D concentrations as well as electrolytes, blood urea nitrogen (BUN), creatinine, thyroid stimulating hormone (TSH), and a 24-hour urine calcium.[154] If any abnormalities are detected, then intake of calcium, vitamin D, and other nutrients associated with bone status should be assessed by periodic dual energy x-ray absorptionmetry (DXA) scans (see Chapter 3).[152-154]

Results of Nutrition Management

Treating patients with CβS deficiency clearly results in a more positive clinical outcome than that seen in untreated patients. However, general experience suggests that late treatment rarely, if ever, completely reverses mental impairment,[19] although treatment has led to behavioral improvement and slowed deterioration in mental capabilities.[131] Yap[78] reported that two late-detected B_6-nonresponsive patients who were placed on nutrition management showed a better mean IQ score (80 and 102) than two late-detected patients who were never treated (IQ 52 and 53).

In a survey by Mulvihill et al.,[72] patients diagnosed and treated before 6 weeks of age showed excellent visual acuity and substantially reduced ocular sequelae than that seen in untreated patients. Burke et al.[73] reported similar findings in 14 infants with CβS deficiency who started treatment in the newborn period. Of these, none developed ectopic lentis after a mean follow up of 8.2 years, compared with a 70% dislocation rate in untreated patients with a similar follow-up period.

Effective treatment of both vitamin B_6-responsive and nonresponsive patients markedly reduced the increased cardiovascular risk associated with classical homocystinuria.[91] Yap et al.[131] evaluated 158 patients from 5 international centers with over 2800 patient years of treatment. Based on the predicted rate of vascular events determined by Mudd et al.,[19] at least 112 vascular events would have been expected if these patients had remained untreated. Instead, only 17 vascular events were recorded in 12 of the 158 patients.[91] In addition, there were no differences in vascular outcomes between the centers, despite minor differences in each clinic's treatment protocol.

However, vascular events have been reported even in treated B_6-responsive patients maintaining long-term plasma-free HCY concentrations below 20 μmol/L. Wilcken and Wilcken[59] reported 2 vascular events in 17 B_6-responsive patients with 281 patient years of treatment. Thus, frequent monitoring in an appropriate cardiovascular clinic is recommended for all patients with classical homocystinuria irrespective of their B_6-responsiveness.

Maternal Homocystinuria

The majority of reported pregnancies have occurred in women with the B_6-responsive form of CβS deficiency.[1] Experience to date suggests that most pregnancies proceed without problems for the mother or infant. However, pregnancy can increase the risk for maternal thromboembolism, especially during the postpartum period.[155-158] Maternal CβS deficiency might also increase the risk of preeclampsia.[159] Limited concern for teratogenicity presently exists, at least in offspring of women who are responsive to B_6, because normal growth and development have been reported in a limited number of cases.[160] Greater risk may occur to the infant from pregnancies in nonresponsive women than in B_6-responsive women; two of eight infants followed long-term developed clinical anomalies, including congenital heart disease in one.[88] Thus, predicting normal outcomes for offspring of pregnancies in B_6-nonresponsive women is still unsure.[88]

Methionine-S-Adenosyltransferase Deficiency

Methionine-S-adenosyltransferase (EC 2.5.1.6) converts MET to SAM, the first step in MET transsulfuration (see Figure 7.1). Two separate genes, MAT1A and MAT2A, have been described. Mutations in MAT1A lead to deficiencies in the combined activity of MATI and MATIII in hepatic tissue.[161] MAT I/III deficiency (OMIM 250850)[13] is the most common genetic cause of persistent isolated hypermethioninemia. Both autosomal recessive and autosomal dominant inheritance have been reported.[162,163] In this disorder, plasma concentrations of MET are typically elevated without associated elevations in HCY[161-166] (see Table 7.1). However, in severe forms of MATI/III, slightly elevated plasma HCY and cystathionine concentrations have been detected.[164,165] Diagnosis of MAT deficiency requires a liver biopsy because reduced enzyme activity in fibroblasts is not detected.[166]

Adverse medical problems are rare in MAT I/III deficiency despite significantly elevated plasma MET concentrations.[161,162,167] Treatment in these cases is not indicated. However, severe MATI/III deficiency can cause demyelination with reduced cognitive function later in childhood.[137,165,168] Treatment with oral adenosylmethionine slowed demyelination and improved neurological function in these patients.[165,168]

S-Adenosylhomocysteine Hydrolase Deficiency

After transsulfuration of SAM to AdoHcy, AdoHcy is further metabolized to HCY and adenosine by S-adenosylhomocysteine hydrolase (EC 3.3.1.1; OMIM 180960)[13] (see Figure 7.1). A single patient with deficiency of this enzyme has been reported.[169] Various biochemical abnormalities, including elevated plasma concentrations of AdoHcy, SAM, and MET were found. This patient exhibited severely delayed psychomotor development, mild hepatic dysfunction, and myopathy with very elevated plasma creatine kinase (CK) concentrations.[169] Delayed myelination and atrophy of white matter were detected by magnetic resonance imaging (MRI). Treatment was attempted with a MET-restricted diet, phosphotidylcholine from egg yolk, and creatine monohydrate. Improvements in biochemical parameters with gradual clinical gains were initially attained; however, long-term effectiveness of this treatment has not been reported.[169]

γ-Cystathionase Deficiency

Following conversion of HCY to cystathionine by cystathionine-β-synthase, cystathionine is converted to CYS by γ-cystathionase (L-cystathionine cysteine-lyase), a B_6-dependent enzyme (see Figure 7.1). Cystathionase deficiency (OMIM 219500)[13] is considered a benign disorder.[2,170,171]

Without B_6 treatment or a MET-restricted diet, these patients excrete from 1000 to 5800 μmol cystathionine daily in urine; plasma cystathionine concentrations are also typically elevated.[2,88,170] Plasma CYS concentration is normal and HCY is absent. To accurately measure cystathionine concentrations in urine, a clean collection is required. Cystathionine can be converted to HCY by bacteria in contaminated samples, which has delayed diagnosis of this disorder.[171] Confirmation of the disorder can be obtained from a cultured lymphoid cell line or liver biopsy, but given the benign nature of this disorder, a biopsy is typically not recommended.[1,171]

γ-cystathionase deficiency can be classified as B_6-responsive or nonresponsive. Responsiveness can be determined by giving 100 mg vitamin B_6 for 2 weeks. If the concentration of cystathionine in urine has not significantly decreased, an additional 100 mg can be administered for an additional 2 weeks.[1] Responsive patients are typically treated with 100 mg vitamin B_6 daily,[172] although the necessity of supplementation has been questioned given the benign nature of this disorder.[2]

S-Adenosylmethionine: Glycine-N-Methyltransferase (GNMT) Deficiency

GNMT (EC 2.1.1.20; defect not shown in Figure 7.1) converts glycine to sarcosine and requires methyl-group transfer from SAM. Deficiency of GNMT (OMIM 606664)[13] was found in two siblings with mild hepatomegaly.[173] Hypermethioninemia and elevated plasma SAM concentrations without elevation in AdoHcy and sarcosine concentrations suggest this disorder. Treatment with a MET-restricted diet and added L-CYS may be beneficial, but little data are available.[173]

5,10-Methylenetetrahydrofolate Reductase (MTHFR) Deficiency

MTHFR (EC 1.5.1.20) converts 5,10-methylenetetrahydrofolate to 5-methyltetrahydrofolate, which is required as a methyl donor for remethylation of HCY to MET (see Figure 7.1). Severe MTHFR deficiency (OMIM 236250)[13] has been described in approximately 100 patients.[2,174-178] When diagnosed in infancy, progressive encephalopathy, apnea, seizures, and microcephaly have been found.[174-176,178] In later childhood and in adults, MTHFR deficiency manifests with ataxic gait, psychiatric disorders, and symptoms related to cardiovascular disease.[2,179] It has been proposed that the symptomology associated with severe MTHFR deficiency is related to cerebral deficiencies of MET and SAM rather than effects related to elevated plasma HCY concentrations.[178]

In patients with severe MTHFR deficiency, plasma elevations of total HCY (often > 100 μmol/L) and decreased MET concentrations are found (see Table 7.1). Homocystinuria is also present, but concentrations are lower than those seen in patients with CβS deficiency. MTHFR activity can be measured in liver, leukocytes, lymphocytes, and cultured fibroblasts.[2]

In patients with the infantile form, treatment with betaine has been successful when initiated from birth.[178,180-182] Later-treated infants (7 to 13 months) showed catch-up growth and marked neurological recovery, but remained delayed in long-term development.[178] Betaine doses used to treat patients with this disorder include 2 to 3 g per day in infants and 6 to 9 g per day in children and adults.[126,178,180-183] Strauss et al.[178] treated five affected children with high-dose betaine at 535 ± 222 mg/kg/day with aspirin every other day. Other therapeutic agents including folic acid, MET, B_6, B_{12}, creatine, and L-carnitine have been prescribed with varying success.[178,183] In addition, patients with severe MTHFR deficiency may be at increased risk for thromboembolism with exposure to nitrous oxide anesthesia.[184]

Methionine Synthase (CBLG) Deficiency (OMIM 250940)[13] and Methionine Synthase Reductase (CBLE) Deficiency (OMIM 236270)[13]

Methionine synthase reductase (MSR; EC 2.1.1.135) activates methionine synthase (MS; EC 2.1.1.13; defect not shown in Figure 7.1), which is necessary for remethylation of HCY to MET (see Figure 7.1). Both enzymes require a cobalamin cofactor; CblG and CblE are required for MS and MSR activity, respectively.[185,186]

Clinical symptoms include developmental delay, hypotonia, seizures, peripheral neuropathy, and visual abnormalities.[185-190] Megaloblastic anemia and cerebral atrophy are typically present. Biochemical indications of these disorders include low-to-normal plasma MET concentrations and elevated HCY concentrations both in plasma and urine without the presence of MMA (see Table 7.1). Patients with cblE and cblG disorders respond to intramuscular hydroxycobalamin with at least partial resolution of their clinical symptoms.[185,190] Folic acid, betaine, MET, and L-carnitine have also been used with varying success.

Other cobalamin defects, cblC, cblD, and cblF, indirectly affect MET synthase activity and are addressed in Chapter 8.

CONCLUSION

Patients with B_6-responsive CβS deficiency tend to show better clinical outcomes than those with B_6-nonresponsive CβS deficiency. However, those with either form of the disorder benefit from early diagnosis and initiation of nutrition management. Widespread institution of MS/MS screening is expected to improve overall diagnosis of nonresponsive cases; however, responsive cases will continue to be missed even with this methodology. Further research to detect and interpret mutation data may prove useful for early detection of all cases with this disorder. Patients with other disorders of the MET-HCY cycle display a wide range of clinical outcomes. Continued research to improve detection and treatment of these enzymatic defects will be necessary to fully understand the spectrum of disorders in sulfur amino acid metabolism.

REFERENCES

1. Mudd SH, Levy HL, Kraus JP. Disorders of transsulfuration. In: Valle D, Beaudet AL, Vogelstein B, eds. *The Metabolic and Molecular Bases of Inherited Disease*. New York, NY: McGraw-Hill Medical, 2007. Available at: http://www.ommbid.com/OMMBID/the_online_metabolic_and_molecular_bases_of_inherited_diseases/b/fulltext/part8/Ch88. Accessed September 1, 2008.
2. Andria G, Fowler B, Sebastio G. Disorders of sulfur amino acid metabolism. In: Fernandes J, Saudubray JM, van den Berghe G, Walter JH, eds. *Inborn Metabolic Disease: Diagnosis and Treatment*. 4th ed. Heidelberg, Germany: Springer Medizin Verlag; 2006:273–282.
3. Storch KJ, Wagner DA, Burke JF, Young VR. Quantitative study in vivo of methionine cycle in humans using (methyl-2H3) and (1-13C) methionine. *Am J Physiol*. 1988;255:E322–E331.
4. Aguilar TS, Benevenga NJ, Harper AE. Effect of dietary methionine level on its metabolism in rats. *J Nutr*. 1974;104:761–771.
5. Griffith OW. Mammalian sulfur amino acid metabolism: an overview. *Methods Enzymol*. 1987;143:366–376.
6. Di Buono M, Wykes LJ, Ball RO, Pencharz PB. Dietary cysteine reduces the methionine requirement in men. *Am J Clin Nutr*. 2001;74:761–766.
7. Baker DH. Comparative species utilization and toxicity of sulfur amino acids. *J Nutr*. 2006;136:1670S–1675S.
8. Shoveller AK, Brunton JA, Pencharz PB, Ball RO. The methionine requirement is lower in neonatal piglets fed parenterally than in those fed enterally. *J Nutr*. 2003;133:1390–1397.
9. Courtney-Martin G, Chapman KP, Moore AM, Kim JH, Ball RO, Pencharz PB. Total sulfur amino acid requirement and metabolism in parenterally fed postsurgical human neonates. *Am J Clin Nutr*. 2008;88:115–124.
10. Carson NA, Neill DW. Metabolic abnormalities detected in a survey of mentally backward individuals in Northern Ireland. *Arch Dis Child*. 1962;37:505–513.
11. Mudd SH, Finkelstein F, Irreverre F, Lester L. Homocystinuria: an enzymatic defect. *Science*. 1964;143:1443–1445.
12. Finkelstein JD, Mudd SH, Laster FIK. Homocystinuria due to cystathionine synthase deficiency: the mode of inheritance. *Science*. 1964;146:785–787.
13. National Center for Biotechnology Information. OMIM™—Online Mendelian Inheritance in Man™ (database). Available at: http://www.ncbi.nlm.nih.gov/sites/entrez?db=omim. Accessed February 2, 2008.
14. Finkelstein JD, Kyle WE, Martin JL, Pick AM. Activation of cystathionine synthase by adenosylmethionine and adenosylethionine. *Biochem Biophys Res Commun*. 1975;66:81–87.
15. Kery V, Poneleit L, Kraus JP. Trypsin cleavage of human cystathionine beta-synthase into an evolutionarily conserved active core: structural and functional consequences. *Arch Biochem Biophys*. 1998;355:222–232.

16. Kraus JP, Janosik M, Kozich V, et al. Cystathionine beta-synthase mutations in homocystinuria. *Hum Mutat*. 1999;13:362–375.
17. Miles EW, Kraus JP. Cystathionine beta-synthase: structure, function, regulation, and location of homocystinuria-causing mutations. *J Biol Chem*. 2004;279: 29871–29874.
18. Fowler B, Kraus J, Packman S, Rosenberg LE. Homocystinuria: evidence for three distinct classes of cystathionine beta-synthase mutants in cultured fibroblasts. *J Clin Invest*. 1978;61:645–653.
19. Mudd SH, Skovby F, Levy HL, et al. The natural history of homocystinuria due to cystathionine beta-synthase deficiency. *Am J Hum Genet*. 1985;37:1–31.
20. Munke M, Kraus JP, Ohura T, Francke U. The gene for cystathionine beta-synthase (CβS) maps to the subtelomeric region on human chromosome 21q and to proximal mouse chromosome 17. *Am J Hum Genet*. 1988;42:550–559.
21. Kraus JP. Biochemistry and molecular genetics of cystathionine beta-synthase deficiency. *Eur J Pediatr*. 1998;157(Suppl 2):S50–S53.
22. Kraus JP, Le K, Swaroop M, et al. Human cystathionine beta-synthase cDNA: sequence, alternative splicing and expression in cultured cells. *Hum Mol Genet*. 1993;2:1633–1638.
23. Moat SJ, Bao L, Fowler B, Bonham JR, Walter JH, Kraus JP. The molecular basis of cystathionine beta-synthase (CβS) deficiency in U.K. and U.S. patients with homocystinuria. *Hum Mutat*. 2004;23:206.
24. Shih VE, Fringer JM, Mandell R, et al. A missense mutation (I278T) in the cystathionine beta-synthase gene prevalent in pyridoxine-responsive homocystinuria and associated with mild clinical phenotype. *Am J Hum Genet*. 1995;57:34–39.
25. Kluijtmans LA, Boers GH, Kraus JP, et al. The molecular basis of cystathionine beta-synthase deficiency in Dutch patients with homocystinuria: effect of CβS genotype on biochemical and clinical phenotype and on response to treatment. *Am J Hum Genet*. 1999;65:59–67.
26 Sebastio G, Sperandeo MP, Panico M, de Franchis R, Kraus JP, Andria G. The molecular basis of homocystinuria due to cystathionine beta-synthase deficiency in Italian families, and report of four novel mutations. *Am J Hum Genet*. 1995; 56:1324–1333.
27. Gallagher PM, Ward P, Tan S, et al. High frequency (71%) of cystathionine beta-synthase mutation G307S in Irish homocystinuria patients. *Hum Mutat*. 1995;6: 177–180.
28. Gallagher PM, Naughten E, Hanson NQ, et al. Characterization of mutations in the cystathionine beta-synthase gene in Irish patients with homocystinuria. *Mol Genet Metab*. 1998;65:298–302.
29. Gaustadnes M, Wilcken B, Oliveriusova J, et al. The molecular basis of cystathionine beta-synthase deficiency in Australian patients: genotype-phenotype correlations and response to treatment. *Hum Mutat*. 2002;20:117–126.
30. Kraus JP, Oliveriusova J, Sokolova J, et al. The human cystathionine beta-synthase (CβS) gene: complete sequence, alternative splicing, and polymorphisms. *Genomics*. 1998;52:312–324.
31. Kim CE, Gallagher PM, Guttormsen AB, et al. Functional modeling of vitamin responsiveness in yeast: a common pyridoxine-responsive cystathionine beta-synthase mutation in homocystinuria. *Hum Mol Genet*. 1997;6:2213–2221.
32. Kruger WD, Wang L, Jhee KH, Singh RH, Elsas LJ. Cystathionine beta-synthase deficiency in Georgia (USA): correlation of clinical and biochemical phenotype with genotype. *Hum Mutat*. 2003;22:434–441.

33. Yap S, Naughten E. Homocystinuria due to cystathionine beta-synthase deficiency in Ireland: 25 years' experience of a newborn screened and treated population with reference to clinical outcome and biochemical control. *J Inherit Metab Dis*. 1998; 21:738–747.
34. Naughten ER, Yap S, Mayne PD. Newborn screening for homocystinuria: Irish and world experience. *Eur J Pediatr*. 1998;157(Suppl 2):S84–S87.
35. Gaustadnes M, Ingerslev J, Rutiger N. Prevalence of congenital homocystinuria in Denmark. *N Engl J Med*. 1999;340:1513.
36. Refsum H, Fredriksen A, Meyer K, Ueland PM, Kase BF. Birth prevalence of homocystinuria. *J Pediatr*. 2004;144:830–832.
37. Chace DH, Hillman SL, Millington DS, Kahler SG, Adam BW, Levy HL. Rapid diagnosis of homocystinuria and other hypermethioninemias from newborns' blood spots by tandem mass spectrometry. *Clin Chem*. 1996;42:349–355.
38. Peterschmitt MJ, Simmons JR, Levy HL. Reduction of false negative results in screening of newborns for homocystinuria. *N Engl J Med*. 1999;341:1572–1576.
39. Whiteman PD, Clayton BE, Ersser RS, Lilly P, Seakins JW. Changing incidence of neonatal hypermethioninaemia: implications for the detection of homocystinuria. *Arch Dis Child*. 1979;54:593–598.
40. Levy H, Naruse H. Early discharge from the newborn nursery: a potential threat to effective newborn screening (Editorial). *Screening*. 1994;3:45–48.
41. Yap S, Rushe H, Howard PM, Naughten ER. The intellectual abilities of early-treated individuals with pyridoxine-nonresponsive homocystinuria due to cystathionine beta-synthase deficiency. *J Inherit Metab Dis*. 2001;24:437–447.
42. Efron ML, Young D, Moser HW, MacCready RA. A simple chromatographic screening test for the detection of disorders of amino acid metabolism. *N Engl J Med*. 1964;270:1378–1383.
43. Guthrie R. Screening for "inborn errors of metabolism" in the newborn infant—a multiple test program. In: Bergsma D, ed. *Human Genetics*. 4th ed. New York, NY: National Foundation—March of Dimes; 1968:92–98.
44. Levy HL, Shih VE, Madigan PM, et al. Hypermethioninemia with other hyperaminoacidemias. Studies in infants on high-protein diets. *Am J Dis Child*. 1969; 117:96–103.
45. Snyderman SE, Sansaricq C. Newborn screening for homocystinuria. *Early Hum Dev*. 1997;48:203–207.
46. Mudd SH, Levy HL. Disorders of transsulfuration. In: Stanbury JB, Wyngaarden JB, Fredrickson DS, Goldstein JL, Brown MS, eds. *The Metabolic Basis of Inherited Disease*. 5th ed. New York, NY: McGraw-Hill; 1983:522–542.
47. Picker JD, Levy HL. Homocystinuria caused by cystathionine beta-synthase deficiency. *Gene Rev*. 2006. Available at: http://www.genetests.org. Accessed September 1, 2008.
48. Boddie AM, Steen MT, Sullivan KM, et al. Cystathionine-beta-synthase deficiency: detection of heterozygotes by the ratios of homocysteine to cysteine and folate. *Metabolism*. 1998;47:207–211.
49. Wiley VC, Dudman NP, Wilcken DE. Interrelations between plasma free and protein-bound homocysteine and cysteine in homocystinuria. *Metabolism*. 1988;37:191–195.
50. Wiley VC, Dudman NP, Wilcken DE. Free and protein-bound homocysteine and cysteine in cystathionine beta-synthase deficiency: interrelations during short- and long-term changes in plasma concentrations. *Metabolism*. 1989;38: 734–739.

51. Mansoor MA, Ueland PM, Aarsland A, Svardal AM. Redox status and protein binding of plasma homocysteine and other aminothiols in patients with homocystinuria. *Metabolism*. 1993;42:1481–1485.
52. Bonham JR, Moat SJ, Allen JC, et al. Free homocystine may be a poor measure of control in homocystinuria. *J Inherit Metab Dis*. 1997;20(Suppl 1):20.
53. Applegarth DA, Vallance HD, Seccombe D. Are patients with homocystinuria being missed? *Eur J Pediatr*. 1995;154:589.
54. Smith KL, Bradley L, Levy HL, Korson MS. Inadequate laboratory technique for amino acid analysis resulting in missed diagnoses of homocystinuria. *Clin Chem*. 1998;44:897–898.
55. McDowell I, Bradley D. Delay in diagnosis of homocystinuria: total rather than free homocysteine is better for screening. *BMJ*. 1997;314:370.
56. Fowler B, Jakobs C. Post- and prenatal diagnostic methods for the homocystinurias. *Eur J Pediatr*. 1998;157(Suppl 2):S88–S93.
57. de Franchis R, Kozich V, McInnes RR, Kraus JP. Identical genotypes in siblings with different homocystinuric phenotypes: identification of three mutations in cystathionine beta-synthase using an improved bacterial expression system. *Hum Mol Genet*. 1994;3:1103–1108.
58. Mudd SH, Levy HL, Skovby F. Disorders of transsulfuration. In: Scriver CR, Beaudet AL, Sly WS, Valle D, eds. *The Metabolic and Molecular Bases of Inherited Disease*. 6th ed. New York, NY: McGraw-Hill; 1989:693–734.
59. Wilcken DE, Wilcken B. The natural history of vascular disease in homocystinuria and the effects of treatment. *J Inherit Metab Dis*. 1997;20:295–300.
60. Perry TL. Homocystinuria. In: Nyhan WL, ed. *Heritable Disorders of Amino Acid Metabolism*. New York, NY: John Wiley & Sons; 1974:395–428.
61. Morrow G III, Barness LA. Combined vitamin responsiveness in homocystinuria. *J Pediatr*. 1972;81:946–954.
62. Wilcken B, Turner B. Homocystinuria. Reduced folate levels during pyridoxine treatment. *Arch Dis Child*. 1973;48:58–62.
63. Nugent A, Hadden DR, Carson NA. Long-term survival of homocystinuria: the first case. *Lancet*. 1998;352:624–625.
64. Schmike RN, McKusick VA, Huang T, Pollack AD. Homocystinuria: studies of 20 families with 38 affected members. *JAMA*. 1965;193:711–719.
65. Beals RK. Homocystinuria: a report of two cases and review of the literature. *J Bone Joint Surg Am*. 1969;51:1564–1572.
66. Welch JP, Clower CG, Schimke RN. The "pink spot" in schizophrenics and its absence in homocystinurics. *Br J Psychiatry*. 1969;115:163–167.
67. Abbott MH, Folstein SE, Abbey H, Pyeritz RE. Psychiatric manifestations of homocystinuria due to cystathionine beta-synthase deficiency: prevalence, natural history, and relationship to neurologic impairment and vitamin B_6-responsiveness. *Am J Med Genet*. 1987;26:959–969.
68. McIlwain H, Poll JD. Adenosine in cerebral homeostatic role: appraisal through actions of homocysteine, colchicine and dipyridamole. *J Neurobiol*. 1986;17:39–49.
69. Flott-Rahmel B, Schurmann M, Schluff P, et al. Homocysteic and homocysteine sulphinic acid exhibit excitotoxicity in organotypic cultures from rat brain. *Eur J Pediatr*. 1998;157(Suppl 2):S112–S117.
70. Schwarz S, Zhou GZ. N-methyl-D-aspartate receptors and CNS symptoms of homocystinuria. *Lancet*. 1991;337:1226–1227.

71. Santhosh-Kumar CR, Hassell KL, Deutsch JC, Kolhouse JF. Are neuropsychiatric manifestations of folate, cobalamin and pyridoxine deficiency mediated through imbalances in excitatory sulfur amino acids? *Med Hypotheses*. 1994;43:239–244.
72. Mulvihill A, Yap S, O'Keefe M, Howard PM, Naughten ER. Ocular findings among patients with late-diagnosed or poorly controlled homocystinuria compared with a screened, well-controlled population. *J AAPOS*. 2001;5:311–315.
73. Burke JP, O'Keefe M, Bowell R, Naughten ER. Ocular complications in homocystinuria—early and late treated. *Br J Ophthalmol*. 1989;73:427–431.
74. Graymore CN. *Biochemistry of the Eye*. London, England: Academic Press; 1970.
75. Cross HE, Jensen AD. Ocular manifestations in the Marfan syndrome and homocystinuria. *Am J Ophthalmol*. 1973;75:405–420.
76. Gerding H. Ocular complications and a new surgical approach to lens dislocation in homocystinuria due to cystathionine-beta-synthetase deficiency. *Eur J Pediatr*. 1998;157(Suppl 2):S94–S101.
77. Labow BI, Greene AK, Upton J. Homocystinuria: an unrecognized cause of microvascular failure. *Plast Reconstr Surg*. 2007;120:6e–12e.
78. Yap S. Classical homocystinuria: vascular risk and its prevention. *J Inherit Metab Dis*. 2003;26:259–265.
79. Celermajer DS, Sorensen K, Ryalls M, et al. Impaired endothelial function occurs in the systemic arteries of children with homozygous homocystinuria but not in their heterozygous parents. *J Am Coll Cardiol*. 1993;22:854–858.
80. Stamler JS, Osborne JA, Jaraki O, et al. Adverse vascular effects of homocysteine are modulated by endothelium-derived relaxing factor and related oxides of nitrogen. *J Clin Invest*. 1993;91:308–318.
81. Tsai JC, Wang H, Perrella MA, et al. Induction of cyclin A gene expression by homocysteine in vascular smooth muscle cells. *J Clin Invest*. 1996;97:146–153.
82. Loscalzo J. The oxidant stress of hyperhomocyst(e)inemia. *J Clin Invest*. 1996;98:5–7.
83. Hofmann MA, Lalla E, Lu Y, et al. Hyperhomocysteinemia enhances vascular inflammation and accelerates atherosclerosis in a murine model. *J Clin Invest*. 2001;107:675–683.
84. Janssen-Heininger YM, Poynter ME, Baeuerle PA. Recent advances towards understanding redox mechanisms in the activation of nuclear factor kappaB. *Free Radic Biol Med*. 2000;28:1317–1327.
85. Ling Q, Hajjar KA. Inhibition of endothelial cell thromboresistance by homocysteine. *J Nutr*. 2000;130:373S–376S.
86. Marchi R, Carvajal Z, Weisel JW. Comparison of the effect of different homocysteine concentrations on clot formation using human plasma and purified fibrinogen. *Thromb Haemost*. 2008;99:451–452.
87. Toohey JI. Homocysteine toxicity in connective tissue: theories, old and new. *Connect Tissue Res*. 2008;49:57–61.
88. Mudd SH, Levy HL, Kraus JP. Disorders of transsulfuration. In: Scriver CR, Beaudet AL, Sly WS, Valle D, eds. *The Metabolic and Molecular Bases of Inherited Disease*. 8th ed. New York, NY: McGraw-Hill; 2001:2007–2056.
89. Lubec B, Fang-Kircher S, Lubec T, Blom HJ, Boers GH. Evidence for McKusick's hypothesis of deficient collagen cross-linking in patients with homocystinuria. *Biochim Biophys Acta*. 1996;1315:159–162.
90. Komrower GM, Lambert AM, Cusworth DC, Westall RG. Dietary treatment of homocystinuria. *Arch Dis Child*. 1966;41:666–671.

91. Wilcken DE, Wilcken B, Dudman NP, Tyrrell PA. Homocystinuria—the effects of betaine in the treatment of patients not responsive to pyridoxine. *N Engl J Med.* 1983;309:448–453.
92. Barber GW, Spaeth GL. Pyridoxine therapy in homocystinuria. *Lancet.* 1967;1: 337–339.
93. Walter JH, Wraith JE, White FJ, Bridge C, Till J. Strategies for the treatment of cystathionine beta-synthase deficiency: the experience of the Willink Biochemical Genetics Unit over the past 30 years. *Eur J Pediatr.* 1998;157(Suppl 2):S71–S76.
94. Poole JR, Mudd SH, Conerly EB, Edwards WA. Homocystinuria due to cystathionine synthase deficiency: studies of nitrogen balance and sulfur excretion. *J Clin Invest.* 1975;55:1033–1048.
95. Mudd SH, Edwards WA, Loeb PM, Brown MS, Laster L. Homocystinuria due to cystathionine synthase deficiency: the effect of pyridoxine. *J Clin Invest.* 1970;49: 1762–1773.
96. Gaull GE, Rassin DK, Sturman JA. Enzymatic and metabolic studies of homocystinuria: effects of pyridoxine. *Neuropaediatriae.* 1969;1:199–226.
97. Hollowell JG Jr, Coryell ME, Hall WK, Findley JK, Thevaos TG. Homocystinuria as affected by pyridoxine, folic acid, and vitamin B_{12}. *Proc Soc Exp Biol Med.* 1968;129:327–333.
98. Bendich A, Cohen M. Vitamin B_6 safety issues. *Ann NY Acad Sci.* 1990;585: 321–330.
99. Ludolph AC, Masur H, Oberwittler C, Koch HG, Ullrich K. Sensory neuropathy and vitamin B_6 treatment in homocystinuria. *Eur J Pediatr.* 1993;152:271.
100. Mpofu C, Alani SM, Whitehouse C, Fowler B, Wraith JE. No sensory neuropathy during pyridoxine treatment in homocystinuria. *Arch Dis Child.* 1991;66: 1081–1082.
101. Institute of Medicine. *Vitamin B_6. Dietary Reference Intakes.* Washington, DC: National Academies Press; 1998:150–195.
102. Shoji Y, Takahashi T, Sato W, Shoji Y, Takada G. Acute life-threatening event with rhabdomyolysis after starting on high-dose pyridoxine therapy in an infant with homocystinuria. *J Inherit Metab Dis.* 1998;21:439–440.
103. Heeley A, Pugh RJ, Clayton BE, Shepherd J, Wilson J. Pyridoxol metabolism in vitamin B_6-responsive convulsions of early infancy. *Arch Dis Child.* 1978;53: 794–802.
104. Bankier A, Turner M, Hopkins IJ. Pyridoxine dependent seizures—a wider clinical spectrum. *Arch Dis Child.* 1983;58:415–418.
105. Kroll JS. Pyridoxine for neonatal seizures: an unexpected danger. *Dev Med Child Neurol.* 1985;27:377–379.
106. Pencharz P. The Hospital for Sick Children, University of Toronto, Toronto, Canada. Personal Communication, 2008.
107. Raguso CA, Regan MM, Young VR. Cysteine kinetics and oxidation at different intakes of methionine and cystine in young adults. *Am J Clin Nutr.* 2000;71: 491–499.
108. Di Buono M, Wykes LJ, Ball RO, Pencharz PB. Total sulfur amino acid requirement in young men as determined by indicator amino acid oxidation with L-(1-13C) phenylalanine. *Am J Clin Nutr.* 2001;74:756–760.
109. Ball RO, Courtney-Martin G, Pencharz PB. The in vivo sparing of methionine by cysteine in sulfur amino acid requirements in animal models and adult humans. *J Nutr.* 2006;136:1682S–1693S.

110. Turner JM, Humayun MA, Elango R, et al. Total sulfur amino acid requirement of healthy school-age children as determined by indicator amino acid oxidation technique. *Am J Clin Nutr.* 2006;83:619–623.
111. Humayun MA, Turner JM, Elango R, et al. Minimum methionine requirement and cysteine sparing of methionine in healthy school-age children. *Am J Clin Nutr.* 2006;84:1080–1085.
112. Acosta PB, Yannicelli S. Protocol 8. Homocystinuria. *Nutrition Support Protocols.* 4th ed. Columbus, OH: Ross Products Division, Abbott Laboratories; 2001:137–165.
113. Otten JJ, Hellwig JP, Meyers LD. *Dietary Reference Intakes: The Essential Guide to Nutrient Requirements.* Washington, DC: National Academies Press; 2006.
114. Grobe H. Homocystinuria (cystathionine synthase deficiency). Results of treatment in late-diagnosed patients. *Eur J Pediatr.* 1980;135:199–203.
115. USDA Agricultural Research Service. Nutrient Data Laboratory. Available at: http://www.nal.usda.gov/fnic/foodcomp/search/. Accessed January 5, 2008.
116. Schuett VE. *Low Protein Food List for PKU.* 2nd ed. Seattle, WA: National PKU News; 2002.
117. Greve LC, Wheeler MD, Green-Burgeson DK, Zorn EM. Breast-feeding in the management of the newborn with phenylketonuria: a practical approach to dietary therapy. *J Am Diet Assoc.* 1994;94:305–309.
118. Lee PJ, Briddon A. A rationale for cystine supplementation in severe homocystinuria. *J Inherit Metab Dis.* 2007;30:35–38.
119. Ajinomoto. *Amino Acid Handbook.* Ajinomoto, Japan: 2004.
120. Andersson HC, Shapira E. Biochemical and clinical response to hydroxocobalamin versus cyanocobalamin treatment in patients with methylmalonic acidemia and homocystinuria (cblC). *J Pediatr.* 1998;132:121–124.
121. Elsas LJ, Acosta PB. Inherited metabolic disease: amino acids, organic acids, and galactose. In: Shils ME, Shike M, Olson J, Ross AC, Caballero B, Cousins RJ, eds. *Modern Nutrition in Health and Disease.* 10th ed. Philadelphia, PA: Lippincott Williams & Wilkins; 2005:909–959.
122. Carey MC, Fennelly JJ, Fitzgerald O. Homocystinuria. II. Subnormal serum folate levels, increased folate clearance and effects of folic acid therapy. *Am J Med.* 1968;45:26–31.
123. Andres E, Loukili NH, Noel E, et al. Vitamin B_{12} (cobalamin) deficiency in elderly patients. *CMAJ.* 2004;171:251–259.
124. Andres E, Affenberger S, Vinzio S, et al. Food-cobalamin malabsorption in elderly patients: clinical manifestations and treatment. *Am J Med.* 2005;118:1154–1159.
125. Surtees R, Bowron A, Leonard J. Cerebrospinal fluid and plasma total homocysteine and related metabolites in children with cystathionine beta-synthase deficiency: the effect of treatment. *Pediatr Res.* 1997;42:577–582.
126. Kishi T, Kawamura I, Harada Y, et al. Effect of betaine on S-adenosylmethionine levels in the cerebrospinal fluid in a patient with methylenetetrahydrofolate reductase deficiency and peripheral neuropathy. *J Inherit Metab Dis.* 1994;17:560–565.
127. Singh RH, Kruger WD, Wang L, Pasquali M, Elsas LJ. Cystathionine beta-synthase deficiency: effects of betaine supplementation after methionine restriction in B_6-nonresponsive homocystinuria. *Genet Med.* 2004;6:90–95.
128. Lawson-Yuen A, Levy HL. The use of betaine in the treatment of elevated homocysteine. *Mol Genet Metab.* 2006;88:201–207.
129. Corkins MR, Shulman RJ. *Pediatric Nutrition in Your Pocket.* Silver Spring, MD: American Society of Parenteral and Enteral Nutrition; 2002:326–337.

130. Schwahn BC, Hafner D, Hohlfeld T, Balkenhol N, Laryea MD, Wendel U. Pharmacokinetics of oral betaine in healthy subjects and patients with homocystinuria. *Br J Clin Pharmacol.* 2003;55:6–13.
131. Yap S, Boers GH, Wilcken B, et al. Vascular outcome in patients with homocystinuria due to cystathionine beta-synthase deficiency treated chronically: a multicenter observational study. *Arterioscler Thromb Vasc Biol.* 2001;21:2080–2085.
132. Matthews A, Johnson TN, Rostami-Hodjegan A, et al. An indirect response model of homocysteine suppression by betaine: optimising the dosage regimen of betaine in homocystinuria. *Br J Clin Pharmacol.* 2002;54:140–146.
133. Yaghmai R, Kashani AH, Geraghty MT, et al. Progressive cerebral edema associated with high methionine levels and betaine therapy in a patient with cystathionine beta-synthase (CβS) deficiency. *Am J Med Genet.* 2002;108:57–63.
134. Devlin AM, Hajipour L, Gholkar A, Fernandes H, Ramesh V, Morris AA. Cerebral edema associated with betaine treatment in classical homocystinuria. *J Pediatr.* 2004;144:545–548.
135. Braverman NE, Mudd SH, Barker PB, Pomper MG. Characteristic MR imaging changes in severe hypermethioninemic states. *AJNR Am J Neuroradiol.* 2005;26: 2705–2706.
136. Carey MC, Donovan DE, Fitzgerald O, McAuley FD. Homocystinuria. I. A clinical and pathological study of nine subjects in six families. *Am J Med.* 1968;45:7–25.
137. Dudman NP, Wilcken DE. Increased plasma copper in patients with homocystinuria due to cystathionine beta-synthase deficiency. *Clin Chim Acta.* 1983;127: 105–113.
138. Yoshida Y, Nakano A, Hamada R, et al. Patients with homocystinuria: high metal concentrations in hair, blood and urine. *Acta Neurol Scand.* 1992;86:490–495.
139. Acosta PB. Personal communication. Atlanta, GA: Ross Products Division, Abbott Laboratories; May 2007.
140. Frost PM. Anaesthesia and homocystinuria. *Anaesthesia.* 1980;35:918–919.
141. Fuks AB, Kaufman E, Galili D, Garfunkel A. Comprehensive dental treatment under general anesthesia for patients with homocystinuria. *ASDC J Dent Child.* 1980;47:340–342.
142. Hargreaves IP, Lee PJ, Briddon A. Homocysteine and cysteine-albumin binding in homocystinuria: assessment of cysteine status and implications for glutathione synthesis? *Amino Acids.* 2002;22:109–118.
143. Levy HL, Shih VE, MacCready RA. Screening for homocystinuria in the newborn and mentally retarded population. In: Carson NAJ, Raine DN, eds. *Inherited Disorders of Sulphur Metabolism.* London, England: Churchill Livingston; 1971:235–244.
144. Gilbert-Barness E, Barness LA. *Clinical Use of Pediatric Diagnostic Tests.* Philadelphia, PA: Lippincott Williams & Wilkins; 2003.
145. Snow C. Laboratory diagnosis of vitamin B_{12} and folate deficiency. *Clin Chem.* 2000;46:1277–1283.
146. Institute of Medicine. *Folate. Dietary Reference Intakes.* Washington, DC: National Academies Press; 1998:196–305.
147. Selhub J, Morris MS, Jacques PF. In vitamin B_{12} deficiency, higher serum folate is associated with increased total homocysteine and methylmalonic acid concentrations. *Proc Natl Acad Sci USA.* 2007;104:19995–20000.
148. Institute of Medicine. *Vitamin B_{12}. Dietary Reference Intakes.* Washington, DC: National Academies Press; 1998:306–356.

149. Klee GG. Cobalamin and folate evaluation: measurement of methylmalonic acid and homocysteine vs vitamin B(12) and folate. *Clin Chem.* 2000;46:1277–1283.
150. Institute of Medicine. *Protein and Amino Acids. Dietary Reference Intakes.* Washington, DC: National Academies Press; 2005:589–768.
151. Clark SF. Iron deficiency anemia. *Nutr Clin Pract.* 2008;23:128–141.
152. Binkley TL, Berry R, Specker BL. Methods for measurement of pediatric bone. *Rev Endocr Metab Disord.* 2008;9:95–106.
153. Panis B, van Kroonenburgh MJ, Rubio-Gozalbo ME. Proposal for the prevention of osteoporosis in paediatric patients with classical galactosaemia. *J Inherit Metab Dis.* 2007;30:982.
154. Blank R. University of Wisconsin, Madison Hospital and Clinics. Personal Communication, 2008.
155. Schulman JD, Mudd SH, Shulman NR, Landvater L. Pregnancy and thrombophlebitis in homocystinuria. *Blood.* 1980;56:326.
156. Constantine G, Green A. Untreated homocystinuria: a maternal death in a woman with four pregnancies. Case report. *Br J Obstet Gynaecol.* 1987;94:803–806.
157. Calvert SM, Rand RJ. A successful pregnancy in a patient with homocystinuria and a previous near-fatal postpartum cavernous sinus thrombosis. *Br J Obstet Gynaecol.* 1995;102:751–752.
158. Luzardo GE, Karlnoski RA, Williams B, Mangar D, Camporesi EM. Anesthetic management of a parturient with hyperhomocysteinemia. *Anesth Analg.* 2008;106: 1833–1836.
159. Rajkovic A, Catalano PM, Malinow MR. Elevated homocyst(e)ine levels with preeclampsia. *Obstet Gynecol.* 1997;90:168–171.
160. Levy HL, Vargas JE, Waisbren SE, et al. Reproductive fitness in maternal homocystinuria due to cystathionine beta-synthase deficiency. *J Inherit Metab Dis.* 2002;25:299–314.
161. Chamberlin ME, Ubagai T, Mudd SH, et al. Methionine adenosyltransferase I/III deficiency: novel mutations and clinical variations. *Am J Hum Genet.* 2000;66: 347–355.
162. Chamberlin ME, Ubagai T, Mudd SH, Levy HL, Chou JY. Dominant inheritance of isolated hypermethioninemia is associated with a mutation in the human methionine adenosyltransferase 1A gene. *Am J Hum Genet.* 1997;60:540–546.
163. Kim SZ, Santamaria E, Jeong TE, et al. Methionine adenosyltransferase I/III deficiency: two Korean compound heterozygous siblings with a novel mutation. *J Inherit Metab Dis.* 2002;25:661–671.
164. Stabler SP, Steegborn C, Wahl MC, et al. Elevated plasma total homocysteine in severe methionine adenosyltransferase I/III deficiency. *Metabolism.* 2002;51: 981–988.
165. Tada H, Takanashi J, Barkovich AJ, Yamamoto S, Kohno Y. Reversible white matter lesion in methionine adenosyltransferase I/III deficiency. *AJNR Am J Neuroradiol.* 2004;25:1843–1845.
166. Gaull GE, Tallan HH, Lonsdale D, Przyrembel H, Schaffner F, von Bassewitz DB. Hypermethioninemia associated with methionine adenosyltransferase deficiency: clinical, morphologic, and biochemical observations on four patients. *J Pediatr.* 1981;98:734–741.
167. Mudd SH, Jenden DJ, Capdevila A, Roch M, Levy HL, Wagner C. Isolated hypermethioninemia: measurements of S-adenosylmethionine and choline. *Metabolism.* 2000;49:1542–1547.

168. Surtees R, Leonard J, Austin S. Association of demyelination with deficiency of cerebrospinal-fluid S-adenosylmethionine in inborn errors of methyl-transfer pathway. *Lancet*. 1991;338:1550–1554.
169. Baric I, Fumic K, Glenn B, et al. S-adenosylhomocysteine hydrolase deficiency in a human: a genetic disorder of methionine metabolism. *Proc Natl Acad Sci USA*. 2004;101:4234–4239.
170. Levy HL, Mudd SH, Uhlendorf BW, Madigan PM. Cystathioninuria and homocystinuria. *Clin Chim Acta*. 1975;58:51–59.
171. Scott CR, Dassell SW, Clark SH, Chiang-Teng C, Swedberg KR. Cystathioninemia: a benign genetic condition. *J Pediatr*. 1970;76:571–577.
172. Berlow S. Studies in cystathioninemia. *Am J Dis Child*. 1966;112:135–142.
173. Mudd SH, Cerone R, Schiaffino MC, et al. Glycine N-methyltransferase deficiency: a novel inborn error causing persistent isolated hypermethioninaemia. *J Inherit Metab Dis*. 2001;24:448–464.
174. Ogier de Baulny H, Gerard M, Saudubray JM, Zittoun J. Remethylation defects: guidelines for clinical diagnosis and treatment. *Eur J Pediatr*. 1998;157(Suppl 2): S77–S83.
175. Fowler B. Genetic defects of folate and cobalamin metabolism. *Eur J Pediatr*. 1998;157(Suppl 2):S60–S66.
176. Sewell AC, Neurich U, Fowler B. Early infantile methylenetetrahydrofolate reductase deficiency: a rare cause of progressive brain atrophy. *J Inherit Metab Dis*. 1998;21:22.
177. Arn PH, Williams CA, Zori RT, Driscoll DJ, Rosenblatt DS. Methylenetetrahydrofolate reductase deficiency in a patient with phenotypic findings of Angelman syndrome. *Am J Med Genet*. 1998;77:198–200.
178. Strauss KA, Morton DH, Puffenberger EG, et al. Prevention of brain disease from severe 5,10-methylenetetrahydrofolate reductase deficiency. *Mol Genet Metab*. 2007;91:165–175.
179. Visy JM, Le Coz P, Chadefaux B, et al. Homocystinuria due to 5,10-methylenetetrahydrofolate reductase deficiency revealed by stroke in adult siblings. *Neurology*. 1991;41:1313–1315.
180. Wendel U, Bremer HJ. Betaine in the treatment of homocystinuria due to 5,10-methylenetetrahydrofolate reductase deficiency. *Eur J Pediatr*. 1984;142: 147–150.
181. Holme E, Kjellman B, Ronge E. Betaine for treatment of homocystinuria caused by methylenetetrahydrofolate reductase deficiency. *Arch Dis Child*. 1989;64: 1061–1064.
182. Ronge E, Kjellman B. Long-term treatment with betaine in methylenetetrahydrofolate reductase deficiency. *Arch Dis Child*. 1996;74:239–241.
183. Abeling NG, van Gennip AH, Blom H, et al. Rapid diagnosis and methionine administration: basis for a favourable outcome in a patient with methylene tetrahydrofolate reductase deficiency. *J Inherit Metab Dis*. 1999;22:240–242.
184. Selzer RR, Rosenblatt DS, Laxova R, Hogan K. Adverse effect of nitrous oxide in a child with 5,10-methylenetetrahydrofolate reductase deficiency. *N Engl J Med*. 2003;349:45–50.
185. Skovby F. Disorders of sulfur amino acids. In: Blau N, Duran M, Blaskovics ME, Gibson KM, eds. *Physician's Guide to the Laboratory Diagnosis of Metabolic Diseases*. 2nd ed. Berlin, Germany: Springer-Verlag; 2002:243–260.

186. Rosenblatt DS, Fenton W. Inherited disorders of folate and cobalamin transport and metabolism. In: Valle D, Beaudet AL, Vogelstein B, eds. *The Metabolic and Molecular Bases of Inherited Disease*. New York, NY: McGraw-Hill Medical; 2007. Available at: http://www.ommbid.com/OMMBID/the_online_metabolic_and_molecular_bases_of_inherited_disease/b/abstract/part17/ch155. Accessed September 15, 2008.
187. Rosenblatt DS, Thomas IT, Watkins D, Cooper BA, Erbe RW. Vitamin B_{12} responsive homocystinuria and megaloblastic anemia: heterogeneity in methylcobalamin deficiency. *Am J Med Genet*. 1987;26:377–383.
188. Harding CO, Arnold G, Barness LA, Wolff JA, Rosenblatt DS. Functional methionine synthase deficiency due to cblG disorder: a report of two patients and a review. *Am J Med Genet*. 1997;71:384–390.
189. Hall CA. Function of vitamin B_{12} in the central nervous system as revealed by congenital defects. *Am J Hematol*. 1990;34:121–127.
190. Shevell MI, Rosenblatt DS. The neurology of cobalamin. *Can J Neurol Sci*. 1992;19:472–486.

Chapter 8

Nutrition Management of Patients with Inherited Disorders of Organic Acid Metabolism

Steven Yannicelli

Propionic Acidemia and Methylmalonic Acidemia

Introduction

Inherited metabolic disorders of propionic acid (PROP; OMIM 606054)[1] and methylmalonic acid (MMA; OMIM 25100)[1] affect approximately 1 in 20,000 to 50,000 infants worldwide but vary dramatically by region.[2,3] Both disorders represent a defect in the body's ability to effectively metabolize isoleucine (ILE), methionine (MET), threonine (THR), valine (VAL), and odd-chain fatty acids (see Figure 8.1). Patients with cobalamin disorders (Cbl-A, OMIM 251100; Cbl-B, OMIM 251110; Cbl-C, OMIM 277400; Cbl-D, OMIM 277410; Cbl-F, OMIM 277380)[1] are subgroups of methylmalonic aciduria due to impaired synthesis of adenosylcobalamin, a coenzyme necessary for the function of methymalonyl-CoA mutase.

The enzymatic defects in the intermediary metabolism of propionyl-CoA result in accumulation of toxic organic compounds. Clinical features include a fulminate neonatal course in severe genotypes, with overwhelming metabolic ketoacidosis, vomiting, lethargy, and coma. PROP and MMA are classified as "intoxication-type" inborn errors of metabolism due to their neonatal presentation; symptoms include metabolic encephalopathy[4,5] and biochemical profile.[6] If untreated, patients will die of multisystem organ failure. Untreated survivors have mental retardation and physical disabilities, including extra-pyramidal movement disorders.

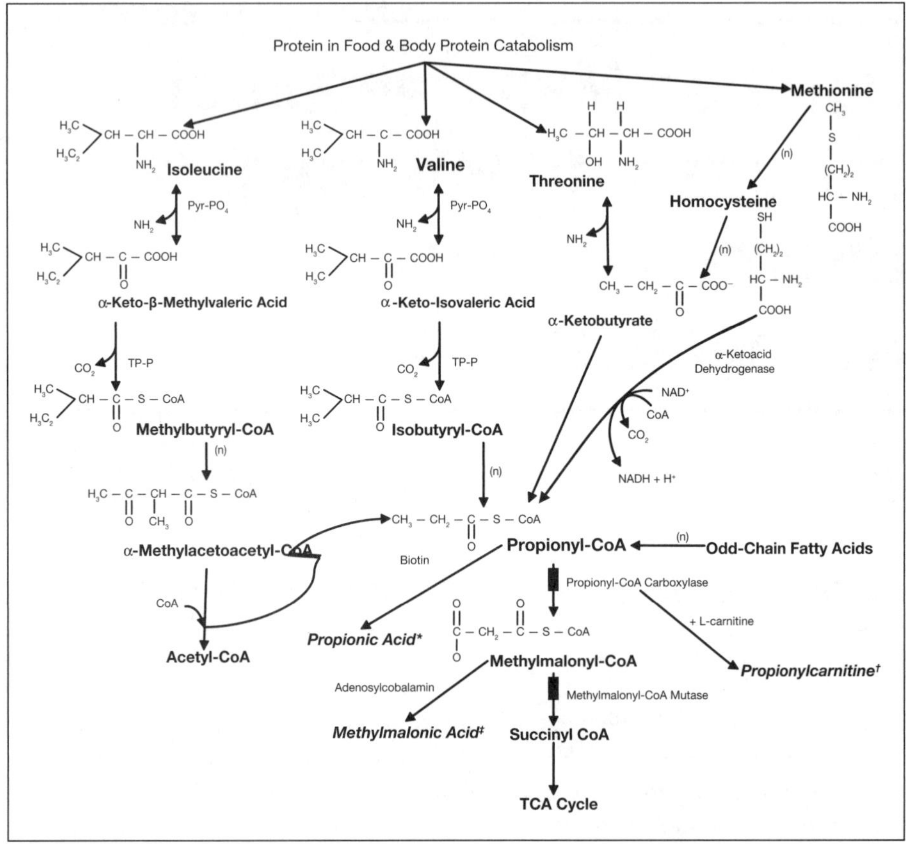

Figure 8.1 *Metabolic Pathways for Isoleucine, Valine, Threonine, Methionine, and Odd-Chain Fatty Acids*

Source: Modified by permission of Elsas LJ, Acosta PB. Inherited metabolic disease: amino acids, organic acids, and galactose. In: Shils ME, Shike M, Olson J, Ross AC, Caballero B, Cousins RJ, eds. *Modern Nutrition in Health and Disease*. 10th ed. Philadelphia, PA: Lippincott Williams & Wilkins; 2005:909–959. Courtesy of Wolters Kluwer Health.

Note: Black bars indicate sites of enzyme defects.

(n) = several steps.

*Accumulates in untreated PROP or MMA.

†Propionylcarnitine found in blood and urine.

‡Accumulates in patients with untreated MMA.

Biochemistry

Through different pathways, and a series of enzymatic steps, the amino acids ILE, MET, THR, and VAL are metabolized to propionyl-CoA and methylmalonyl-CoA for entry into the Krebs cycle via succinyl-CoA (see

Figure 8.1). Odd-chained fatty acids, either via β-oxidation or exogenous sources, are oxidized to propionyl-CoA. Propionyl-CoA is ordinarily carboxylated to D-methylmalonyl-CoA via propionyl-CoA carboxylase (PCC; EC 6.4.1.3), a biotin-dependent enzyme (see Figure 8.1). D-methylmalonyl-CoA is then epimerized to L-methylmalonyl-CoA, which is converted to succinyl-CoA by methylmalonyl-CoA mutase (MCM; EC 5.4.99.2), a cobalamin-dependent cytosolic enzyme. Stable isotope studies in patients with PROP or MMA show that approximately 50% of propionate arises from amino acid catabolism, 25% from gut bacteria, and 25% from odd-chain fatty acid oxidation.[7,8]

PROP results from a defect in mitochondrial PCC required for conversion of propionyl-CoA to L-methylmalonyl-CoA (see Figure 8.1). PCC is composed of α subunits (PCCA), which function to bind biotin, and β subunits (PCCB).[9] There is little evidence that a biotin-responsive form, which would influence the phenotype of the disease, exists. However, one patient with PROP was reported to have demonstrated increased $^{13\text{-}}CO_2$ production (in vitro) during biotin treatment.[10]

MMA is due either to a defect in the mutant MCM apoenzyme or impaired synthesis of adenosylcobalamin, the coenzyme for MCM. A defect in conversion of methylmalonyl-CoA to succinyl-CoA results in accumulation of plasma and urine methylmalonic acid, methylcitric acid, and 3-hydroxypropionic acid with urinary excretion of these acids. Several autosomal recessive mutations within genes for the mutase and for cobalamin coenzymes have been identified.[11] Defects in the gene for the mutase are most common.

Molecular Biology

PROP and MMA result from single gene defects in the propionate pathway, and both disorders are inherited by an autosomal recessive mode. A wide spectrum of clinical expression exists in patients with PROP or MMA, as with other inherited metabolic disorders (IMDs), due in part to gene polymorphisms. For this reason, a direct relationship between genotype and phenotype and phenotype with metabolite is not absolute. Alpha and beta subunits of PCC are encoded in the PCCA and PCCB genes, respectively. Nearly 100 identified mutations are present in the PCCA and PCCB genes.[12]

Mutations in MMA are categorized as either Mut^0, a nonfunctional mutase, or Mut^-, a structurally altered mutase with small affinity for the adenosylcobalamin coenzyme. Over 170 mutations have been reported,[13,14] and the majority of mutations in the MCM gene are either missense or nonsense[14,15] (see Chapter 1). Multiple variations in mutations occur at the MCM locus.[11] Genotype/phenotype correlations are difficult to determine because of the many allelic interactions in the MCM gene.[16]

Newborn Screening

Early screening, diagnosis, and nutrition management provide promise to reduce morbidity and mortality. Screening for these disorders is either required by law or universally offered in the majority of states.[17] See Chapter 2 for a review of newborn screening for IMDs by tandem mass spectrometry (MS/MS). Screening for PROP and MMA are by evaluation of C3-acylcarnitine in collected blood spots using MS/MS technology.

Diagnosis

Follow-up diagnostic studies are required to confirm whether the patient has PROP or MMA, and consist of plasma, urine organic acids, and plasma amino acids, including homocysteine. Enzyme activity may be quantitated using skin fibroblasts. A mutation can occur in either the PCCA or PCCB gene and mutated genes may be determined by complementation studies in fibroblast cell lines.[12] Algorithms are available to assist in screening and diagnosis of organic acidemias.[18]

Patients with PROP or MMA present in the neonatal period with clinical symptoms of vomiting, lethargy, failure to thrive, and coma if not diagnosed and treated within the first week of life. Clinical presentation is heterogeneous and symptoms vary among patients partly due to severity of the defective enzyme. Plasma amino acid analysis shows significantly elevated glycine (GLY) concentration and possibly ILE, MET, and THR, and to a lesser extent, VAL. In patients with cobalamin defects, elevated concentrations of plasma and urine homocystine (homocystinuria) are found. Hypoglycemia, hyperammonemia, and a high anion gap, indicative of significant metabolic acidosis, are routinely found. Hyperammonemia can contribute to clinical symptoms[19,20] and is triggered by catabolism with associated elevations in plasma propionic acid metabolites.[21] Ketotic hyperglycinemia is the pathognomonic finding in patients with PROP or MMA. Neutropenia and thrombocytopenia may also be present in patients with severe genotypes.[22-24]

Urine contains large amounts of acylcarnitine esters (propionyl-carnitine) and organic acid esters of propionate or methylmalonate, which vary dependent on severity of genotype. Patients with MMA may have urine methylmalonic acid concentrations as low as 10 mmol/mol creatinine in mild variants to greater than 20,000 mmol/mol creatinine in severe genotypes.[25] A comprehensive review of 30 patients with propionic acidemia indicated that the most specific diagnostic metabolites were methylcitric-, 3-hydroxypropionic-, and 2-methyl-3-oxovaleric acids.[26] These authors also reported increased plasma and urine lysine concentrations. Prenatal diagnosis using stable isotope dilution gas chromatography/mass spectroscopy quantitation of amniotic methylcitrate concentrations has been reported.[27]

Patients with mild genotypes may present later in infancy or even early childhood. Nutrition history in these late-onset patients often shows an infant who was breast fed with an accompanying failure to thrive. In these patients, naturally low-protein content of human milk as compared to proprietary infant formula (see Appendix B) may prevent early clinical presentation. Frequently, either consumption of excess intact protein or onset of an infectious illness will result in an acute presentation requiring immediate medical intervention.

Pseudo-MMA secondary to vitamin B_{12} deficiency has been reported in infants who were human milk fed by vegan, B_{12}-deficient mothers.[28,29] In both reports, symptoms resolved with pharmacologic doses of cobalamin. Some newborns with vitamin B_{12} deficiency are now identified by newborn screening.[30]

Outcomes if Untreated

Untreated patients with severe, early-onset PROP or MMA often expire of overwhelming multi-organ system failure. The toxic effects of accumulated organic acids are devastating to organs and especially the brain, resulting in both severe debilitation and death. Patients with mild phenotypes, who present in late infancy or early toddler years, often suffer growth and development delays[31] or may expire secondary to acute infection.

Nutrition Management

The goal of nutrition management of PROP or MMA is to reduce toxic tissue concentrations of organic compounds while aggressively supporting anabolism, normal growth, and nutrition status. Goals of nutrition management are to

1. Provide all essential nutrients to promote normal physical and mental development.
2. Maintain adequate intakes of restricted ILE, MET, THR, VAL, and other essential nutrients to support anabolism and prevent deficiencies.
3. Supplement L-carnitine to help promote excretion of toxic acyl compounds and to prevent secondary deficiency.
4. Provide pharmacologic amounts of coenzyme (vitamin B_{12} in some forms of MMA; biotin in PROP) to enhance any residual enzyme activity.
5. Limit fasting and maintain adequate hydration.
6. Provide aggressive medical and nutrition intervention during critical illness.
7. Manage acid:base status to help avoid acidosis.

Table 8.1 *Components of Nutrition Management for Patients with PROP or MMA*

Nutrients	*Source*
ILE, MET, THR, VAL	Proprietary infant formula, expressed human milk, cow's milk, beikost, table foods
Other essential and nonessential amino acids (protein equivalent); majority of macro- and micronutrients	Medical foods
Energy	Nonprotein energy sources: carbohydrate modules, carbohydrate–fat modules, fats/oils, sugar, very-low-protein foods (see Appendix E)
Fluid	Water, energy-supplemented beverages
L-carnitine (100 to 300 mg/kg/day)	Oral L-carnitine (pharmaceutical grade); intravenous L-carnitine during acute illness
Biotin (coenzyme for patients with PROP only; 5 to 10 mg/day)	Oral biotin (pharmaceutical grade)
Cobalamin (B_{12}) for patients with cobalamin defects (MMA subgroup; 1 to 2 mg/day)	Hydroxycobalamin (IV, oral)

Table 8.1 provides a list of components for nutrition management of patients with PROP or MMA.

Nutrient Requirements

Isoleucine, Methionine, Threonine, Valine

Firm requirements for ILE, MET, THR, and VAL have not been established for patients with PROP or MMA although some recommendations have been previously published.[32-34] Polymorphisms in the defective genes in PROP and MMA may influence tolerance to ILE, MET, THR, and VAL. Adequacy of these restricted essential amino acids can be estimated based on the patient's plasma concentrations of amino acids, protein status indices, and growth. Queen et al.[35] reported sufficient growth in one 3-year-old patient with PROP consuming intakes of the following (mg/kg body weight): ILE 46, MET 28, THR 41, and VAL 56). Yannicelli et al.[36] reported similar amino acid intakes by patients, most of whom were infants, with the exception of ILE, which was greater than that reported by Queen et al.[35] Table 8.2 gives recommended ILE, MET, THR, and VAL intakes for age and weight in infancy and per day after infancy.

Table 8.2 ***Recommended Daily Nutrient Intakes for Patients with PROP or MMA***

	Nutrients					
Age	***ILE***	***MET***	***THR***	***VAL***	***Protein****	***Energy***
Infants, mo	(mg/kg)	(mg/kg)	(mg/kg)	(mg/kg)	(g/kg)	(kcal/kg)
0.0 < 0.5	110–60	50–20	125–50	105–60	2.75–3.50	125–145
0.5 < 1.0	90–40	40–15	75–20	80–40	2.50–3.25	115–140
Children, yr	(mg/day)	(mg/day)	(mg/day)	(mg/day)	(g/kg)	(kcal/day)
1 < 4	485–735	275–390	415–600	550–830	1.80–2.60	900–1800
4 < 7	630–960	360–510	540–780	720–1080	1.60–2.00	1300–2300
7 < 11	715–1090	410–580	610–885	815–1225	1.55–1.85	1600–2800
Female, yr						
11 < 15	965–1470	390–780	830–1195	1105–1655	1.50–1.80	1500–2800
15 < 19	965–1470	275–780	830–1195	1105–1655	1.45–1.75	1200–2800
> 19	925–1410	265–750	790–1145	790–1585	1.45–1.75	1400–2400
Male, yr						
11 < 15	540–765	290–765	810–1170	1080–1515	1.45–1.75	2000–3200
15 < 19	670–950	475–950	1010–1455	1345–2015	1.45–1.75	2100–3200
> 19	1175–1190	475–950	1010–1455	1345–2015	1.45–1.75	2000–3000

Sources:

Acosta PB, Yannicelli S. Protocol 13. Propionic or methylmalonic acidemia. *Nutrition Support Protocols*. 4th ed. Columbus, OH: Ross Products Division, Abbott Laboratories; 2001.

Acosta PB. Nutrition support of inborn errors of metabolism. In: Queen Samour P, Helm KK, Lang CE, eds. *Handbook of Pediatric Nutrition*. 2nd ed. Rockville, MD: Aspen; 1999:243–292.

Elsas LJ, Acosta PB. Inherited metabolic disease: amino acids, organic acids, and galactose. In: Shils ME, Shike M, Olson J, Ross AC, Caballero B, Cousins RJ, eds. *Modern Nutrition in Health and Disease*. 10th ed. Philadelphia, PA: Lippincott Williams & Wilkins; 2005:909–959.

FAO/WHO/UNU. *Expert Consultation on Energy and Protein Requirements*. WHO technical report series; No. 724. Geneva, Switzerland: World Health Organization; 1985:71–112.

North KN, Korson MS, Gopal YR, et al. Neonatal-onset propionic acidemia: neurologic and developmental profiles, and implications for management. *J Pediatr*. 1995;126:916–922.

Ogier de Baulny H, Saudubray JM. Branched-chain organic aciduria. In: Fernandes J, Saudubray JM, van den Berghe G, eds. *Inborn Metabolic Diseases. Diagnosis and Treatment*. 3rd ed. Berlin, Germany: Springer-Verlag; 2000:197–212.

Otten JJ, Hellwig JP, Meyers LD. *Dietary Reference Intakes: The Essential Guide to Nutrient Requirements*. Washington, DC: National Academies Press; 2006:197–201.

Queen PM, Fernhoff PM, Acosta PB. Protein and essential amino acid requirements in a child with propionic acidemia. *J Am Diet Assoc*. 1981;79:562–565.

Touati G, Valayannopoulos V, Mention K, et al. Methylmalonic and propionic acidurias: management without or with a few supplements of specific amino acid mixture. *J Inherit Metab Dis*. 2006;29:288–298.

FAO/WHO/UNU. *Expert Consultation on Protein and Amino Acid Requirements in Human Nutrition*. WHO technical report series; No 935. Geneva, Switzerland: World Health Organization; 2002.

Yannicelli S, Acosta PB, Velazquez A, et al. Improved growth and nutrition status in children with methylmalonic or propionic acidemia fed an elemental medical food. *Mol Genet Metab*. 2003;80:181–188.

Note: Actual requirements may differ and must be based on patient's phenotype, biochemistries, protein status, and growth. For patients with failure to thrive, calculate protein and energy on "ideal" weight for age.
*Protein may differ if hyperammonemia is present or renal function is impaired. If the patient fails to grow linearly normally, see recommended intakes in Chapter 3, Table 3.1.

Providing adequate intakes of ILE, MET, THR, and VAL is important to support plasma and tissue concentrations required for protein synthesis and prevent deficiency. Patients may present with low plasma concentrations of ILE and VAL,[36-38] often requiring long-term supplementation (100 mg/day).[37] The reason for suboptimal plasma and tissue concentrations is not well known, and oftentimes significant amounts of L-ILE supplementation (10 mg L-ILE/mL solution) are required to normalize plasma concentrations. Despite intakes that would appear adequate for normal children, a large number of patients may still not reach minimum plasma reference ILE concentrations.[36] Over-restriction of ILE can cause classic deficiency signs and symptoms in patients with PROP or MMA (see Figure 8.2).[39,40]

When filling the prescription for patients with PROP or MMA, approximately one-half of the total prescribed protein may be derived from intact protein if the amount of ILE, MET, THR, and VAL supplied is not excessive. The remainder will be obtained from medical foods. Adequate intact protein must be prescribed to help support growth and prevent deficiencies in the essential restricted amino acids.

Avoid dietary sources of odd-chain fatty acids in nutrition management of patients with PROP or MMA. Fat from ruminants such as milk fat, butter,

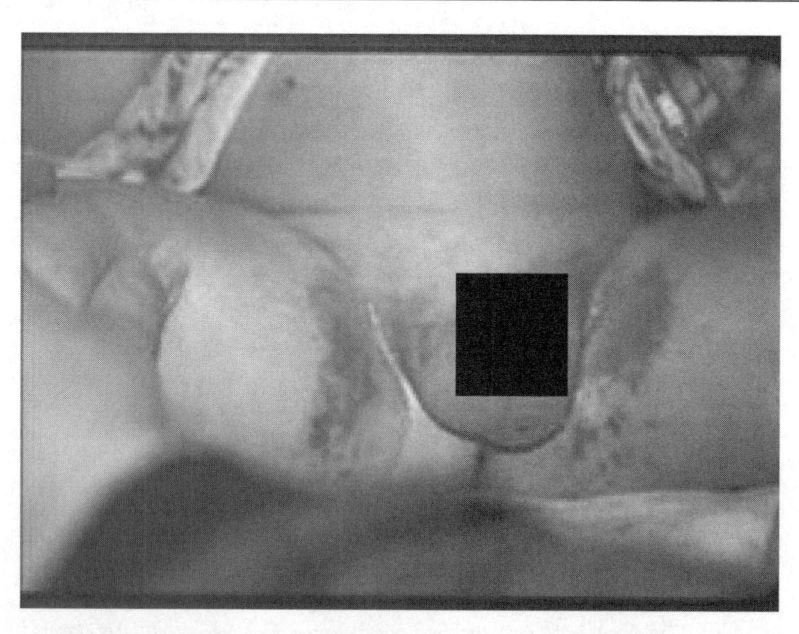

Figure 8.2 *Clinical Sign of Isoleucine deficiency*

Courtesy of Dr. Rani Singh, Emory University, Atlanta, Georgia. September 24, 2008.

cream,[41] and lard as well as from some marine oils[42] contribute odd-chain fatty acids to the diet. Catabolism is a major source of endogenous odd-chain fatty acids and should be avoided. Propionic acid is often added to foods to retard spoilage.

Protein

Total protein recommendation is higher than the dietary reference intakes (DRIs)[43] when the majority of protein is supplied by free amino acids[36] (see Table 8.2 and Chapter 3, Table 3.1). Adequate protein intake is essential to prevent protein insufficiency and support linear growth in patients with inherited metabolic disorders.[44] However, patients with MMA and renal disease may require lower total protein than normal persons to help preserve renal function.[45] Hypoproteinemia can occur with protein over-restriction[37,46] while sufficient total protein from intact protein and medical foods can normalize protein status indices.[36-38] Titrating restricted amino acid intakes to maintain targeted plasma concentrations and careful monitoring can lead to normal protein status indices.[36,38]

Nutrition management of PROP or MMA requires use of free amino acid-based medical foods. Medical foods may contribute up to half of daily total protein prescription, depending, in part, on genotype, disease severity, and tolerance to restricted amino acids.

Fat and Essential Fatty Acids

Essential fatty acid deficiency has been described in patients with organic acidemias.[47] Vlaardingerbroek et al.[48] reported lower plasma erythrocyte concentrations of docosahexaenoic acid (DHA; 22:6 n-3) but not arachidonic acid (ARA; 20:4 n-6) in patients with inborn errors of amino acid metabolism compared with healthy controls. Overall essential fatty acid status between patients with an IMD and the control group did not differ significantly. In the patients with organic acidemias, the major source of fatty acids was from either low-protein food products or special low-protein preparations (approximately 20% contribution). Essential fatty acid should be monitored in these patients.

DHA administration (25 mg/kg/day) to children with MMA (Mut^0) decreased plasma triacylglycerol concentrations that may be elevated.[49] Plasma DHA concentrations also increased significantly ($p=0.005$) after administration of supplemental DHA. Plasma DHA and ARA concentrations did not differ between controls and treated patients with MMA at baseline. See Chapter 3, Table 3.1, for recommended intakes of fat and essential fatty acids.

Energy and Fluid

Energy requirement and resting energy expenditure have been reported lower than predicted for age and gender during the well-state in patients.[50,51]

Lower than normal energy expenditure by patients with PROP or MMA may be due to decreased lean body mass,[50,52] mental retardation, decreased physical activity, or decreased protein intake. In the study by Feillet et al.,[50] however, resting energy expenditure was not related to protein intake. Yannicelli et al.[36] reported increased mean weight centiles in infants and toddlers with PROP or MMA despite energy intakes lower than recommended for age.

To support sufficient growth, energy intakes at or greater than 100% of recommended intakes for age are required, especially by infants and young children, when metabolic crises are a common problem. Importantly, during illness, resting energy expenditure increases,[53] necessitating excess energy intake to prevent catabolism and decompensation. See Table 8.1 for recommended energy intakes for age, but if weight gain is inadequate, see Chapter 3, Table 3.1.

Fasting, as previously noted, must be avoided in patients with PROP or MMA because it leads to increased production of odd-chain fatty acids, causing increased plasma and urine concentrations of toxic metabolites.[54] Endogenous odd-chain fatty acid oxidation also contributes to propionate production in patients with PROP or MMA.[7]

Maintaining adequate hydration is essential in patients with PROP or MMA to prevent dehydration and promote excretion of offending metabolites. Some patients may have a low renal concentrating capacity and not tolerate hyperosmolar feeds. Consequently, care must be taken to avoid hyperosmotic medical food mixtures and to provide sufficient free water. A minimum of 1.5 mL/kcal for infants and 1.0 mL/kcal for children and adults is recommended.[55] Recommended osmolality of medical food mixtures for infants is <450 mOsm/L; for children, <750 mOsm/L; and adults, <1000 mOsm/L. Additional water is required during intermittent febrile illnesses and with increased stool loss.

Minerals and Vitamins

Trace element deficiency has been reported in patients with PROP or MMA.[56] To avoid deficiencies in patients dependent on elemental diets, mineral and vitamin intakes are recommended at greater than 100% of DRIs for age (see Chapter 3, Table 3.1). For this reason, frequent monitoring of nutrient intake from all sources is essential. Ensuring diet adherence is important in maintaining adequate mineral and vitamin intakes because some patients may not consume all the prescribed medical food mixture, the major source of nutrients.

Matern et al.[57] reported two cases of thiamine deficiency in patients with propionic acidemia. In both patients, initial clinical presentation with severe lactic acidosis worsened because of thiamine deficiency. One patient was on parenteral nutrition without added vitamins and minerals. This patient responded within 5 hours to 11 mg/kg body weight of intravenous thiamine by reduction in metabolic acidosis. Thiamine is an essential coenzyme in pyruvate dehydrogenase, the rate-limiting enzyme in entry of pyruvate into the Krebs cycle. Inhibition of pyruvate dehydrogenase can result in shunting pyruvate to lactic acid. Children with either PROP or MMA who require parenteral nutrition should receive adequate amounts of vitamins and minerals to prevent deficiency.

Lactic acidosis, along with multi-organ failure, has been reported in a 7-year-old patient with Mut$^-$ MMA secondary to glutathione deficiency.[58] This child responded to high dose vitamin C (ascorbic acid) at 2 g per day (120 mg/kg) for 2 weeks. Ascorbate, glutathione, and vitamin E are important intracellular antioxidants. Treacy and others[58] reported low plasma amino acid concentrations despite this patient receiving 1.3 g protein/kg/day.

Patients with organic acidemias are at risk for fractures from osteopenia and osteoporosis.[37,59] Reasons for the increased risk include protein insufficiency[60] and chronic metabolic acidosis,[61] as well as insufficient mineral and vitamin intakes (calcium and vitamin D) and reduced weight-bearing physical activity.[62] In one patient, intervention with G-tube feedings resulted in improved bone status.[37]

Other Therapies

Secondary carnitine deficiency is common in patients with organic acidemias.[63,64] Carnitine conjugates with toxic acyl-CoA compounds of each disorder and is excreted in the urine. L-carnitine supplementation is essential in the majority of patients with organic acidemias to replenish depleted tissue stores and to enhance detoxification. Additional L-carnitine above that in medical foods may be required. Administration greater than 300 mg/kg/day can cause a fishy odor due to overproduction of methylamines.[65]

A trial of oral biotin (10 to 20 mg/day) is recommended for patients with PROP.[66,67] Patients with cobalamin-responsive MMA require intramuscular injections of vitamin B_{12} (1 to 2 mg/day), as hydroxycobalamin, which is the primary therapy in patients with cobalamin defects and required to reduce plasma methylmalonic acid, homocysteine, and homocystine.[25]

Metronidazole (Flagyl®; Pfizer Inc., New York City, New York) has been used to reduce gut bacteria that synthesize propionate in patients with excessive plasma propionic acid concentrations.[68,69] Gut propionate may be a significant source of plasma propionate and should be controlled to reduce absorption. Metronidazole is not benign and may induce diarrhea, sometimes severe, and use must be carefully monitored. Some clinicians have recommended 20 mg/kg/day for intermittent treatment.[70]

Soluble fiber supplementation may be effective in relieving constipation in patients with PROP or MMA (E. Jurecki, personal communication, June 12, 2008). Relief of constipation is important in helping reduce accumulated gut propionate. When prescribing fiber, sufficient fluid should be given to promote gut motility. If constipation is severe, laxatives may be given to stimulate bowel movement.

Bicitra® (sodium citrate; Ortho-McNeil Pharmaceutical, Inc., Raritan, New Jersey) is often prescribed as a urine alkalizing agent in patients with PROP or MMA. Dosage is based on medical condition and response to therapy. A liquid preparation can be made and given by G-tube.

Patients with a cobalamin C defect will require betaine (Cystadane®, betaine anhydrous; Accredo Health Group, Inc., Memphis, Tennessee), and other methyl group donors involved with enhancing remethylation of homocysteine to methionine (see Chapter 7, Figure 7.1). Betaine administration of 100 to 200 mg/kg/day and a minimum of 400 μg of folic acid are used.[71]

Medical Foods

Intact protein alone will provide insufficient nitrogen, essential amino acids, and energy for growth. Using DRIs[72] or FAO/WHO/UNU[73,74] to establish a safe protein intake is not ideal because neither is indicated for patients with chronic diseases. In patients with PROP or MMA, intermittent infections with concomitant catabolism result in constant stress necessitating increased protein intake. These factors plus genetic and environmental factors all influence protein requirements.[75] Food sources (fruits, grains, and vegetables) in the diets of patients with PROP or MMA contain proteins of poor biologic value and may be difficult to digest. For these reasons, medical foods are indicated in the diet prescription of patients with severe PROP or MMA (see Table 8.3).

Patients with less severe phenotypes of these disorders, including patients with cobalamin-responsive disorders, may tolerate a somewhat higher intact protein intake without use of medical foods than those with severe genotypes. For early-treated patients with cobalamin-responsive disorders, introducing a medical food to acquire its taste may help with compliance later in life if a stricter diet is required for management.

Use of medical foods in treatment of PROP or MMA is not universally recognized.[38,76] Although there is agreement that medical foods provide essential micro- and macronutrients, some clinicians argue that intact protein intake alone may be adequate if provided at safe levels.[73,74] An informal survey among clinicians from 15 metabolic centers in 26 European countries showed lack of consensus.[76] The issue is that although medical foods provide a good source of nitrogen and other nutrients and support growth,[36,77] there

Table 8.3 ***Formulation, Nutrient Composition, and Sources of Medical Foods for Patients with Propionic Acidemia or Methylmalonic Acidemia (per 100 g powder)***

Medical Foods	Modified Nutrient(s) (mg/100 g)	Protein Equiv[a] (g/100 g, source)	Fat (g/100 g, source)	Carbohydrate (g/100 g, source)	Energy (kcal/100 g/kJ/100 g)	Linoleic Acid/ α-Linolenic Acid (mg/100 g)
			Abbott Nutrition[b]			
Propimex®-1	MET 0, VAL 0 ILE 120, THR 100 L-carnitine 900 Taurine 40	15 Amino acids[c]	21.7 High oleic safflower, coconut, soy oils	53.0 Corn syrup solids	480/2006	3500/350
Propimex®-2	MET 0, VAL 0 ILE 240, THR 200 L-carnitine 1800 Taurine 50	30 Amino acids[c]	14.0 High oleic safflower, coconut, soy oils	35.0 Corn syrup solids	410/1714	2200/225
			Mead Johnson Nutritionals[d]			
OA1®	MET 0, VAL 0 ILE 0, THR 0 L-carnitine 0 Taurine 0	15.7 Amino acids[c]	26.0 Palm olein, soy, coconut, high oleic safflower oils	51.0 Corn syrup solids, sugar, modified cornstarch, maltodextrin	500/2090	4500/380
OA2®	MET 0, VAL 0 ILE 0, THR 0 L-carnitine ND Taurine ND	21.0 Amino acids[c]	9.0 Soy oil	59.0 Corn syrup solids, sugar, modified cornstarch, maltodextrin	410/1714	4600/608

(continues)

Table 8.3 ***Formulation, Nutrient Composition, and Sources of Medical Foods for Patients with Propionic Acidemia or Methylmalonic Acidemia (per 100 g powder)***, *Continued*

Medical Foods	**Modified Nutrient(s) (mg/100 g)**	**Protein Equiv[a] (g/100 g, source)**	**Fat (g/100 g, source)**	**Carbohydrate (g/100 g, source)**	**Energy (kcal/100 g/kJ/100 g)**	**Linoleic Acid/ α-Linolenic Acid (mg/100 g)**
			Nutricia North America			
XMTVI Analog®	MET 0, VAL 0 ILE trace, THR 0 L-carnitine 10 Taurine 20	13.0 Amino acids[c]	20.9 High oleic safflower, coconut, soy oils	59.0 Corn syrup solids, galactose	475/1985	3025/ND
XMTVI Maxamaid®	MET 0, VAL 0 ILE trace, THR 0 L-carnitine 20 Taurine 40	25.0 Amino acids[c]	<0.1	56.0 Sugar, corn syrup solids	324/1354	0/0
XMTVI Maxamum®	MET 0, VAL 0 ILE trace, THR 0 L-carnitine 39 Taurine 140	40.0 Amino acids[c]	<1.0	34.0 Sugar, corn syrup solids	305/1275	0/0
Milupa OS2®	MET 0, VAL 0 ILE 0, THR 0 L-carnitine 0 Taurine 0	56.0 Amino acids[c]	0.0	18.9 Sugar	300/1254	0/0

(continues)

Table 8.3 ***Formulation, Nutrient Composition, and Sources of Medical Foods for Patients with Propionic Acidemia or Methylmalonic Acidemia (per 100 g powder)***, *Continued*

Medical Foods	Modified Nutrient(s) (mg/100 g)	Protein Equiv[a] (g/100 g, source)	Fat (g/100 g, source)	Carbohydrate (g/100 g, source)	Energy (kcal/100 g/kJ/100 g)	Linoleic Acid/ α-Linolenic Acid (mg/100 g)
Vitaflo US LLC[f]						
MMA/PA Express™	MET 0, VAL 0 ILE 0, THR 0 L-carnitine added Taurine added	42.0 Amino acids[c]	<0.5	15 Sugar, starch, dried glucose syrup	302/1260	0/0
MMA/PA Gel™	MET 0, VAL 0 ILE 0, THR 0 L-carnitine added Taurine 217	42.0 Amino acids[c]	<0.5	43.0 Sugar, starch, dried glucose syrup	342/1428	0/0

Source: Data supplied by each company.

Notes: ND = no data.

Values listed, although accurate at time of publication, are subject to change. The most current information may be obtained by referring to product labels.

[a]Protein equivalent, g = g nitrogen × 6.25.

[b]Abbott Nutrition, 625 Cleveland Avenue, Columbus, Ohio, 43215. 800-551-5838.

[c]All except glycine are in the L-form.

[d]Mead Johnson Nutritionals, 2400 West Lloyd Expressway, Evansville, Indiana 47721. 800-457-3550.

[e]Nutricia North America, PO Box 117, Gaithersburg, Maryland, 20884. 800-365-7354.

[f]Vitaflo US LLC, 123 East Neck Road, Huntington, New York 11743. 888-848-2356.

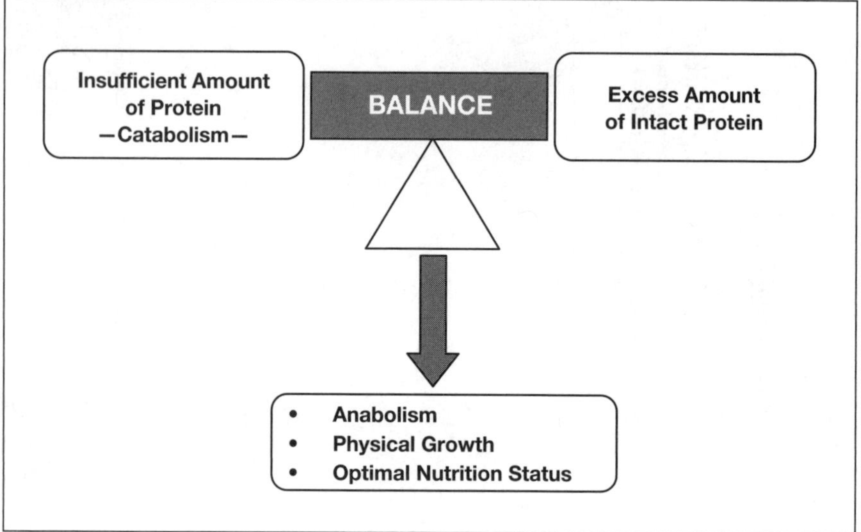

Figure 8.3 *Optimal Balance Should Be Provided Between Protein Intake and Endogenous Catabolism in Patients with Organic Acidemias*

are few studies on dosage and long-term outcomes. Regardless, providing a balance between excess and insufficient restricted amino acids, and protein for optimal growth and protein anabolism, must be assessed on an individual basis (see Figure 8.3).

Initiation of Nutrition Management and During Critical Illness or Following Trauma

Newborns with either suspected PROP or MMA require immediate medical and nutrition intervention while laboratory results are pending. Aggressive intervention is required during metabolic decompensation to reduce catabolism and inhibit plasma accumulation of toxic organic metabolites and ammonia. In severe cases, hemodialysis is indicated to remove toxic compounds.

Symptoms are typically triggered by infections, protracted fasting, or exposure to excess intact protein loads containing ILE, MET, THR, and VAL. Metabolic acidosis and decompensation occur frequently in infancy and childhood with some tolerance developing with maturity. During acute crisis, all sources of protein containing ILE, MET, THR, and VAL must be removed from the diet. Intravenous (IV) glucose and electrolytes at approximately 150 mL/kg/24 hours are required to provide a glucose infusion rate (GIR) of 10 mg/kg/min.[6] Aggressive nutrition intervention providing 120 to 150 kcal/kg/24 hours is required to promote anabolism, attenuate catabolism, and help reduce blood concentrations of toxic precursors. IV lipids may be added via peripheral or central lines at 2 to 3 g/kg/day. A combination of parenteral and enteral nutrition should be instituted as tolerated by the patient within 24 to 48 hours to prevent deficiency of ILE, MET, THR, and VAL. If using standard parenteral solutions, initiate protein at 0.5 g/kg/day and increase as tolerated, not to exceed the prescribed amount of ILE, MET, THR, and VAL. If long-term parenteral nutrition is required, tailored solutions are available (see Appendix D). Patients should be transitioned to oral feeds and nutrition management, which includes medical foods designed for PROP and MMA (see Table 8.3) and intact protein to provide ILE, MET, THR, and VAL, as soon as possible, to promote anabolism. During acute crises and transition to oral feeds, plasma amino acid concentrations should be monitored daily until the patient is stable. The goal is to maintain plasma ILE, MET, THR, and VAL concentrations in treatment ranges for long-term care. See Assessment of Nutrition Management, page 303, for concentrations to maintain.

Once the neonate has been stabilized and a diagnosis confirmed, disorder-specific therapy should be initiated without delay. Peripheral parenteral nutrition alone will not provide sufficient energy or protein to enhance anabolism. Small drip feeds of an enteral medical food mixture without ILE, MET, THR, and VAL delivered into the gastrointestinal (GI) tract should be provided as soon as the patient is stable and has bowel sounds. Introduction of oral ILE, MET, THR, and VAL as intact protein and energy is vital for anabolism.[33] Detailed information on nutrition and medical intervention during acute crises is given in Table 8.4, as a guide only.[6,78]

Long-Term Nutrition Management

Intact protein sources of ILE, MET, THR, and VAL for infants are either proprietary infant formulas or human milk (see Appendix B). As children age, ILE, MET, THR, and VAL may be supplied by low-protein foods (fruits, vegetables, and grains). For patients who are G-tube dependent, intact protein will be obtained from whole milk, soy milk (see Appendix B), and other liquids containing protein. In many cases, G-tube feedings are required for long-term care. For nutrient contents of foods, see references 32 and 79.

Use of human milk (see Appendix B) as a source of ILE, MET, THR, and VAL has been reported in infants with organic acidemias.[80-82] Due to the feeding difficulties in these patients, "on-demand" feeding is not recommended. In one patient, direct sucking was terminated after several months because of onset of two acute metabolic crises.[81] S. Yannicelli had a similar experience in one patient who had two episodes of metabolic decompensation along with failure to thrive over a 3-month period. If human milk is prescribed,

Table 8.4 *Emergency Treatment*

Acute Intervention

- **Goal:** Treat decompensation and inhibit catabolism.
  - Stop all intact protein for 24 to 48 hours.
  - Begin IV glucose + insulin and IV lipid therapy.
  - Monitor electrolytes frequently.
  - Treat metabolic acidosis aggressively.
  - Give IV L-carnitine (100 to 300 mg/kg/day) to help remove toxic metabolites.
- Maintain plasma sodium concentrations in normal range (see Chapter 3, Table 3.7).

Transition to Enteral Feeds

- **Goal:** Enhance protein anabolism and growth.
  - Provide high energy feeds (120 to 150 kcal/kg/day).
  - Initiate medical food free of or low in ILE, MET, THR, and VAL.
  - Gradually increase intact protein, as tolerated. Start at 0.5 g/kg/day within 24 to 48 hours once patient is stabilized. Transition to full oral feeds with prescribed medical food (see Table 8.3).
- Supplement L-ILE or L-VAL, if needed, to maintain plasma treatment ranges.
- MMA: Vitamin B_{12}, 1 to 2 mg/week as intramuscular hydroxy (OH)-cobalamin for cobalamin-deficient patients.
- PROP: Oral biotin 10 to 20 mg/day.

expressed milk is recommended because it can be accurately measured and intake carefully monitored. A sample diet for a 1-month-old infant with either PROP or MMA is given in Table 8.5.

Nonprotein energy sources may be required and may be derived from either carbohydrate–fat modules or single-nutrient modules with only fat or carbohydrate (see Appendix C). This is especially true for the G-tube dependent patients. For patients who can feed orally, very-low-protein foods (see Appendix E) are available for additional energy. It is important not to overfeed the non-ambulatory patient who may have decreased energy requirements because of decreased physical activity.

Challenges in Providing Adequate Nutrients

Frequent infections and vomiting provide a challenge to treating patients with PROP or MMA who are prone to recurrent infections resulting in metabolic decompensation, which over time leads to organic failure to thrive (see Figure 8.4).[22-24] Infections occur in approximately 80% of patients despite aggressive therapy.[83] With frequent illness, patients often

Table 8.5 *Diet for a 1-Month-Old Infant with PROP Weighing 4.1 kg*

	Amount	ILE (mg)	MET (mg)	THR (mg)	VAL (mg)	Carnitine (mg)	Protein (g)	Energy (kcal)
Similac® Advance® powder	66 g	380	182	386	422	5	7.20	347
XMTVI Analog® powder	55 g	38	0	0	0	6	7.20	261
L-carnitine (100 mg/mL)	4.0 mL	0	0	0	0	400	0.00	0
Total		418	182	386	422	411	14.40	608
Per kg body weight		102	44	94	103	100	3.50	148

Notes: Add water to yield 752 mL (~ 25 fluid oz).
Feed every 2 to 3 hours.
See Table 8.2 for recommended nutrient intakes.
If infant fails to grow normally linearly, see Chapter 3, Table 3.1.

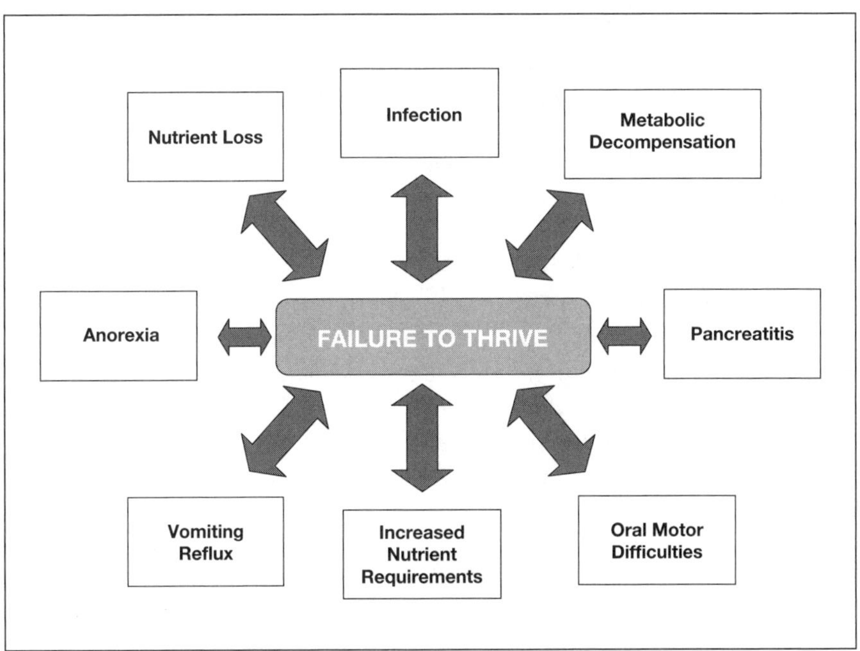

Figure 8.4 *Complications Associated with Failure to Thrive in Patients with PROP or MMA*

do not receive adequate quantities of nutrients required for growth and may require tailored parenteral nutrition.[84] Many patients suffer through a vicious cycle of illness and poor feeding, especially during infancy and early childhood.

During mid to late infancy, the majority of patients with a severe genotype for PROP or MMA develop feeding difficulties including anorexia and poor suck. Anorexia and food refusal may be both organic and behavioral. Hyman et al.[85] hypothesized that physiologic anorexia may be the result of altered serotonin metabolism in patients with organic acidemias. In patients with cancer, manipulating brain tryptophan (TRP) concentrations reduced anorexia and increased food intake.[86] Physiologic anorexia is more likely related to multifactorial interactions between brain biochemistry and peripheral metabolism and has been reported in animals to result from severe deficiency of essential amino acids.[87,88]

New Approaches to Therapy

In vitro studies have shown that certain forms of mutant PCC genes increase their activity in response to chemical chaperones. Chaperones are small molecules of an altered form of the PCC gene that may help increase the activity of the defective enzyme by modifying protein folding.[89] Chaparones may hold promise for future management in patients with PROP.

N-acetylglutamate (NAG) is an endogenous essential cofactor for conversion of ammonia to urea. Deficiency of NAG causes hyperammonemia and occurs in patients with PROP or MMA through inhibition of its rate-limiting enzyme, N-acetylglutamate synthase (NAGS), by methylmalonic and propionic acid.[20] Carbamyglu® (N-carbamyl glutamate), an experimental medication, has been shown effective in reducing plasma ammonia concentrations.[90,91] Further studies are warranted, but this novel adjunct therapy may show promise in patients with PROP or MMA.

Patients with PROP or MMA have been reported to have below normal concentrations of growth hormone.[52,92] Growth hormone therapy has been used in patients with PROP to promote anabolism and has resulted in accelerated growth and improved protein tolerance.

Successful liver and/or renal transplantations in a few patients have resulted in better quality of life but have not prevented neurological and various visceral complications.[93,94] Liver and liver–kidney transplantation can eliminate the risk of severe metabolic ketoacidosis, but it does not cure the disease.[95] Biochemical phenotype is still evident after transplantation and some patients continue to exhibit disease progression. One patient who had a liver transplant developed renal failure, requiring a second transplantation.[96] Nor does liver transplantation guarantee correction of growth retardation often found in these patients.[97] Risks and benefits of medical treatment versus transplantation should be assessed in any patient who is a potential candidate.[94,98]

For patients with severe anorexia, G-tubes are medically indicated for long-term nutrition intervention to improve growth and nutrition status.[36,37] Dysphagia and a hyperactive gag reflex, both of which decrease oral nutrient intakes, are common in these patients. Feeding difficulties pose long-term challenges to clinicians in treating patients with PROP or MMA.

Assessment of Nutrition Management

Approaches to monitoring patients with PROP or MMA are varied and clinic-specific.[99] Despite lack of consensus on methods of monitoring, careful follow up is essential in meeting nutrition management goals. When prescribing any nutrition management, clinicians must ensure adequate nutrient intakes. Scholl-Burgi et al.[100] reported that greater than 50% of diet diaries indicated below-prescribed amounts of protein intake by 8 patients with PROP. Reasons for intakes less than prescribed could be secondary to purposeful non-adherence due to concern among parents of excess protein and their failure to adjust diet based on growth and eating habits. Thus, nutrient intakes from frequent diet diary entries should be assessed.

Monitoring amino acid intakes and plasma amino acid concentrations is important for ongoing patient care and required to ensure adequate nutrition management and prevention of protein malnutrition. Plasma concentrations should be maintained in the low normal to normal range for age. Suggested treatment concentrations are given in Table 8.6.[32,34,101-104]

Plasma GLY concentrations are not a reliable indicator for assessing clinical status of patients with PROP or MMA, and North et al.[37] noted that plasma GLY concentrations did not correlate with metabolic control. Interestingly, plasma GLY concentrations were low during times of metabolic acidosis and high during the well-state. Yannicelli et al.[36] reported an inverse correlation between plasma GLY concentrations and energy intake, and others found acid base status and plasma GLY concentration to be related.[105] Subnormal concentrations of the branched-chain amino acids are associated with increased plasma GLY and alanine concentrations.[77] Despite issues surrounding interpretation of elevated concentrations of plasma GLY, lowering of concentrations suggests improved metabolic control.

Two mutations, called CblC and CblD, causing impaired synthesis of both adenosylcobalamin and methylcobalamin, result in defective activity of both methylmalonyl-CoA mutase and methionine synthase (see Figures 7.1 and 8.1). For patients with cobalamin C/D deficiency, plasma MET concentrations may be below reference ranges. L-methionine supplementation

Table 8.6 ***Recommended Selected Plasma Amino Acid Concentrations for Patients with Propionic or Methylmalonic Acidemia***

Amino Acid	*Reference Ranges (μmol/L)**
Glycine	115–290
Isoleucine	25–105
Methionine	18–45
Threonine	45–250
Valine	65–250

Sources:

Acosta PB, Yannicelli S. Protocol 13. Propionic or methylmalonic acidemia. *Nutrition Support Protocols*. 4th ed. Columbus, OH: Ross Products Division, Abbott Laboratories; 2001.

Applegarth DA, Edelstein AD, Wong LT, Morrison BJ. Observed range of assay values for plasma and cerebrospinal fluid amino acid levels in infants and children aged 3 months to 10 years. *Clin Biochem*. 1979;12:173–178.

Elsas LJ, Acosta PB. Inherited metabolic disease: amino acids, organic acids, and galactose. In: Shils ME, Shike M, Olson J, Ross AC, Caballero B, Cousins RJ, eds. *Modern Nutrition in Health and Disease*. 10th ed. Philadelphia, PA: Lippincott Williams & Wilkins; 2005:909–959.

MacLean WC Jr, Placko RP, Graham GG. Fasting plasma free amino acids of infants and children consuming cow milk proteins. *Johns Hopkins Med J*. 1978;142:147–151.

Meites S. *Pediatric Clinical Chemistry. Reference (Normal) Values*. Washington, DC: American Association for Clinical Chemistry; 1989.

Soldin SJ, Brugnara C, Gunter KC, Wong EC. *Pediatric Reference Intervals*. 7th ed. Washington, DC: AAAC Press; 2007.

*Check with local laboratory for normal reference ranges for age.

(approximately 35 to 50 mg/kg/day) may be required to normalize plasma concentrations. Plasma total homocysteine concentrations should be monitored in patients with cobalamin C/D deficiency. Plasma concentrations are difficult to maintain in the normal range; therefore a realistic concentration is near 50 μmol/L.

Micronutrients and essential fatty acid intakes should be assessed as needed. Chemically defined medical foods used for patients with an IMD can affect the bioavailability of macro and trace elements, including iron, copper, selenium, and zinc. Inadequate nutrient intakes may result in deficiencies[56,57,106,107] and periodic assessment of mineral status is recommended. Table 8.7 outlines routine nutrition assessment guidelines for patients with

Table 8.7 ***Suggested Nutrition Assessment Parameters during Long-Term Management of Patients with PROP, MMA, or GAI***

Assessment	***Quantitated Parameters***	***Frequency***
Growth	Length/height, head circumference, weight (age-dependent)*	Monthly for infants to 12 months of age; as needed thereafter
Nutrient adequacy	3-day diet diaries prior to blood or urine collection	Before each blood test or as needed
Protein status indices	Total protein, albumin, transthyretin (prealbumin)*	Every 3 months for infants to 12 months of age; every 6 months thereafter or as needed
Plasma amino acids	Full amino acid profile*	Weekly or biweekly for 0 to 4 months of age; weekly for 4 to 12 months; as needed thereafter
Organic acids (blood, urine)	Organic acid profile; acylcarnitine esters*	Monthly or more frequently for infants; as needed thereafter.
Blood ammonia (PROP or MMA only)	Blood ammonia	Monthly or more frequently for infants; monthly or quarterly thereafter, as needed. Obtain when either plasma amino acids or organic acids are quantitated.
Serum carnitine	Free and esters (bound)*	As needed to monitor status

Note: Frequency of tests may differ based on patients' clinical status and specific clinical protocols. *Obligatory assessment parameters. Additional nutrition assessments may include essential fatty acids and trace elements. Other tests may be indicated as needed for patient management. See Chapter 3, *Evaluation of Nutrition Status*, Tables 3.7 and 3.9.

PROP or MMA. Other assessment guidelines can be found in Chapter 3, Table 3.7.

Plasma or serum ammonia concentrations should be maintained in the normal range for age. For infants, normal ammonia concentration is < 74 μmol/L; for children 1 to 4 years it is < 68 μmol/L, depending on the laboratory and method used (see Chapter 3, Table 3.7).[104]

Measurement of urine methylmalonic acid to monitor medical and nutrition management is variable and not wholly reliable. Multiple factors affect urine organic acid concentrations, including intact protein intake, vitamin B_{12} status, renal function, and health status.[25] Plasma methylmalonic acid concentrations may better reflect methylmalonic acid metabolism than urine.[95] Normal plasma concentrations are below 0.27 μmol/L, but this is not achievable in patients with MMA. For patients with PROP or MMA, management is aimed at maintaining plasma organic acids at concentrations that support optimal clinical outcomes.

Home Monitoring

Parents and caregivers must be counseled on how to monitor their children's clinical status and diet regimen daily. Measurement of daily urine ketones (Ketostix® Reagent Strips, Bayer Health Care, Morristown, New Jersey) is required to assess clinical status and impending ketosis that may occur without obvious clinical signs. Urine ketones should be maintained at zero to trace concentrations. Assessment of feeding tolerance by the patient is essential because an initial sign of a clinical problem is vomiting. Parents should be taught to provide alternate feeds in response to either a change in clinical status or increased urinary ketones.

During infancy and early childhood metabolic decompensation can occur with standard immunizations and mild trauma, which in normal children would be well tolerated with minor insult. Oral and live immunizations may cause clinical decompensation in patients with organic acidemias with neutropenia or thrombocytopenia. Careful planning is required by the clinician to offset any major adverse event secondary to basic pediatric management.

All patients with an IMD in whom illness or stress can cause metabolic decompensation must have an emergency letter with the following information: name of disease, symptoms, and consequences of metabolic decompensation; and treatment strategies, including plan for stabilization, type and amount of IV fluids, administration of detoxifying or coenzyme therapy, and metabolic physician contact information for transfer or consultation.

Results of Nutrition Management

Until recently, patients with severe forms of PROP or MMA rarely reached adolescence or adulthood. Aggressive medical intervention, effective chronic nutrition management, and in some cases liver transplantation,[108] have resulted in patients living longer, more healthful lives than previously achieved. Mental development and cognition may be normal depending on severity of disease.[109] In spite of advances in medical and nutrition intervention, the majority of patients still suffer from chronic, debilitating symptoms. Cobalamin-responsive patients with MMA have better clinical outcomes compared to patients with severe mutase deficiency but are still at risk for neurologic complications.[110]

Disease severity, enzyme function, and age at presentation correlate with clinical outcome.[93,111] Patients with Mut^- MMA have a milder clinical course than those patients with Mut^0 MMA. Patients who present later in life often have a milder enzyme defect, are more clinically stable, and tolerate more intact protein than those who present as neonates.[70,112] For Mut^0 or Mut^- MMA, dystonia, developmental delay, and chronic renal failure have been reported,[113,114] with the latter requiring transplantation. Chronic renal failure is a severe complication in patients with MMA. The exact pathophysiology of renal failure is not known but it may share similar pathomechanisms with the nervous system.[114] Hypotheses include methylmalonic acid as a nephrotoxin[115,116] and disturbances in mitochondrial function.[114,117]

Patients who survive the neonatal course and who are undergoing chronic management may later develop complications including cardiomyopathy, heart failure,[45,118-120] and pancreatitis.[121,122] Mardach et al.[119] reported fatal cardiomyopathy in one patient with low total and free cardiac carnitine concentrations despite normal plasma free carnitine concentrations while receiving L-carnitine. These authors noted that this patient was not adherent to her diet prescription. Disparity between plasma and tissue carnitine concentrations have been reported, with low tissue concentrations and adequate plasma concentrations.[123] However, one patient with heart failure showed resolution of symptoms within 24 hours after increased L-carnitine administration (125 mg/kg/24 hours).[118]

Developmental delay and cognitive impairment may still be evident in patients with PROP or MMA despite appropriate management.[45,70,93,112] In milder forms of disease, normal cognition has been reported, despite a moderately severe clinical course.[109]

Early intervention and adequate nutrition management can result in normal growth and outcome in patients with PROP or MMA.[36,37,45,70] Nonetheless, malnutrition and growth retardation are still frequently reported in these patients and adversely affect clinical outcome. Clinical symptoms of metabolic decompensation, including hyperammonemia and metabolic acidosis, have been reported as a consequence of protein over-restriction and subsequent malnutrition.[45,70,93] Long-term protein-energy malnutrition can lead to a decline in mental and physical development.[124]

Yannicelli et al.[36] reported improved growth and protein status indices in infants and toddlers receiving a medical food. In this study, patients with improved linear growth had protein intakes greater than 120% of FAO/WHO/UNU recommendations[73] and energy intakes greater than 100% of recommended for age. Patients with limited growth in this study consumed protein and energy at or below FAO/WHO/UNU recommendations.

Maternal Methylmalonic or Propionic Acidemia

Several case reports of successful pregnancy have been reported in women with mild MMA[125-127] or PROP[128] managed by diet. One pregnancy in a woman with cobalamin A MMA was also reported.[129] In the patient with cobalamin A disease, intramuscular injections of cobalamin throughout pregnancy resulted in good fetal outcome and reduction of plasma and urine methylmalonate concentrations, while in one case, fetal outcome was good despite elevated plasma and urine methylmalonate concentrations.[126] Reviews on pregnancies and issues in patients with an IMD are available by Koch et al.[130] and Lee.[131] For suggested protein and energy intakes in pregnancy, see Chapter 3, Table 3.1.

Glutaric Aciduria Type 1

Introduction

Glutaric aciduria Type 1 (GAI; OMIM 231670)[1] is one of a few organic acidurias that have been classified as "cerebral" because of its overwhelming cerebral involvement. The disorder was first described by Goodman and colleagues[132] and reported as a distinct encephalopathic disorder in 1991.[133] Patients often appear normal at birth and thrive during the first half of infancy. Between 6 and 18 months of age, onset of an acute infectious illness often results in overwhelming encephalopathy causing permanent neurologic impairment.[134]

Prevalence of GAI is approximately 1:50,000 live births but varies between 1:30,000 to 1:100,000.[135,136] In Old Order Amish (Lancaster, Pennsylvania) and in the Saulteaux-Ojibway Indians (Canada) the incidence is much higher.[137-139] An increased incidence has also been reported in the Lumbee Native American tribe (North Carolina).[140] Clinical variability among patients with GAI is broad.[137]

Biochemistry

GAI is an autosomal recessive disorder of lysine (LYS), hydroxylysine (OH-LYS), and tryptophan (TRP) metabolism (see Figure 8.5). A defect in activity of the mitochondrial enzyme, glutaryl-CoA dehydrogenase (GCDH; EC 1.3.99.7), results in incomplete oxidation of LYS, OH-LYS, and TRP leading to elevated plasma glutaric acid, OH-glutaric acid, and, to a lesser amount, glutaconic acid concentration. GCDH catalyzes oxidative decarboxylation of glutaryl-CoA to crotonyl-CoA. GCDH is flavin-dependent and riboflavin supplementation is indicated as adjunct therapy. Electrons from mitochondrial GCDH and other flavoprotein dehydrogenases are transferred to ubiquinone in the electron transport chain by electron transfer flavoprotein (ETF).[141]

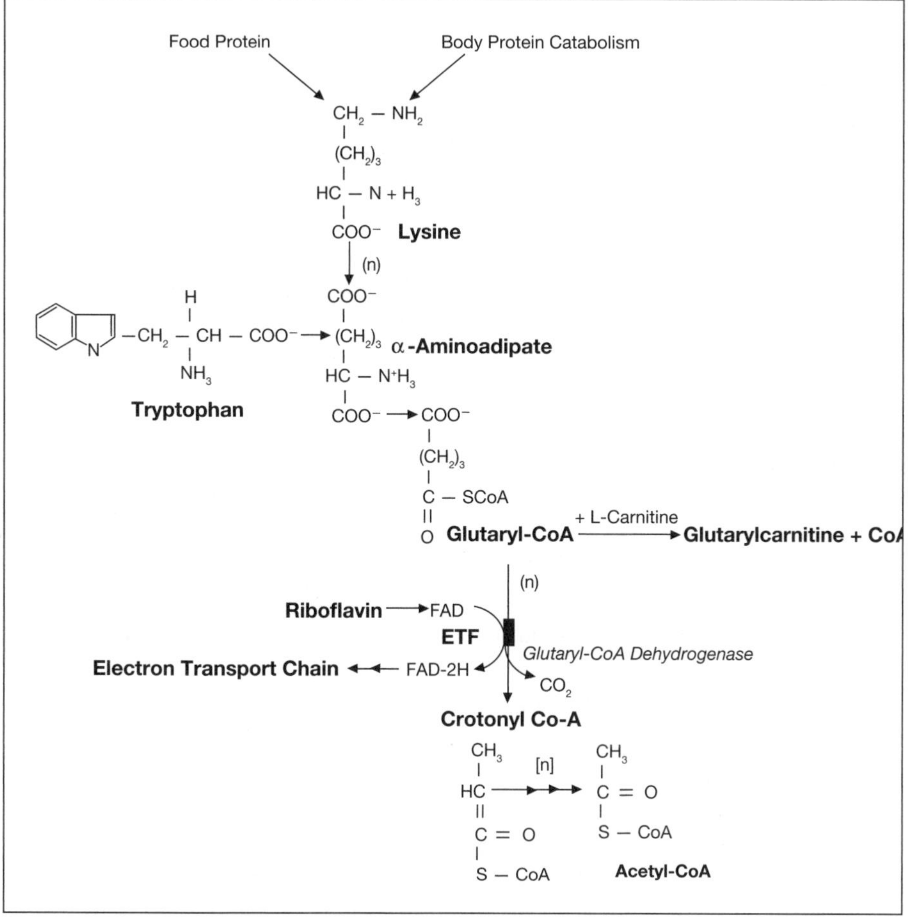

Figure 8.5 *Metabolism of Lysine and Tryptophan*

Source: Modified by permission of Elsas LJ, Acosta PB. Inherited metabolic disease: amino acids, organic acids, and galactose. In: Shils ME, Shike M, Olson J, Ross AC, Caballero B, Cousins RJ, eds. *Modern Nutrition in Health and Disease.* 10th ed. Philadelphia, PA: Lippincott Williams & Wilkins; 2005:909–959. Courtesy of Wolters Kluwer Health.

Notes: Black bar indicates enzyme defect.

(n) = indicates several steps in metabolism.

ETF is the electron transfer factor.

A defect in GCDH results in accumulation of glutaric acid, 3-OH glutaric acid, and glutarylcarnitine in body fluids. Patients may be classified based on urinary metabolite excretion as either high excretors (urine glutaric acid >100 mmol/mol creatinine) or low excretors (urine glutaric acid <100 mmol/mol creatinine).[136,142] More than 50% of patients with GAI are classified as high excretors.[136] Patients who are high excretors excrete both glutaric acid (mean 3134 mmol/mol creatinine) and 3-OH glutaric acid (mean 618 mmol/mol creatinine) in high concentrations compared to low excretors (20 mmol/mol creatinine; 153 mmol/mol creatinine, respectively). Patients classified as low excretors may show normal urine glutaric acid concentration and only moderately elevated urine 3-OH glutaric acid concentration. Urine excretion of metabolites may vary among patients and during times of acute crises compared to the well-state.[143]

Elevated brain LYS concentrations may be precursors for toxic organic acids. Study of a GAI murine model has shown that accumulation in immature brain precipitates production of glutaric acid resulting in injury.[144] This finding may provide a model for different approaches to treatment, especially during times of acute crises.

Molecular Biology

Genetic variance in GAI is well known and can be, in part, related to biochemical phenotype (see Chapter 1). The GCDH gene is localized on chromosome 19p13.2.[145] Certain mutations (V400M and R227P) are found frequently in patients with normal urine glutaric acid excretion.[143] Over 150 mutations in the GCDH gene have been identified.[134,143,146] A number of different mutations have been associated with residual enzyme activity. Patients with nearly 30% residual enzyme activity are homozygous for M263V or compound heterozygosity for R227P and V400M.[136] The most common European mutation is R402W, with other specific mutations found in Old Order Amish and Ogibway Indians of Canada. Patients homozygous for R402W excrete large amounts of glutaric acid and 3-OH glutaric acid and have little or no enzyme activity.[143]

Genotype/phenotype correlations in patients with GAI have not been established. Lindner et al.[136] reported no relationship between disease severity and either molecular or biochemical findings. They also reported that a majority of patients (64%) who were classified as low excretors had severe phenotypes in comparison with 51% of high excretors.[136] Lack of genotype/phenotype correlation poses a challenge to clinicians in counseling families and in nutrition management.

Newborn Screening

GAI has been included as one of 29 IMDs on the core panel for expanded newborn screening.[147] Implementation of newborn screening by MS/MS identifies newborns who may be affected with GAI (see Chapter 2). Early detection and diagnosis provide a means for medical and nutrition intervention before onset of acute encephalopathy, thereby preventing lifelong neurologic impairment. Newborn screening for GAI requires estimating the amount of

C5-dicarboxylic (DC; glutaryl) carnitine, an acylcarnitine intermediate in dried blood spots obtained between 24 to 72 hours postnatally.

Diagnosis

Clinical evaluation and additional diagnostic tests are essential for confirmatory diagnosis and include quantitating urine glutaric acid, 3-OH glutaric acid, and glutarylcarnitine. Patients with GAI (low excretors) not detected by newborn screening have been reported.[148,149] Other patients may excrete either only glutaric acid or 3-OH glutaric acid with variation in glutarylcarnitine excretion.[142,149,150] In some cases, the risk of not detecting low excretors necessitates additional confirmatory testing.[149,150]

If analysis of organic acids is not confirmatory, then additional tests should be completed on urine glutarylcarnitine, blood and cerebrospinal fluid (CSF) 3-OH glutaric acid, and enzyme assay from skin fibroblasts. Optional confirmatory tests include molecular analysis of the GCDH gene.[147] Algorithms are available to clinicians to assist in screening and diagnosis of organic acidemias.[18]

Physical examination shows macrocephaly, progressive ataxia, myoclonic jerks, acute encephalopathy, and psychomotor retardation. Neuroradiologic examination may reveal basal ganglia anomaly, brain atrophy, and progressive demyelinization. Macrocephaly is found in about 75% of patients.[150] Clinical symptoms may include vomiting, fever, and failure to thrive. Diagnostic measures also include assessing plasma amino acids, plasma and urine organic acids, and free and acylated carnitine. Morton et al.[138] reported urinary glutaric acid to be an effective diagnostic biomarker in the Old Order Amish population. Other biochemical findings include decreased free plasma carnitine concentrations with significantly elevated plasma and urine acylcarnitines, specifically glutarylcarnitine.[151] Plasma LYS and TRP concentrations vary and may be only slightly elevated.

Differential diagnosis includes mitochondrial disorders and glutaric aciduria type II, a distinct disease. One study using a GAI murine model showed that proton nuclear magnetic resonance spectroscopy of brain glutamate and γ-aminobutyric acid might be another diagnostic marker. Both of these analytes were reported as depleted in the GAI murine brain, and inversely correlated with glutaric acid accumulation.[144] Consensus guidelines for diagnosis of patients with GAI have been published.[152]

Outcomes if Untreated

GAI is a catastrophic disease in patients with a severe genotype who are not treated, and in absence of newborn screening, patients with a severe phenotype clinically present with acute encephalopathic crisis often by late infancy to early toddler years. Permanent damage to the striatum results in severe dystonia and dyskinesis movement disorders. Idiopathic cerebral palsy has been diagnosed in some patients prior to identification of GAI.[138] Persistent elevated brain glutaric acid concentrations are toxic early in life, but not in later life.[138] Children who avoid encephalopathic crisis during the first 5 years of life remain asymptomatic throughout life.[134] Animal models are now available[144] that may help unravel the pathology and lead to improved medical and nutrition intervention. Death may result at any time during a significant acute episode. Cognition is preserved in the majority of patients regardless of age at clinical presentation.

Exact pathophysiology of GAI has not been elucidated, but has been attributed to neurotoxic accumulation of glutaric acid, quinolinic acid, and 3-hydroxy (OH) glutaric acid.[153-155] Sauer[156] hypothesized that glutaric acid and 3-OH glutaric acid may be synthesized de novo and become trapped in brain tissue. A thorough review of the suggested pathogenesis of GAI and other IMDs can be found in reference 157.

Nutrition Management

The goal of nutrition management is to promote normal growth and development and reduce risk of onset of encephalopathic crisis. In patients who have had a neurologic insult, the goals will be to prevent malnutrition and further neurologic deterioration.[158] Restriction of the essential amino acids LYS and TRP, and medical foods free of LYS and TRP, are the cornerstones of nutrition management.[153,158] A LYS- and TRP-restricted diet can minimize risk of malnutrition and promote growth and development in infants and children birth to 6 years of age.[153,158,159] After 6 years of age, a diet based on intact protein restriction alone has been proposed.[153,159] The best approach for patients greater than 6 years of age is not well-known, but considering the concerns of malnutrition and feeding difficulties, continuation of LYS and TRP restriction using medical food is suggested. Nutrition management should be tailored to each patient for optimal clinical outcome.

The LYS- and TRP-restricted diet requires prescribed amounts of intact protein (sources of LYS and TRP; see Appendix B) and medical foods free of LYS and TRP to provide the majority of protein, energy, and micronutrients. Table 8.8 describes the components of nutrition management of patients with GAI.

Nutrient Requirements

LYS and TRP requirements in patients with GAI are not well established and are based on clinical experience and anecdotal data. Requirements vary

Table 8.8 *Components for Nutrition Management of Patients with GAI*

Nutrients	*Source (examples)*
LYS and TRP (Intact protein)	Proprietary infant formula or expressed human milk, cow's milk, beikost, and table foods; prescribed grains, fruits, and vegetables
Other essential and nonessential amino acids (g protein equivalent = nitrogen, g × 6.25)	LYS-, TRP-free medical foods
Energy	Nonprotein energy sources: carbohydrate modules, carbohydrate–fat modules, sugar, very-low-protein foods
Fluid	Water, energy-supplemented beverages
L-carnitine	Oral L-carnitine (pharmaceutical grade); IV L-carnitine during acute illness
Riboflavin (100 to 200 mg/day with food)	Oral riboflavin (pharmacologic grade)

based on genotype and residual enzyme activity, as well as age, growth rate, nutrient adequacy, and health status. Table 8.9 lists recommended intakes for beginning management of patients with GAI.

One early report showed that reducing LYS (50 mg/kg/day) in a 5-month-old infant reduced plasma and urine concentrations of glutaric acid.[160] Despite improved biochemical markers, clinical manifestations did not improve. This finding has been reported by others.[158,161-163] Effects of LYS reduction on decreasing urine organic acids may not always reflect plasma or cerebrospinal fluid concentrations.[162] The lack of relationship between plasma and brain concentrations poses a challenge to clinicians in identifying proper biochemical biomarkers to use in managing patients. Notwithstanding, early diagnosis and intervention prior to acute encephalopathic crisis offer hope to patients who would otherwise suffer lifelong debilitating disease.

Published estimates of LYS and TRP requirements[164-169] may not apply to all patients with GAI, but recommendations found in the DRIs[72] may be used until adequate data are available. Requirements will differ from patient to patient and can be assessed only by frequent monitoring of plasma amino acid concentrations, growth, and other biomarkers for nutrition status (see Chapter 3, Table 3.7). Care must be taken not to over-restrict TRP; a major concern among metabolic clinicians. According to Hoffmann,[170] TRP contributes ≤20% of glutaric acid production, and excessive restriction is not warranted because over-restriction may cause deficiency and poor growth. The issue of restricting TRP is controversial due in part to concern of over-restriction and lack of specific and sensitive plasma analysis.

Table 8.9 ***Recommended Daily Nutrient Intakes for Patients with Glutaric Aciduria Type I***

Age (yr)	*Lysine (mg/kg)*	*Tryptophan (mg/kg)*	*Protein (g/kg)*	*Energy (kcal/kg)*
0.0 < 0.5	70–100	10–25	2.75–3.50	125–145
0.5 < 1.0	55–70	10–20	2.50–3.25	140–115
				(kcal/day)
1 < 4	50–80	8–12	1.80–2.60	900–1800
4 < 7	40–70	8–12	1.60–2.00	1300–2300
7 < 11	35–65	5–10	1.55–1.85	1600–2800
Female				
11 < 15	35–40	5–8	1.50–1.80	1500–2800
15 < 19	33–40	4–6	1.45–1.75	1200–2800
> 19	30–40	4–6	1.45–1.75	1400–2400
Male				
11 < 15	35–40	5–8	1.45–1.75	2000–3200
15 < 19	33–45	6–8	1.45–1.75	2100–3200
> 19	30–40	4–6	1.45–1.75	2000–3000

Sources:

Acosta PB, Yannicelli S. Protocol 9. Glutaric acidemia type I or 2-ketoadipic aciduria. *Nutrition Support Protocols*. 4th ed. Columbus, OH: Ross Products Division, Abbott Laboratories; 2001.

Clark HE, Kenney MA, Goodwin AF, Goyal K, Mertz ET. Effect of certain factors on nitrogen retention and lysine requirements of adult human subjects. IV. Total nitrogen intake. *J Nutr*. 1963;81:223–229.

Clark HE, Mertz ET, Kwong EH, Howe JM, Delong DC. Amino acid requirements of men and women. I. Lysine. *J Nutr*. 1957;62:71–82.

FAO/WHO/UNU. *Expert Consultation on Energy and Protein Requirements*. WHO technical report series; No. 724. Geneva, Switzerland: World Health Organization; 1985:71–112.

Fisher H, Brush MK, Griminger P. Reassessment of amino acid requirements of young women on low nitrogen diets. 1. Lysine and tryptophan. *Am J Clin Nutr*. 1969;22:1190–1196.

Otten JJ, Hellwig JP, Meyers LD. *Dietary Reference Intakes: The Essential Guide to Nutrient Requirements*. Washington, DC: National Academies Press; 2006:197–201.

Snyderman SE, Norton PM, Fowler DI, Holt LE. The essential amino acid requirements of infants: lysine. *AMA J Dis Child*. 1959;97:175–185.

Tome D, Bos C. Lysine requirement through the human life cycle. *J Nutr*. 2007;137:1642S–1645S.

FAO/WHO/UNU. *Expert Consultation on Protein and Amino Acid Requirements in Human Nutrition*. WHO technical report series; No. 935. Geneva, Switzerland: World Health Organization; 2002.

Note: Actual requirements may differ based on patient's phenotype, biochemical status, and growth. If patients fail to grow normally linearly, see Chapter 3, Table 3.1. Patients with GAI who are nonambulatory will require a lower energy intake than ambulatory patients. If the patient is obese, protein prescription should be based on 50th percentile weight for age.

Kahler and Iafolla[171] reported that LYS intake of 90 mg/kg/day by 1 infant was prescribed for growth. However, energy intake (80 kcal/kg/day) was poor and negatively affected growth. Hoffmann et al.[133] reported LYS and TRP intakes by 11 patients with GAI. With the exception of 2 patients, intakes that achieved optimal reduction of urinary glutaric acid excretion with no sign of malnutrition were similar to those noted in Table 8.9. Yannicelli et al.[158] reviewed LYS and TRP intakes by infants and children treated pre- and postneurologic crises. Intakes and clinical and biochemical results varied greatly among patients.

Protein

Intact protein restriction alone, without a specific LYS and TRP precription or medical foods, has been reported in patients with GAI with mixed success.[138,172-174] LYS and TRP restriction in combination with medical foods has been more effective than restriction of intact protein alone in reducing frequency of acute encephalopathic crisis.[134] For this reason, and to prevent malnutrition, a LYS- and TRP-restricted diet using medical foods is the preferred diet strategy.[152,159]

Over-restriction of protein can lead to malnutrition and deficiency.[175,176] Hoffmann and associates[175] reported a case study of a 5-year-old patient with GAI who developed acrodermatitis acidemia after 6 weeks of ingesting 0.5 g protein and 75 kcal/kg/day. These authors also reported hypoalbuminemia and below-normal plasma concentrations of ILE, selenium, zinc, and pyridoxine. Resolution of symptoms occurred with diet modification. Almost identical clinical signs were reported in a 5-year-old Turkish patient with GAI.[176] In neither of these case studies were signs of malnutrition associated with GAI, and were most likely due to iatrogenic causes.

Fat and Essential Fatty Acids

DRIs have been published[72] and are noted in Chapter 3, Table 3.1. Essential fatty acids, linoleic and α-linolenic are also given. Because some medical foods for children and adults do not contain fat, sources of essential fatty acids may be required in the diet (see Appendix F).

Energy and Fluid

Patients with GAI and neurological impairment may have lower energy requirements than patients who are not impaired.[177-179] Non-ambulation, muscle atrophy, and below-normal activity all contribute to decreased resting energy expenditures. Published equations and mathematical formulas for calculating energy expenditure are based on healthy individuals and may overestimate the needs of the physically challenged patient. For accuracy and individualized energy recommendation, clinicians could measure by indirect calorimetry. As this may not be readily available, titrating energy needs to support growth and prevent malnutrition is recommended. Patients with GAI who have intermittent fever will require more energy than those without fever. See Table 8.9 for guidelines on energy requirements.

Adequate hydration is essential to maintain fluid balance and promote excretion of toxic metabolites. Patients with involuntary muscle contractions will require increased fluids[161] over those without muscle contractions. Adequate fluid is also essential during periods of intermittent illness, especially if the patient is febrile. Strict attention to electrolytes is important. Care must be taken to avoid hyperosmotic medical food mixtures and to provide sufficient free water. A minimum of 1.5 mL/kcal of water for infants and 1.0 mL/kcal of water for children and adults is recommended.[55] Osmolality of medical food mixtures for infants is <450 mOsm/L; for children, <750 mOsm/L; and adults, <1000 mOsm/L. Additional water is required during intermittent febrile illnesses and with increased stool loss.

Minerals and Vitamins

Mineral and vitamin intakes from the medical food mixture and other foods must meet at least 100% of DRIs for age[43,72] to prevent deficiency and support growth and development. If patients are obtaining a majority of their nutrients from a medical food, intakes greater than 100% of DRIs[43,72] are required secondary to poor absorption. Alexander et al.[180] reported that a number of minerals were poorly absorbed by patients ingesting an elemental diet. See Chapter 3, Table 3.1 for suggested intakes of minerals and vitamins that should prevent deficiencies if adequate medical food is ingested.

Preformed niacin should be prescribed to meet at least 100% of DRIs for age[43,72] due to TRP restriction. Under normal conditions, niacin can be synthesized de novo from TRP (i.e., 60 mg TRP = 1 niacin equivalent).[43]

Pharmacologic doses of riboflavin (vitamin B_2; 100 to 200 mg/day) should be tried in all patients. Brandt et al.[181] reported neurologic improvement and reduced urinary glutaric acid excretion in 1 patient, while protein restriction (1.0 g/kg/day) plus riboflavin (20 mg/kg/day) reduced urinary glutaric acid to non-detectable concentrations and improved ataxia in a 3 year old.[182] Chalmers et al.[183] described a riboflavin-responsive patient with S139L and P248L mutation of GCDH in whom in vitro analysis of GCDH showed 20% residual activity. In this 14-week-old patient, riboflavin alone, 25 mg three times daily (TID) and later 50 mg (TID) significantly increased excretion of glutaric acid, with some reduction in 3-OH glutaric acid. Introduction of a LYS-restricted diet further increased urine excretion of glutaric acid and 3-OH glutaric acid. At the time of publication, the patient was 21 years of age and clinically and neurologically normal.

High-dose riboflavin can cause serious gastric distress. Dosage studies in healthy adults showed that a single dose of 27 mg riboflavin was maximally absorbed.[184] For these reasons, 15 to 25 mg of riboflavin should be administered throughout the day and is best absorbed if given with food.[72] Parents should be informed that a side effect of high-dose riboflavin is a change in urine color to yellow–orange. Riboflavin is highly water insoluble and should not be administered intravenously.

L-carnitine supplementation (100 to 300 mg/kg/day) is required to replenish tissue carnitine concentrations, facilitate urinary excretion of glutarylcarnitine, and prevent carnitine deficiency. Valproic acid, an anticonvulsant, can result in secondary carnitine deficiency.[185,186] Carnitine has an important cellular function in the rate-limiting step in mitochondrial β-oxidation of long-chain fatty acids and in esterifying toxic acyl-CoA metabolites. L-carnitine administration should be titrated until normal plasma free concentrations are attained (≥ 30 μmol/L; check with a reference laboratory for their normal reference ranges). Oral L-carnitine absorption is approximately 20%, and high doses are known to result in gastrointestinal effects, including a fishy odor due to production of gut methylamines.[65] Another side effect is diarrhea. Reducing the oral L-carnitine dosage helps eliminate side effects.

Adjunct therapies, including supplementation of antioxidants and creatine monohydrate, are infrequently prescribed for use in patients with GAI.[187] Use of these compounds, as well as other neuroprotective agents, is not recommended for routine use.[152]

LYS- and TRP-Free Medical Foods

Medical foods, free of LYS and TRP, often comprise the majority of the patient's total daily protein intake.[158] Medical foods contain free amino acids, carbohydrates, minerals and vitamins, and may contain fat. Dependence on medical foods requires total amounts of protein equivalent (nitrogen, g × 6.25) greater than the DRIs for age (see Chapter 3).[43] Use of medical foods is nearly universally accepted for nutrition management of patients with GAI who have been diagnosed and treated from the neonatal period and before neurologic crisis.[76,134] See Table 8.10 for GAI-specific medical foods.

Intact Protein

Infants with GAI may use either human milk or proprietary infant formula (see Appendix B) as their source of restricted LYS and TRP. For accuracy in assessing intake, human milk should be expressed and added to the entire medical food mixture. Direct sucking (demand feeding) is not a choice when managing patients with organic acidurias.[82] Concerns over maintaining good metabolic control and inability for the infant to suck, if ill, are two practical difficulties. In addition to immunologic properties of human milk and bioactive compounds, it contains less LYS per gram of protein than proprietary formulas (6.6% versus 8.0%, respectively). TRP content of human milk is not significantly higher compared to proprietary infant formula (1.7% versus 1.57%, respectively). Consequently, more intact high biological value protein could be prescribed.

As the infant ages, proprietary infant formula or human milk will be replaced by prescribed beikost (baby food) consisting of fats, fruits, grains, vegetables, and very-low-protein food products and, later, low-protein table

Table 8.10 ***Formulation, Nutrient Composition, and Sources of Medical Foods for Patients with Glutaric Aciduria Type I (per 100 g powder)***

Medical Foods	*Modified Nutrient(s) (mg/100 g)*	*Protein Equiv[a] (g/100 g, source)*	*Fat (g/100 g, source)*	*Carbohydrate (g/100 g, source)*	*Energy (kcal/100 g/kJ/100 g)*	*Linoleic Acid/ α-Linolenic Acid (mg/100 g)*
Abbott Nutrition[b]						
Glutarex®-1	LYS 0, TRP 0 L-carnitine 900 Taurine 40	15.0 Amino acids[c]	21.7 High oleic safflower, coconut, soy oils	53.0 Corn syrup solids	480/2006	3500/350
Glutarex®-2	LYS 0, TRP 0 L-carnitine 1800 Taurine 50	30.0 Amino acids[c]	14.0 High oleic safflower, coconut, soy oils	35.0 Corn syrup solids	410/1714	2200/225
Mead Johnson Nutritionals[d]						
GA®	LYS 0, TRP 0 L-carnitine ND Taurine ND	15.1 Amino acids[c]	26.0 Palm olein, soy, coconut, high oleic safflower oils	52.0 Corn syrup solids, sugar, modified cornstarch, maltodextrin	500/2090	4500/380
Nutricia North America[e]						
XLYS, XTRP Analog®	LYS 0, TRP 0 L-carnitine 10 Taurine 20	13.0 Amino acids[c]	20.9 High oleic safflower, coconut, soy oils	59.0 Corn syrup solids	475/1985	3025/ND
XLYS, XTRP Maxamaid®	LYS 0, TRP 0 L-carnitine 20 Taurine 140	25.0 Amino acids[c]	<0.3	56.0 Sugar, corn syrup solids	324/1354	0/0

(continues)

Table 8.10 ***Formulation, Nutrient Composition, and Sources of Medical Foods for Patients with Glutaric Aciduria Type I (per 100 g powder)***, *Continued*

Medical Foods	***Modified Nutrient(s) (mg/100 g)***	***Protein Equiv[a] (g/100 g, source)***	***Fat (g/100 g, source)***	***Carbohydrate (g/100 g, source)***	***Energy (kcal/100 g/kJ/100 g)***	***Linoleic Acid/ α-Linolenic Acid (mg/100 g)***
XLYS Maxamum®	LYS 0, TRP 0 L-carnitine 39 Taurine 140	40.0 Amino acids[c]	<1.0	34.0 Sugar, corn syrup solids	305/1693	0/0
			Vitaflo US LLC[f]			
GA Gel®	LYS 0, TRP 0 L-carnitine 46 Taurine 90	42.0 Amino acids[c]	0.0	43.0 Sugar, starch, dried glucose syrup	342/1430	0/0

Notes: ND = no data.

Values listed, although accurate at time of publication, are subject to change. The most current information may be obtained by referring to product labels.

Data supplied by each company.

[a]g protein equivalent = g nitrogen × 6.25.

[b]Abbott Nutrition, 625 Cleveland Avenue, Columbus, Ohio, 43215. 800-551-5838.

[c]All except glycine are in the L-form.

[d]Mead Johnson Nutritionals, 2400 West Lloyd Expressway, Evansville, Indiana 47721. 800-457-3550.

[e]Nutricia North America, PO Box 117, Gaithersburg, Maryland 20884. 800-365-7354.

[f]Vitaflo US LLC, 123 East Neck Road, Huntington, New York 11743. 888-848-2356.

foods. High biologic value proteins (eggs, fish, meat, and poultry) are avoided because of their high content of LYS and TRP. In tube-dependent patients, either cow's milk (see Appendix B) or other protein-containing liquid formulas are provided as sources of LYS and TRP. LYS, TRP, protein, and energy content of foods may be found in reference 169. For more extensive information on nutrient content of foods, access the United States Department of Agriculture database.[79]

Initiation of Nutrition Management and Management During Critical Illness or Following Trauma

During acute crises prompt, aggressive medical intervention is required.[6,152,153] Approaches to treatment of patients with GAI are similar to those of other intoxication organic acidemias. The major goal is to prevent encephalopathic crises during illness by reducing catabolism.[153,161,163,188,189] Adequate fluid is essential to prevent dehydration, especially if vomiting, diarrhea, and decreased fluid intake are evident. Dehydration may lead to acidosis, electrolyte imbalance, and may precipitate acute encephalopathic crisis.[134,161]

Initially, dietary LYS, TRP, and total protein must be eliminated (usually 24 to 48 hours) until organic acids are reduced and the patient is stable.[153] IV glucose (10% solution) and electrolytes at approximately 150 mL/kg/24 hours to provide a GIR of 10 mg/kg/min[6,78,189] should be administered. Aggressive nutrition intervention providing between 120 to 150 kcal/kg/24 hours is required to promote anabolism and attenuate catabolism. Kolker et al.[153] recommended energy intakes at approximately 120% DRIs.[6] Energy intakes fewer than 120 kcal/kg/24 hours are not sufficient to significantly reduce blood concentrations of toxic precursors. Intravenous lipids can be added via peripheral or central lines at 2 to 3 g/kg/day. A combination of parenteral and enteral nutrition should be used as tolerated. Oral riboflavin supplementation (100 to 200 mg/day) given with food and in 15 to 25 mg portions several times a day is initiated.

Sources of LYS and TRP may be introduced as the patient stabilizes. Intact protein should be initiated as soon as possible (within 24 to 48 hours) to prevent deficiency and promote anabolism.[153] Protein may be given via total parenteral nutrition or orally.[171] Standard parenteral solutions may be used temporarily until transition to full oral feeds. Guidelines vary as to how much protein to offer initially. If using standard parenteral solutions, initiate protein at approximately 0.8 g/kg/day and increase as tolerated, but do not exceed the prescribed LYS and TRP. If long-term parenteral nutrition is necessary, tailored solutions are available (see Appendix D). A comprehensive review of emergency medical and nutrition management may be found in reference 153.

Long-Term Nutrition Management

Once the neonate has been stabilized, transition to full oral feeds as tolerated. Long-term (chronic) nutrition management for the neonate will include all components noted above. Table 8.9 includes recommended intakes for age. Intake of sufficient nutrients is difficult to maintain in patients who are neurologically impaired. Reflux, nausea, vomiting, spasticity, choreoathetosis, oral-motor dysfunction, non-ambulation, intermittent fevers, and constipation pose challenges to clinicians. For these patients, long-term G-tube feedings are usually required and will be limited to liquid preparations of medical food mixtures including most, it not all, of the components noted in Table 8.8. Antiemetics may be prescribed and valproic acid may be administered for seizures, and may depress appetite as well as enhance urinary loss of carnitine.[123] Drug-nutrient interactions must be assessed in all patients to ensure no long-term negative effects on nutrition status. A diet for a 4-month-old infant weighing 4.1 kg is given in Table 8.11.

Assessment of Nutrition Management

Laboratory monitoring of blood and urine organic acids is required to ensure adequate nutrition and health status. Because of the complexity of the disease and the variable phenotypes, there are no reliable biomarkers that truly reflect the clinical status of patients with GAI.[187] Unlike patients with other organic acidurias, patients with GAI might excrete high concentrations of glutaric and 3-OH glutaric acids but be in relatively good health. During

Table 8.11 ***Medical Food Mixture for a 4-Month-Old Infant with GAI Weighing 6.1 kg***

	Amount	*LYS (mg)*	*TRP (mg)*	*Carnitine (mg)*	*Protein (g)*	*Energy (kcal)*
Similac® Advance® powder with iron	48 g	430	84	4	5.2	252
XLYS, XTRP Analog® powder	113 g	0	0	11	14.6	537
L-carnitine (100 mg/mL)	6.0 mL	0	0	600	0.0	0
Water to make*						
Total		430	84	614	19.6	789
Per kg body weight		70	14	101	3.0	129

Notes: Feed every 3 hours.
See Table 8.9 for recommended daily intakes.
If infant does not grow normally linearly, see Chapter 3, Table 3.1.
*Add water to yield 945 mL (~32 fluid oz).

nutrition management, the goal is to maintain plasma glutaric acid concentrations in treatment range <250 ng/mL.[149] Concentrations vary and may not accurately reflect status. Morton et al.[138] reported plasma glutaric acid concentrations ranging from 4.8 to 14.2 μmol/L (nL 0 to 5.6 μmol/L) and urinary glutaric acid concentrations from 12.5 to 196 mg/g creatinine (nL 0.5 to 8.4 mg/g creatinine) by Amish patients. High excretors and low excretors may respond to nutrition management differently, making it difficult to adjust the diet.[161,188,190] Moreover, urine organic acid concentrations do not correlate well with cerebral spinal fluid concentrations.[134] Overall, lack of correlation between genotype and phenotype provides a challenge to effective nutrition management.

Assessment of nutrition management should be aimed toward maintaining growth and nutrition status[152,158] (see Chapter 3). Prevention of malnutrition is paramount,[152,158,159] and careful monitoring of the concentrations of plasma amino acids, including LYS, TRP, and protein status, will help ensure adherence to the nutrition prescription. Plasma LYS and TRP should be maintained at near normal concentrations: LYS 45 to 90 μmol/L.[101-104] Not all laboratories quantitate plasma TRP concentration that is essential to prevent TRP deficiency. Low plasma TRP concentrations may result in sleep irregularity,[191,192] weight loss, and impaired nitrogen retention.[33]

Protein status indices should be assessed regularly (see Chapter 3, Table 3.7). Measurement of transthyretin (prealbumin) is recommended as a sensitive marker of current protein status. Arnold et al.[44] reported that low plasma concentrations of transthyretin, but not albumin, significantly correlated with impaired hematopoiesis and poor growth in treated children with phenylketonuria (PKU). Routine monitoring of iron and protein status is recommended for children treated for an IMD (see Chapter 3, Table 3.7).

Deficient trace mineral and vitamin intakes and plasma concentrations have been reported in children consuming elemental formulas.[56,180,193] Thus, routine assessment of adequacy of mineral and vitamin intakes is required (see Chapter 3, Tables 3.7 and 3.9).

Home Monitoring

Parents and caregivers must be counseled on how to carefully monitor their child's clinical status and daily diet. Measurement of urine ketones using Ketostix® Reagent Strips (Bayer Health Care, Morristown, New Jersey) is recommended to assess impending ketosis that may occur without obvious clinical symptoms. Urine ketones should be maintained at zero to trace concentrations. Additionally, assessment of feeding tolerance is essential because an initial sign of clinical problems is vomiting. Parents should be taught to provide appropriate feeds in response to either a change in clinical status or increased urinary ketones.

Parents and caregivers should be taught to monitor hydration status, especially if the patient is dysarthric and cannot communicate. Simple signs of dehydration include dry mouth, decreased urine output, lethargy, and poor skin elasticity.

All patients with an IMD in which illness or stress cause metabolic decompensation require an emergency letter with the following information: name of disease, symptoms and consequences of metabolic decompensation, treatment strategies including plan for stabilization, type and amount of IV fluids, administration of detoxifying or coenzyme therapy, and metabolic physician contact information for transfer or consultation.

Recommended biochemical monitoring during hospital admission for acute illness includes complete blood count, electrolytes, blood gases, plasma glucose, urine ketones, serum creatinine and urea, plasma free and acyl carnitines, and C-reactive protein.[152] Additional blood analyses may be indicated based on the clinical situation.

Outcomes of Nutrition Management

Early diagnosis and aggressive medical and nutrition management will positively affect outcome in patients with GAI. Researchers have reported near-normal development in many patients treated neonatally.[142,158,163,173] However, even with newborn screening, early diagnosis and medical and nutrition management, one-third of patients do not respond and still suffer from brain injury,[188] while early diagnosis and treatment can reduce neurologic complications in some patients.[194,195] Asymptomatic newborns with screened and carefully managed GAI may have significantly reduced basal ganglia injury from approximately 90 to 35%.[188] The long-term benefit to patients of newborn screening, early diagnosis, and nutrition management is still being determined.

Iafolla and Kahler[162] first reported positive clinical outcomes in a patient diagnosed and managed with a LYS- and TRP-restricted diet using medical food prior to onset of acute encephalopathic crisis. Boneh et al.[173] provided evidence that newborn screening and diagnosis with early and aggressive medical and nutrition management could prevent severe neurologic complications. Early nutrition and medical therapy also supported normal to high cognitive function and gross motor skills.[173]

Patients who develop acute encephalopathy before or during treatment may suffer permanent loss of motor function, but retain cognitive skills despite nutrition intervention. Patients with late onset GAI may suffer chronic neurologic deterioration even without onset of encephalopathy.[143,195] Nutrition management has had mixed results on clinical outcome.[158] Dyskinesia and gross motor delay[196] continue in most patients but some show improvement, even if modest.[138,158,161] Brandt et al.[181] reported that nutrition management improved motor activity and decreased hyperkinesia in three patients with late-treated GAI. In contrast, others have reported no improvement in clinical course after instituting a LYS-restricted diet.[160] Reduction in urinary excretion of glutaric acid and 3-OH glutaric acid may not occur after initiation of the diet.[138,161]

Maternal Glutaric Aciduria Type 1

Offspring born to women with undiagnosed maternal GAI (MGA1) have been reported.[197,198] Mothers were found to have GAI from the newborn screen of their offspring. Crombez et al.[197] reported two women with undiagnosed GAI who were identified by low plasma carnitine in their offspring. Evaluation of the mothers showed low plasma carnitine and acylcarnitine concentrations that were in the normal range but urine glutaric acid and 3-OH glutaric acid excretion that were elevated. Offspring were normal and mothers were in good health, except for intermittent fatigue.[197] In the other reported cases, 2 infants born to untreated mothers had structural changes in the brain at 4 months of age, but overall normal physical and neurologic development at ages 2 and 5 years.[198]

Biotin Response Multiple Carboxylase Deficiency

Introduction

Biotinidase deficiency (BD; OMIM 253260)[1] (late-onset multiple carboxylase deficiency) is an autosomal recessive inherited disorder in which the body cannot reutilize biotin, an essential nutrient.[199] Partial and profound BD occurs in approximately 1 in 60,000 newborns. Patients with partial BD often do not develop clinical symptoms, but this is not universal.[200]

Holocarboxylase synthetase (HCS) deficiency (OMIM 235270)[1] is a severe metabolic disorder of the biotin-responsive multiple carboxylases. HCS deficiency was initially described as early-onset multiple carboxylase deficiency because onset of symptoms usually presented early in life, in comparison with BD. Patients with less severe HCS deficiency and later disease onset may present with metabolic acidosis and broad spectrum organic acidurias. Both HCS deficiency and BD may be distinguished by a serum biotinidase assay.

Biochemistry

Biotin is an essential nutrient and functions as a coenzyme in four important carboxylation reactions involved in fatty acid synthesis, gluconeogenesis, and amino acid catabolism[201,202] (see Figure 8.6). In nature, biotin exists in free and protein-bound forms, the latter being the most common food form. Biotinidase is required to liberate protein-bound food sources for use by the body. The lack of free endogenous biotin can result in metabolic acidosis, coma, and death.

The biotin-dependent carboxylases that have been identified in humans are propionyl-CoA carboxylase (PCC), methylcrotonyl-CoA carboxylase (MCC), pyruvate carboxylase (PC), and two forms of acetyl-CoA carboxylase (isoforms ACC-1 and ACC-2).[202] With exception of ACC-2, all other carboxylases are mitochondrial enzymes. Holocarboxylase synthetase (EC 6.3.1.10) catalyzes the incorporation of biotin into the active carboxylases.[203,204] The

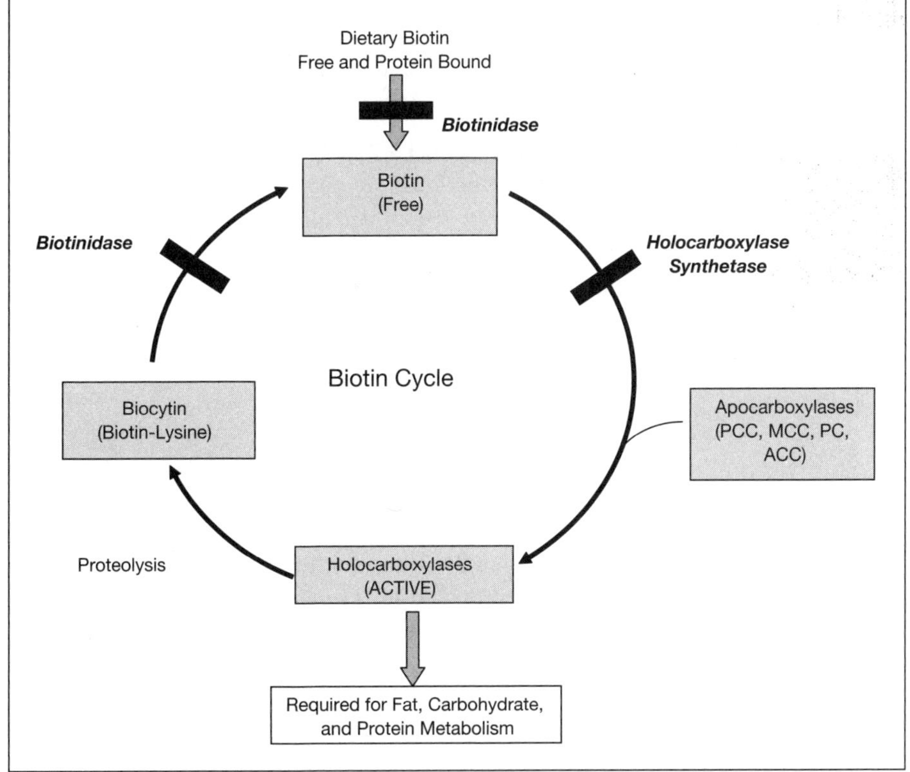

Figure 8.6 *Biotin Cycle*

Note: Black bars indicate sites of enzyme defects.

biotinylation of these carboxylases is essential for enzyme activation. A defect in activation has serious metabolic and clinical consequences and is potentially lethal.[201]

Molecular Biology

Profound BD results when biotinidase activity is <10% of normal while partial BD results when biotinidase activity is between 10 and 30% of normal activity.[205] Normal serum biotinidase activity is reported as between 6.30 and 10.54 nmol/min/mL[206] and normal ranges may differ among laboratories.[200] Over 100 mutations that cause BD have been reported[207,208] and in patients with profound BD, 13 novel mutations have been identified. Mutations in the HCS gene vary significantly among ethnic groups.[204] In Europeans, the predominant mutation is IVS10+5G to A, whereas in Japanese there are several distinct mutations. Over 20 mutations in the HCS gene and approximately 30 mutations in biotinidase have been reported (see Chapter 1).[209] In patients with profound BD no direct genotype/phenotype correlations have been reported.[210]

Newborn Screening

Neonatal screening for biotinidase and HCS deficiencies has been effective in preventing death and irreversible brain damage. Newborn screening may be inconclusive and follow up with a confirmatory diagnosis is essential to prevent irreversible morbidity.[211] Screening for these disorders is either required by law or offered in the majority of states.[17] See Chapter 2 for a review of newborn screening for inherited metabolic disorders.

Diagnosis

Signs and symptoms of biotinidase and HCS deficiencies may appear from early infancy up until 10 years of age.[209] Age at presentation is dependent, in part, on genotype.[212] Yang et al.[204] reported patients with the Japanese HCS mutation present neonatally. Non-Japanese patients with HCS deficiency present later in infancy at a median age of 9 months. Symptomatic patients may present with ketolactic acidosis and organic aciduria with elevated concentrations of 3-hydroxyisolvaleric acid, 3-methylcrotonylglycine, 3-hydroxypropionate, methylcitrate, and lactate.[213] In patients with HCS deficiency, respiratory symptoms are the most common initial clinical finding.[209] One late-treated patient with HCS deficiency had an initial clinical presentation of diabetic ketoacidosis.[214]

Patients with HCS deficiency often present with characteristic features of multiple carboxylase deficiency, while patients with BD have variable clinical presentations.[209] Plasma biotin concentrations are normal in patients with HCS deficiency.[209,214] Confirmatory diagnosis of serum biotinidase activity is required in patients with suspected multiple carboxylase deficiencies, in part because of indistinguishable clinical symptoms between HCS deficiency and BD.

Prenatal diagnosis of BD or HCS deficiency, using enzymatic and molecular analyses of biotinidase activity in either chorionic fluid or amniotic fluid, has been described,[206,210,215] and reported prenatal diagnosis in one patient with HCS deficiency completed by means of enzyme assays from amniotic fluid and confirmed postnatally by fibroblast studies.[215] Biotin therapy (10 mg/day) was started in the pregnant mother at 20 weeks gestation. Algorithms are available to clinicians to assist in screening and diagnosis of organic acidemias.[18]

Outcomes if Untreated

Untreated and late-treated patients with profound BD may develop vision and hearing loss, alopecia, dermatitis, and irreversible neurologic deficits.[209,212,216,217] Some patients may also develop candidiasis, a fungal infection. Patients with partial BD may suffer from alopecia, dermatitis, and hypotonia, but usually only during times of infection and acute illness. Audio-visual deficits and neurologic damage have not been reported in patients with HCS deficiency.[209]

Weber et al.[217] reported delay in attaining developmental milestones in patients with BD who had residual enzyme activity less than 1% and not detected by newborn screening. Differences were reported in communication skills, daily living skills, and socialization between patients identified through newborn screening compared to those who were not detected, despite some enzyme activity.

Hearing loss may occur in approximately 76% of untreated patients with BD.[218] Biotin therapy can halt further hearing loss, but the loss is not reversible.[218,219] Genotype/phenotype correlation for hearing loss has been reported in patients who are homozygous for specific biotinidase mutations.[220]

Nutrition Management

Biotin is a water-soluble vitamin found in small amounts in a wide variety of foods, and liver contains one of the highest concentrations (100 μg/100 g), while fruits and vegetables contain roughly 1 μg/100 g.[72] Daily adequate intakes for biotin range from 5 μg (normal infants 0 through 6 months) to 30 μg for adults and women during pregnancy and lactation. Biotin requirements may be met by food sources and gut bacteria synthesis. However, patients with biotin-responsive multiple carboxylase deficiencies do not consume sufficient amounts of biotin to supply requirements. There is no tolerable Upper Limit (UL) suggested for biotin. The UL is defined as "the highest level of intake likely to pose no risk of adverse effects for almost all people."[72]

The cornerstone of nutrition management is oral biotin administration, which must be started immediately after diagnosis is confirmed. Patients should be treated with biotin regardless of residual enzyme activity or genotype.[218] Treatment with biotin is recommended even for patients with partial BD.[200] The required dose is dependent on severity of the enzyme defect. Most patients show significant improvement in clinical symptoms and correction of biochemical manifestations at pharmacologic doses ranging between 10 to 20 mg/day.[201] Higher doses (up to 100 mg/day) may be required in some patients.[201,221,222] Biotin toxicity has not been reported in patients provided daily oral doses of up to 200 mg and 20 mg IV.[72] Lifelong biotin supplementation is necessary.

Predicting who will respond to biotin therapy is not clear-cut based on biochemical and molecular data.[212] For this reason, it is recommended that all infants identified by newborn screening and confirmed with profound BD be treated.[218]

Results of Nutrition Management

Biotin-responsive patients with biotinidase or HSC deficiency have good clinical outcomes.[209] Patients with partial response may have some skin and neurologic difficulties later in life.

Newborn screening, diagnosis, and biotin treatment have had a profound positive effect on patient outcomes. Patients with biotin-responsive BD, identified by newborn screening and diagnosed and treated early in infancy, have significantly better outcomes compared to late-treated patients.[208,212,217] Late-treated (symptomatic) patients with BD have hearing impairment, optic atrophy, developmental delay, and neurologic damage, none of which have been found in early biotin-treated patients.[217]

Assessment of Specific Aspects of Nutrition Management

Patients with BD or HCS deficiency should be monitored for biotin adequacy. Families and patients should be counseled to look for visual signs of biotin deficiency, including dermatitis and hair changes; prolonged biotin deficiency can result in alopecia. Quantitation of serum biotin concentrations may be warranted when clinical signs of deficiency are visible. Normal serum biotin concentrations in healthy adults are between 34 to 89 ng/mL.[223] However, in normal healthy adults made biotin deficient, serum biotin concentrations did not decrease significantly after 20 days. Mock et al.[223] reported that increased urinary 3-hydroxyisovaleric acid excretion and decreased excretion of biotin were sensitive indicators of biotin status.

Maternal Biotinidase Deficiency

One case has been published of a 20-year-old female who presented at 22 weeks gestation.[224] Upon clinic presentation the patient had been compliant in taking her biotin supplementation (10 mg daily). Biotin supplementation was increased to 15 mg twice daily throughout pregnancy, which was similar to her prescribed dose during puberty. A normal infant was born and met developmental milestones at 3 months of age.

CONCLUSION

With expanded newborn screening, early diagnosis, and aggressive medical and nutrition management, many patients with an organic acidemia now have an improved quality of life. Nutrition management is still the primary approach to treatment. Newborn screening, diagnosis, and therapy have been instrumental in avoiding lifelong medical problems, neurologic complications, and in some cases, death. Compliance to daily biotin administration is imperative to the health and well-being of patients with carboxylase deficiencies. Biotin supplementation does not cure the disease and monitoring and long-term follow up are essential.

REFERENCES

1. National Center for Biotechnology Information. OMIM™—Online Mendelian Inheritance in Man™ (database). Available at: http://www.ncbi.nlm.nih.gov/sites/entrez?db=omim. Accessed February 2, 2008.
2. Schoen EJ, Baker JC, Colby CJ, To TT. Cost-benefit analysis of universal tandem mass spectrometry for newborn screening. *Pediatrics*. 2002;110:781–786.
3. Ciske JB, Hoffman G, Hanson K, et al. Newborn screening in Wisconsin: program overview and test addition. *WMJ*. 2000;99:38–42.
4. Cohn RM, Roth KS. Hyperammonemia, bane of the brain. *Clin Pediatr (Phila)*. 2004;43:683–689.
5. Felipo V, Butterworth RF. Neurobiology of ammonia. *Prog Neurobiol*. 2002;67:259–279.
6. Prietsch V, Lindner M, Zschocke J, Nyhan WL, Hoffmann GF. Emergency management of inherited metabolic diseases. *J Inherit Metab Dis*. 2002;25:531–546.

7. Sbai D, Narcy C, Thompson GN, et al. Contribution of odd-chain fatty acid oxidation to propionate production in disorders of propionate metabolism. *Am J Clin Nutr*. 1994;59:1332–1337.
8. Leonard JV. Stable isotope studies in propionic and methylmalonic acidaemia. *Eur J Pediatr*. 1997;156(Suppl 1):S67–S69.
9. Ogier de Baulny H, Saudubray JM. Branched-chain organic aciduria. In: Fernandes J, Saudubray JM, van den Berghe G, eds. *Inborn Metabolic Diseases. Diagnosis and Treatment*. 3rd ed. Berlin, Germany: Springer-Verlag; 2000:197–212.
10. Barshop BA, Yoshida I, Ajami A, et al. Metabolism of 1-13C-propionate in vivo in patients with disorders of propionate metabolism. *Pediatr Res*. 1991;30:15–22.
11. Chandler RJ, Venditti CP. Genetic and genomic systems to study methylmalonic acidemia. *Mol Genet Metab*. 2005;86:34–43.
12. Desviat LR, Perez B, Perez-Cerda C, Rodriguez-Pombo P, Clavero S, Ugarte M. Propionic acidemia: mutation update and functional and structural effects of the variant alleles. *Mol Genet Metab*. 2004;83:28–37.
13. Lempp TJ, Suormala T, Siegenthaler R, et al. Mutation and biochemical analysis of 19 probands with mut^0 and 13 with mut^- methylmalonic aciduria: identification of seven novel mutations. *Mol Genet Metab*. 2007;90:284–290.
14. Worgan LC, Niles K, Tirone JC, et al. Spectrum of mutations in mut methylmalonic acidemia and identification of a common Hispanic mutation and haplotype. *Hum Mutat*. 2006;27:31–43.
15. Peters HL, Wood L, Benoist JF. Development of pharmacological therapy to treat methylmalonic aciduria (MMA) resulting from mutase deficiency. *J Inherit Metab Dis*. 2007;30(Suppl 1):34A.
16. Janata J, Kogekar N, Fenton WA. Expression and kinetic characterization of methylmalonyl-CoA mutase from patients with the mut^- phenotype: evidence for naturally occurring interallelic complementation. *Hum Mol Genet*. 1997;6:1457–1464.
17. National Newborn Screening and Genetics Resource Center. National Newborn Screening Status Report, updated September 16, 2008. Available at: http://genes-r-us.uthscsa.edu/nbsdisorders.pdf. Accessed September 19, 2008.
18. American College of Medical Genetics. Newborn screening ACT sheets and confirmatory algorithms. Available at: http://www.acmg.net/resources/policies/ACT/condition-analyte-links.htm. Accessed February 27, 2008.
19. Coude FX, Sweetman L, Nyhan WL. Inhibition by propionyl-coenzyme A of N-acetylglutamate synthetase in rat liver mitochondria: a possible explanation for hyperammonemia in propionic and methylmalonic acidemia. *J Clin Invest*. 1979;64:1544–1551.
20. Stewart PM, Walser M. Failure of the normal ureagenic response to amino acids in organic acid-loaded rats. Proposed mechanism for the hyperammonemia of propionic and methylmalonic acidemia. *J Clin Invest*. 1980;66:484–492.
21. Filipowicz HR, Ernst SL, Ashurst CL, Pasquali M, Longo N. Metabolic changes associated with hyperammonemia in patients with propionic acidemia. *Mol Genet Metab*. 2006;88:123–130.
22. Inoue S, Krieger I, Sarnaik A, Ravindranath Y, Fracassa M, Ottenbreit MJ. Inhibition of bone marrow stem cell growth in vitro by methylmalonic acid: a mechanism for pancytopenia in a patient with methylmalonic acidemia. *Pediatr Res*. 1981;15:95–98.
23. Stork LC, Ambruso DR, Wallner SF, et al. Pancytopenia in propionic acidemia: hematologic evaluation and studies of hematopoiesis in vitro. *Pediatr Res*. 1986;20:783–788.

24. Raby RB, Ward JC, Herrod HG. Propionic acidaemia and immunodeficiency. *J Inherit Metab Dis*. 1994;17:250–251.
25. Fowler B, Leonard JV, Baumgartner MR. Causes of and diagnostic approach to methylmalonic acidurias. *J Inherit Metab Dis*. 2008;31:350–360.
26. Lehnert W, Sperl W, Suormala T, Baumgartner ER. Propionic acidaemia: clinical, biochemical and therapeutic aspects: experience in 30 patients. *Eur J Pediatr*. 1994;153:S68–S80.
27. Inoue Y, Ohse M, Shinka T, Kuhara T. Prenatal diagnosis of propionic acidemia by measuring methylcitric acid in dried amniotic fluid on filter paper using GC/MS. *J Chromatogr B Analyt Technol Biomed Life Sci*. 2008;870:160–163.
28. Higginbottom MC, Sweetman L, Nyhan WL. A syndrome of methylmalonic aciduria, homocystinuria, megaloblastic anemia and neurologic abnormalities in a vitamin B_{12}-deficient breast-fed infant of a strict vegetarian. *N Engl J Med*. 1978; 299:317–323.
29. Specker BL, Miller D, Norman EJ, Greene H, Hayes KC. Increased urinary methylmalonic acid excretion in breast-fed infants of vegetarian mothers and identification of an acceptable dietary source of vitamin B-12. *Am J Clin Nutr*. 1988; 47:89–92.
30. Campbell CD, Ganesh J, Ficicioglu C. Two newborns with nutritional vitamin B_{12} deficiency: challenges in newborn screening for vitamin B_{12} deficiency. *Haematologica*. 2005;90:ECR45.
31. Ampola MG. *Metabolic Diseases in Pediatric Practice*. Boston, MA: Little, Brown & Company; 1982:119–140.
32. Acosta PB, Yannicelli S. Protocol 13. Propionic or methylmalonic acidemia. *Nutrition Support Protocols*. 4th ed. Columbus, OH: Ross Products Division, Abbott Laboratories; 2001.
33. Acosta PB. Nutrition support of inborn errors of metabolism. In: Queen Samour P, Helm KK, Lang CE, eds. *Handbook of Pediatric Nutrition*. 2nd ed. Rockville, MD: Aspen; 1999:243–292.
34. Elsas LJ, Acosta PB. Inherited metabolic disease: amino acids, organic acids, and galactose. In: Shils ME, Shike M, Olson J, Ross AC, Caballero B, Cousins RJ, eds. *Modern Nutrition in Health and Disease*. 10th ed. Philadelphia, PA: Lippincott Williams & Wilkins; 2005:909–959.
35. Queen PM, Fernhoff PM, Acosta PB. Protein and essential amino acid requirements in a child with propionic acidemia. *J Am Diet Assoc*. 1981;79:562–565.
36. Yannicelli S, Acosta PB, Velazquez A, et al. Improved growth and nutrition status in children with methylmalonic or propionic acidemia fed an elemental medical food. *Mol Genet Metab*. 2003;80:181–188.
37. North KN, Korson MS, Gopal YR, et al. Neonatal-onset propionic acidemia: neurologic and developmental profiles, and implications for management. *J Pediatr*. 1995;126:916–922.
38. Touati G, Valayannopoulos V, Mention K, et al. Methylmalonic and propionic acidurias: management without or with a few supplements of specific amino acid mixture. *J Inherit Metab Dis*. 2006;29:288–298.
39. Lane TN, Spraker MK, Parker SS. Propionic acidemia manifesting with low isoleucine generalized exfoliative dermatosis. *Pediatr Dermatol*. 2007;24: 508–510.
40. De Raeve L, De Meirleir L, Ramet J, Vandenplas Y, Gerlo E. Acrodermatitis enteropathica-like cutaneous lesions in organic aciduria. *J Pediatr*. 1994;124: 416–420.

41. Mulder H, Walstra P. *The Milk Fat Globule. Emulsion Science Applied to Milk Products and Comparable Foods*. Farnham Royal, Bucks, England: Commonwealth Agricultural Bureaux; 1974:25–32.
42. Paradis M, Ackman RG. Localization of a marine source of odd chain-length fatty acids. I. The amphipod *Pontoporeia femorata* (kroyer). *Lipids*. 1976; 11:863–870.
43. Trumbo P, Schlicker S, Yates AA, Poos M. Dietary reference intakes for energy, carbohydrate, fiber, fat, fatty acids, cholesterol, protein and amino acids. *J Am Diet Assoc*. 2002;102:1621–1630.
44. Arnold GL, Vladutiu CJ, Kirby RS, Blakely EM, Deluca JM. Protein insufficiency and linear growth restriction in phenylketonuria. *J Pediatr*. 2002;141:243–246.
45. Baumgarter ER, Viardot C. Long-term follow-up of 77 patients with isolated methylmalonic acidaemia. *J Inherit Metab Dis*. 1995;18:138–142.
46. Luder AS, Yannicelli S, Green CL. Normal growth and development with unrestricted protein intake after severe infantile propionic acidaemia. *J Inherit Metab Dis*. 1989;12:307–311.
47. Sanjurjo P, Ruiz JI, Montejo M. Inborn errors of metabolism with a protein-restricted diet: effect on polyunsaturated fatty acids. *J Inherit Metab Dis*. 1997;20: 783–789.
48. Vlaardingerbroek H, Hornstra G, de Koning TJ, et al. Essential polyunsaturated fatty acids in plasma and erythrocytes of children with inborn errors of amino acid metabolism. *Mol Genet Metab*. 2006;88:159–165.
49. Aldamiz-Echevarria L, Sanjurjo P, Elorz J, et al. Effect of docosahexaenoic acid administration on plasma lipid profile and metabolic parameters of children with methylmalonic acidaemia. *J Inherit Metab Dis*. 2006;29:58–63.
50. Feillet F, Bodamer OA, Dixon MA, Sequeira S, Leonard JV. Resting energy expenditure in disorders of propionate metabolism. *J Pediatr*. 2000;136:659–663.
51. Thomas JA, Bernstein LE, Greene CL, Koeller DM. Apparent decreased energy requirements in children with organic acidemias: preliminary observations. *J Am Diet Assoc*. 2000;100:1074–1076.
52. Marsden D, Barshop BA, Capistrano-Estrada S, et al. Anabolic effect of human growth hormone: management of inherited disorders of catabolic pathways. *Biochem Med Metab Biol*. 1994;52:145–154.
53. Bodamer OA, Hoffmann GF, Visser GH, et al. Assessment of energy expenditure in metabolic disorders. *Eur J Pediatr*. 1997;156(Suppl 1):S24–S28.
54. Thompson GN, Chalmers RA. Increased urinary metabolite excretion during fasting in disorders of propionate metabolism. *Pediatr Res*. 1990;27:413–416.
55. MacLean W, Graham G. *Pediatric Nutrition in Clinical Practice*. Menlo Park, CA: Addison-Wesley; 1982.
56. Yannicelli S, Hambidge KM, Picciano MF. Decreased selenium intake and low plasma selenium concentrations leading to clinical symptoms in a child with propionic acidaemia. *J Inherit Metab Dis*. 1992;15:261–268.
57. Matern D, Seydewitz HH, Lehnert W, Niederhoff H, Leititis JU, Brandis M. Primary treatment of propionic acidemia complicated by acute thiamine deficiency. *J Pediatr*. 1996;129:758–760.
58. Treacy E, Arbour L, Chessex P, et al. Glutathione deficiency as a complication of methylmalonic acidemia: response to high doses of ascorbate. *J Pediatr*. 1996;129: 445–448.
59. Talbot JC, Gummerson NW, Kluge W, Shaw DL, Groves C, Lealman GT. Osteoporotic femoral fracture in a child with propionic acidaemia presenting as non-accidental injury. *Eur J Pediatr*. 2006;165:496–497.

60. Orwoll ES. The effects of dietary protein insufficiency and excess on skeletal health. *Bone*. 1992;13:343–350.
61. Krieger NS, Sessler NE, Bushinsky DA. Acidosis inhibits osteoblastic and stimulates osteoclastic activity in vitro. *Am J Physiol*. 1992;262:F442–F448.
62. Bounds W, Skinner J, Carruth BR, Ziegler P. The relationship of dietary and lifestyle factors to bone mineral indexes in children. *J Am Diet Assoc*. 2005;105: 735–741.
63. Chalmers RA, Stacey TE, Tracey BM, et al. L-carnitine insufficiency in disorders of organic acid metabolism: response to L-carnitine by patients with methylmalonic aciduria and 3-hydroxy-3-methylglutaric aciduria. *J Inherit Metab Dis*. 1984;7(Suppl 2):109–110.
64. Di Donato S, Rimoldi M, Garavaglia B, Uziel G. Propionylcarnitine excretion in propionic and methylmalonic acidurias: a cause of carnitine deficiency. *Clin Chim Acta*. 1984;139:13–21.
65. Rehman HU. Fish odor syndrome. *Postgrad Med J*. 1999;75:451–452.
66. Barnes ND, Hull D, Balgobin L, Gompertz D. Biotin-responsive propionicacidaemia. *Lancet*. 1970;2:244–245.
67. Wolf B, Hsia YE. Biotin responsiveness in propionicacidaemia. *Lancet*. 1978;2:901.
68. Bain MD, Jones M, Borriello SP, et al. Contribution of gut bacterial metabolism to human metabolic disease. *Lancet*. 1988;1:1078–1079.
69. Thompson GN, Walter JH, Bresson JL, et al. Sources of propionate in inborn errors of propionate metabolism. *Metabolism*. 1990;39:1133–1137.
70. van der Meer SB, Poggi F, Spada M, et al. Clinical outcome and long-term management of 17 patients with propionic acidaemia. *Eur J Pediatr*. 1996;155:205–210.
71. Verhoef P, de Groot LC. Dietary determinants of plasma homocysteine concentrations. *Semin Vasc Med*. 2005;5:110–123.
72. Otten JJ, Hellwig JP, Meyers LD. *Dietary Reference Intakes: The Essential Guide to Nutrient Requirements*. Washington, DC: National Academies Press; 2006:197–201.
73. FAO/WHO/UNU. *Expert Consultation on Energy and Protein Requirements*. WHO technical report series; No. 724. Geneva, Switzerland: World Health Organization. 1985;71–112.
74. FAO/WHO/UNU. *Expert Consultation on Protein and Amino Acid Requirements in Human Nutrition*. WHO technical report series; No 935. Geneva, Switzerland: World Health Organization. 2002.
75. Reeds PJ, Garlick PJ. Protein and amino acid requirements and the composition of complementary foods. *J Nutr*. 2003;133:2953S–2961S.
76. Walter JH, MacDonald A. The use of amino acid supplements in inherited metabolic disease. *J Inherit Metab Dis*. 2006;29:279–280.
77. Yannicelli S. Nutrition therapy of organic acidaemias with amino acid-based formulas: emphasis on methylmalonic and propionic acidaemia. *J Inherit Metab Dis*. 2006;29:281–287.
78. Yannicelli S, Camp K. Enteral and parenteral nutrition therapy in inherited metabolic disease. In: Baker SS, Baker RD, Davis AM, eds. *Pediatric Nutrition Support*. Sudbury, MA: Jones and Bartlett; 2007:409–431.
79. USDA Agricultural Research Service. Available at: http://www/nal.usda.gov/fnic/foodcomp/search. Accessed September 16, 2008.
80. Huner G, Baykal T, Demir F, Demirkol M. Breastfeeding experience in inborn errors of metabolism other than phenylketonuria. *J Inherit Metab Dis*. 2005;28:457–465.
81. Gokcay G, Baykal T, Gokdemir Y, Demirkol M. Breast feeding in organic acidaemias. *J Inherit Metab Dis*. 2006;29:304–310.

82. MacDonald A, Depondt E, Evans S, et al. Breast feeding in IMD. *J Inherit Metab Dis*. 2006;29:299–303.
83. Al Essa M, Rahbeeni Z, Jumaah S, et al. Infectious complications of propionic acidemia in Saudia Arabia. *Clin Genet*. 1998;54:90–94.
84. Kahler SG, Millington DS, Cederbaum SD, et al. Parenteral nutrition in propionic and methylmalonic acidemia. *J Pediatr*. 1989;115:235–241.
85. Hyman SL, Porter CA, Page TJ, Iwata BA, Kissel R, Batshaw ML. Behavior management of feeding disturbances in urea cycle and organic acid disorders. *J Pediatr*. 1987;111:558–562.
86. Rossi-Fanelli F, Laviano A. Role of brain tryptophan and serotonin in secondary anorexia. *Adv Exp Med Biol*. 2003;527:225–232.
87. Plata-Salaman CR. Central nervous system mechanisms contributing to the cachexia-anorexia syndrome. *Nutrition*. 2000;16:1009–1012.
88. Gietzen DW, Hao S, Anthony TG. Mechanisms of food intake repression in indispensable amino acid deficiency. *Annu Rev Nutr*. 2007;27:63–78.
89. Jiang H, Rao KS, Yee VC, Kraus JP. Characterization of four variant forms of human propionyl-CoA carboxylase expressed in Escherichia coli. *J Biol Chem*. 2005;280:27719–27727.
90. Touma EH, Rashed M. Carbamyglu effective in lowering hyperammonemia in a 3-year old propionic acidemia patient. *J Inherit Metab Dis*. 2007;30(Suppl 1):35A.
91. Tuchman M, Caldovic L, Daikhin Y, et al. N-carbamylglutamate markedly enhances ureagenesis in N-acetylglutamate deficiency and propionic acidemia as measured by isotopic incorporation and blood biomarkers. *Pediatr Res*. 2008;64: 213–217.
92. Al Owain M, Freehauf C, Bernstein L, Kappy M, Thomas J. Growth hormone deficiency associated with methylmalonic acidemia. *J Pediatr Endocrinol Metab*. 2004;17:239–243.
93. Ogier de Baulny H, Benoist JF, Rigal O, Touati G, Rabier D, Saudubray JM. Methylmalonic and propionic acidaemias: management and outcome. *J Inherit Metab Dis*. 2005;28:415–423.
94. Sokal EM. Liver transplantation for inborn errors of liver metabolism. *J Inherit Metab Dis*. 2006;29:426–430.
95. Chandler RJ, Sloan J, Fu H, et al. Metabolic phenotype of methylmalonic acidemia in mice and humans: the role of skeletal muscle. *BMC Med Genet*. 2007;8:64.
96. Nyhan WL, Gargus JJ, Boyle K, Selby R, Koch R. Progressive neurologic disability in methylmalonic acidemia despite transplantation of the liver. *Eur J Pediatr*. 2002;161:377–379.
97. Morioka D, Kasahara M, Takada Y, et al. Living donor liver transplantation for pediatric patients with inheritable metabolic disorders. *Am J Transplant*. 2005; 5:2754–2763.
98. Barshes NR, Vanatta JM, Patel AJ, et al. Evaluation and management of patients with propionic acidemia undergoing liver transplantation: a comprehensive review. *Pediatr Transplant*. 2006;10:773–781.
99. Zwickler T, Lindner M, Aydin HI, et al. Diagnostic work-up and management of patients with isolated methylmalonic acidurias in European metabolic centres. *J Inherit Metab Dis*. 2008;31:361–367.
100. Scholl-Burgi S, Grissenauer G, Fendl A, Baumgartner S, Konstantopoulou V, Skladal D. Dietary therapy in propionic acidemia: recommended versus real protein supply. *J Inherit Metab Dis*. 2004;27:43A.

101. Meites S. *Pediatric Clinical Chemistry. Reference (Normal) Values*. Washington, DC: American Association for Clinical Chemistry; 1989.
102. MacLean WC Jr, Placko RP, Graham GG. Fasting plasma free amino acids of infants and children consuming cow milk proteins. *Johns Hopkins Med J*. 1978; 142:147–151.
103. Applegarth DA, Edelstein AD, Wong LT, Morrison BJ. Observed range of assay values for plasma and cerebrospinal fluid amino acid levels in infants and children aged 3 months to 10 years. *Clin Biochem*. 1979;12:173–178.
104. Soldin SJ, Brugnara C, Gunter KC, Wong EC. *Pediatric Reference Intervals*. 7th ed. Washington, DC: AAAC Press; 2007.
105. Al Hassnan ZN, Boyadjiev SA, Praphanphoj V, et al. The relationship of plasma glutamine to ammonium and of glycine to acid-base balance in propionic acidaemia. *J Inherit Metab Dis*. 2003;26:89–91.
106. Gropper SS, Acosta PB, Clarke-Sheehan N, Wenz E, Cheng M, Koch R. Trace element status of children with PKU and normal children. *J Am Diet Assoc*. 1988; 88:459–465.
107. Reilly C, Barrett JE, Patterson CM, Tinggi U, Latham SL, Marrinan A. Trace element nutrition status and dietary intake of children with phenylketonuria. *Am J Clin Nutr*. 1990;52:159–165.
108. Kayler LK, Merion RM, Lee S, et al. Long-term survival after liver transplantation in children with metabolic disorders. *Pediatr Transplant*. 2002;6:295–300.
109. Varvogli L, Repetto GM, Waisbren SE, Levy HL. High cognitive outcome in an adolescent with mut$^-$ methylmalonic acidemia. *Am J Med Genet*. 2000;96:192–195.
110. Nicolaides P, Leonard J, Surtees R. Neurological outcome of methylmalonic acidaemia. *Arch Dis Child*. 1998;78:508–512.
111. Dionisi-Vici C, Deodato F, Roschinger W, Rhead W, Wilcken B. "Classical" organic acidurias, propionic aciduria, methylmalonic aciduria and isovaleric aciduria: long-term outcome and effects of expanded newborn screening using tandem mass spectrometry. *J Inherit Metab Dis*. 2006;29:383–389.
112. van der Meer SB, Poggi F, Spada M, et al. Clinical outcome of long-term management of patients with vitamin B_{12}-unresponsive methylmalonic acidemia. *J Pediatr*. 1994;125:903–908.
113. Rutledge SL, Geraghty M, Mroczek E, Rosenblatt D, Kohout E. Tubulointerstitial nephritis in methylmalonic acidemia. *Pediatr Nephrol*. 1993;7:81–82.
114. Morath MA, Okun JG, Muller IB, et al. Neurodegeneration and chronic renal failure in methylmalonic aciduria—a pathophysiological approach. *J Inherit Metab Dis*. 2008;31:35–43.
115. Kashtan CE, Abousedira M, Rozen S, Manivel JC, McCann M, Tuchman M. Chronic administration of methylmalonic acid (MMA) to rats causes proteinuria and renal tubular injury [abstract]. *Pediatr Res*. 1998;1998:409.
116. Schmitt CP, Mehls O, Trefz FK, Horster F, Weber TL, Kolker S. Reversible end-stage renal disease in an adolescent patient with methylmalonic aciduria. *Pediatr Nephrol*. 2004;19:1182–1184.
117. Mirandola SR, Melo DR, Schuck PF, Ferreira GC, Wajner M, Castilho RF. Methylmalonate inhibits succinate-supported oxygen consumption by interfering with mitochondrial succinate uptake. *J Inherit Metab Dis*. 2008;31: 44–54.
118. Azar MR, Shakiba M, Tafreshi RI, Rashed MS. Heart failure in a patient with methylmalonic acidemia. *Mol Genet Metab*. 2007;92:188.

119. Mardach R, Verity MA, Cederbaum SD. Clinical, pathological, and biochemical studies in a patient with propionic acidemia and fatal cardiomyopathy. *Mol Genet Metab*. 2005;85:286–290.
120. Massoud AF, Leonard JV. Cardiomyopathy in propionic acidaemia. *Eur J Pediatr*. 1993;152:441–445.
121. Burlina AB, Dionisi-Vici C, Piovan S, et al. Acute pancreatitis in propionic acidaemia. *J Inherit Metab Dis*. 1995;18:169–172.
122. Kahler SG, Sherwood WG, Woolf D, et al. Pancreatitis in patients with organic acidemias. *J Pediatr*. 1994;124:239–243.
123. Shapira Y, Gutman A. Muscle carnitine deficiency in patients using valproic acid. *J Pediatr*. 1991;118:646–649.
124. Fanjiang G, Kleinman RE. Nutrition and performance in children. *Curr Opin Clin Nutr Metab Care*. 2007;10:342–347.
125. Deodato F, Rizzo C, Boenzi S, Baiocco F, Sabetta G, Dionisi-Vici C. Successful pregnancy in a woman with mut$^-$ methylmalonic acidaemia. *J Inherit Metab Dis*. 2002;25:133–134.
126. Diss E, Iams J, Reed N, Roe DS, Roe C. Methylmalonic aciduria in pregnancy: a case report. *Am J Obstet Gynecol*. 1995;172:1057–1059.
127. Wasserstein MP, Gaddipati S, Snyderman SE, Eddleman K, Desnick RJ, Sansaricq C. Successful pregnancy in severe methylmalonic acidaemia. *J Inherit Metab Dis*. 1999;22:788–794.
128. van Calcar SC, Harding CO, Davidson SR, Barness LA, Wolff JA. Case reports of successful pregnancy in women with maple syrup urine disease and propionic acidemia. *Am J Med Genet*. 1992;44:641–646.
129. Boneh A, Greaves RF, Garra G, Pitt JJ. Metabolic treatment of pregnancy and post-delivery period in a patient with cobalamin A disease. *Am J Obstet Gynecol*. 2002;187:225–226.
130. Koch R, Acosta PB, Williams JC. Nutritional therapy for pregnant women with a metabolic disorder. *Clin Perinatol*. 1995;22:1–14.
131. Lee PJ. Pregnancy issues in inherited metabolic disorders. *J Inherit Metab Dis*. 2006;29:311–316.
132. Goodman SI, Markey SP, Moe PG, Miles BS, Teng CC. Glutaric aciduria; a "new" disorder of amino acid metabolism. *Biochem Med*. 1975;12:12–21.
133. Hoffmann GF, Trefz FK, Barth PG, et al. Glutaryl-coenzyme A dehydrogenase deficiency: a distinct encephalopathy. *Pediatrics*. 1991;88:1194–1203.
134. Kolker S, Garbade SF, Greenberg CR, et al. Natural history, outcome, and treatment efficacy in children and adults with glutaryl-CoA dehydrogenase deficiency. *Pediatr Res*. 2006;59:840–847.
135. Kyllerman M, Steen G. Glutaric aciduria. A "common" metabolic disorder? *Arch Fr Pediatr*. 1980;37:279.
136. Lindner M, Kolker S, Schulze A, Christensen E, Greenberg CR, Hoffmann GF. Neonatal screening for glutaryl-CoA dehydrogenase deficiency. *J Inherit Metab Dis*. 2004;27:851–859.
137. Haworth JC, Booth FA, Chudley AE, et al. Phenotypic variability in glutaric aciduria type I: report of fourteen cases in five Canadian Indian kindreds. *J Pediatr*. 1991;118:52–58.
138. Morton DH, Bennett MJ, Seargeant LE, Nichter CA, Kelley RI. Glutaric aciduria type I: a common cause of episodic encephalopathy and spastic paralysis in the Amish of Lancaster County, Pennsylvania. *Am J Med Genet*. 1991;41:89–95.

139. Naylor EW, Chace DH. Automated tandem mass spectrometry for mass newborn screening for disorders in fatty acid, organic acid, and amino acid metabolism. *J Child Neurol*. 1999;14(Suppl 1):S4–S8.
140. Basinger AA, Booker JK, Frazier DM, Koeberl DD, Sullivan JA, Muenzer J. Glutaric acidemia type 1 in patients of Lumbee heritage from North Carolina. *Mol Genet Metab*. 2006;88:90–92.
141. Goodman SI, Frerman FE. Organic acidemias due to defects in lysine oxidation: 2-ketoadipic acidemia and glutaric acidemia. In: Scriver CR, Beaudet AL, Sly WS, Valle D, eds. *The Molecular Basis of Inherited Disease*. 6th ed. New York, NY: McGraw-Hill; 1989:845–853.
142. Baric I, Wagner L, Feyh P, Liesert M, Buckel W, Hoffmann GF. Sensitivity and specificity of free and total glutaric acid and 3-hydroxyglutaric acid measurements by stable-isotope dilution assays for the diagnosis of glutaric aciduria type I. *J Inherit Metab Dis*. 1999;22:867–881.
143. Busquets C, Merinero B, Christensen E, et al. Glutaryl-CoA dehydrogenase deficiency in Spain: evidence of two groups of patients, genetically and biochemically distinct. *Pediatr Res*. 2000;48:315–322.
144. Zinnanti WJ, Lazovic J, Housman C, et al. Mechanism of age-dependent susceptibility and novel treatment strategy in glutaric acidemia type I. *J Clin Invest*. 2007; 117:3258–3270.
145. Fu Z, Wang M, Paschke R, Rao KS, Frerman FE, Kim JJ. Crystal structures of human glutaryl-CoA dehydrogenase with and without an alternate substrate: structural bases of dehydrogenation and decarboxylation reactions. *Biochemistry*. 2004;43:9674–9684.
146. Goodman SI, Stein DE, Schlesinger S, et al. Glutaryl-CoA dehydrogenase mutations in glutaric acidemia (type I): review and report of thirty novel mutations. *Hum Mutat*. 1998;12:141–144.
147. American College of Medical Genetics. Newborn screening: toward a uniform screening panel and system. *Genet Med*. 2006;8(Suppl 1):1S–252S.
148. Smith WE, Millington DS, Koeberl DD, Lesser PS. Glutaric acidemia, type I, missed by newborn screening in an infant with dystonia following promethazine administration. *Pediatrics*. 2001;107:1184–1187.
149. Gallagher RC, Cowan TM, Goodman SI, Enns GM. Glutaryl-CoA dehydrogenase deficiency and newborn screening: retrospective analysis of a low excretor provides further evidence that some cases may be missed. *Mol Genet Metab*. 2005;86:417–420.
150. Lindner M, Ho S, Fang-Hoffmann J, Hoffmann GF, Kolker S. Neonatal screening for glutaric aciduria type I: strategies to proceed. *J Inherit Metab Dis*. 2006;29:378–382.
151. Tortorelli S, Hahn SH, Cowan TM, Brewster TG, Rinaldo P, Matern D. The urinary excretion of glutarylcarnitine is an informative tool in the biochemical diagnosis of glutaric acidemia type I. *Mol Genet Metab*. 2005;84:137–143.
152. Kolker S, Christensen E, Leonard JV, et al. Guideline for the diagnosis and management of glutaryl-CoA dehydrogenase deficiency (glutaric aciduria type I). *J Inherit Metab Dis*. 2007;30:5–22.
153. Kolker S, Greenberg CR, Lindner M, Muller E, Naughten ER, Hoffmann GF. Emergency treatment in glutaryl-CoA dehydrogenase deficiency. *J Inherit Metab Dis*. 2004;27:893–902.
154. Sauer SW, Okun JG, Fricker G, et al. Intracerebral accumulation of glutaric and 3-hydroxyglutaric acids secondary to limited flux across the blood–brain barrier constitute a biochemical risk factor for neurodegeneration in glutaryl-CoA dehydrogenase deficiency. *J Neurochem*. 2006;97:899–910.

155. Zinnanti WJ, Lazovic J, Wolpert EB, et al. A diet-induced mouse model for glutaric aciduria type I. *Brain*. 2006;129:899–910.
156. Sauer SW. Biochemistry and bioenergetics of glutaryl-CoA dehydrogenase deficiency. *J Inherit Metab Dis*. 2007;30:673–680.
157. Kolker S, Sauer SW, Hoffmann GF, Muller I, Morath MA, Okun JG. Pathogenesis of CNS involvement in disorders of amino and organic acid metabolism. *J Inherit Metab Dis*. 2008.
158. Yannicelli S, Rohr F, Warman ML. Nutrition support for glutaric acidemia type I. *J Am Diet Assoc*. 1994;94:183–188,191.
159. Muller E, Kolker S. Reduction of lysine intake while avoiding malnutrition—major goals and major problems in dietary treatment of glutaryl-CoA dehydrogenase deficiency. *J Inherit Metab Dis*. 2004;27:903–910.
160. Whelan DT, Hill R, Ryan ED, Spate M. L-glutaric acidemia: investigation of a patient and his family. *Pediatrics*. 1979;63:88–93.
161. Hoffmann GF, Athanassopoulos S, Burlina AB, et al. Clinical course, early diagnosis, treatment, and prevention of disease in glutaryl-CoA dehydrogenase deficiency. *Neuropediatrics*. 1996;27:115–123.
162. Iafolla AK, Kahler SG. Megalencephaly in the neonatal period as the initial manifestation of glutaric aciduria type I. *J Pediatr*. 1989;114:1004–1006.
163. Monavari AA, Naughten ER. Prevention of cerebral palsy in glutaric aciduria type 1 by dietary management. *Arch Dis Child*. 2000;82:67–70.
164. Clark HE, Mertz ET, Kwong EH, Howe JM, Delong DC. Amino acid requirements of men and women. I. Lysine. *J Nutr*. 1957;62:71–82.
165. Clark HE, Kenney MA, Goodwin AF, Goyal K, Mertz ET. Effect of certain factors on nitrogen retention and lysine requirements of adult human subjects. IV. Total nitrogen intake. *J Nutr*. 1963;81:223–229.
166. Fisher H, Brush MK, Griminger P. Reassessment of amino acid requirements of young women on low nitrogen diets: 1. Lysine and tryptophan. *Am J Clin Nutr*. 1969;22:1190–1196.
167. Snyderman SE, Norton PM, Fowler DI, Holt LE. The essential amino acid requirements of infants: lysine. *AMA J Dis Child*. 1959;97:175–185.
168. Tome D, Bos C. Lysine requirement through the human life cycle. *J Nutr*. 2007; 137:1642S–1645S.
169. Acosta PB, Yannicelli S. Protocol 9. Glutaric acidemia type I or 2-ketoadipic aciduria. *Nutrition Support Protocols*. 4th ed. Columbus, OH: Ross Products Division, Abbott Laboratories; 2001.
170. Hoffmann GF. Disorders of lysine catabolism and related cerebral organic acid disorder. In: Fernandes J, Saudubray JM, van den Berghe G, eds. *Inborn Metabolic Diseases. Diagnosis and Treatment*. 3rd ed. Berlin, Germany: Springer-Verlag; 2000:243–253.
171. Kahler SG, Iafolla AK. Effect of dietary alteration and parenteral nutrition in glutaric aciduria type I (glutaryl-CoA dehydrogenase deficiency). *J Human Genet*. 1988;43(Suppl 1):A9.
172. Amir N, el Peleg O, Shalev RS, Christensen E. Glutaric aciduria type I: clinical heterogeneity and neuroradiologic features. *Neurology*. 1987;37:1654–1657.
173. Boneh A, Beauchamp M, Humphrey M, Watkins J, Peters H, Yaplito-Lee J. Newborn screening for glutaric aciduria type I in Victoria: treatment and outcome. *Mol Genet Metab*. 2008;94:287–291.
174. Lipkin PH, Roe CR, Goodman SI, Batshaw ML. A case of glutaric acidemia type I: effect of riboflavin and carnitine. *J Pediatr*. 1988;112:62–65.

175. Hoffmann GF, Happle R, Kolker S. Acrodermatitis acidaemia secondary to "overtreatment" and protein deficiency. *J Inherit Metab Dis*. 2006;29:173–174.
176. Niiyama S, Koelker S, Degen I, Hoffmann GF, Happle R, Hoffmann R. Acrodermatitis acidemica secondary to malnutrition in glutaric aciduria type I. *Eur J Dermatol*. 2001;11:244–246.
177. Hogan SE. Energy requirements of children with cerebral palsy. *Can J Diet Pract Res*. 2004;65:124–130.
178. Stallings VA, Zemel BS, Davies JC, Cronk CE, Charney EB. Energy expenditure of children and adolescents with severe disabilities: a cerebral palsy model. *Am J Clin Nutr*. 1996;64:627–634.
179. Taylor SB, Shelton JE. Caloric requirements of a spastic immobile cerebral palsy patient: a case report. *Arch Phys Med Rehabil*. 1995;76:281–283.
180. Alexander JW, Clayton BE, Delves HT. Mineral and trace-metal balances in children receiving normal and synthetic diets. *Q J Med*. 1974;169:80–111.
181. Brandt NJ, Gregersen N, Christensen E, Gron IH, Rasmussen K. Treatment of glutaryl-CoA dehydrogenase deficiency (glutaric aciduria). Experience with diet, riboflavin, and GABA analogue. *J Pediatr*. 1979;94:669–673.
182. Chaves-Carballo E, Frank LM. Glutaric aciduria type I responsive to riboflavin. *Neurology*. 1988;38(Suppl 1):293–294.
183. Chalmers RA, Bain MD, Zschocke J. Riboflavin-responsive glutaryl CoA dehydrogenase deficiency. *Mol Genet Metab*. 2006;88:29–37.
184. Zempleni J, Galloway JR, McCormick DB. Pharmacokinetics of orally and intravenously administered riboflavin in healthy humans. *Am J Clin Nutr*. 1996;63:54–66.
185. Hug G, McGraw CA, Bates SR, Landrigan EA. Reduction of serum carnitine concentrations during anticonvulsant therapy with phenobarbital, valproic acid, phenytoin, and carbamazepine in children. *J Pediatr*. 1991;119:799–802.
186. Opala G, Winter S, Vance C, Vance H, Hutchison HT, Linn LS. The effect of valproic acid on plasma carnitine levels. *Am J Dis Child*. 1991;145:999–1001.
187. Muhlhausen C, Hoffmann GF, Strauss KA, et al. Maintenance treatment of glutaryl-CoA dehydrogenase deficiency. *J Inherit Metab Dis*. 2004;27:885–892.
188. Strauss KA, Puffenberger EG, Robinson DL, Morton DH. Type I glutaric aciduria, part 1: natural history of 77 patients. *Am J Med Genet C Semin Med Genet*. 2003; 121C:38–52.
189. Ogier de Baulny H. Management and emergency treatments of neonates with a suspicion of inborn errors of metabolism. *Semin Neonatol*. 2002;7:17–26.
190. Greenberg CR, Prasad AN, Dilling LA, et al. Outcome of the first 3-years of a DNA-based neonatal screening program for glutaric acidemia type 1 in Manitoba and northwestern Ontario, Canada. *Mol Genet Metab*. 2002;75:70–78.
191. Arnulf I, Konofal E, Merino-Andreu M, et al. Parkinson's disease and sleepiness: an integral part of PD. *Neurology*. 2002;58:1019–1024.
192. Arnulf I, Quintin P, Alvarez JC, et al. Mid-morning tryptophan depletion delays REM sleep onset in healthy subjects. *Neuropsychopharmacology*. 2002;27: 843–851.
193. Fujimoto W, Inaoki M, Fukui T, Inoue Y, Kuhara T. Biotin deficiency in an infant fed with amino acid formula. *J Dermatol*. 2005;32:256–261.
194. Bijarnia S, Wiley V, Carpenter K, Christodoulou J, Ellaway CJ, Wilcken B. Glutaric aciduria type I: outcome following detection by newborn screening. *J Inherit Metab Dis*. 2008;31:503–507.
195. Kulkens S, Harting I, Sauer S, et al. Late-onset neurologic disease in glutaryl-CoA dehydrogenase deficiency. *Neurology*. 2005;64:2142–2144.

196. Kyllerman M, Skjeldal OH, Lundberg M, et al. Dystonia and dyskinesia in glutaric aciduria type I: clinical heterogeneity and therapeutic considerations. *Mov Disord.* 1994;9:22–30.
197. Crombez EA, Cederbaum SD, Spector E, et al. Maternal glutaric acidemia, type I identified by newborn screening. *Mol Genet Metab*. 2008;94:132–134.
198. Garcia P, Martins E, Diogo L, et al. Outcome of three cases of untreated maternal glutaric aciduria type I. *Eur J Pediatr*. 2008;167:569–573.
199. Wolf B, Grier RE, Allen RJ, Goodman SI, Kien CL. Biotinidase deficiency: the enzymatic defect in late-onset multiple carboxylase deficiency. *Clin Chim Acta.* 1983;131:273–281.
200. Laszlo A, Schuler EA, Sallay E, et al. Neonatal screening for biotinidase deficiency in Hungary: clinical, biochemical and molecular studies. *J Inherit Metab Dis.* 2003;26:693–698.
201. Pacheco-Alvarez D, Solorzano-Vargas RS, Del Rio AL. Biotin in metabolism and its relationship to human disease. *Arch Med Res*. 2002;33:439–447.
202. Gravel RA, Narang MA. Molecular genetics of biotin metabolism: old vitamin, new science. *J Nutr Biochem*. 2005;16:428–431.
203. Wolf B. Disorders of biotin metabolism. In: Scriver CR, Beaudet AL, Sly WS, Valle D, eds. *The Metabolic and Molecular Bases of Inherited Disease*. 8th ed. New York, NY: McGraw-Hill; 2001:3935–3962.
204. Yang X, Aoki Y, Li X, et al. Structure of human holocarboxylase synthetase gene and mutation spectrum of holocarboxylase synthetase deficiency. *Hum Genet.* 2001;109:526–534.
205. Moslinger D, Stockler-Ipsiroglu S, Scheibenreiter S, et al. Clinical and neuropsychological outcome in 33 patients with biotinidase deficiency ascertained by nationwide newborn screening and family studies in Austria. *Eur J Pediatr*. 2001;160:277–282.
206. Malvagia S, Morrone A, Pasquini E, et al. First prenatal molecular diagnosis in a family with holocarboxylase synthetase deficiency. *Prenat Diagn*. 2005;25:1117–1119.
207. Hymes J, Stanley CM, Wolf B. Mutations in BTD causing biotinidase deficiency. *Hum Mutat*. 2001;18:375–381.
208. Wolf B, Jensen KP, Barshop B, et al. Biotinidase deficiency: novel mutations and their biochemical and clinical correlates. *Hum Mutat*. 2005;25:413.
209. Baumgarter ER, Suormala T. Biotin-responsive multiple carboxylase deficiency. In: Fernandes J, Saudubray JM, van den Berghe G, eds. *Inborn Metabolic Diseases: Diagnosis and Treatment*. Berlin, Germany: Springer-Verlag; 2000:272–282.
210. Pomponio RJ, Hymes J, Pandya A, et al. Prenatal diagnosis of heterozygosity for biotinidase deficiency by enzymatic and molecular analyses. *Prenat Diagn*. 1998;18:117–122.
211. Hoffman TL, Simon EM, Ficicioglu C. Biotinidase deficiency: the importance of adequate follow-up for an inconclusive newborn screening result. *Eur J Pediatr*. 2005;164:298–301.
212. Moslinger D, Muhl A, Suormala T, Baumgartner R, Stockler-Ipsiroglu S. Molecular characterisation and neuropsychological outcome of 21 patients with profound biotinidase deficiency detected by newborn screening and family studies. *Eur J Pediatr*. 2003;162(Suppl 1):S46–S49.
213. Seymons K, De Moor A, De Raeve H, Lambert J. Dermatologic signs of biotin deficiency leading to the diagnosis of multiple carboxylase deficiency. *Pediatr Dermatol*. 2004;21:231–235.

214. Hou JW. Biotin responsive multiple carboxylase deficiency presenting as diabetic ketoacidosis. *Chang Gung Med J*. 2004;27:129–133.
215. Suormala T, Fowler B, Jakobs C, et al. Late-onset holocarboxylase synthetase-deficiency: pre- and post-natal diagnosis and evaluation of effectiveness of antenatal biotin therapy. *Eur J Pediatr*. 1998;157:570–575.
216. Navarro PC, Guerra A, Alvarez JG, Ortiz FJ. Cutaneous and neurologic manifestations of biotinidase deficiency. *Int J Dermatol*. 2000;39:363–365.
217. Weber P, Scholl S, Baumgartner ER. Outcome in patients with profound biotinidase deficiency: relevance of newborn screening. *Dev Med Child Neurol*. 2004;46:481–484.
218. Wolf B. Children with profound biotinidase deficiency should be treated with biotin regardless of their residual enzyme activity or genotype. *Eur J Pediatr*. 2002;161:167–168.
219. Welling DB. Long-term follow-up of hearing loss in biotinidase deficiency. *J Child Neurol*. 2007;22:1055.
220. Sivri HS, Genc GA, Tokatli A, et al. Hearing loss in biotinidase deficiency: genotype-phenotype correlation. *J Pediatr*. 2007;150:439–442.
221. Baumgartner ER, Suormala T. Multiple carboxylase deficiency: inherited and acquired disorders of biotin metabolism. *Int J Vitam Nutr Res*. 1997;67:377–384.
222. Wolf B, Hsia YE, Sweetman L, et al. Multiple carboxylase deficiency: clinical and biochemical improvement following neonatal biotin treatment. *Pediatrics*. 1981;68:113–118.
223. Mock NI, Malik MI, Stumbo PJ, Bishop WP, Mock DM. Increased urinary excretion of 3-hydroxyisovaleric acid and decreased urinary excretion of biotin are sensitive early indicators of decreased biotin status in experimental biotin deficiency. *Am J Clin Nutr*. 1997;65:951–958.
224. Hendriksz CJ, Preece MA, Chakrapani A. Successful pregnancy in a treated patient with biotinidase deficiency. *J Inherit Metab Dis*. 2005;28:791–792.

Chapter 9

Nutrition Management of Patients with Inherited Disorders of Galactose Metabolism

Phyllis B. Acosta

INTRODUCTION

Since the report of the first patient with galactosuria (galactosemia), who expired with a diagnosis of cirrhosis (reported in Nadler et al.[1]), reports of two other forms of galactoremia have been published.[2,3] Galactosuria was ultimately named galactosemia (OMIM 230400)[4] due to elevated galactose in the blood. The usual clinical presentation of patients with a deficiency of galactose-1-phosphate uridyltransferase deficiency (GALT; EC 2.7.7.12) includes hepatic, renal, gastrointestinal, eye, and immune manifestations. Feeding difficulties, vomiting, and diarrhea occur very early in the neonatal period after the introduction of lactose, and jaundice, hepatomegaly, and clotting abnormalities soon appear.[5] Cataracts were seen at or within a few days of birth in some patients.[6] During early infancy a number of children with galactosemia were noted to have recurring bacterial infections[1] and Levy et al.[7] reported sepsis due to *E. coli* in very young infants with galactosemia.

Galactokinase (GALK; EC 2.7.1.6) deficiency (OMIM 230200)[2] presents with cataracts that are identical to those found in patients with GALT deficiency.[8] Some patients with GALK deficiency have presented with pseudotumor cerebri.[9]

Deficiency of uridine disphosphate galactose-4-epimerase (GALE; OMIM 230350)[2] may occur in the erythrocytes, resulting in a lack of symptoms, while patients with a generalized, severe form of GALE (EC 5.1.3.2) deficiency present in a similar fashion to those patients with GALT deficiency.

Biochemistry

Galactose (GAL), a sugar found largely in the lactose of human milk, cow's milk, and many proprietary infant formulas, supplies 38 to 41% of the energy ingested by infants.[10] Ingested lactose is hydrolyzed in the small intestine by β-galactosidase (lactase), which extends through the luminal surface of the microvilli. The resulting glucose and galactose are rapidly absorbed from the intestine by a sodium-coupled energy-dependent system.[11]

Galactose must be converted to glucose in order to be used for energy purposes, and this takes place via the Leloir pathway that occurs primarily in the liver (see Figure 9.1). Following the entrance of GAL into the cell by a permease, it is phosphorylated into galactose-1-phosphate (GAL-1-P) by galactokinase (GALK). Galactose-1-phosphate uridyltransferase deficiency (GALT) is the second enzyme in the Leloir pathway, and its deficiency leads to classic galactosemia. Two reactions occur by which uridine disphosphate (UDP) glucose binds and releases GAL-1-P. Subsequently, the uridine monophosphate (UMP)-GALT complex binds GAL-1-P, releases UDP-GAL, and frees GALT for another set of reactions. UDP-GAL and UDP-glucose are interconverted by epimerase (see Figure 9.1). UDP-GAL and UDP-GLU are important for the synthesis of glycolipids and glycoproteins.

Molecular Biology

A genetic basis for GALT deficiency was first suggested by Goppert in 1917,[12] reported by Komrower in 1969,[12] and later by Mason and Turner in 1935.[13] GALT deficiency was first demonstrated in erythrocytes of patients with galactosemia in 1956[14] and subsequently in white cells,[15] liver,[16] and fibroblasts,[17] and its absence has been suspected in brain cells.[18]

All forms of galactosemia are inherited as autosomal recessive disorders (see Chapter 1). The gene encoding GALT is located on chromosome 9p13 and bridges 4.3 kb of DNA arranged on 11 exons.[5] Leslie and coworkers cloned the GALT gene in 1992.[19] Over 180 different mutations in the GALT gene have been identified.[20]

A number of common mutations have been reported in different ethnic groups including Q188R in Caucasians, in which the glutamine in Q188R is changed into arginine. Over 50% of African Americans who have galactosemia usually have the S135L mutation in which serine replaces leucine. The mutations that occur determine the amount of activity of the GALT enzyme and the galactosylation of lipids and proteins. Patients with mutations that result in >2% GALT activity appear to have fewer long-term effects

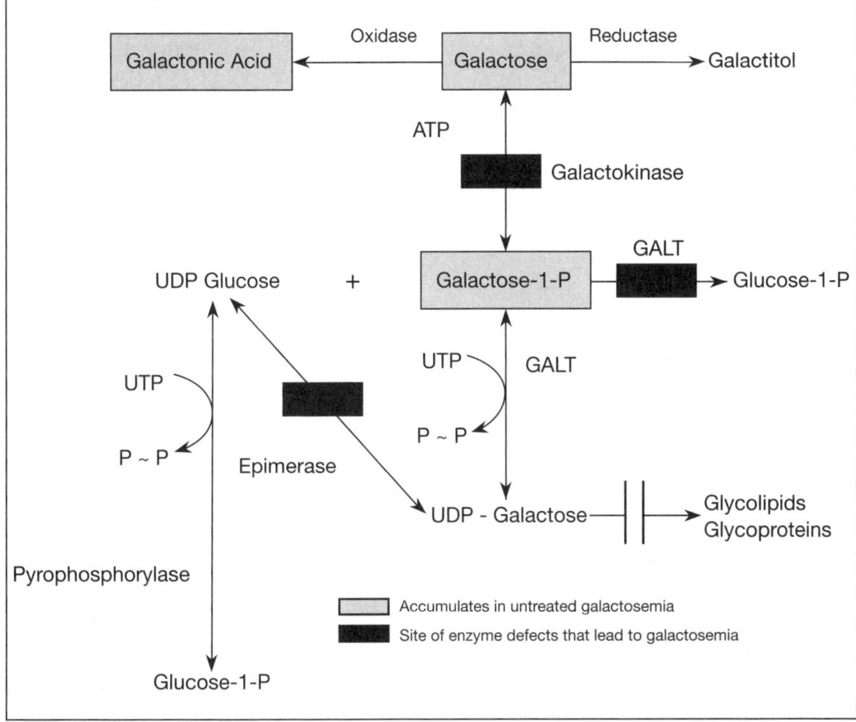

Figure 9.1 *Metabolic Blocks in Galactose Metabolism that Lead to Galactosemia*

Source: Modified by permission of Elsas LJ, Acosta PB. Inherited metabolic disease: amino acids, organic acids, and galactose. In: Shils ME, Shike M, Olson J, Ross AC, Caballero B, Cousins RJ, eds. *Modern Nutrition in Health and Disease*. 10th ed. Philadelphia, PA: Lippincott Williams & Wilkins; 2005:909–959. Courtesy of Wolters Kluwer Health.

Note: Classical galactosemia is caused by GALT deficiency.

compared to those found that result in <2% GALT activity in patients. For more information on molecular biology of GALT deficiency, see reference 21.

Newborn Screening

The most common screening for galactosemia is the Beutler fluorescent test.[22] Erythrocytes from dried blood are incubated on filter paper with a mixture of UDP-GLU, GLU-6-P dehydrogenase, and NADP, while erythrocytes from normal individuals that contain GALT and phosphoglucomutase produce GLU-1-P, GLU-6-P, and fluorescent NADPH through the reaction of excess GLU-6-P dehydrogenase. If heat has inactivated this reaction, as may occur in summer, GLU-1-P is added to differentiate between heat inactivation that included endogenous phosphoglucomutase and GALT deficiency alone.[21]

Positive screening results occur with classic (G/G) GALT deficiency and with variants of GALT that are themolabile, such as Duarte/galactosemia (D/G) compound heterozygote. Confirmation of a positive Beutler screening test result requires quantitative enzyme activity and quantitation of erythrocyte GAL and GAL-1-P content.

Diagnosis

A combined analysis of the GALT biochemical phenotype and molecular genotype is important for diagnosis, therapy, prognosis, and genetic counseling.[23-25] A test of total body oxidation of GAL to expired CO_2 is the method of choice for prognosis.

All lactose should be immediately removed from the diets of patients with a positive Beutler test while enzyme diagnosis and family work-up proceed. Fresh, sterile, heparinized blood should be sent to a laboratory experienced in enzyme, analyte, and molecular analyses. Both patient and parents should be evaluated for biochemical phenotype and molecular genotype. Diagnosis of the specific enzymatic cause occurs through measurement of activity of the enzymes involved in GAL metabolism.[21] Because the Q188R allele occurs in 70% of Caucasians with galactosemia, it is important to identify it.[24,26,27] The Duarte allele (314D) has a characteristic pattern when isoelectric focusing is used to study the GALT enzyme. Therapy may only be needed in patients who have enzyme activity of < 25%. Factors that suggest the need for therapy include an erythrocyte GAL-1-P > 2 mg/dL, hepatotoxicity, or plasma galactitol of 20 mmol/mol creatinine.[21]

Galactose-1-phosphate uridyltransferase is expressed both in amniotic fluid cells and in chorionic villi. Consequently, GALT deficiency can be detected prenatally by both direct enzyme assay and DNA analysis if the mutations are known.[28]

Incidence of GALT deficiency has been reported to range from 1 in 10,000 to 1 in 30,000 live births,[21] and Bosch et al. estimated that in Western Europe, the incidence is between 1 in 23,000 and 1 in 44,000.[29]

Outcomes if Untreated

The first patient reported with GALK deficiency was 9 years of age.[3] A second patient was reported by Thalhammer et al. in Vienna.[30] Nuclear cataracts became apparent at the age of 3.5 weeks before treatment was initiated in 1 patient. Though blind, neither of these patients demonstrated any mental retardation. Bosch et al. reported that of 32 patients reported with GALK deficiency, 24 (75%) had cataracts.[31] Segal et al. reported in addition to cataracts, mental retardation in 2 brothers. By 8 years of age, the first brother had few scorable intelligence test (IQ) results. As early as 2 years of age, the second brother had no scorable IQ test results.[32] Bosch et al.[31] reported only 1 additional child with mental retardation with GALK deficiency of 43 patients.

Nadler reported that infants with GALT deficiency often expired with liver failure.[1] Vomiting or diarrhea occurred in about 80%, cataracts in about 49%, and growth retardation in height and weight (< 3 percentile) in 25%. All had IQ below that of their normal siblings with a specific learning difficulty in mathematics, and about 40% had anemia.

Few patients with GALE deficiency have been reported. Those that have been reported have been classified into benign, severe, or peripheral form in the past but now appear to be a continuum of one disease.[33,34]

Nutrition Management

Goals of therapy in patients with galactosemia are to prevent symptoms while supplying required energy, protein, and other nutrients for normal growth and development. Treatment, which is life-saving in GALT-deficient infants, should begin as early in life as possible and should delete as much galactose as possible from the diet of infants and children. Adequate studies have not been reported on these patients to determine energy and protein requirements for optimal growth. Due to the fact that these patients must be fed soy protein isolate rather than casein, they may require more energy and protein than normal infants, children, and adults (see Chapter 3, Table 3.1), due to the rapid digestion of the soy protein and the accumulation of GAL-1-P.

The opinion of many healthcare professionals who work with patients with a deficiency of GALK, GALT, or GALE is that a diet restricted in galactose should be used to manage the patients for life, although recently many have questioned the necessity for strict deletion of GAL by the adult. Initiation of restriction of GAL in the GALK-deficient patient often results in resorption of cataracts, while in the GALT-deficient patient during the neonatal period, cataracts and renal, brain, and immune dysfunction are reversed and accumulated GAL metabolites are decreased.[35] Endocrine abnormalities and hypoglycosylation are present in female GALT-deficient patients. The hypoglycosylation is diet-dependent and could worsen when GAL intake increases either because of poor compliance or diet liberalization.[36,37] Several theories have been proposed to explain the poor outcomes in patients with GALT deficiency. These include in utero fetal damage, damage before nutrition intervention, over- or under-restriction of GAL, de novo GAL synthesis,[38] or a deficiency of uridine disphosphate galactose (UDP-GAL).[39] However, oral uridine administration has not been beneficial in spite of normalization of erythrocyte UDP-GAL concentrations.[40]

In 1999, the Galactosemia Steering Group of the United Kingdom published their recommendations for nutrition management of patients with galactosemia. Foods such as meats, fruits, and legumes are suggested to be insignificant sources of galactose by the Galactosemia Steering Group, and soy protein isolate powdered formulas replace human milk or infant formula containing GAL.[41]

Bosch and coworkers in The Netherlands reported that 1 adolescent patient with classical GALT deficiency tolerated up to 600 mg galactose daily, but this patient may have had a greater capacity to dispose of galactose by pathways unknown.[42]

Nutrient Requirements

Galactose

In the past, recommended nutrition management consisted of rigid exclusion of as much GAL as possible from the diets of patients with GALT deficiency.[43] Galactose exclusion was also found to be important in treatment of patients with GALK deficiency to prevent cataracts, while those with GALE deficiency were thought to require the addition of measured/prescribed amounts of GAL to the GAL-restricted diet.[44] With the accumulation of knowledge on intake and in vivo synthesis of large amounts of GAL, more rapid decline of erythrocyte GAL-1-P concentrations in patients whose whole body oxidation (WBO) is > 2%, the ubiquity of GAL in foods,[45] and the report that one GALT-deficient patient has normal IQ without restriction of GAL,[46] the question has been raised about the necessity of more than moderate restriction of GAL intake beyond early life when its restriction prevents death.

While infants ingest more GAL per unit of body weight than adults, de novo synthesis of GAL appears to be greater in younger than in older individuals with or without GALT deficiency. Berry et al.,[47] using 1-13-C-galactose, analyzed the apparent GAL appearance rate (GAR) in GALT-deficient patients and control subjects. Assuming that the GAL synthesis rate remained constant[48] for 24 hours as during the study period, its maximum synthesis is described in patients and controls less than and greater than 18 years of age with and without a priming dose of GAL. Control children and adults appeared to synthesize significantly less GAL than children and adults with GALT deficiency, and Schadewaldt et al.[49] verified decreased GAL synthesis with age in patients with GALT deficiency.

Glucose intake appears to decrease serum GAL concentrations in some normal individuals. Normal volunteer adult males were each given 0.5 g GAL kg BW orally with various amounts of oral or intravenous glucose. Oral glucose intake at 750 mg/kg body weight (BW) reduced the mean area under the serum GAL curve by 75%, with smaller oral glucose loads leading to lower declines in the serum GAL response curves.[50] Insulin administration alone did not lower serum GAL concentrations in subjects in the study. Whether ongoing intakes of oral glucose (or sucrose) would have long-term effects on serum GAL concentrations and outcomes of patients with GALT deficiency is unknown. Urinary GAL excretion did not increase with increased intakes of glucose.

Oxidation of whole body GAL to CO_2, as measured in the breath test, provides information on WBO capacity. When 1-13-GAL conversion to 13-CO_2 was measured for 2 hours after administration of 1-13-C-GAL to 37 patients 3 to 48 years old with GALT deficiency (no detectable erythrocyte GALT activity) and to control subjects 3 to 37 years old, 11 patients with Q188R/Q188R genotype, 7 patients with one mutant Q188R allele and a second mutant allele as L195P, E308K, V151A, M142K, or Q344K, and 1 patient with a mutant Q285N/unknown genotype eliminated $< 2\%$ of a bolus of 1-C-13-galactose as 13-CO_2. When patients had one mutant Q188R allele and either a mutant 314D or S135L as the second allele or mutant K284N/N314D or other rarer mutant genotypes, galactose metabolism was normal as measured by the breath test.[51]

Of interest is the report that rates of decline in erythrocyte GAL-1-P differed in patients with differing classical genotypes. For example, patients all receiving the same nutrition management, whose genotype was Q188R/Q188R, had an erythrocyte GAL-1-P concentration at 5 to 8 months of age of 4.9 mg/dL while patients with a genotype of Q188R/other had an erythrocyte GAL-1-P concentration at the same age of 3.3 mg/dL, and those with other/other of 2.5 mg/dL. Decline of erythrocyte GAL-1-P concentration from that found at diagnosis in the neonatal period was found to be more rapid in patients with nonclassical genotypes.[52] Those patients with $< 2\%$ WBO of 1-13-C-GAL to 13-CO_2 had the slowest decline in erythrocyte GAL-1-P. Zlatunich and Packman reported that early treatment of a GALT-deficient patient with an elemental formula containing no GAL caused a rapid decrease in erythrocyte GAL-1-P concentration.[53]

Energy and Fluid

Energy needs of patients with galactosemia are likely greater than suggested for normal subjects[54] since growth in both weight and length/height of the GALT-deficient patient is reported to be less than that of normal children of the same age and gender.[55] Whether the rapidly digested soy protein isolate fed in very low-GAL proprietary infant formulas leads to a greater energy requirement as found in infants fed free amino acid formulas is not known.[56,57]

If adequate weight gain for age is not achieved by infants with galactosemia ingesting energy intakes recommended in Chapter 3, Table 3.1, energy intake should be increased to amounts required to achieve daily weight gains within the ranges suggested by Fomon et al.[58] Carefully plotting patients' weights on Centers for Disease Control (CDC) growth charts[59] is also useful in determining adequacy of growth. Recommended energy intakes based on below average weight and height for age may continue to lead to poor weight gain (see Chapter 3), and energy intakes (see Chapter 4, Feeding for Catch-Up Growth) may need to be given in amounts suggested for catch-up growth.

Fluid requirements are 1.5 mL/kcal ingested for the infant and decline to about 1.0 mL/kcal ingested for the adult (see Chapter 3, Table 3.1). Thirst is considered an adequate guide to intake for older children and in adults. Vomiting, diarrhea, and very warm environmental temperatures without the availability of air conditioning may increase fluid requirements considerably.

Protein

Protein requirements of infants with galactosemia fed soy protein isolate (a rapidly digested protein) formulas are likely to be somewhat greater than those required by infants fed casein-predominant formulas to achieve normal growth in supine length (see Chapter 3, Table 3.1) and should be at least 3.75 g protein per 100 kcal to supply 15% of energy intake for infants. Table 3.1 suggests protein intakes that, along with increased energy intakes, should help support normal growth in patients with galactosemia.

Fats and Essential Fatty Acids

Proprietary infant formulas made with soy protein isolate contain fat and essential fatty acids (see Appendix B). For recommended daily intakes, see Chapter 3, Table 3.1.

Minerals and Vitamins

Hypergonadotropic hypogonadism was first reported in female patients with GALT deficiency in 1981.[60] Later, Kaufman et al.[61] reported that all of 40 patients (3.4 to 44.2 years of age) had bone densities below those of control subjects. All female patients, and especially those not given estrogen–progestin replacement therapy, had a bone density significantly below normal controls. Calcium intake was below recommended by patients but correlated positively with bone density in both females and males.

Forty Dutch children (3 to 17 years of age; 27 females, 13 males) with GALT deficiency on nutrition management were evaluated for bone mineral density (BMD), nutrient intakes, and serum concentrations of a number of nutrients and bone metabolism markers.[62] Mean BMD Z-scores (measured by dual energy x-ray absorptiometry, DXA) of the lumbar spine and femoral neck were significantly below normal. All patients had intakes of calcium, magnesium, zinc, vitamin D, and protein that met the Recommended Dietary Allowances (RDAs). Patients with GALT deficiency had significantly below normal concentrations of IGF-1, carboxylated osteocalcin, N-terminal telopeptide, and C-terminal telopeptide, suggesting decreased bone metabolism. When these GALT-deficient patients received daily supplements of 750 mg calcium, 1.0 mg vitamin K_1, and 10 μg vitamin D_3 or a placebo, in addition to the nutrients in the diet, after 2 years only the prepubertal children receiving supplements had increased concentrations of carboxylated osteocalcin and a significant increase in the bone mineral content of the lumbar spine.[63] Recommendations for preventing osteoporosis in patients over 3 years of age with GALT deficiency include use of the above supplements, estrogen administration to females, adequate physical activity, and routine DXAs to assess bone mineral content.[64] Studies of bone mineralization of children with GALT deficiency under 3 years of age have not been reported. Consequently, whether supplemental calcium, vitamin D_3, and vitamin K_1, in addition to usual intake, are required prior to 3 years of age is not known. The recommended intakes given in Chapter 3, Table 3.1, for infants per 100 kcal fall significantly below the recommendations of Panis et al.[64] Until more studies are published on mineral and vitamin takes that result in excellent bone status, the recommended intakes for infants in Table 3.1 should be fed.

Foods

Human Milk, Proprietary Infant Formulas, Cow's Milk, and Milk Products

Human milk, proprietary infant formulas containing added lactose, and cow's milk have long been thought to be the primary sources of galactose in the diet. Human milk contains 6 to 8% lactose, cow's milk 3 to 4%, and proprietary infant formulas 7%. Human milk contains, on average, 33.5 g galactose per liter, while proprietary infant formulas such as Enfamil® Lipil® (Mead Johnson Nutritionals, Evansville, Indiana) and Similac® Advance® (Abbott Nutrition, Columbus, Ohio) contain about 36.0 g per liter and cow's milk about 26.0 g per liter[10,65-67] (see Table 9.1).

The 3.5 kg newborn infant, when ingesting 500 mL human milk consumes about 20 times more GAL per unit of body weight than does the 55 kg adult ingesting 500 mL of cow's milk daily (see Figure 9.2). These milks must be replaced by powdered soy protein isolate formulas free of carrageenan (27% GAL) and very low in GAL or by an elemental infant formula (EleCare®, Abbott Nutrition, Columbus, Ohio; NeoCate®, Nutricia North America, Gaithersburg, Maryland) free of lactose or GAL.

Powdered formulas containing soy protein isolate contain about 14 mg of GAL per liter in the form of raffinose and stachyose; that is, oligosaccharides that contain GAL. At one time, it was thought that these oligosaccharides yielded free GAL on hydrolysis in the intestine. It is now believed that the human intestine has no enzymes to hydrolyze these oligosaccharides. Thus, they may be safely used for feeding infants and children with galactosemia. Similac Isomil® and Go and Grow™ Soy Based powder formula (Abbott Nutrition, Columbus, Ohio), Enfamil ProSobee® Lipil® (Mead Johnson, Evansville, Indiana) may be used by children and adults who require an

Table 9.1 ***Approximate Lactose and Galactose in One Liter of Human Milk, Selected Proprietary Infant Formulas, and Cow's Milk***

Milk or Formula	*Lactose (g/L)*	*Galactose (g/L)*
Human milk, mature	67.0	33.5
Enfamil® Lipil®	73.7	36.8
Similac® Advance®	73.0	36.5
Cow's milk, 3.3% fat	52.0	26.0

Sources:

Abbott Nutrition. Similac® Advance. Available at: http://abbottnutrition.com/products.aspx?pid=44. Accessed May 28, 2008.

Mead Johnson Nutritionals. *Pediatric Products Handbook*. Evansville, IN: Mead Johnson & Company; 2004:8–13.

Pennington JAT. *Bowes and Church's Food Values of Portions Commonly Used.* 17th ed. Philadelphia, PA: Lippincott Williams & Wilkins; 1998:222.

Picciano MF, McDonald SS. Lactation. In: Shils ME, Shike M, Olson J, Ross AC, Caballero B, Cousins RJ, eds. *Modern Nutrition in Health and Disease.* 10th ed. Philadelphia, PA: Lippincott Williams & Wilkins; 2005:784–796.

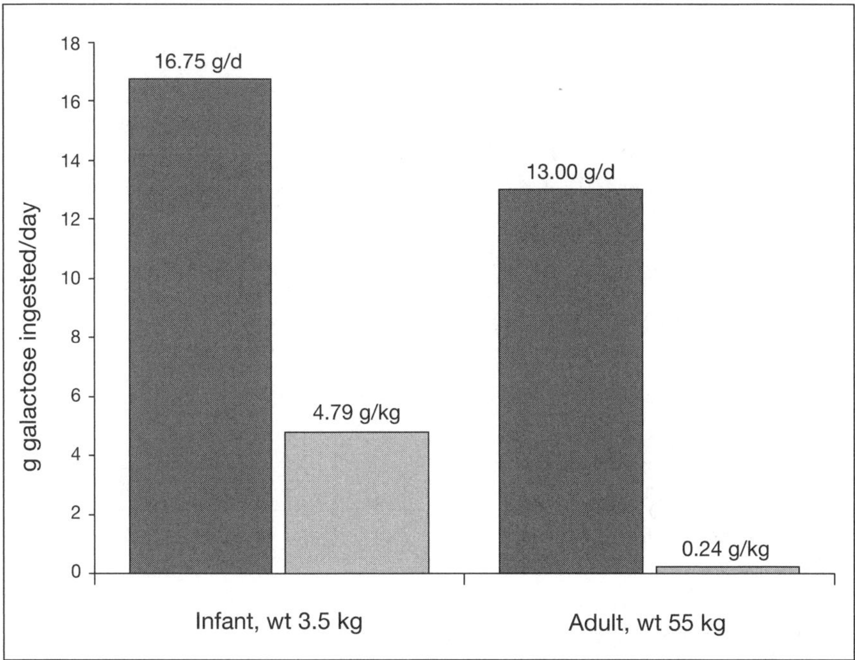

Figure 9.2 *Intake of Galactose per Day and per Kilogram of Body Weight by Infants Ingesting 500 mL of Human Milk and by Adults Ingesting 500 mL of Cow's Milk*

almost GAL-free formula. Casein hydrolysates such as Alimentum® (Abbott Nutrition, Columbus, Ohio), Nutramigen, and Pregestimil (Mead Johnson, Evansville, Indiana; see Appendix B) have been treated to remove lactose but may still contain small amounts of GAL (< 37 mg/L). Liquid Alimentum also contains carrageenan. Alimentum powder contains xanthan gum as stabilizer, and while the casein hydrolysate contains < 37 mg GAL/L, the xanthan gum provides no bioavailable GAL. Lactose-free infant formulas may contain up to as much as 75 mg GAL/L and should be avoided by infants with GALT deficiency.

While lactose is found in whey, it is also found in large amounts in sweetened condensed milk, condensed whey, nonfat dry milk, sweet dry whey, dried acid whey, modified whey solids, and in any other food in which milk, milk products, or whey is found.[68] Whey is also used in many foods such as baked goods, sweet goods, breads, crackers, dry mixes, confections, icings, jams, apple butter, batter mix, and processed cheese foods. α, β, and γ casein each contain different amounts of galactose, while whole casein may have up to 184 mg/100 g.[69]

Cheddar cheese quality and GAL content are dependent on the behavior of *Streptococcus thermophilus* in combination with *Lactococcus lactis* subsp cremoris or subsq lactis mesophilic starters in experimental cheddar cheese.[70] Harvey et al. reported considerable amounts of lactose and GAL in aged cheddar cheese (see Table 9.2).[71]

Hard grated cheeses that contain sugars may be contaminated with whey or soft cheese. Uncontaminated hard cheeses, on average, contain signifi-

Table 9.2 ***Maximum Lactose and Galactose in Cheese***

Cheese	*Lactose (mg/100 g)*	*Free Galactose (mg/100 g)*	*Total Galactose (mg/100 g)*
Hard Cheese[a]			
Imported Parmesan	10	30	35
Domestic Parmesan	10	30	35
Pecorino Romano	10	20	25
Domestic Romano	0	10	10
Domestic Romano[b]	0	56	56
Soft Cheese			
Whey Ricotta	3640	70	1890
Milk Ricotta	3020	50	1560
Mozzarella	1360	1190	1870
Cheddar	298	24	322
Processed American	10	80	85
Provolone	0	40	40
Washed Curd	0	20	20
Swiss	0	10	10

Sources:

Harvey CD, Jenness R, Morries HA. Gas chromatographic quantitation of surgars and non-volatile water soluble-organic acids in commercial cheddar cheese. *J Dairy Sci*. 1981;61:1648–1654.

Michel V, Martley FG. Streptococcus thermophilus in cheddar cheese—production and fate of galactose. *J Dairy Res*. 2001;68:317–325.

Pollman RM. Ion chromatographic determination of lactose, galactose, and dextrose in grated cheese using pulsed amperometric detection. *J Assoc Off Anal Chem*. 1989;72:425–428.

[a]Hard grated cheeses that contain sugars may be contaminated with whey or soft cheese.

[b]Made by an alternative procedure used by two US manufacturers.

cantly less total GAL (< 56 mg/100 g) than soft cheeses. Milk ricotta, whey ricotta, and mozzarella contain up to 1980 g GAL/100 g, while processed American provolone and Swiss cheeses contain < 100 mg/100 g.[72]

Beikost (Baby Foods)

Cereals, fruits, and vegetables may contain differing amounts of galactose depending on variety, soil, amount of water supply, ripeness, length of storage, and time and method of preparation and these differences may be as much as tenfold.[73,74]

Enzymes are required to digest galactose in other forms than lactose, and cooking yields, in some foods, relatively large amounts of free GAL. α-galactosidases, enzymes that digest carbohydrates with GAL in α-linkages, are found in human tissues and are probably responsible for the degradation of tissue galactosylcerebrosides, galactosylsulfatides, and gangliosides. α-gangliosidases also appear to be distributed in many plant tissues.[75] Bean-O® is an α-galactosidase isolated from *Aspergillus niger* and marketed by AkPharma, Inc. (Pleasantville, New Jersey) as a food enzyme that reduces gas formation from many vegetables.[21] α-galactosidases can hydrolyze the terminal GAL attached to digalactosyldiacylglycerol, yielding GAL and monogalactosyldiacylglycerol.[75]

β-galactosidases are found in many foods, including apples, pears, peppers, tomatoes, and cocoa beans.[75] The human intestine also contains β-galactosidases.[76] The β-galactosidases in the human intestine digest lactose, but also have heterogenous activity on compounds with GAL in β-1,4 linkages.[76] β-galactosidase preparations from *E. coli* release GAL from ferulic acid and from monogalactosyldiacylglycerols.[75] Galactolipids in foods are hydrolyzed by human pancreatic lipolytic enzymes and duodenal contents.[77]

Of the BeechNut, Gerber, and Heinz baby cereals analyzed, none except Gerber rice with banana had more than 3.5 ± 0.3 mg/100 g (mean ± SEM) of free GAL.[78] However, none of the bound galactose was reported in any of the cereals.[78] Gropper and coworkers reported free GAL in baby fruits and vegetables varying from none detected in Gerber and Heinz apricots and Heinz peaches to 58.54 ± 7.80 mg/100 mg (mean ± SEM) in Gerber squash, while BeechNut squash contained 0.88 ± 0.34 mg/100 g.[79] Some Gerber and Heinz 2nd baby foods were also reported by Gropper et al., and fruits and vegetables supplying greater than or equal to 10 mg galactose per 100 g serving are reported.[80] Both free and bound galactose in baby food meats (beef, chicken, ham, lamb, turkey, and veal) have been reported and, while free galactose in Gerber's chicken was only 31 ± 10 mg/100 g, in lamb bound galactose was 137 ± 16 mg/100 g.

Table Cereals, Fruits, and Vegetables

Gross and Acosta were the first to report in the medical literature that fruits and vegetables were sources of free galactose from their cell walls.[45] This GAL may be present in the free form or in several different bound forms, such as arabinogalactan I and II, feruloylated D-galactose, galactan, galactinol, galactolipids, raffinose, stachyose, verbascose, and rhamnogalacturonan I and II.[75]

Glycolipids in cereal grains have been analyzed, and the galactose content of corn has been found to yield up to 1% of the molar ratio.[81] Rye grain, especially that from Canada, was found to have up to 16 ± 1% SD of its weight as galactose.[82] The hemicellulose portion of rice was found to range from 1 to 5% galactose.[83] According to Carter and coworkers, wheat flour lipids also contain GAL in galactolipids, monogalactosyl, and digalactosyl fractions with the monogalactose present at 71% and the digalactose fraction present at 84%.[84] Other cereal grains such as oatmeal and millet are likely to contain galactose as a part of their cell walls. Oat seeds were found to contain a galactolipid consisting of one molecule of avenoleic acid, two molecules of linoleic acid, two molecules of GAL, and one molecule of glycerol.[85]

According to Aspinall, arabinogalactans I are characterized by linear β-2-4 D galactan chains that may be digested and absorbed.[86] Apricots, peaches, pears, and apples were first analyzed for GAL content in 1955, and peaches, pears, and apples were found to contain free GAL.[87]

According to Gross and Acosta,[45] 100 g each ingested daily of cucumber, pear, plum, and tomato could potentially provide approximately 500 mg of total galactose (soluble + cell wall galactan). Berry et al. reported that the effects of fruits and vegetables on erythrocyte GAL-1-P concentration and urinary galactitol were minimal. However, other than the 50 g pure GAL fed 4 times daily, the amounts of GAL ingested in food for each of the 3 days of study were 45.2 ± 1.4, 33.9 ± 1.9, and 37.3 ± 10.5 g (mean ± SEM), respectively.[88]

Dried Beans and Peas

Various forms of GAL are found in a number of different dried beans and peas and include arabinogalactan I and II, galactan, galactinol, galactolipids, galactopinitols, raffinose, and rhamnogalacturonan I and II.[75] In addition to free GAL released from cell walls by cooking, the possibility of gut microorganisms releasing GAL is also possible. Dried beans, after boiling for 2.5 hours, yielded from 42 mg/100 g (pinto beans) to 444 mg/100 g (garbanzo beans) when cooking water was included. Holton reported that when legumes were incorporated in the diet of patients with GALT deficiency, mean erythrocyte GAL-1-P concentration increased appreciably. On the other hand, three of the four patients with GALT deficiency fed a diet containing no legumes had a decline in erythrocyte GAL-1-P.[89] More than likely, all dried beans and peas contain significant amounts of GAL.

Organ Meats and Meats

Galactosylcerebrosides, galactosyl sulfatides, gangliosides, lactosylceramides, and lactosyl sulfatides are found in brain, kidney, liver, and spleen and are ubiquitous but low in most tissues. According to Wiesman et al., they may contribute 0.5 to 1.0% of GAL to the diet.[90] These compounds are constantly turned over in living organisms and in patients with GALT deficiency, and the free GAL liberated is metabolized to GAL-1-P or other metabolites such as galactitol.[91]

Cured and Fermented Foods

A number of foods routinely ingested are previously cured or fermented. Bacteria are used for both processes, and acids produced by some bacteria preserve foods including, among others, legumes, miso, natto, pickles, sauerkraut, and some soy sauces. Cerbullis[92] reported the freeing of GAL in cocoa beans during their processing for cocoa and chocolate. Yokotsuka[93] reported that fermented soy sauce contained 170 mg of free GAL per 100 g. Twenty-four hours of fermentation increased monosaccharides and sucrose in cow peas by about 73%.[94]

Free and Bound Galactose in Food and Drugs

Hash browned potatoes and some other prepared foods were found by Smith and associates to contain added lactose, and some chefs sprinkle meat with lactose before frying for faster and better browning.[95] Lactulose, used to treat hyperammonemia, contains GAL.[21] Calcium lactobionate, the active ingredient in Neocalglucon,® is a liquid calcium supplement that is a substrate of β-galactosidase and yields free galactose.[96] Of interest is the fact that pharmaceutical companies are free to use any carbohydrate they wish as excipient in both over-the-counter and prescription drugs.[97]

Alternative Approaches to Therapy

Because long-term outcomes of nutrition management have not been as successful as predicted in the early years, alternative approaches to therapy are now being sought. At present, some investigators are evaluating GALK inhibitors as possible therapy since they hypothesized that elimination of GAL-1-P production will relieve GALT-deficient cells from GAL toxicity.[98]

Assessment of Specific Aspects of Nutrition Management

Erythrocyte GAL-1-P concentration is the primary indicator of adequacy of nutrition management in patients with GALT deficiency and is considered excellent if below 2 mg/dL.[99] However, it may not be possible to attain this concentration if the patient has the Q188R/Q188R mutation.[52] Other analytes suggested for assessment include erythrocyte and urinary galactitol and galactonate.[100-102] For other aspects of assessment of nutrition management, see Chapter 3.

Results of Nutrition Management

Cognitive

Komrower and Lee reported a mean IQ score of 84 in 32 GALT-deficient patients who were 6.75 years of age and had "good" control, while the 22 patients who were 8.75 years of age who had "moderate" or "poor" control had a mean IQ score of 77.[103] Early diagnosis and excellent control of erythrocyte GAL-1-P concentrations in patients has been reported to result in better outcomes than in those patients who are diagnosed late or have poor control,[104] although outcomes may be more dependent on genotype than control.[105] For example, children with GALT deficiency and language disorders have a four to six times greater risk for language impairment than children with early speech disorders of unknown origin.[106] Total body oxidation of galactose to CO_2 in expired air is reported to reflect genotype in patients with galactosemia as well as predict verbal dyspraxia.[107] Elsas et al. had previously reported that homozygosity for Q188R mutations in the GALT gene is a significant risk factor for developmental verbal dyspraxia but that erythrocyte GAL-1-P concentrations greater than 3.28 mg/dL prevent this relationship.[108]

In a report of 83 patients born between 1955 and 1989, 78 of whom were homozygous and 5 of whom were compound heterozygous, neurological abnormalities such as ataxia (n = six), intention tremor (n = 11), and microcephaly (n = 10) were reported. Of the 66 patients greater than 3 years of age, 43 had speech disturbances and 29 had arithmetic deficits or problems with visual perception. IQ declined with age. Concentrations of erythrocyte GAL-1-P, UDP-GAL, and plasma and urinary galactitol did not correlate with IQ.[109] Children and adolescents homozygous for the Q188R mutation functioned within the low average IQ range, and had less developed executive functions than healthy age- and gender-matched controls.[110] Recent studies of glucose metabolism in 20- to 40-year-old patients reported significant abnormalities in brain regions that may be associated with the neuropsychological deficits reported in patients with galactosemia.[111]

Endocrine Function

In 1979, Kaufman et al. reported that 8 of 12 female patients over 13 years of age who had been managed with a GAL-restricted diet had hypergonadotropic hypogonadism.[112] Subsequently, this group found that the frequency of hypergonadotropic hypogonadism was higher in females in whom nutrition management was delayed.[60] Kaufman et al. also found that ovarian function was correlated with activity of GALT and that a patient with some activity had a lower concentration of erythrocyte GAL-1-P and higher concentrations of UDP-GLU and UDP-GAL in hemoglobin than patients with no GALT activity.[60,113] Some risk factors for premature ovarian failure in females with GALT deficiency were reported to be a genotype of Q188R/Q188R, a mean erythrocyte GAL-1-P concentration of > 3.5 mg/dL during treatment, and recovery of $^{13}CO_2$ from whole body ^{13}C-GAL oxidation of < 5%.[25]

The secondary hypoglycosylation disorders seen in patients with GALT deficiency often improve but do not disappear when GAL is removed from the diet. Berger et al. reported low blood thyroxine concentrations in two untreated infants that rose to normal on GAL removal from the diet.[114] Hypoglycosylated follicle stimulating hormone, unable to activate cyclic adenosylmonophosphate (AMP), was found in some GALT deficient females.[115,116] Later, the defective galactosylation of serum transferrin was found to improve in patients receiving a GAL-restricted diet.[36] These and other reports led to a study of 25 females and 12 males (5 to 19 years of age) with GALT deficiency (0.35 ± 0.23 mean ± SD µmol/hr/g hemoglobin, similar to activity found in homozygotes for the Q188R mutation), assessing concentrations of urinary GAL, galactitol, erythrocyte GAL-1-P, serum growth hormone (GH), leutinizing hormone (LH), follicle stimulating hormone (FSH), prolactin, estradiol, free T_4, testosterone, androstenedione, insulin-like growth factor (IGF-1), and insulin growth factor binding protein (IGFBP-3).[37]

Of the panel of analytes assessed in patients with GALT deficiency, two females had increased concentrations of GH and most girls had low normal

IGF-1 and IGFBP-3, while boys had normal concentrations. Three of 18 female patients not on estradiol supplementation and 2 of 6 on estradiol supplementation had increased FSH and LH concentrations. Concentrations of serum testosterone and sex-hormone-binding globulin were normal in all except two female patients receiving estradiol supplementation, while androstenedione and dihydroepiandrosterone (DHEAS) were normal in all patients. Prolactin serum concentrations were normal in 35 of 37 patients and serum TSH concentrations in 34 of 37 patients. Hypoglycosylation was suggested to be responsible for abnormalities found and could worsen if GAL intake was increased for any reason.[37]

Growth

Growth of children with a deficiency of GALK or GALE has not been reported, although Bosch et al.[31] found that 3 of 43 infants with GALK deficiency were small for gestational age at birth. Nadler et al. reported in 1969 that of 45 patients with GALT deficiency, 27 were less than the 10th percentile for height and weight at diagnosis and about half remained below the 10th percentile after many years of nutrition management.[1] In 1990, a report of growth in 281 patients with GALT deficiency managed with diet since an early age suggested that although growth was delayed during childhood and early adolescence, it frequently continued through the late teens, resulting in normal heights for age. Weight for height in the early years of life were not as reduced as height for age.[104] Panis et al. reported that 40 Dutch children 3 to 17 years of age on a GAL-restricted diet had significantly decreased height and weight Z-scores.[62] This group of 40 GALT-deficient patients was later reported to have normal birth length, head circumference, and weight, and 5 children grew beyond the age of 18 years.[55]

Bone Metabolism

In late 1993, Kaufman et al. reported that 40 GALT deficient patients, 3.4 to 44.2 years of age, had decreased bone density when compared to age- and gender-matched controls. The suggestion was made that the decreased sex steroids, low calcium intake, and possibly a defect in galactosylation of the collagen matrix of the bone resulted in the decreased bone density.[61] Five male and 6 female patients 2 to 18 years of age with GALT deficiency undergoing GAL restriction were found to have significantly decreased bone mineral density in relation to control subjects. Calcium intake, plasma calcium, phosphorus, parathyroid hormone (PTH), bone alkaline phosphatase, vitamin D metabolites, and osteocalcin concentrations were all normal. Only the blood concentrations of N-terminal telopeptide found in type I collagen were found to be significantly lower in patients than controls, suggesting decreased bone resorption.[117] This group subsequently reported data from 40 patients (3 to 17 years of age) with GALT deficiency undergoing GAL restriction. These Dutch patients were said to ingest recommended intakes of calcium, magnesium, zinc, vitamin D, and protein and had normal concentrations of previously reported analytes as well as 17-β-estradiol. Only concentrations of N-terminal and C-terminal telopeptides were significantly below those found in control subjects.[62]

A group of Spanish investigators reported that urinary markers of bone resorption and bone mineral density were within the normal range in six children with GALT deficiency. The suggestion was made that adequate intakes of protein and minerals and a healthy lifestyle could prevent major changes in bone metabolism.[118] Data of 62 children (5.9 ± 2.7 years, mean ± SD) and adolescents (15.6 ± 2.4 years) with GALT deficiency under good control since diagnosis as neonates were compared to data of 70 normal children. While concentrations of bone markers in the younger patients were lower than in controls, slightly higher concentrations were found in the adolescent patients. Normally, bone turnover markers decrease from childhood to adolescence with a decline during aging.[119] Further studies are needed to determine whether higher intakes of protein, minerals, and vitamins as well as tighter control of concentrations of erythrocyte GAL-1-P, if possible, and long-term administration of sex steroids and exercise would alter bone mineral density.

Maternal GALT Deficiency

While premature ovarian failure and infertility have been reported in patients with GALT deficiency even when a GAL-restricted diet is begun in infancy, some patients have produced normal children. The first report was of a black American woman, diagnosed at 4 months of age with growth failure, hepatomegaly, cataracts, a nonglucose-reducing substance in the urine, and GALT deficiency. She was subsequently found to have lactase deficiency. Only at 5 months of gestation was this GAL-restricted patient found to have an elevated concentration of erythrocyte GAL-1-P. Pregnancy and delivery were normal and the infant was clinically normal.[120] A survey of pregnancies in GALT-deficient women reported 50 pregnancies with the genotype reported only in 10. Four of the 10 women were homozygous for Q188R.[121] For suggested nutrient intakes during pregnancy, see Chapter 3, Table 3.1.

CONCLUSION

While newborn screening, early diagnosis, and nutrition management have prevented death in the infant with galactosemia, adverse effects have not been totally prevented. The expectation is that continuing scientific research will find alternative therapies for improving long-term outcomes in patients with galactosemia.

REFERENCES

1. von Reuss A. Zuckerausscheidung im säulingsalter. *Wien med Wschr*. 1908;59:799 in Nadler HL, Inouye T, Hsia DYY. Classical galactosemia: a study of fifty-five cases. In: Hsia DYY, ed. *Galactosemia*. Springfield, IL: Charles C Thomas; 1969: 127–139.
2. Gitzelmann R. Deficiency of erythrocyte galactokinase in a patient with galactose diabetes. *Lancet*. 1965;2:670–671.
3. Gitzelmann R, Steinmann B, Mitchell B, Hargis E. Uridine diphosphate galactose-4-epimerase deficiency. IV. Report of eight cases in three families. *Helv Pediatr Acta*. 1976;31:441–452.
4. National Center for Biotechnology Information. OMIM™—Online Mendelian Inheritance in Man™ (database). Available at: http://www.ncbi.nlm.nih.gov/sites/entrez?db=omim. Accessed February 2, 2008.
5. Bosch AM. Classical galactosaemia revisited. *J Inherit Metab Dis*. 2006;29:516–525.
6. Cordes FC. Galactosemia cataracts: a review. *Am J Ophthalmol*. 1960;50:1151.
7. Levy HL, Sepe SJ, Shih VE, Vawter GF, Klein JO. Sepsis due to Escherichia coli in neonates with galactosemia. *N Engl J Med*. 1977;297:823–825.
8. Holton JB, Walter JH, Tyfield LA. Galactosemia. In: Scriver CR, Beaudet AL, Sly WS, Valle D, eds. *The Metabolic and Molecular Bases of Inherited Disease*. 8th ed. New York, NY: McGraw-Hill; 2001:1553–1587.
9. Huttenlocher PR, Hillman RE, Hsia YE. Pseudotumor cerebri in galactosemia. *J Pediatr*. 1970;76:902–905.
10. Picciano MF, McDonald SS. Lactation. In: Shils ME, Shike M, Olson J, Ross AC, Caballero B, Cousins RJ, eds. *Modern Nutrition in Health and Disease*. 10th ed. Philadelphia, PA: Lippincott Williams & Wilkins; 2005:784–796.
11. Gray GM. Carbohydrate digestion and absorption. Role of the small intestine. *N Engl J Med*. 1975;292:1225–1230.
12. Goppert F. Galactosemia. *Klin Wschr* 1917;54:473 in Komrower GM, The seven ages of galactosemia. In: Hsia DYY, ed. *Galactosemia*. Springfield, IL: Charles C Thomas; 1969:5–12.
13. Mason HH, Turner ME. Chronic galactosemia. *Am J Dis Child*. 1935;50:359.
14. Kalckar HM, Anderson EP, Isselbacher KJ. Galactosemia, a congenital defect in a nucleotide transferase. *Biochim Biophys Acta*. 1956;20:262–268.
15. Weinberg AN. Detection of congenital galactosemia and the carrier state using galactose C^{14} and blood cells. *Metabolism*. 1961;10:728–734.
16. Anderson EP, Isselbacher KJ, Kalckar HM. Defect in uptake of galactose-1-phosphate into liver nucleotides in congenital galactosemia. *Science*. 1957;125:113–114.

17. Krooth RS, Weinberg AN. Studies on cell lines developed from the tissues of patients with galactosemia. *J Exp Med*. 1961;113:1155–1171.
18. Crome L. A case of galactosaemia with the pathological and neuropathological findings. *Arch Dis Child*. 1962;37:415–421.
19. Leslie ND, Immerman EB, Flach JE, Florez M, Fridovich-Keil JL, Elsas LJ. The human galactose-1-phosphate uridyltransferase gene. *Genomics*. 1992;14:474–480.
20. Tyfield L, Carmichael D. The Galactose-1-Phosphate Uridyltrasnferase Mutation Analysis Database Home Page (GALTdb). Available at: www://ich.bris.ac.uk/galtdb/. Accessed May 9, 2008.
21. Elsas LJ, Acosta PB. Inherited metabolic disease: amino acids, organic acids, and galactose. In: Shils ME, Shike M, Olson J, Ross AC, Caballero B, Cousins RJ, eds. *Modern Nutrition in Health and Disease*. 10th ed. Philadelphia, PA: Lippincott Williams & Wilkins; 2005:909–959.
22. Beutler E, Baluda MC. A simple spot screening test for galactosemia. *J Lab Clin Med*. 1966;68:137–141.
23. Elsas LJ, Langley S, Steele E, et al. Galactosemia: a strategy to identify new biochemical phenotypes and molecular genotypes. *Am J Hum Genet*. 1995;56:630–639.
24. Elsas LJ, Langley S, Paulk EM, Hjelm LN, Dembure PP. A molecular approach to galactosemia. *Eur J Pediatr*. 1995;154:S21–S27.
25. Guerrero NV, Singh RH, Manatunga A, Berry GT, Steiner RD, Elsas LJ. Risk factors for premature ovarian failure in females with galactosemia. *J Pediatr*. 2000; 137:833–841.
26. Lai K, Willis AC, Elsas LJ. The biochemical role of glutamine 188 in human galactose-1-phosphate uridyltransferase. *J Biol Chem*. 1999;274:6559–6566.
27. Elsas LJ, Fridovich-Keil J, Leslie ND. Galactosemia: a molecular approach to the enigma. *Int Pediatr*. 1993;8:101–109.
28. Elsas LJ. Prenatal diagnosis of galactose-1-phosphate uridyltransferase (GALT)-deficient galactosemia. *Prenat Diagn*. 2001;21:302–303.
29. Bosch AM, Ijlst L, Oostheim W, et al. Identification of novel mutations in classical galactosemia. *Hum Mutat*. 2005;25:502.
30. Thalhammer O, Gitzelmann R, Pantlitschko M. Hypergalactosemia and galactosuria due to galactokinase deficiency in a newborn. *Pediatrics*. 1968;42:441–445.
31. Bosch AM, Bakker HD, van Gennip AH, van Kempen JV, Wanders RJ, Wijburg FA. Clinical features of galactokinase deficiency: a review of the literature. *J Inherit Metab Dis*. 2002;25:629–634.
32. Segal S, Rutman JY, Frimpter GW. Galactokinase deficiency and mental retardation. *J Pediatr*. 1979;95:750–752.
33. Timson DJ. The structural and molecular biology of type III galactosemia. *IUBMB Life*. 2006;58:83–89.
34. Chhay JS, Vargas CA, McCorvie TJ, Fridovich-Keil JL, Timson DJ. Analysis of UDP-galactose 4-epimerase mutations associated with the intermediate form of type III galactosaemia. *J Inherit Metab Dis*. 2008;31:108–116.
35. Ridel KR, Leslie ND, Gilbert DL. An updated review of the long-term neurological effects of galactosemia. *Pediatr Neurol*. 2005;33:153–161.
36. Charlwood J, Clayton P, Keir G, Mian N, Winchester B. Defective galactosylation of serum transferrin in galactosemia. *Glycobiology*. 1998;8:351–357.
37. Rubio-Gozalbo ME, Panis B, Zimmermann LJ, Spaapen LJ, Menheere PP. The endocrine system in treated patients with classical galactosemia. *Mol Genet Metab*. 2006;89:316–322.

38. Berry GT, Nissim I, Lin Z, Mazur AT, Gibson JB, Segal S. Endogenous synthesis of galactose in normal men and patients with hereditary galactosaemia. *Lancet.* 1995;346:1073–1074.
39. Ng WG, Xu YK, Kaufman FR, Donnell GN. Deficit of uridine diphosphate galactose in galactosaemia. *J Inherit Metab Dis.* 1989;12:257–266.
40. Manis FR, Cohn LB, McBride-Chang C, Wolff JA, Kaufman FR. A longitudinal study of cognitive functioning in patients with classical galactosaemia, including a cohort treated with oral uridine. *J Inherit Metab Dis.* 1997;20:549–555.
41. Walter JH, Collins JE, Leonard JV. Recommendations for the management of galactosaemia. UK Galactosaemia Steering Group. *Arch Dis Child.* 1999;80:93–96.
42. Bosch AM, Bakker HD, Wenniger-Prick LJMdB, Wanders RJ, Wijburg FA. High tolerance for oral galactose in classical galactosaemia: dietary implications. *Arch Dis Child.* 2004;89:1034–1036.
43. Koch R, Acosta P, Ragsdale N, Donnell G. Nutrition in the treatment of galactosemia. *J Am Diet Assoc.* 1963;43:216–222.
44. Holton JB, Gillett MG, MacFaul R, Young R. Galactosaemia: a new severe variant due to uridine diphosphate galactose-4-epimerase deficiency. *Arch Dis Child.* 1981;56:885–887.
45. Gross KC, Acosta PB. Fruits and vegetables are a source of galactose: implications in planning the diets of patients with galactosaemia. *J Inherit Metab Dis.* 1991;14:253–258.
46. Panis B, Bakker JA, Sels JP, Spaapen LJ, van Loon LJ, Rubio-Gozalbo ME. Untreated classical galactosemia patient with mild phenotype. *Mol Genet Metab.* 2006;89:277–279.
47. Berry GT, Moate PJ, Reynolds RA, et al. The rate of de novo galactose synthesis in patients with galactose-1-phosphate uridyltransferase deficiency. *Mol Genet Metab.* 2004;81:22–30.
48. Huidekoper HH, Bosch AM, van der Crabben SN, Sauerwein HP, Ackermans MT, Wijburg FA. Short-term exogenous galactose supplementation does not influence rate of appearance of galactose in patients with classical galactosemia. *Mol Genet Metab.* 2005;84:265–272.
49. Schadewaldt P, Kamalanathan L, Hammen HW, Wendel U. Age dependence of endogenous galactose formation in Q188R homozygous galactosemic patients. *Mol Genet Metab.* 2004;81:31–44.
50. Williams CA, Phillips T, Macdonald I. The influence of glucose on serum galactose levels in man. *Metabolism.* 1983;32:250–256.
51. Berry GT, Singh RH, Mazur AT, et al. Galactose breath testing distinguishes variant and severe galactose-1-phosphate uridyltransferase genotypes. *Pediatr Res.* 2000;48:323–328.
52. Singh RH, Kennedy MJ, Jonas CR, Dembure P, Elsas LJ. Whole body oxidation and galactosemia genotype: prognosis for galactose tolerance in the first year of life. *J Inherit Metab Dis.* 2003;26:123A.
53. Zlatunich CO, Packman S. Galactosaemia: early treatment with an elemental formula. *J Inherit Metab Dis.* 2005;28:163–168.
54. Otten JJ, Hellwig JP, Meyers LD, eds. *Dietary Reference Intakes: The Essential Guide to Nutrient Requirements.* Washington, DC: National Academies Press, 2006.
55. Panis B, Gerver WJ, Rubio-Gozalbo ME. Growth in treated classical galactosemia patients. *Eur J Pediatr.* 2007;166:443–446.

56. Pratt EL, Snyderman SE, Cheung MW, et al. The threonine requirement of the normal infant. *J Nutr*. 1955;56:231–251.
57. Rose WC. Amino acid requirements of man. *Fed Proc*. 1949;8:546–552.
58. Fomon SJ, Haschke F, Ziegler EE, Nelson SE. Body composition of reference children from birth to age 10 years. *Am J Clin Nutr*. 1982;35:1169–1175.
59. National Center for Health Statistics. 2000 CDC Growth Charts: United States. Available at: http://www.cdc.gov/growthcharts/. Accessed January 4, 2008.
60. Kaufman FR, Kogut MD, Donnell GN, Goebelsmann U, March C, Koch R. Hypergonadotropic hypogonadism in female patients with galactosemia. *N Engl J Med*. 1981;304:994–998.
61. Kaufman FR, Loro ML, Azen C, Wenz E, Gilsanz V. Effect of hypogonadism and deficient calcium intake on bone density in patients with galactosemia. *J Pediatr*. 1993;123:365–370.
62. Panis B, Forget PP, van Kroonenburgh MJ, et al. Bone metabolism in galactosemia. *Bone*. 2004;35:982–987.
63. Panis B, Vermeer C, van Kroonenburgh MJ, et al. Effect of calcium, vitamins K1 and D3 on bone in galactosemia. *Bone*. 2006;39:1123–1129.
64. Panis B, van Kroonenburgh MJ, Rubio-Gozalbo ME. Proposal for the prevention of osteoporosis in paediatric patients with classical galactosaemia. *J Inherit Metab Dis*. 2007;30:982.
65. Mead Johnson Nutritionals. *Pediatric Products Handbook*. Evansville, IN: Mead Johnson & Company; 2004:8–13.
66. Abbott Nutrition. Similac® Advance. Available at: http://abbottnutrition.com/products.aspx?pid=44. Accessed May 28, 2008.
67. Pennington JAT. *Bowes and Church's Food Values of Portions Commonly Used*. 17th ed. Philadelphia, PA: Lippincott Williams & Wilkins; 1998:222.
68. Nickerson TA. Why use lactose and its derivatives in foods? *Food Tech*. 1978;32:40–46.
69. Reynolds LM, Henneberry GO, Baker BE. Studies on casein II. The carbohydrate moiety of casein. *J Dairy Sci*. 1959;42:1464–1471.
70. Michel V, Martley FG. Streptococcus thermophilus in cheddar cheese—production and fate of galactose. *J Dairy Res*. 2001;68:317–325.
71. Harvey CD, Jenness R, Morries HA. Gas chromatographic quantitation of surgars and non-volatile water soluble-organic acids in commercial cheddar cheese. *J Dairy Sci*. 1981;61:1648–1654.
72. Pollman RM. Ion chromatographic determination of lactose, galactose, and dextrose in grated cheese using pulsed amperometric detection. *J Assoc Off Anal Chem*. 1989;72:425–428.
73. Scaman CH, Jim VJ, Hartnett C. Free galactose concentrations in fresh and stored apples (*Malus domestica*) and processed apple products. *J Agric Food Chem*. 2004;52:511–517.
74. Hartnett C, Kim HO, Scaman CH. Effect of processing on galactose in selected fruits. *Can J Diet Pract Res*. 2007;68:46–50.
75. Acosta PB, Gross KC. Hidden sources of galactose in the environment. *Eur J Pediatr*. 1995;154:S87–S92.
76. Asp NG. Human small-intestinal-galactosidases: separation and characterization of three forms of an acid-galactosidase. *Biochem J*. 1971;121:299–308.
77. Andersson L, Bratt C, Arnoldsson KC, et al. Hydrolysis of galactolipids by human pancreatic lipolytic enzymes and duodenal contents. *J Lipid Res*. 1995;36:1392–1400.

78. Gross KC, Weese SJ, Johnson J, Gropper SS. Soluble galactose content of selected baby food. Cereal and juices. *J Food Comp Anal*. 1995;8:319–323.
79. Gropper SS, Gross KC, Olds SJ. Galactose content of selected fruit and vegetable baby foods: implications for infants on galactose-restricted diets. *J Am Diet Assoc*. 1993;93:328–330.
80. Gropper SS, Weese JO, West PA, Gross KC. Free galactose content of fresh fruits and strained fruit and vegetable baby foods: more foods to consider for the galactose-restricted diet. *J Am Diet Assoc*. 2000;100:573–575.
81. Minka S, Laurent G, Brunteau M, Pivot V, Michel G. Isolation and composition of glycolipids from corn flour. *Food Chem*. 1991;39:329–336.
82. Bengtson S, Andersson R, Westerlund E, Aman P. Content, structure and viscosity of soluble arabino-xylans in rye grain from several countries. *J Sci Food Agric*. 1992;58:531–537.
83. Bevenue A, Williams KT. Rice analysis. Hemicellulose components of rice. *Agric Food Chem*. 1956;4:1014–1017.
84. Carter HE, McCleur RH, Slifer ED. Lipids of wheat flour. I. Characterization of galactosylglycerol components. *J Am Chem Soc*. 1956;78:3735–3738.
85. Hamberg M, Liepinsh E, Otting G, Griffiths W. Isolation and structure of a new galactolipid from oat seeds. *Lipids*. 1998;33:355–363.
86. Aspinall GO. Chemistry of Cell Wall Polysaccharides. In: Preiss J, ed. *The Biochemistry of Plants*. New York, NY: Academic Press; 1980:473–500.
87. Ash ASF, Reynolds TM. Water-soluble constituents of fruit. II. An examination of the sugars and polyols of apricots, peaches, pears, and apples by paper chromatography. *Aust J Chem*. 1955;8:276–279.
88. Berry GT, Palmieri M, Gross KC, et al. The effect of dietary fruits and vegetables on urinary galactitol excretion in galactose-1-phosphate uridyltransferase deficiency. *J Inherit Metab Dis*. 1993;16:91–100.
89. Holton JB. Galactosemia. In: Schaub J, van Hoof F, Vis HL, eds. *Inborn Errors of Metabolism*. New York, NY: Raven Press; 1991:169–180.
90. Wiesmann UN, Rose-Beutler B, Schluchter R. Leguminosae in the diet: the raffinose-stachyose question. *Eur J Pediatr*. 1995;154:S93–S96.
91. Segal S. The enigma of galactosemia. *Int Pediatr*. 1992;7:75–82.
92. Cerbullis J. Sugars in Caracas cocoa beans. *Arch Biochem Biophys*. 1954;449–450.
93. Yokotsuka T. Soy sauce biochemistry. *Adv Food Res*. 1986;30:195–329.
94. Akinyele IO, Akinlosotu A. Effect of soaking, dehulling and fermentation on oligosaccharides and nutrient content of cow peas. *Food Chem*. 1991;41:43–53.
95. Smith JS, Villalobos MC, Kottemann CM. Quantitative determination of sugars in various food products. *J Food Sci*. 1986;51:1373–1375.
96. Harju M. Lactobionic acid as a substrate of β-galactosidases. *Milchwissenschaft*. 1990;45:411–415.
97. Kumar A, Weatherly MR, Beaman DC. Sweeteners, flavorings, and dyes in antibiotic preparations. *Pediatrics*. 1991;87:352–360.
98. Wierenga KJ, Lai K, Buchwald P, Tang M. High-throughput screening for human galactokinase inhibitors. *J Biomol Screen*. 2008;13:415–423.
99. Donnell GN, Bergren WR, Perry G, Koch R. Galactose-1-phosphate in galactosemia. *Pediatrics*. 1963;31:802–810.
100. Wehrli SL, Berry GT, Palmieri M, Mazur A, Elsas L III, Segal S. Urinary galactonate in patients with galactosemia: quantitation by nuclear magnetic resonance spectroscopy. *Pediatr Res*. 1997;42:855–861.

101. Ficicioglu C, Yager C, Segal S. Galactitol and galactonate in red blood cells of children with the Duarte/galactosemia genotype. *Mol Genet Metab*. 2005;84:152–159.
102. Yager CT, Chen J, Reynolds R, Segal S. Galactitol and galactonate in red blood cells of galactosemic patients. *Mol Genet Metab*. 2003;80:283–289.
103. Komrower GM, Lee DH. Long-term follow-up of galactosaemia. *Arch Dis Child*. 1970;45:367–373.
104. Waggoner DD, Buist NR, Donnell GN. Long-term prognosis in galactosaemia: results of a survey of 350 cases. *J Inherit Metab Dis*. 1990;13:802–818.
105. Shield JP, Wadsworth EJ, MacDonald A, et al. The relationship of genotype to cognitive outcome in galactosaemia. *Arch Dis Child*. 2000;83:248–250.
106. Potter NL, Lazarus JA, Johnson JM, Steiner RD, Shriberg LD. Correlates of language impairment in children with galactosaemia. *J Inherit Metab Dis*. 2008;31:524–532.
107. Webb AL, Singh RH, Kennedy MJ, Elsas LJ. Verbal dyspraxia and galactosemia. *Pediatr Res*. 2003;53:396–402.
108. Robertson A, Singh RH, Guerrero NV, Hundley M, Elsas LJ. Outcomes analysis of verbal dyspraxia in classic galactosemia. *Genet Med*. 2000;2:142–148.
109. Schweitzer S, Shin Y, Jakobs C, Brodehl J. Long-term outcome in 134 patients with galactosaemia. *Eur J Pediatr*. 1993;152:36–43.
110. Antshel KM, Epstein IO, Waisbren SE. Cognitive strengths and weaknesses in children and adolescents homozygous for the galactosemia Q188R mutation: a descriptive study. *Neuropsychology*. 2004;18:658–664.
111. Dubroff JG, Ficicioglu C, Segal S, Wintering NA, Alavi A, Newberg AB. FDG-PET findings in patients with galactosaemia. *J Inherit Metab Dis*. 2008;31:533–539.
112. Kaufman F, Kogut MD, Donnell GN, Koch H, Goebelsmann U. Ovarian failure in galactosaemia. *Lancet*. 1979;2:737–738.
113. Kaufman FR, Xu YK, Ng WG, Donnell GN. Correlation of ovarian function with galactose-1-phosphate uridyl transferase levels in galactosemia. *J Pediatr*. 1988;112:754–756.
114. Berger HM, Vlasveld L, van Gelderen HH, Ruys JH. Low serum thyroxine (T_4) concentrations in babies with galactosemia. *J Pediatr*. 1983;103:930–932.
115. Prestoz LL, Couto AS, Shin YS, Petry KG. Altered follicle stimulating hormone isoforms in female galactosaemia patients. *Eur J Pediatr*. 1997;156:116–120.
116. Combarnous Y. Molecular basis of the specificity of binding of glycoprotein hormones to their receptors. *Endocr Rev*. 1992;13:670–691.
117. Rubio-Gozalbo ME, Hamming S, van Kroonenburgh MJ, Bakker JA, Vermeer C, Forget PP. Bone mineral density in patients with classic galactosaemia. *Arch Dis Child*. 2002;87:57–60.
118. Fernandez Espuelas C, Manjon Llorente G, Gonzalez Lopez JM, Ruiz-Echarri MP, Baldellou Vazquez A. Bone mineral turnover and bone densitometry in patients with a high-risk diet: hyperphenylalaninemia and galactosemia. *An Pediatr (Barc)*. 2005;63:224–229.
119. Gajewska J, Ambroszkiewicz J, Radomyska B, et al. Serum markers of bone turnover in children and adolescents with classic galactosemia. *Adv Med Sci*. 2008; 53:214–220.
120. Roe TF, Hallatt JG, Donnell GN, Ng WG. Childbearing by a galactosemic woman. *J Pediatr*. 1971;78:1026–1030.
121. Gubbels CS, Land JA, Rubio-Gozalbo ME. Fertility and impact of pregnancies on the mother and child in classic galactosemia. *Obstet Gynecol Surv*. 2008;63:334–343.

Chapter 10

Nutrition Management of Patients with Inherited Disorders of Mitochondrial Fatty Acid Oxidation

Melanie B. Gillingham

INTRODUCTION

Fatty acid oxidation (FAO) defects are a family of at least 22 different inherited genetic disorders in the mitochondrial fatty acid oxidation pathway. Most of the disorders have an increasingly broad range of recognized phenotypes (see Chapter 1) from mild to severe. Severe phenotypes typically present in infancy with catastrophic episodes of fasting or illness-induced hypoketotic hypoglycemia. The most common clinical presentation of all patients with FAO disorders is relatively uniform: nausea, vomiting, somnolence, and hepatic encephalopathy, indistinguishable from Reye syndrome, progressing to coma and often death.[1] Cardiomyopathy is a frequent life-threatening complication of acute metabolic decompensation in many patients with an FAO defect. FAO defects may also present in patients as sudden infant death; as many as one-third of the initial episodes may be fatal.[2] Children who survive an initial metabolic crisis may suffer recurrent decompensation episodes prior to diagnosis and develop chronic disability including muscular hypotonia and developmental delay. Alternately, patients with mild phenotypes of FAO deficiency may not present until adolescence or adulthood, and these cases typically present as exercise intolerance with recurrent episodes of rhabdomyolysis and myoglobinuria. A few affected cases may remain permanently asymptomatic.

Collectively, patients with an FAO defect appear to be relatively common (up to 1 out of 9,000 births in some populations). All are inherited in an autosomal recessive pattern, and specific gene defects have been identified for most of the disorders. The biochemical hallmark of all patients with an FAO disorder is an abnormal response to fasting characterized by low ketone production in the face of increased energy demands. The consequence is fasting hypoglycemia, often in association with severe acidosis secondary to the inappropriate accumulation of intermediate metabolites of fatty acid oxidation.

Biochemistry

The process of mitochondrial fatty acid β-oxidation is depicted in Figure 10.1. The first and rate-limiting step of long-chain fatty acid oxidation is conducted by carnitine palmitoyltransferase 1 (CPT-1; step 1). CPT-1 catalyzes the conversion of a long-chain fatty acyl CoA to a fatty acylcarnitine. CPT-1 is highly regulated by its allosteric inhibitor, malonyl-CoA. In the presence of adequate glucose, cytosolic malonyl-CoA concentrations rise and inhibit CPT-1 activity. During periods of fasting or prolonged exercise, malonyl-CoA concentrations decrease and the inhibition of CPT-1 is released. In the presence of active CPT-1, the acylcarnitine conjugates are then transported into the mitochondria by carnitine:acylcarnitine translocase (step 2). Once inside the matrix, the reaction is reversed by CPT-2 and free carnitine, and a long-chain fatty acyl-CoA is reformed (step 3).

Long-chain fatty acid oxidation represents the major pathway for adenosine triphosphate (ATP) synthesis from fatty acids because > 95% of dietary fatty acids in the diet as well as the majority of endogenous lipid stores are long-chain fatty acids. Oxidation of medium- and short-chain fatty acids (SCFAs) is primarily from the successful oxidation of long-chain fats to shorter chain lengths and/or the oxidation of SCFAs from colonic fermentation. The average diet contains little medium- or SCFAs (< 5% of total lipid) unless specifically supplemented with medium chain triglycerides (MCTs). Transport of medium- ($C_{6\text{-}10}$) and short-chain ($C_{4\text{-}6}$) fatty acids into the mitochondria does not absolutely require L-carnitine, although the carnitine shuttle system may contribute to mitochondrial uptake of these substrates.

Once inside the mitochondria, fatty acid β-oxidation occurs in a repeating four-enzyme cycle, each "spiral" of the cycle releasing one molecule of acetyl-CoA (steps 4–7). The first reaction is performed by one of five acyl-CoA dehydrogenases; the choice of enzyme is dependent upon the structure and chain length of the fatty acid substrate. Straight-chain fatty acids of 12 to

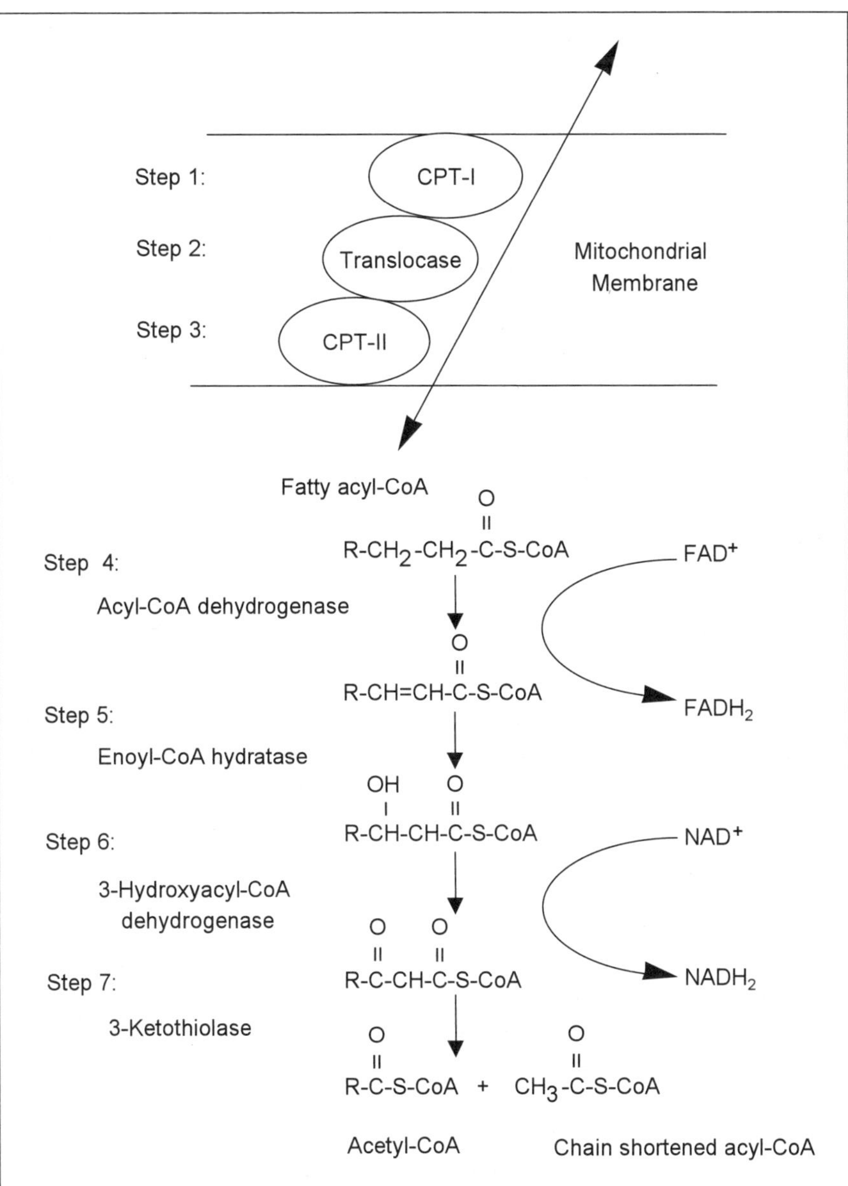

Figure 10.1 *Fatty Acid β-Oxidation*

Source: Courtesy of Oxford University Press. Reprinted with permission from Ekvall SW, Ekvall VK, eds. *Pediatric Nutrition in Chronic Diseases and Developmental Disorders*. 2nd ed. Oxford, United Kingdom: Oxford University Press; 2005.

Note: CoA, coenzyme A; CPT-1, -2, carnitine palmitoyl transferase-1, -2; FAD^+ flavin adenine dinucleotide; $FADH_2$, FAD; NAD^+ nicotinamide adenine dineucleotide.

18 carbons in length ($C_{12\text{-}18}$) are metabolized by very-long-chain acyl-CoA dehydrogenase (VLCAD), an enzyme that is bound to the inner mitochondrial membrane. Long-chain branched or desaturated fatty acids are likely substrates for long-chain acyl-CoA dehydrogenase (LCAD), an enzyme found within the mitochondrial matrix, but the physiological importance of this enzyme in humans is questionable. To date, no deficiency disorder of LCAD has been identified in humans.[1] Long-chain fatty acids may also be dehydrogenated by a newly identified enzyme, acyl-CoA dehydrogenase 9 (ACAD9), that has a substrate preference for polyunsaturated fatty acids and is the primary acyl-CoA dehydrogenase expressed in the central nervous system.[3,4] ACAD9 deficiency was recently described in three patients.[5] Chain-shortened fatty acids become substrates for either medium-chain ($C_{6\text{–}12}$; MCAD) or short-chain ($C_{4\text{–}6}$; SCAD) acyl-CoA dehydrogenases. All these reactions require riboflavin in the form of flavin adenine dinucleotide (FAD) as a coenzyme and provide reducing equivalents (FADH). FADH is coupled directly to ATP synthesis through electron transfer flavoprotein (ETF) and ETF:CoQ oxidoreductase (ETF:QO) to coenzyme Q of the electron transport chain.

Three further enzymatic steps (steps 5–7) complete one cycle, leaving a fatty acyl-CoA two carbons shorter for further β-oxidation. For long-chain fatty acids, steps 5 to 7 are catalyzed by a single membrane-bound enzyme complex called mitochondrial trifunctional protein (TFP). TFP catalyzes the long-chain enoyl-CoA hydratase, long-chain 3-hydroxyacyl-CoA dehydrogenase, and long-chain ketothiolase activities. For shorter fatty acids, a series of distinct mitochondrial matrix proteins individually catalyze the remaining steps of the β-oxidation cycle. These enzymes include crotonase or short-chain enoyl-CoA hydratase, and medium/short-chain 3-hydroxyacyl-CoA dehydrogenase (M/SCHAD) that are responsible for steps 5 (hydration) and 6 (dehydration) of both medium- and SCFAs.[1] Niacin in the form of niacin adenine dineucleotide (NAD) is a required coenzyme for both the LCHAD function of trifunctional protein and M/SCAD activity. Reducing equivalents (NADH) generated in this step (3-hydroxyacyl-CoA dehydrogenase) are coupled to Complex I of the electron transport chain and used to generate ATP. Human deficiency of M/SCHAD has been reported and was previously referred to as short-chain 3-hydroxyacyl-CoA dehydrogenase or SCHAD deficiency. More recently this disorder has been termed 3-hydroxyacyl-CoA dehydrogenase (HAD) deficiency.[6]

The final cleavage step (step 7) is catalyzed by medium-chain 3-ketoacyl-CoA thiolase (MKAT) for medium-chain fatty acids and by short-chain 3-ketoacyl-CoA thiolase (SKAT) for SCFAs.[1] The product for each cycle of the FAO system is a chain-shortened fatty acid and one molecule of acetyl-CoA. In the liver and muscle, acetyl-CoA generated through fatty acid oxidation is a substrate for the citric acid cycle, sparing glycogen and preventing glucose depletion. Acetyl-CoA generated from fatty acid oxidation is also necessary for the liver to make ketone bodies during periods of fasting. Ketone bodies are released into circulation and provide an alternative fuel for tissues such as the brain.

Molecular Biology

All of the enzymes involved in the FAO system, their associated gene (see Chapter 1), OMIM number,[7] and chromosome location are listed in Table 10.1. CPT-1 has three isoforms, products of three separate genes. CPT-1a is the isoform expressed in liver, kidney, brain, fibroblasts, and leukocytes. CPT-1b is the isoform expressed in muscle and white adipose tissue. CPT-1c was recently identified and is localized to brain and testes.[8] While both CPT-1a and CPT-1b readily form acylcarnitines and are inhibited (90% decrease in enzyme activity) by malonyl-CoA in culture, CPT-1c does not appear to form acylcarnitines.[9] The function and purpose of this isoform remains to be established. To date all cases of CPT-1 deficiency in humans are due to inherited defects of the CPT-1a gene. No cases of CPT-1b or CPT-1c deficiency have been identified. Multiple mutations in the CPT-1a gene have been described.[10] Recently, a common mutation in CPT-1a has been noted in the Alaska Native and First Nations population of Canada. Identified infants are homozygous for the same DNA sequence variant (c.1436C→T), which results in the substitution of a conserved proline at amino acid 479 with leucine (P479L). The clinical phenotype of this common variant is unknown at this time.

The mature VLCAD protein contains 20 exons and is bound to the inner mitochondrial membrane. More than 80 different mutations spanning the VLCAD gene have been reported and no common mutation has been identified.[11] ACAD9 contains 22 exons and has two predominant isoforms due to alternative splicing of the mRNA; one isoform is localized to the mitochondria and one to the cytoplasm of cells expressing ACAD9.[5] Because only three patients with ACAD9 deficiency have been reported, common mutations have not yet been described.

Mitochondrial trifunctional protein is a heteroctomer comprised of four α and four β subunits encoded by two different genes, both located on chromosome 2p23(11). The long-chain acyl-CoA hydratase and the long-chain hydroxyacyl-CoA dehydrogenase activity are encoded in the α subunit and the long-chain acyl-CoA ketothiolase activity is encoded in the β subunit. Isolated LCHAD deficiency results from the selective loss of LCHAD activity and relative preservation of hydratase and ketothiolase activity. A common

Table 10.1 *Enzymes of the Fatty Acid Oxidation Pathway*

Enzyme	*OMIM Number*	*Gene Location*
Carnitine palmityltransferase-1A (CPT1A)	600528	11q13
Carnitine palmityltransferase-1B (CPT1B)	601987	22qter
CPT1C	608846	19q13.33
Carnitine/acylcarnitine translocase (CACT)	212138	3p21.31
Carnitine palmityltransferase-2 (CPT2)	600650	1p32
Very long-chain acyl-CoA dehydrogenase (VLCAD)	609575	17p13
Acyl-CoA dehydrogenase 9 (ACAD9)	611126	3q26
Long-chain acyl-CoA dehydrogenase (LCAD)	201460	2q34-q35
Mitochondrial trifunctional protein (TFP)	600890 (α subunit) 143450 (β subunit)	2p23
Medium-chain acyl-CoA dehydrogenase (MCAD)	607008	1p31
Medium-chain 3-ketoacyl-CoA thiolase (MCKAT)	602199	
Short-chain acyl-CoA dehydrogenase (SCAD)	201470	12q22-qter
Short-chain enoyl-CoA hydratase (SCEH)	602292	10q26.2-q26.3
M/Short-chain 3-hydroxyacyl-CoA dehydrogenase (SCHAD)	300256	Xp11.2
Short-chain 3-ketoacyl-CoA thiolase (SCKAT) or β-ketothiolase	607809	11q22.3-q23.1

Source: National Center for Biotechnology Information. OMIM™—Online Mendelian Inheritance in Man™ (database). Available at: http://www.ncbi.nlm.nih.gov/sites/entrez?db=omim. Accessed February 2, 2008.

Note: Enzymes of the mitochondrial fatty acid β-oxidation pathway. Online Mendelian Inheritance in Man, OMIM, is a searchable database of known inherited diseases and their associated genes. Chromosome location gives the known chromosome that particular gene is mapped to.

missense mutation, (c.1528G→C) accounts for about 87% of the alleles in LCHAD deficiency.[12] This common mutation decreases LCHAD activity but does not alter the amount of protein expression of either mitochondrial trifunctional protein (MTP) subunit. Other mutations in both the α and β subunits have been shown to result in the loss of all three enzyme activities and TFP deficiency. These mutations appear to lead to destabilization of the heterodimer and selective degradation of the protein.[13,14]

Medium-chain acyl-CoA dehydrogenase deficiency (MCADD) is the most common defect in patients with an FAOD. In 1990, a common mutation in the MCAD gene, a c.985A→G point mutation, was identified resulting in a lysine to glutamic acid substitution at position 304 of the mature protein. This missense mutation was subsequently shown to account for approximately 90% of the alleles in identified patients.[15] Other point mutations have been identified in the first 11 of 12 exons, but the 985A>G point mutation still accounts for the majority of disease-causing alleles.[11] The c.985A→G mutation results in decreased but not absent expression of the mutant protein due to defective protein folding.[15]

Two common mutations in the SCAD gene have been described (c.511C→T and c.625G→A), but population studies have found that up to 14% of the general population is homozygous or compound heterozygous for these common missense mutations.[16] This observation combined with the new finding that many infants identified by newborn screening remain asymptomatic has led to considerable debate about the clinical relevance of the common mutations and presentation of patients with true SCAD deficiency. Multiple, other rare mutations have also been described. Patients with SCAD deficiency present with primarily neuromuscular symptoms and are characterized by increased ethylmalonic aciduria. The variations in the SCAD gene, both common and rare mutations, appear to be susceptibility genes that together with other environmental factors may result in symptomatic SCAD deficiency.[15]

Approximately five patients with short-chain hydroxyacyl-CoA dehydrogenase (SCHAD) deficiency have been described in the literature. The mutations in the SCHAD gene among these patients is heterogeneous with multiple unique missense mutations described among different families.[17]

Newborn Screening and Diagnosis

The advent of tandem mass spectroscopy for newborn screening has changed the way many patients are being identified. Each specific FAO defect is associated with a unique blood acylcarnitine profile (see an example in Table 10.2). Most U.S. states screen acylcarnitine profiles from a blood spot as part of the newborn screening program (see Chapter 2). Tandem mass spectroscopy newborn screening can detect affected children presymptomatically and, with proper nutrition management and medical treatment, prevent catastrophic illness and death.[18-20] Once a specific FAO defect has been suggested by screening laboratory studies, further tests must be performed to confirm the diagnosis. Confirmatory tests may include additional acylcarnitine

Table 10.2 ***A Comparison of Plasma Acylcarnitine Profile in Subjects with Different FAO Disorders***

	CPT2i	*CPT2a*	*VLCAD*	*LCHAD*	*TFP*	*MCAD*	*SCAD*	*Normal Range*
C:0				37.17				6.29–27.73
C:2	11.37	4.27	1.99	14.06	9.64	1.53	15.37	1.83–27.57
C3	0.35	0.28	0.26	0.80	0.20	0.12	0.38	0.08–1.77
C4	0.16 0.03	0.11 0.00	0.16 0.00	0.25	0.41 0.01	0.06	1.20 0.02	0.06–1.05
C5	0.06	0.14	0.13	0.24	0.11	0.10	0.57	0.05–0.62
C4-OH		0.00	0.00	0.06	0.01	0.00		0.01–0.50
C6	0.67	0.04	0.00	0.10	0.07	0.30		0.01–0.22
C5-OH		0.00	0.00	0.05	0.03	0.03	0.04	0.01–0.11
C6-OH		0.00	0.00	0.02	0.05			0.00–0.18
C8:1	0.02	0.16	0.05	0.12	0.14	0.12		0.02–0.90
C8	1.00	0.09	0.00	0.15	0.32	1.55	0.14	0.01–0.44
C10:2		0.14		0.03	0.05		0.02	0.00–0.11
C10:1	0.13		0.06	0.20	0.12	0.29	0.11	0.01–0.45
C:10	5.91		0.04	0.29	0.12 0.03	0.22	0.27	0.02–0.90
C10:1-OH				0.05	0.03			0.00–0.11

(continues)

Table 10.2 ***A Comparison of Plasma Acylcarnitine Profile in Subjects with Different FAO Disorders**, Continued*

	CPT2i	***CPT2a***	***VLCAD***	***LCHAD***	***TFP***	***MCAD***	***SCAD***	***Normal Range***
C5-DC		0.00		0.21	0.16			0.00–0.09
C12:1		0.12	0.06	0.76	0.19	0.03	0.09	0.00–0.36
C12		0.23	0.10	0.78	0.20	0.03	0.10	0.02–0.34
C12:1-OH				0.15	0.05			0.00–0.05
C12-OH				0.22	0.08			0.00–0.08
C14:2	0.08	0.05	0.51	1.07	0.15	0.00	0.02	0.01–0.12
C14:1	0.06	0.10	1.76	2.21	0.32	0.04	0.08	0.01–0.34
C14	0.16	0.19	0.32	0.62	0.13	0.00	0.06	0.01–0.14
C14:1-OH		0.03	0.00	0.17	0.06	0.00	0.01	0.00–0.17
C14-OH		0.00	0.00	0.25	0.04	0.00		0.00–0.04
C16:1	0.10			0.37	0.04			0.00–0.20
C16	1.44	0.57	0.29	0.43	0.09	0.08	0.20	0.04–0.51
C16:1-OH			0.00	0.35	0.04	0.00	0.03	0.00–0.35
C16-OH		0.00	0.00	0.60	0.05	0.00	0.02	0.00–0.06

(continues)

Table 10.2 *A Comparison of Plasma Acylcarnitine Profile in Subjects with Different FAO Disorders,* Continued

	CPT2i	*CPT2a*	*VLCAD*	*LCHAD*	*TFP*	*MCAD*	*SCAD*	*Normal Range*
C18:2	0.51	0.36	0.17	0.41	0.06	0.00	0.09	0.00–0.30
C18:1	0.74	0.93	0.33	0.50	0.12	0.06	0.13	0.03–0.44
C18	0.72			0.17	0.05		0.07	0.01–0.11
C18:2-OH	0.02	0.00		0.17	0.02	0.00	0.01	0.00–0.05
C18:1-OH	0.02	0.00		0.72	0.04	0.00	0.01	0.00–0.03
C18-OH				0.47	0.03		0.01	0.00–0.04

Notes: Data are expressed as μmol/L.
Analysis completed at the Biochemical Genetics Laboratory, Mayo Clinic, Rochester, Minnesota.
Representative acylcarnitine profiles from patients with various FAO disorders.

profiles on blood spots or plasma, direct enzymatic assays in liver, peripheral blood lymphocytes, or cultured skin fibroblasts or mutation analysis. Some fatty acid oxidation defects, namely MCAD or LCHAD deficiencies, are associated with specific disease-causing mutations in the gene that encodes the enzyme in question. Mutation analysis, when available, is easy and quick to perform, less expensive than enzymatic testing, and absolutely diagnostic if the patient is homozygous for a common mutation. The common mutations associated with these conditions are responsible for most but not all cases, so negative findings on a specific mutation analysis do not definitively rule out these disorders. Some cases may be missed by newborn screening and present symptomatically later in life. As with newborn screening, the majority of FAO defects are detected by studies of plasma acylcarnitine profiles in patients presenting with Reye syndrome, myopathy, cardiomyopathy, unexplained liver disease, or hypoglycemia. Urine organic dicarboxycylic aciduria is also suggestive of an FAO disorder. Specific profiles observed in urine organic acids or acylcarnitine profiles suggest specific defects in FAO metabolism that warrant further confirmatory testing.

Outcomes if Untreated

Medium-chain acyl-CoA dehydrogenase deficiency is the most common defect in fatty acid oxidation. The typical acute clinical presentation of the patient includes fasting- or illness-induced hypoketotic hypoglycemia, often associated with metabolic acidosis and hepatocellular dysfunction that can progress to full-blown Reye syndrome. Chronically, cardiomyopathy and/or signs of muscle carnitine depletion such as weakness or hypotonia can also occur and may be accompanied by fatigue or lethargy. The most severe presentation is of sudden death in the first months of life or even within the first few days after birth, presumably due to hypoglycemia. On the other hand, some patients who are MCAD deficient may never become symptomatic. The reason some cases never develop symptoms is unknown but is hypothesized to be because these persons never develop carnitine depletion together with sufficient stress to induce a metabolic crisis, or because they carry mutations with relatively mild physiologic effects. Avoidance of fasting with administration of high carbohydrate supplements during periods of illness or stress prevents most episodes of metabolic decompensation.[21]

Short-chain acyl-CoA dehydrogenase deficiency can cause failure to thrive, recurrent vomiting with or without hypoglycemia and/or ketosis, hypotonia, marked developmental delay, seizures, and early demise. Symptomatic SCAD deficiency is very rare and is characterized by urinary ethylmalonic acid excretion.[22]

3-hydroxyacyl-CoA dehydrogenase deficiency has a similar presentation to SCADD including hypoglycemia, hypotonia, and seizures. Even with frequent high-carbohydrate meals, episodes of hypoglycemia and hyperinsulinemia may occur.[23,24] Diagnosis and metabolic status of HAD deficiency must be measured using plasma-free 3-hydroxy fatty acid profiles because short- and medium-chain 3-hydroxy fatty acids do not form acylcarnitine conjugates.[25,26]

Defects in carnitine-dependent transport of long-chain fatty acids into the mitochondria include carnitine transport defects, carnitine palmitoyl transferase 1 deficiency (CPT-1), CPT-2 deficiency, and carnitine/acylcarnitine translocase deficiency. Muscle depletion of carnitine presents with hypotonia or weakness, cardiac depletion causes cardiomyopathy, and hepatocellular depletion can cause hepatic steatosis or fulminant Reye syndrome, any of which can be precipitated during stress or minor starvation.

Carnitine palmitoyl transferase 1a deficiency (CPT-1a) causes symptomatic fasting hypoketotic hypoglycemia and occasionally hepatocellular damage. The heart and muscle are rarely involved because CPT-1a is the liver isoform of the enzyme. One case of CPT-1 deficiency with muscle pain and rhabdomyolysis in a previously asymptomatic adult has been reported in the literature.[10] In CPT-1 deficiency, total and free plasma carnitine concentrations are characteristically elevated; this observation is unique among all known fatty acid oxidation defects and is otherwise seen only in association with carnitine supplementation or renal insufficiency.[27]

In CPT-2 deficiency, an infantile form presents with severe hypoglycemia, myopathy, and cardiomyopathy leading to death.[27] Plasma-free carnitine concentration is low with elevated acylcarnitines. A milder form presents with lipid myopathy, recurrent rhabdomyolysis, and myoglobinuria in young adults. Carnitine/acylcarnitine translocase deficiency is clinically similar to infantile CPT-2 deficiency. Patients often present in the neonatal or infant period with severe hypoketotic hypoglycemia, hyperammonemia due to liver failure, and elevated acylcarnitine concentrations associated with intercurrent illness.[28]

Very-long-chain acyl-CoA-dehydrogenase deficiency has two different clinical phenotypes. The severe phenotype is characterized by hypertrophic cardiomyopathy with pericardial effusion very early in life often resulting in early demise with or without treatment. The mild phenotype presents as hypoketotic hypoglycemia with recurrent myopathy and rhabdomyolysis similar to MCAD and LCHAD deficiencies. During acute illness there are characteristic increases in plasma long-chain acylcarnitine concentrations.[29]

ACAD9 deficiency can include hypoketotic hypoglycemia, liver failure, and cardiomyopathy but also includes some neurological symptoms such as cerebral stroke.[5]

Long-chain 3-hydroxyacyl-CoA dehydrogenase deficiency (selective loss of the LCHAD activity within TFP) and mitochondrial trifunctional protein deficiency (loss of all three enzymatic functions) have very similar presentation and clinical course. Like MCADD, children typically present with hypoketotic hypoglycemia, associated with metabolic acidosis, hepatocellular dysfunction, and cardiomyopathy. Elevated plasma long-chain hydroxy acylcarnitine concentrations are diagnostic of LCHAD or TFP deficiency and are useful in monitoring nutrition management of the disorder. Pigmentary retinopathy and vision loss during childhood and progressive peripheral neuropathy are complications specific to LCHAD/TFP deficiency that are not observed in the other FAO disorders.[30] Not all patients experience all complications of the disease. While the underlying etiology of the hypoketotic hypoglycemia appears to be a deficiency of energy from depleted carbohydrate stores, the etiology of the other complications is not completely understood. A depletion of energy or the toxic effects of the accumulation of potentially toxic metabolic products are thought to be causative. Thus, the primary goal of nutrition management is to provide adequate energy and minimize accumulation of potentially toxic metabolites such as hydroxyacylcarnitines and hydroxy fatty acids (see Table 10.2).

Nutrition Management

Optimal nutrition management of patients with disorders of most of the FAs has not been studied in a systematic manner and is generally based upon anecdotal experience. The primary goal of nutrition management in all patients with an FAO defect is to minimize fatty acid oxidation by avoiding fasting and providing adequate nonfat energy during stress, either orally or parenterally if needed. Provision of adequate energy and frequent feeding should be initiated in infants suspected of having an FAO disorder prior to confirmation of the diagnosis.

Avoid Fasting

Healthy infants and children adapt to fasting by increasing hepatic gluconeogenesis and mobilizing fat stores for ketogenesis, in order to maintain adequate blood concentrations of substrates for systemic energy production. However, a fatty acid oxidation disorder reduces the capacity to utilize free fatty acids (FFAs) for energy and ketone production. In addition, the reduced ability to oxidize fatty acids for ATP production impairs hepatic gluconeogenesis. Normal gluconeogenesis depends on adequate acetyl-CoA as substrate and uses ATP to synthesize glucose; the block in FAO impairs the production of the necessary substrate (acetyl-CoA) and energy (ATP) for glucose synthesis in the liver. This is compounded by the increased systemic need for glucose resulting from the lack of ketones, ultimately leading to hypoglycemia. Controlled fasting has been used diagnostically in patients suspected to have a disorder of fatty acid oxidation, and also for the development of guidelines for the treatment of patients with a known FAO disorder.[31]

A fasting test in two patients with classic CPT-1a deficiency (9 months and 19 months old) demonstrated a markedly increased FFA/ketone ratio (7 and 40, normal = 0.8), and hypoglycemia (40 and 27 mg/dL) after 20 hours of fasting.[31] Several studies have reported the results of fasting in patients with MCADD, the most common of the FAO disorders.[31-34] Based on an analysis of 35 fasting studies performed on 31 patients with MCADD, a maximum duration of fasting of 8 hours between 6 months and 1 year of age, 10 hours in the second year of life, and 12 hours thereafter has been recommended.[32] These authors defined a safe duration of fasting as the period during which no clinical symptoms (lethargy, vomiting, sweating, tachycardia) or hypoglycemia (glucose < 47 mg/dL) were observed. Significantly, in 6 out of 35 fasting tests in patients with MCADD, clinical symptoms were observed before hypoglycemia was noted, consistent with the generally held belief that blood glucose concentrations are a poor indicator of metabolic status in patients with an FAO disorder. Because lethargy, sweating, or tachycardia may precede hypoglycemia, blood glucose monitoring may not be helpful in the management of these disorders and provide a false sense of security to families. Other fasting studies have used abnormal metabolites such as an increase in plasma acylcarnitine concentration as an end point. Plasma long-chain acylcarnitine concentrations increased dramatically after a 12-hour fast in a 10-year-old patient with VLCAD deficiency, and plasma long-chain hydroxyacylcarnitine concentrations rose after 6 hours of fasting in a toddler with LCHAD deficiency.[35,36] Plasma glucose concentrations remained normal during these controlled fasts and the effects of elevated plasma acylcarnitine concentrations on clinical outcomes are not completely understood.

In general, the results of controlled fasting studies in patients with an FAO disorder suggest that fasting > 12 hours should be avoided. The necessity of more specific fasting guidelines is debatable; most healthy children will choose to eat frequently, approximately every 6 to 8 hours. However, many U.S. metabolic centers use the following guidelines: infants less than 4 months of age should not exceed 4 hours; between 5 and 12 months, an additional hour can be added for each month.[37,38] Nutrition management that includes avoidance of fasting and frequent high-carbohydrate meals for the routine management of all patients with an FAO disorder prevents most episodes of metabolic decompensation. It is important to note that all controlled fasting studies have been conducted in healthy subjects. The majority of episodes of metabolic decompensation in patients with an FAO disorder occur with intercurrent illness or prolonged exercise. The ability of patients with an FAO disorder to tolerate fasting during illness or stress is significantly reduced.

Nutrient Requirements

Fat and Essential Fatty Acids

Restricting fat intake in patients with defects in short- or medium-chain fatty acid oxidation does not appear to be beneficial. A study among patients with SCAD deficiency found fat restriction did not improve the clinical course.[39] To date, there has been no study examining the effects of a low-fat diet on clinical outcomes in patients with MCADD. In practice, many metabolic centers in the United States recommend that patients with MCADD consume a moderately low-fat diet (30% of total energy from fat) similar to a heart-healthy diet while others do not recommend a specific restriction in fat intake. Research establishing the clinical benefit of fat restriction in patients with MCADD is needed.

Restricting fat intake decreases the accumulation of potentially toxic metabolites such as acylcarnitines among patients with a deficiency of CPT-2, LCHAD, TFP, or VLCAD.[35,40-42] In addition, supplemental MCT provides an alternate energy source downstream of the enzymatic block and decreases long-chain fatty acid (LCFA) oxidation.[30,41,43-45] (MCT supplementation should not be given to patients with medium- or short-chain FAO defects.) Patients with LCHAD or TFP deficiency consuming 10% of energy from LCFA and 10 to 20% of energy from MCT have significantly lower plasma hydroxylated acylcarnitine concentrations than those consuming more LCFA or less MCT (see Figure 10.2).[41]

While the relationship between increasing long-chain fat intake and increasing circulating plasma acylcarnitine concentrations is well established, the effects of lowering plasma acylcarnitine concentrations on long-term outcomes has not been determined. To date, restricting fat intake and lowering long-chain plasma acylcarnitine concentrations in patients with VLCAD or CPT-2 deficiency has not been correlated with improvement in clinical outcomes such as a decreased incidence of rhabdomyolysis. However, lower plasma hydroxyacylcarnitine concentrations in patients with LCHAD or TFP deficiency are associated with improved retinal function and slower progression of chorioretinopathy (see Figure 10.3).[46] Patients with LCHAD and TFP deficiency who maintained lower plasma hydroxyacylcarnitine concentrations had significantly better vision and slower progression of chorioretinopathy over 4 years of follow up than those patients who failed to lower those concentrations.

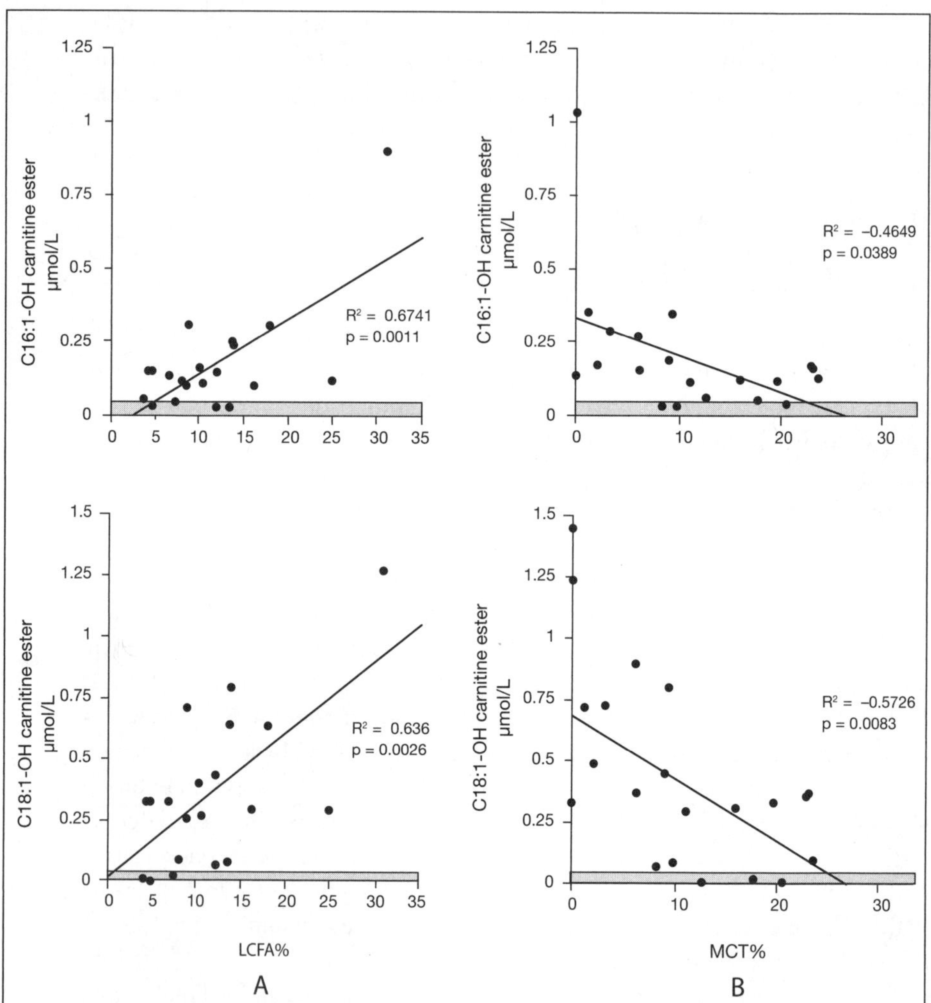

Figure 10.2 *Association Between Fat Intake and Plasma Hydroxyacylcarnitine Concentrations in Patients with LCHAD or TFP Deficiency*

Source: Gillingham MB, Connor WE, Matern D, et al. Optimal dietary therapy of long-chain 3-hydroxyacyl-CoA dehydrogenase deficiency. *Mol Genet Metab.* 2003; 79:114–123.

Note: Percent of energy from long-chain fatty acids positively correlated (A) and energy from medium-chain triglycerides negatively correlated (B) with plasma hydroxyacylcarnitines in 10 subjects with LCHAD deficiency.

Biochemical essential fatty acid deficiency has been diagnosed in treated patients with LCHAD, TFP, or VLCAD deficiency although overt clinical symptoms of deficiency have not always been documented.[30,41,47] Patients with long-chain FAO defects on low-fat diets are at high risk for essential fatty acid deficiency, and plasma fatty acid concentrations should be regularly

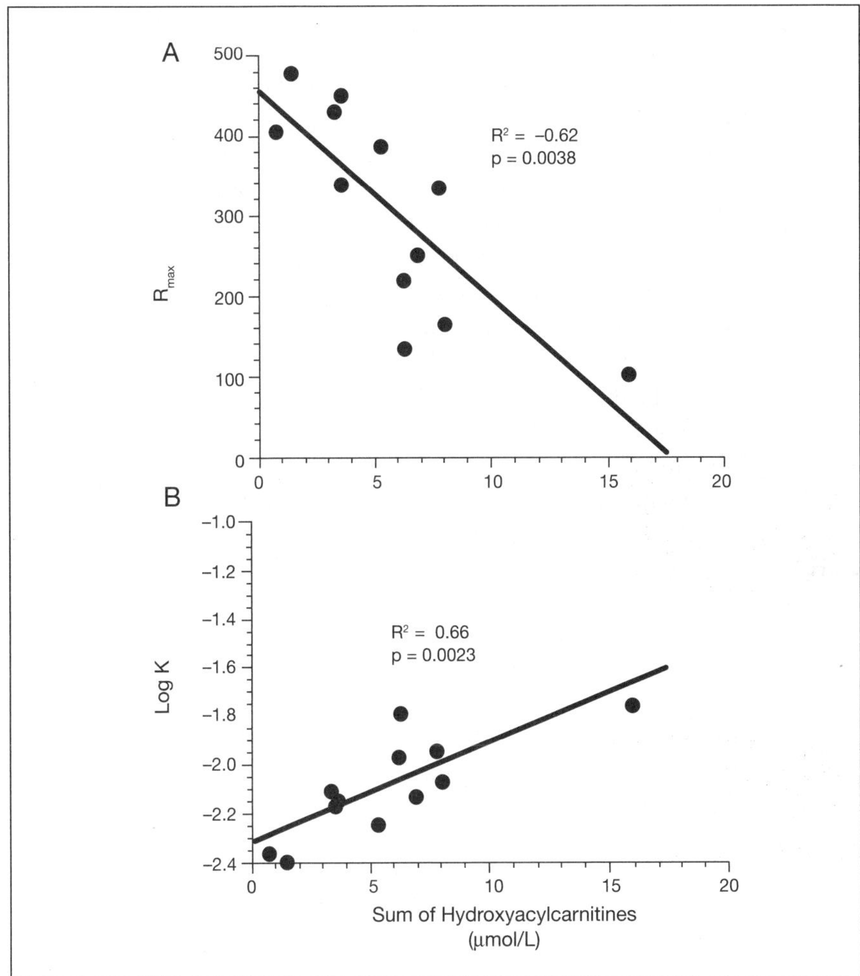

Figure 10.3 *Correlation of Plasma Hydroxyacylcarnitines and Overall Retinal Function*

Source: Gillingham MB, Weleber RG, Neuringer M, et al. Effect of optimal dietary therapy upon visual function in children with long-chain 3-hydroxyacyl-CoA dehydrogenase and trifunctional protein deficiency. *Mol Genet Metab.* 2005;86:124–133.

Note: A negative correlation exists between cumulative hydroxyacylcarnitine concentration (μmol/L) and the maximal ERG response (R_{max}; A) and retinal sensitivity (log K; B) in 13 children with LCHAD or TFP deficiency ($R^2 = 0.66$; $p = 0.002$). Low retinal sensitivity = –1.0; high retinal sensitivity = –2.4 log units.

monitored, preferably by a quantitative method.[48] Providing 4% of energy as linoleic acid (C18:2-n6) and 0.6% as α-linolenic acid (C18:3-n3) normalized plasma concentrations of essential fatty acids in two children with VLCADD.[47] Thus, saturated LCFA intake from prepared foods should be minimized and the majority of the LCFA intake should be provided by oils rich in essential fatty acids (see Figure 10.4). In addition to preventing EFA deficiency, ingesting more polyunsaturated fatty acids and decreasing consumption of saturated fat may lower plasma acylcarnitine concentrations. A recent study in cultured fibroblasts of patients with VLCAD, LCHAD, or TFP deficiency suggested linoleic and α-linolenic produced significantly fewer plasma acylcarnitines than oleic (18:1) and palmitic (C16:0) acids.[49] Soybean and walnut oils are good sources of both linoleic and α-linolenic acid and provide a nice balance between the n-6 and n-3 fatty acids. Corn oil is high in linoleic acid but has almost no n-3 fatty acids. Flaxseed oil provides primarily α-linolenic acid with little n-6 fatty acids.

A specific deficiency of docosahexaenoic acid (C22:6n-3; DHA) has been noted in some children with LCHAD, TFP, or VLCAD deficiency.[30,47] DHA is an essential component of cell membranes and is necessary for normal retinal and brain functions. Whether the cause of the DHA deficiency is related to the low-fat diet or to altered synthesis of DHA from its precursor α-linolenic acid is not known. Supplementing the diets of children with LCHAD, TFP, or VLCAD deficiency with preformed DHA (60 mg/day for

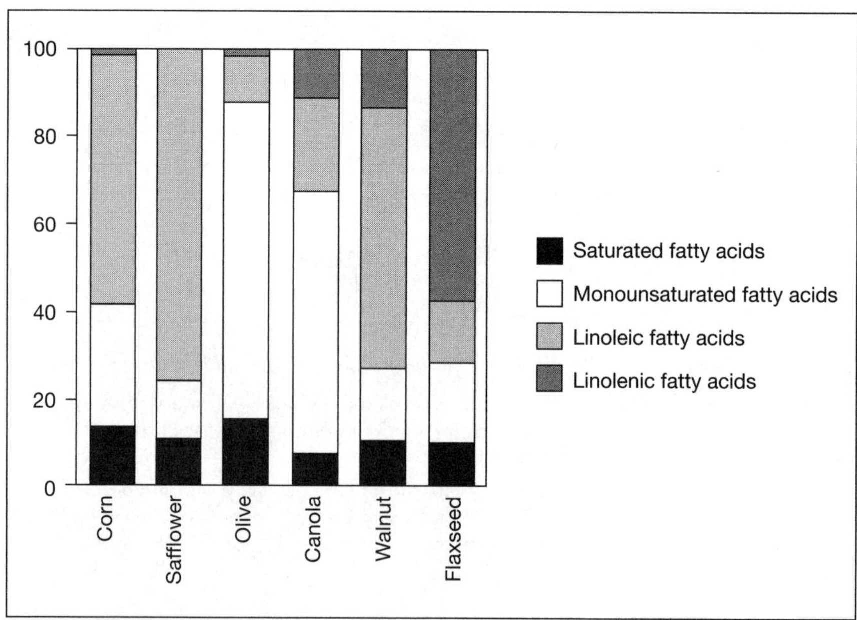

Figure 10.4 *Fatty Acid Composition of Several Edible Oils*

Source: Courtesy of Oxford University Press. Reprinted with permission from Ekvall SW, Ekvall VK, eds. *Pediatric Nutrition in Chronic Diseases and Developmental Disorders*. 2nd ed. Oxford, United Kingdom: Oxford University Press; 2005.

infants and toddlers; 100 mg/day for children and adults) will normalize plasma DHA concentrations and may slow progression of pigmentary retinopathy and/or peripheral neuropathy in patients with LCHAD/TFP deficiency.[46,50,51]

At rest, skeletal muscle burns free fatty acids almost exclusively (85 to 90% of total energy).[52] During exercise, muscle glycogen stores provide the majority of energy during the initial 20 minutes. Thereafter, the ratio of energy from stored carbohydrate and fatty acids is dependent on the intensity of the exercise. At low or moderate exercise intensity, fatty acids provide as much as 60% of the required energy for exercise.[53] Patients with long-chain FAO disorders including VLCAD, LCHAD, TFP, or CPT-2 deficiency often have recurrent episodes of exercise-induced rhabdomyolysis. Rhabdomyolysis may be related to an energy deficit in skeletal muscle resulting from the inability to oxidize LCFAs. Standard treatment has been a low-fat, high-carbohydrate diet designed to maximize energy production from glucose oxidation. Patients with CPT-2 deficiency have been shown to have a lower heart rate and perceived exertion (Borg scale) with an increased duration of exercise when given carbohydrates intravenously or orally prior to exercise.[54,55] Carbohydrates before and during exercise may help prevent the onset of exercise-induced rhabdomyolysis.

Alternatively, fatty acid supplements that bypass the block in long-chain FAO may prove to be beneficial. The use of MCT as a performance-enhancing energy substrate has been studied in athletes. Trained adult athletes given MCT while exercising oxidized 72% of the MCT dose during that bout of exercise.[56] Oral MCT is rapidly absorbed into the circulatory system (< 20 minutes) and preferentially oxidized by liver and muscle.[57,58] We tested the hypothesis that MCT given immediately prior to exercise would improve exercise tolerance in patients with LCHAD or TFP deficiency.[59] Patients had significantly lower heart rates and plasma hydroxyacylcarnitine concentrations with higher ketone synthesis (see Figure 10.5) when given MCT prior to a moderate-intensity treadmill exercise test than patients who were not given MCT. Similarly, a recent case report concluded that MCT prior to exercise lowered muscle pain and the incidence of rhabdomyolysis in a patient with VLCAD deficiency.[60] Oral MCT supplementation with or without carbohydrates immediately prior to exercise may improve exercise tolerance among patients with VLCAD, LCHAD/TFP, or CPT-2 deficiency.

Protein

Many children with an FAO defect become obese, possibly due to low-fat, high-carbohydrate diets that are fed frequently to prevent hypoglycemia. Because of the obesity, a short-term (6 days) high-protein diet (30% of

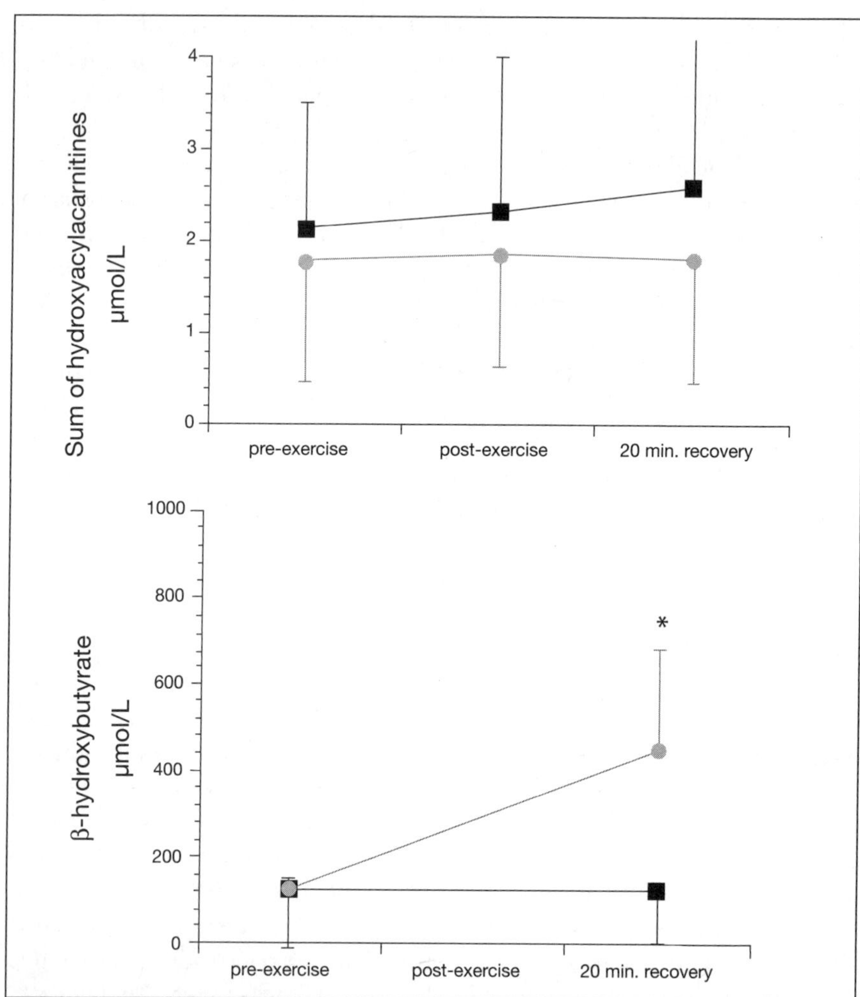

Figure 10.5 *MCT Prior to Exercise-Lowered Post-Exercise Hydroxyacylcarntines and Increased Ketones*

Source: Gillingham MB, Scott B, Elliott D, Harding CO. Metabolic control during exercise with and without medium-chain triglycerides (MCT) in children with long-chain 2-hydroxyacyl-CoA dehydrogenase (LCHAD or trifunctional protein (TFP) deficiency. *Mol Genet Metab.* 2006;89:58–63.

Notes: Mean (± standard deviation) of sum of plasma long-chain hydroxyacylcarnitine concentrations and of plasma β-hydroxybutyrate concentration prior to, and following, moderate intensity exercise and after 20 minutes of recovery in nine children with LCHAD or TFP deficiency.

■ Represent concentration during the exercise test pretreated with orange juice alone.

● Represent levels during the exercise test pretreated with orange juice + MCT.

There was no significant difference between tests pre- or post-exercise.

There was significantly lower plasma hydroxyacylcarnitine concentration after 20 minutes of recovery when patients were pretreated with orange juice + MCT.

* Indicates a significant difference between the two tests at $p \leq 0.05$.

energy, 135 to 180 g/day) was fed to nine patients with LCHAD or TFP deficiency. Patients ranged from 7 to 14 years of age. Energy content of diets was approximately 110 to 120% of patients' estimated energy needs. Data obtained were compared to results found when patients were ingesting only 11% of energy as protein and 67% as carbohydrate. While patients were on the high-protein diet, energy consumption averaged 50 kcal/day lower ($p = 0.02$) and resting energy expenditure ~170 kcal/day higher ($p = 0.05$) than while on the high-carbohydrate diet.[61] Whether the high-protein intake is applicable to all patients with an FAOD has not been evaluated nor are data available as to whether a somewhat lower protein intake would be beneficial long term.

Energy and Fluid

Excess energy intake that leads to obesity should be avoided. However, adequate energy must be supplied to help prevent hypoglycemia and support growth. The range of energy intake recommended in Chapter 3, Table 3.1 is likely to supply the needs of the patient with an FAOD. If physical activity is low, energy intake should be prescribed to prevent obesity.

Fluid intake provided should be 1.5 mL/kcal for the infant and about 1.0 mL/kcal for older children and adults (see Chapter 3, Table 3.1).

Minerals and Vitamins

Mineral intakes should meet dietary reference intakes (DRIs) for age.[62] Treated children with LCHAD, TFP, or VLCAD deficiency are also at risk for fat-soluble vitamin deficiency because of the stringent LCFA restriction. A review of the nutrient intake of 10 children with LCHAD or TFP deficiency found adequate intakes of vitamins A and D related to the regular consumption of 2 to 3 cups of skim milk per day.[41] Intake of skim milk provides a low-fat source of protein and B vitamins, and vitamins A and D and should be encouraged. However, vitamin D intake may appear adequate by diet analysis but patients can have a biochemical deficiency defined as plasma 1-25-dihydroxy vitamin D of < 30 ng/ml. Recent studies have found that very little vitamin D is present in supplemented nonfat milk when purchased in the store and that much of the U.S. population is vitamin D deficient.[63] In response to this, the American Academy of Pediatrics recently increased the recommended intake of vitamin D. Routine supplementation of vitamin D in northern latitudes for all children, and especially for children on fat-restricted diets, is advisable.

Based on diet records, the intakes of vitamins E and K were approximately 50% of the DRIs.[62] Children with LCHAD, TFP, or VLCAD deficiency should take a daily multivitamin and mineral supplement that includes vitamin E. Vitamin E deficiency has been noted in patients with LCHAD or TFP deficiency while they were consuming a multivitamin containing the Recommended Dietary Allowance (RDA) for vitamin E (personal communication, Dr. Maret Traber, Linus Pauling Institute, Corvallis, Oregon, October 28, 2008). Additional vitamin E may be necessary and should be consumed with meals to enhance the absorption of the vitamin. Vitamin K is not routinely included in multivitamins. To date there have been no reports of prolonged bleeding time or other coagulopathies due to vitamin K deficiency in patients with long-chain FAO disorders. However, given the growing evidence of the role of vitamin K in bone health and potentially in glucose homeostasis, a separate vitamin K supplement may be warranted. Further research on fat-soluble vitamin status in patients with FAO disorders is needed.

B Vitamins

All of the acyl-CoA dehydrogenase enzymes utilize riboflavin as a coenzyme. There are reports of patients with specific SCAD mutations responding to riboflavin supplementation. High doses of riboflavin (25 mg/day) appear to improve clinical symptoms in some but not all genotypes.[39,64] Riboflavin is extremely insoluble and should be given orally with food for best absorption.[62] Niacin is the required coenzyme for the LCHAD function of TFP and for HAD. However, there are no reports of (1) supplemental niacin improving residual enzyme activity or (2) niacin deficiency in these disorders. Niacin supplementation above normal requirements does not appear to be warranted.

L-Carnitine

Carnitine is found in meat and dairy products or synthesized in vivo from lysine and methionine in the liver. Carnitine deficiency is rare but can occur in liver or kidney disease, malnutrition, and malabsorption. No primary defect of carnitine synthesis is currently known. The term "primary deficiency" is reserved for patients in whom there is a defect in the uptake of carnitine into cells. Such carnitine transport defects may be paracellular or tissue specific in myocytes, renal tubular cells or, rarely, hepatocytes. L-carnitine supplementation in patients with acute carnitine deficiency syndromes, such as cardiomyopathy secondary to a defect in cellular carnitine transporter, is life saving.[65] Treatment for carnitine transport defects consists of L-carnitine supplementation of 25 to 350 mg/kg/day; occasionally higher doses are warranted.

L-carnitine (50 to 300 mg/kg/day orally or 50 to 100 mg/kg/day IV) is often prescribed for other disorders of FAO to prevent plasma carnitine deficiency and to enhance urinary excretion of toxic fatty acid oxidation intermediates as carnitine conjugates, but few controlled trials of L-carnitine supplementation have been performed to prove its clinical efficacy.[66] In patients with MCAD deficiency, carnitine supplementation does increase the urinary excretion of medium-chain acylcarnitine moieties but this has not been shown to improve symptoms precipitated by fasting or acute illness.[34,66,67] L-carnitine supplementation also impairs the formation of medium-chain glycine conjugates, which is the major pathway of excretion for potentially toxic medium-chain metabolites, suggesting that long-term L-carnitine supplementation may not be beneficial.[66]

L-carnitine supplementation in children with long-chain FAO defects is controversial. Some clinicians are concerned that L-carnitine supplementation will increase plasma concentrations of potentially toxic acylcarnitines while others believe L-carnitine supplementation will improve the excretion of these abnormal metabolites. Two reports of patients with LCHAD/TFP deficiency concluded that L-carnitine supplementation was not associated with decreased incidence of metabolic decompensation or lower plasma hydroxylated acylcarnitines but did not cause obvious harm either.[2,30] However, L-carnitine supplementation in children with the infantile form of VLCADD complicated by severe cardiomyopathy appears to be life saving.[68,69]

L-carnitine supplementation in patients with CPT-1 deficiency is not indicated because patients have increased plasma free carnitine and low acylcarnitine concentrations specific to this FAO disorder.

Medical Foods

Infants with medium- and short-chain disorders should consume breast milk or routinely prescribed proprietary infant formulas free of MCTs. Infants with long-chain FAO disorders benefit from an MCT-containing formula providing an energy source that bypasses the block in long-chain FAO. Several formulas and products are now available. A comparison of these products was complied by the Genetic Metabolic Dietitians International (GMDI) and is available on their website (http://www.gmdi.org), and formulation, selected composition, and sources are given in Table 10.3.

Intact Foods

Foods to supply essential fatty acids, protein, and energy to the child and adult include restricted amounts of fat sources given in Appendix F as well as cereals, fruits, and vegetables, and low-fat meats, poultry, and fish. Foods should not be fried during preparation. While many clinicians believe fat restriction is unnecessary, it helps control obesity.

Table 10.3 ***Formulation, Selected Nutrient Composition, and Sources of Medical Foods (Per 100 Grams of Powder) for Patients with Disorders of Fatty Acid Oxidation***

Medical Foods	***Modified Nutrient(s) (g/100 g)***	***Protein Equiv (g/100 g, source)***	***Fat (g/100 g, source)***	***Carbohydrate (g/100 g, source)***	***Energy (kcal/100 g/kJ/100 g)***	***Linoleic Acid/ α-Linolenic Acid (mg/100 g)***
			Mead Johnson Nutritionals[a]			
Pregestimil Lipil®	Medium chain fatty acids 75.3, L-carnitine added, Taurine added	14.0 Casein hydrolysate, L-amino acids	28.0 MCT, soy, high oleic vegetable, single cell oils (ARA, DHA)	51.0 Corn syrup solids, dextrose, modified corn starch	500/2090	5200/590
Portagen®	Medium chain fatty acids 19.1, L-carnitine added, Taurine added	16.5 Casein hydrolysate	22.0 MCT, corn oils	54.0 Corn syrup solids, sugar	470/1965	1620/ND
			Nutricia[b]			
Monogen®	Medium chain fatty acids 10.6, L-carnitine added, Taurine added	11.4 Whey protein concentrate, L-amino acids	11.8 Fractionated coconut, walnut oils	68.0 Corn syrup solids	424/1772	473/101

(continues)

Table 10.3 ***Formulation, Selected Nutrient Composition, and Sources of Medical Foods (Per 100 Grams of Powder) for Patients with Disorders of Fatty Acid Oxidation,*** *Continued*

Medical Foods	Modified Nutrient(s) (g/100 g)	Protein Equiv (g/100 g, source)	Fat (g/100 g, source)	Carbohydrate (g/100 g, source)	Energy (kcal/100 g/kJ/100 g)	Linoleic Acid/ α-Linolenic Acid (mg/100 g)
			Vitaflo US LLC[c]			
Lipistart™	Medium chain fatty acids 17.0, L-carnitine added, Taurine added	14.1 Whey protein isolate, sodium caseinate	21.7 Fractionated coconut, soy oils	56.0 Dried glucose syrup	466/1948	1767/246

Notes: ND = no data.

Values listed, although accurate at time of publication, are subject to change. The most current information may be obtained by referring to product labels.

Data supplied by each company.

[a]Mead Johnson Nutritionals, 2400 West Lloyd Expressway, Evansville, Indiana 47721. 800-457-3550. http://www.MeadJohnson.com.

[b]Nutricia North America, PO Box 117, Gaithersburg, Maryland 20884. 800-365-7354; Canada, 4515 Dobrin Street, St. Laurent, QC H4R 2L8. http://www.Nutricia-NA.com.

[c]Vitaflo US LLC, 123 East Neck Road, Huntington, New York 11743. 888-848-2356. http://www.VitaflowUSA.com.

Initiation of Nutrition Management and During Illness or Following Trauma

Intervention during illness is crucial and can be life saving in patients with an FAO disorder. Illness increases energy requirements while decreasing appetite and potentially increasing energy and fluid loss from emesis and diarrhea, resulting in a negative energy balance. Increasing intake of fluid and carbohydrate is essential during illness or stress. Managing an illness at home should include frequent intake of sweetened beverages or fruit juices containing approximately 2.5 g of carbohydrate per fluid oz, and monitoring the patient for symptoms of metabolic decompensation.[37] Should the patient develop lethargy, a decline in mental status, or hypoglycemia, emergency care should be initiated immediately. Intravenous (IV) treatment with 10% dextrose and electrolytes infused at 1.5 maintenance fluid rate is recommended to maintain normoglycemia. Caregivers should be provided an emergency letter to present to the emergency healthcare personnel and should be educated on the importance of quick action during illness. Examples of an emergency letter can be found on the FAOD parent support website at http://www.foodsupport.org.

Metabolic acidosis is a common complication of metabolic decompensation in FAO disorders and is most often associated with elevated blood lactate concentrations. Acidosis is diagnosed by a low blood pH (< 7.35) measured in arterial blood gases. In lactic acidosis, the anion gap can be elevated (anion gap = $Na^+ - (Cl^- + HCO_3^-) > 16$ mmol/L). After initiating acute treatment with IV glucose and fluids, blood gases may be monitored to document the acidosis has resolved.

Nighttime hypoglycemia can occur in some patients with an FAO disorder and is a major concern for parents. The risk of nighttime hypoglycemia appears to diminish as the child ages and most patients can safely sleep through the night after age 4 years. For continued concern about nighttime hypoglycemia, both uncooked cornstarch at bedtime or overnight tube feedings have been used to provide a continuous source of carbohydrate. Uncooked cornstarch (1 g/kg) given at bedtime has been used successfully in patients with both long-chain and short-chain FAO disorders.[23,39,70,71]

In most medical facilities, anesthesia for routine surgical procedures requires fasting of at least 6 hours to minimize the risk of aspiration. Fasting prior to surgery places patients with FAO disorders at risk for metabolic decompensation. We have successfully used the following protocol for anesthesia with good outcomes in patients with LCHAD or TFP deficiency.[46] Prior to the procedure, solid foods are withheld for 6 hours and patients are given clear liquids (4 to 6 fl oz of apple juice or other carbohydrate-containing beverage) approximately 2 hours before the procedure. At the initiation of anesthesia, an IV infusion of 10% dextrose and electrolytes is begun at maintenance fluid rate and continued until the patient is able to consume liquids orally. A lipid-based anesthesia has been used successfully with no increase in post-procedure plasma acylcarnitine concentrations and no adverse effects.

New Approaches to Therapy

Energy production in the tricarboxcylic acid cycle (TCA) and the electron transport chain is dependent upon maintaining mitochondrial pools of TCA intermediates. Several investigators have suggested that TCA intermediates may become depleted in patients with long-chain FAO disorders. Substrates that increase the TCA intermediate pools are termed "anaplerotic." Anaplerotic therapy has been suggested as a way to increase energy metabolism in patients with long-chain FAO disorders. Heptanoate (C7:0) is oxidized by enzymes of the medium-chain FAO pathway to two acetyl-CoAs and one propionyl-CoA. Propionate is anaplerotic and can be converted to succinate. Three observational studies using triheptanoate supplements as anaplerotic therapy in metabolic disorders have been published.[72-74] The studies by Roe et al. compared biochemical and physical outcomes of patients with a variety of FAO disorders and specifically in CPT-2 deficiency before and after treatment with triheptanoate.[73,74] The authors report significant improvement in cardiomyopathy and decreased frequency and severity of rhabdomyolysis when patients were supplemented with triheptanoate. Plasma concentrations of C4 and C5 ketones were higher and disease-specific acylcarnitine concentrations were lower in patients on trihepatanoate therapy than in those who were not. However, the study did not directly compare equal amounts of MCT and triheptanoate; the amount of triheptanoate administered was much greater than the amount of MCT consumed on standard therapy. The observed results could be due to increased total energy intake and/or increased energy from a medium-chain fat (C7) and not necessarily the specific effects of triheptanoate. In another report, a patient with pyruvate carboxylase deficiency was supplemented with triheptanoate resulting in rapid and significant improvement of biochemical outcomes.[72] Research comparing isocaloric amounts of MCT and triheptanoate are needed to determine the benefit of C7 over traditional MCT oil.

Assessment of Nutrition Management

The practice of routine biochemical and laboratory monitoring of patients with FAO disorders varies widely across centers in the United States. Biochemical monitoring of patients with MCAD deficiency should consist of routine laboratory tests.[37] Acylcarnitine profiles or urine organic acids are not indicated during follow up. For patients with long-chain FAO disorders in which a low-fat, MCT-supplemented diet is prescribed, routine monitoring should include acylcarnitine profiles, plasma fatty acid profiles, and potentially fat soluble vitamin concentrations.[38] The goal of the fat-restricted diet with MCT administration is to normalize acylcarnitine profiles as much as possible. A sum of the abnormal plasma acylcarnitine species is a helpful clinical tool to assess diet management. For VLCAD, a sum of the long-chain C14:0, C16:0, C16:1, C18:0, C18:1, and C18:2 plasma acylcarnitine esters can be calculated. For LCAHD/TFP deficiency, a sum of the long-chain plasma hydroxyacylcarnitines C16:0-OH, C16:1-OH, C18:0-OH, C18:1-OH, and C18:2-OH can be calculated. In our experience, a sum of long-chain species < 2 μmol/L is considered good metabolic control. For some patients, this is easily achieved and for others it can be quite challenging. Comparing the sum over time within a patient is the most helpful marker of routine metabolic control.

Results of Nutrition Management

Newborn screening for disorders of fatty acid oxidation, leading to diagnosis and nutrition management, has only been instituted in a large part of the United States within the last few years. Consequently, reports on outcomes in patients diagnosed and treated from the neonatal period are few. Further complicating outcomes is the fact that some patients do not develop symptoms even without nutrition management.

Iafolla et al.[75] reported outcomes of 97 of 120 surviving children with MCADD treated for an average of 2.6 years. Age of onset of symptoms and diagnosis are unclear. All patients were advised to avoid fasting. Seventy-four percent received L-carnitine, 63% were fed a low-fat diet, 2 patients were given glycine, and 1 was given riboflavin. Muscle weakness was found in 16%, seizures in 14%, failure to thrive (< 3rd percentile in height and weight for age) in 10%, and cerebral palsy in 9%. Of the 73 children > 2 years of age, 40% had an abnormal psychodevelopment screening test and speech disabilities were found in 22% with attention deficit disorders in 11%.

Of the 34 patients in New South Wales identified with MCADD following newborn screening and diagnosis, all caregivers were advised to minimize fasting. Thus, the correlation between genotype and phenotype could not be determined. The authors stated that "both environmental and epigenetic influences must be involved in the variations seen in clinical effects."[76]

Fourteen children with LCAD or TFP deficiency between 1 and 12 years of age were followed for 2 to 5 years while being given 65 to 130 mg DHA daily as part of a fat-restricted diet supplemented with MCT and L-carnitine. The data obtained suggested that patients with LCHAD deficiency should follow a diet with about 10% of energy as long-chain fat, ≥ 10% of energy as MCT, and moderate DHA supplementation that may improve visual acuity.[46] Growth of 10 Swedish patients with LCHADD was reported. Patients were managed with restricted long-chain fat intake, 20% of energy as MCT, and administration of linoleic and α-linolenic acids and DHA. At 4 years of age the median height Z-score mean was 0 (range –1.5 to 2.0) and the median body mass index (BMI) Z-score mean 1.25 (range –2.0 to 2.25). The BMI suggested a tendency to overweight.[77]

Eight patients with SCAD deficiency were all diagnosed within the first month of life except 1 who was diagnosed at 9 months. Three of the patients received a fat-restricted diet and all received frequent feeds. None received L-carnitine. Presently, the patients all have normal development (15 months to 4 years) with 1 patient having a delay in language at 26 months.[78]

Clearly, further research on the effects of early diagnosis and management of patients with FAODs requires completion to ascertain their lifelong results.

Maternal Fatty Acid Oxidation Disorders

Mothers carrying fetuses affected by certain FAO defects have a frequent incidence of late-pregnancy disorders including preeclampsia, HELLP syndrome (hemolysis, elevated liver enzymes, low platelets), and acute fatty liver of pregnancy (AFLP).[79-84] The incidence of maternal HELLP and AFLP syndrome is particularly high in mothers carrying fetuses with LCHAD/TFP deficiency, but it has been documented in pregnancies in which the fetus was subsequently diagnosed with other FAO defects as well.[85-87] Why the affected fetus is toxic to the heterozygote mother is unknown, but studies suggest the placenta performs substantial fatty acid oxidation and may produce potentially toxic metabolites that would be filtered into the mother's circulation.[88,89]

CONCLUSION

For patients with any defect in FAO metabolism, preventing fasting is the key component of nutrition management. Early treatment with IV fluids and dextrose during illness is recommended when oral intake is poor. Restricting fat intake improves some clinical and biochemical outcomes in patients with long-chain FAO disorders but has not been studied in other disorders. If fat is severely restricted, the diet should be supplemented to prevent fat-soluble vitamin and essential fatty acid deficiencies. L-carnitine supplementation remains controversial.

REFERENCES

1. Rinaldo P, Matern D, Bennett MJ. Fatty acid oxidation disorders. *Annu Rev Physiol*. 2002;64:477–502.
2. Saudubray JM, Martin D, DeLonlay P, et al. Recognition and management of fatty acid oxidation defects: a series of 107 patients. *J Inherit Metab Dis*. 1999;22: 488–502.
3. Ensenauer R, He M, Willard JM, et al. Human acyl-CoA dehydrogenase-9 plays a novel role in the mitochondrial beta-oxidation of unsaturated fatty acids. *J Biol Chem*. 2005;280:32309–32316.
4. Oey NA, Ruiter JP, Ijlst L, et al. Acyl-CoA dehydrogenase 9 (ACAD 9) is the long-chain acyl-CoA dehydrogenase in human embryonic and fetal brain. *Biochem Biophys Res Commun*. 2006;346:33–37.
5. He M, Rutledge SL, Kelly DR, et al. A new genetic disorder in mitochondrial fatty acid beta-oxidation: ACAD9 deficiency. *Am J Hum Genet*. 2007;81:87–103.
6. He XY, Yang SY. 3-hydroxyacyl-CoA dehydrogenase (HAD) deficiency replaces short-chain hydroxyacyl-CoA dehydrogenase (SCHAD) deficiency as well as medium- and short-chain hydroxyacyl-CoA dehydrogenase (M/SCHAD) deficiency as the consensus name of this fatty acid oxidation disorder. *Mol Genet Metab*. 2007;91:205–206.
7. National Center for Biotechnology Information. OMIM™—Online Mendelian Inheritance in Man™ (database). Available at: http://www.ncbi.nlm.nih.gov/sites/entrez?db=omim. Accessed February 2, 2008.
8. Wolfgang MJ, Kurama T, Dai Y, et al. The brain-specific carnitine palmitoyltransferase-1c regulates energy homeostasis. *Proc Natl Acad Sci USA*. 2006;103: 7282–7287.
9. Price N, van der LF, Jackson V, et al. A novel brain-expressed protein related to carnitine palmitoyltransferase I. *Genomics*. 2002;80:433–442.
10. Brown NF, Mullur RS, Subramanian I, et al. Molecular characterization of L-CPT I deficiency in six patients: insights into function of the native enzyme. *J Lipid Res*. 2001;42:1134–1142.
11. Gregersen N, Andresen BS, Corydon MJ, et al. Mutation analysis in mitochondrial fatty acid oxidation defects: exemplified by acyl-CoA dehydrogenase deficiencies, with special focus on genotype-phenotype relationship. *Hum Mutat*. 2001;18: 169–189.

12. Ijlst L, Ruiter JP, Hoovers JM, Jakobs ME, Wanders RJ. Common missense mutation G1528C in long-chain 3-hydroxyacyl-CoA dehydrogenase deficiency. Characterization and expression of the mutant protein, mutation analysis on genomic DNA and chromosomal localization of the mitochondrial trifunctional protein alpha subunit gene. *J Clin Invest*. 1996;98:1028–1033.
13. Spiekerkoetter U, Khuchua Z, Yue Z, Bennett MJ, Strauss AW. General mitochondrial trifunctional protein (TFP) deficiency as a result of either alpha- or beta-subunit mutations exhibits similar phenotypes because mutations in either subunit alter TFP complex expression and subunit turnover. *Pediatr Res*. 2004;55:190–196.
14. Spiekerkoetter U, Sun B, Khuchua Z, Bennett MJ, Strauss AW. Molecular and phenotypic heterogeneity in mitochondrial trifunctional protein deficiency due to beta-subunit mutations. *Hum Mutat*. 2003;21:598–607.
15. Gregersen N, Andresen BS, Bross P. Prevalent mutations in fatty acid oxidation disorders: diagnostic considerations. *Eur J Pediatr*. 2000;159 (Suppl 3):S213–S218.
16. Pedersen CB, Kolvraa S, Kolvraa A, et al. The ACADS gene variation spectrum in 114 patients with short-chain acyl-CoA dehydrogenase (SCAD) deficiency is dominated by missense variations leading to protein misfolding at the cellular level. *Hum Genet*. 2008;124:43–56.
17. Bennett MJ, Russell LK, Tokunaga C, et al. Reye-like syndrome resulting from novel missense mutations in mitochondrial medium- and short-chain l-3-hydroxyacyl-CoA dehydrogenase. *Mol Genet Metab*. 2006;89:74–79.
18. Hintz SR, Matern D, Strauss A, et al. Early neonatal diagnosis of long-chain 3-hydroxyacyl coenzyme a dehydrogenase and mitochondrial trifunctional protein deficiencies. *Mol Genet Metab*. 2002;75:120–127.
19. Matern D, Strauss AW, Hillman SL, Mayatepek E, Millington DS, Trefz FK. Diagnosis of mitochondrial trifunctional protein deficiency in a blood spot from the newborn screening card by tandem mass spectrometry and DNA analysis. *Pediatr Res*. 1999;46:45–49.
20. Rinaldo P, Matern D. Disorders of fatty acid transport and mitochondrial oxidation: challenges and dilemmas of metabolic evaluation. *Genet Med*. 2000;2:338–344.
21. Wilson CJ, Champion MP, Collins JE, Clayton PT, Leonard JV. Outcome of medium chain acyl-CoA dehydrogenase deficiency after diagnosis. *Arch Dis Child*. 1999; 80:459–462.
22. Corydon MJ, Gregersen N, Lehnert W, et al. Ethylmalonic aciduria is associated with an amino acid variant of short-chain acyl-coenzyme A dehydrogenase. *Pediatr Res*. 1996;39:1059–1066.
23. Clayton PT, Eaton S, Aynsley-Green A, et al. Hyperinsulinism in short-chain L-3-hydroxyacyl-CoA dehydrogenase deficiency reveals the importance of beta-oxidation in insulin secretion. *J Clin Invest*. 2001;108:457–465.
24. Filling C, Keller B, Hirschberg D, et al. Role of short-chain hydroxyacyl CoA dehydrogenases in SCHAD deficiency. *Biochem Biophys Res Commun*. 2008;368: 6–11.
25. Jones PM, Burlina AB, Bennett MJ. Quantitative measurement of total and free 3-hydroxy fatty acids in serum or plasma samples: short-chain 3-hydroxy fatty acids are not esterified. *J Inherit Metab Dis*. 2000;23:745–750.
26. Treacy EP, Lambert DM, Barnes R, et al. Short-chain hydroxyacyl-coenzyme A dehydrogenase deficiency presenting as unexpected infant death: a family study. *J Pediatr*. 2000;137:257–259.

27. Brivet M, Boutron A, Slama A, et al. Defects in activation and transport of fatty acids. *J Inherit Metab Dis*. 1999;22:428–441.
28. Lopriore E, Gemke RJ, Verhoeven NM, et al. Carnitine-acylcarnitine translocase deficiency: phenotype, residual enzyme activity and outcome. *Eur J Pediatr*. 2001; 160:101–104.
29. Vianey-Saban C, Divry P, Brivet M, et al. Mitochondrial very-long-chain acyl-coenzyme A dehydrogenase deficiency: clinical characteristics and diagnostic considerations in 30 patients. *Clin Chim Acta*. 1998;269:43–62.
30. Gillingham M, van Calcar S, Ney D, Wolff J, Harding C. Dietary management of long-chain 3-hydroxyacyl-CoA dehydrogenase deficiency (LCHADD): a case report and survey. *J Inherit Metab Dis*. 1999;22:123–131.
31. Bonnefont JP, Specola NB, Vassault A, et al. The fasting test in paediatrics: application to the diagnosis of pathological hypo- and hyperketotic states. *Eur J Pediatr*. 1990;150:80–85.
32. Derks TG, van Spronsen FJ, Rake JP, van der Hilst CS, Span MM, Smit GP. Safe and unsafe duration of fasting for children with MCAD deficiency. *Eur J Pediatr*. 2007;166:5–11.
33. Stanley CA, Hale DE, Coates PM, et al. Medium-chain acyl-CoA dehydrogenase deficiency in children with non-ketotic hypoglycemia and low carnitine levels. *Pediatr Res*. 1983;17:877–884.
34. Treem WR, Stanley CA, Goodman SI. Medium-chain acyl-CoA dehydrogenase deficiency: metabolic effects and therapeutic efficacy of long-term L-carnitine supplementation. *J Inherit Metab Dis*. 1989;12:112–119.
35. Costa CG, Dorland L, de Almeida IT, Jakobs C, Duran M, Poll-The BT. The effect of fasting, long-chain triglyceride load and carnitine load on plasma long-chain acylcarnitine levels in mitochondrial very long-chain acyl-CoA dehydrogenase deficiency. *J Inherit Metab Dis*. 1998;21:391–399.
36. Halldin MU, Forslund A, von Dobeln U, Eklund C, Gustafsson J. Increased lipolysis in LCHAD deficiency. *J Inherit Metab Dis*. 2007;30:39–46.
37. Frazier D. Medium chain acyl CoA dehydrogenase deficiency (MCADD) nutrition guidelines (patient care guidelines). 2008. Available at: http://www.gmdi.org/guidelines. Accessed February 10, 2008.
38. Rohr F, van Calcar S. Very long chain acyl CoA dehydrogenase deficiency (VLCADD) nutrition guidelines. Available at: http://www.gmdi.org/guidelines. Accessed February 10, 2008.
39. Tein I, Haslam RH, Rhead WJ, Bennett MJ, Becker LE, Vockley J. Short-chain acyl-CoA dehydrogenase deficiency: a cause of ophthalmoplegia and multicore myopathy. *Neurology*. 1999;52:366–372.
40. Bonnefont JP, Djouadi F, Prip-Buus C, Gobin S, Munnich A, Bastin J. Carnitine palmitoyltransferases 1 and 2: biochemical, molecular and medical aspects. *Mol Aspects Med*. 2004;25:495–520.
41. Gillingham MB, Connor WE, Matern D, et al. Optimal dietary therapy of long-chain 3-hydroxyacyl-CoA dehydrogenase deficiency. *Mol Genet Metab*. 2003;79: 114–123.
42. Spiekerkotter U, Schwahn B, Korall H, Trefz FK, Andresen BS, Wendel U. Very-long-chain acyl-coenzyme A dehydrogenase (VLCAD) deficiency: monitoring of treatment by carnitine/acylcarnitine analysis in blood spots. *Acta Paediatr*. 2000; 89:492–495.

43. Duran M, Wanders RJ, de Jager JP, et al. 3-hydroxydicarboxylic aciduria due to long-chain 3-hydroxyacyl-coenzyme A dehydrogenase deficiency associated with sudden neonatal death: protective effect of medium-chain triglyceride treatment. *Eur J Pediatr*. 1991;150:190–195.
44. Moore R, Glasgow JF, Bingham MA, et al. Long-chain 3-hydroxyacyl-coenzyme A dehydrogenase deficiency—diagnosis, plasma carnitine fractions and management in a further patient. *Eur J Pediatr*. 1993;152:433–436.
45. Van Hove JL, Kahler SG, Feezor MD, et al. Acylcarnitines in plasma and blood spots of patients with long-chain 3-hydroxyacyl-coenzyme A dehydrogenase defiency. *J Inherit Metab Dis*. 2000;23:571–582.
46. Gillingham MB, Weleber RG, Neuringer M, et al. Effect of optimal dietary therapy upon visual function in children with long-chain 3-hydroxyacyl CoA dehydrogenase and trifunctional protein deficiency. *Mol Genet Metab*. 2005;86:124–133.
47. Ruiz-Sanz JI, Aldamiz-Echevarria L, Arrizabalaga J, et al. Polyunsaturated fatty acid deficiency during dietary treatment of very long-chain acyl-CoA dehydrogenase deficiency: rescue with soybean oil. *J Inherit Metab Dis*. 2001;24:493–503.
48. Lagerstedt SA, Hinrichs DR, Batt SM, Magera MJ, Rinaldo P, McConnell JP. Quantitative determination of plasma c8-c26 total fatty acids for the biochemical diagnosis of nutritional and metabolic disorders. *Mol Genet Metab*. 2001;73:38–45.
49. Roe CR, Roe DS, Wallace M, Garritson B. Choice of oils for essential fat supplements can enhance production of abnormal metabolites in fat oxidation disorders. *Mol Genet Metab*. 2007;92:346–350.
50. Harding C, Gillingham M, van Calcar S, Wolff J, Verhoeve J, Mills M. Effects of docosahexaenoic acid (DHA) supplementation upon retinal function in children with long chain 3-hydroxyacyl-CoA dehydrogenase deficiency. 36th Annual Symposium of the Society for the Study of Inborn Errors of Metabolism. York, England. 1998.
51. Tein I, Vajsar J, MacMillan L, Sherwood WG. Long-chain L-3-hydroxyacyl-coenzyme A dehydrogenase deficiency neuropathy: response to cod liver oil. *Neurology*. 1999;52:640–643.
52. Wahren J. Glucose turnover during exercise in man. *Ann NY Acad Sci*. 1977;301: 45–55.
53. Romijn JA, Coyle EF, Sidossis LS, et al. Regulation of endogenous fat and carbohydrate metabolism in relation to exercise intensity and duration. *Am J Physiol*. 1993;265:E380–E391.
54. Orngreen MC, Ejstrup R, Vissing J. Effect of diet on exercise tolerance in carnitine palmitoyltransferase II deficiency. *Neurology*. 2003;61:559–561.
55. Orngreen MC, Olsen DB, Vissing J. Exercise tolerance in carnitine palmitoyltransferase II deficiency with IV and oral glucose. *Neurology*. 2002;59:1046–1051.
56. Jeukendrup AE, Saris WH, Schrauwen P, Brouns F, Wagenmakers AJ. Metabolic availability of medium-chain triglycerides coingested with carbohydrates during prolonged exercise. *J Appl Physiol*. 1995;79:756–762.
57. Odle J. New insights into the utilization of medium-chain triglycerides by the neonate. Observations from a piglet model. *J Nutr*. 1997;127:1061–1067.
58. Odle J, Benevenga NJ, Crenshaw TD. Utilization of medium-chain triglycerides by neonatal piglets: II. Effects of even- and odd-chain triglyceride consumption over the first 2 days of life on blood metabolites and urinary nitrogen excretion. *J Anim Sci*. 1989;67:3340–3351.

59. Gillingham MB, Scott B, Elliott D, Harding CO. Metabolic control during exercise with and without medium-chain triglycerides (MCT) in children with long-chain 3-hydroxy acyl-CoA dehydrogenase (LCHAD) or trifunctional protein (TFP) deficiency. *Mol Genet Metab*. 2006;89:58–63.
60. Salmenniemi U, Ruotsalainen E, Pihlajamaki J, et al. Multiple abnormalities in glucose and energy metabolism and coordinated changes in levels of adiponectin, cytokines, and adhesion molecules in subjects with metabolic syndrome. *Circulation*. 2004;110:3842–3848.
61. Gillingham MB, Purnell JQ, Jordan J, Stadler D, Haqq AM, Harding CO. Effects of higher dietary protein intake on energy balance and metabolic control in children with long-chain 3-hydroxy acyl-CoA dehydrogenase (LCHAD) or trifunctional protein (TFP) deficiency. *Mol Genet Metab*. 2007;90:64–69.
62. Otten JJ, Hellwig JP, Meyers LD. *Dietary Reference Intakes: The Essential Guide to Nutrient Requirements*. Washington, DC: National Academies Press; 2006.
63. Holick MF. Vitamin D deficiency. *N Engl J Med*. 2007;357:266–281.
64. Kmoch S, Zeman J, Hrebicek M, Ryba L, Kristensen MJ, Gregersen N. Riboflavin-responsive epilepsy in a patient with SER209 variant form of short-chain acyl-CoA dehydrogenase. *J Inherit Metab Dis*. 1995;18:227–229.
65. Pierpont ME, Breningstall GN, Stanley CA, Singh A. Familial carnitine transporter defect: a treatable cause of cardiomyopathy in children. *Am Heart J*. 2000;139: S96–S106.
66. Rinaldo P, Schmidt-Sommerfeld E, Posca AP, Heales SJ, Woolf DA, Leonard JV. Effect of treatment with glycine and L-carnitine in medium-chain acyl-coenzyme A dehydrogenase deficiency. *J Pediatr*. 1993;122:580–584.
67. Schmidt-Sommerfeld E, Penn D, Kerner J, Bieber LL, Rossi TM, Lebenthal E. Quantitation of urinary carnitine esters in a patient with medium-chain acyl-coenzyme A dehydrogenase deficiency: effect of metabolic state and L-carnitine therapy. *J Pediatr*. 1989;115:577–582.
68. Brown-Harrison MC, Nada MA, Sprecher H, et al. Very long-chain acyl-CoA dehydrogenase deficiency: successful treatment of acute cardiomyopathy. *Biochem Mol Med*. 1996;58:59–65.
69. Cox GF, Souri M, Aoyama T, et al. Reversal of severe hypertrophic cardiomyopathy and excellent neuropsychologic outcome in very-long-chain acyl-coenzyme A dehydrogenase deficiency. *J Pediatr*. 1998;133:247–253.
70. Birkebaek NH, Simonsen H, Gregersen N. Hypoglycaemia and elevated urine ethylmalonic acid in a child homozygous for the short-chain acyl-CoA dehydrogenase 625G > A gene variation. *Acta Paediatr*. 2002;91:480–482.
71. Stoler JM, Sabry MA, Hanley C, Hoppel CL, Shih VE. Successful long-term treatment of hepatic carnitine palmitoyltransferase I deficiency and a novel mutation. *J Inherit Metab Dis*. 2004;27:679–684.
72. Mochel F, DeLonlay P, Touati G, et al. Pyruvate carboxylase deficiency: clinical and biochemical response to anaplerotic diet therapy. *Mol Genet Metab*. 2005;84: 305–312.
73. Roe CR, Sweetman L, Roe DS, David F, Brunengraber H. Treatment of cardiomyopathy and rhabdomyolysis in long-chain fat oxidation disorders using an anaplerotic odd-chain triglyceride. *J Clin Invest*. 2002;110:259–269.
74. Roe CR, Yang BZ, Brunengraber H, Roe DS, Wallace M, Garritson BK. Carnitine palmitoyltransferase II deficiency: successful anaplerotic diet therapy. *Neurology*. 2008;71:260–264.

75. Iafolla AK, Thompson RJ Jr, Roe CR. Medium-chain acyl-coenzyme A dehydrogenase deficiency: clinical course in 120 affected children. *J Pediatr*. 1994;124:409–415.
76. Waddell L, Wiley V, Carpenter K, et al. Medium-chain acyl-CoA dehydrogenase deficiency: genotype-biochemical phenotype correlations. *Mol Genet Metab*. 2006; 87:32–39.
77. Bieneck Haglind C, Ask S, Halldin M, et al. Growth in 10 Swedish patients with long-chain 3OH-acyl-CoA dehydrogenase (LCHAD) deficiency. *J Inherit Metab Dis*. 2008;31(Suppl 1):30A.
78. Waisbren SE, Levy HL, Noble M, et al. Short-chain acyl-CoA dehydrogenase (SCAD) deficiency: an examination of the medical and neurodevelopmental characteristics of 14 cases identified through newborn screening or clinical symptoms. *Mol Genet Metab*. 2008;95:39–45.
79. Ibdah JA, Bennett MJ, Rinaldo P, et al. A fetal fatty-acid oxidation disorder as a cause of liver disease in pregnant women. *N Engl J Med*. 1999;340:1723–1731.
80. Isaacs JD Jr, Sims HF, Powell CK, et al. Maternal acute fatty liver of pregnancy associated with fetal trifunctional protein deficiency: molecular characterization of a novel maternal mutant allele. *Pediatr Res*. 1996;40:393–398.
81. Schoeman MN, Batey RG, Wilcken B. Recurrent acute fatty liver of pregnancy associated with a fatty-acid oxidation defect in the offspring. *Gastroenterology*. 1991;100:544–548.
82. Treem WR, Shoup ME, Hale DE, et al. Acute fatty liver of pregnancy, hemolysis, elevated liver enzymes, and low platelets syndrome, and long chain 3-hydroxyacyl-coenzyme A dehydrogenase deficiency. *Am J Gastroenterol*. 1996;91:2293–2300.
83. Tyni T, Ekholm E, Pihko H. Pregnancy complications are frequent in long-chain 3-hydroxyacyl-coenzyme A dehydrogenase deficiency. *Am J Obstet Gynecol*. 1998; 178:603–608.
84. Wilcken B, Leung KC, Hammond J, Kamath R, Leonard JV. Pregnancy and fetal long-chain 3-hydroxyacyl coenzyme A dehydrogenase deficiency. *Lancet*. 1993; 341:407–408.
85. Ibdah JA, Yang Z, Bennett MJ. Liver disease in pregnancy and fetal fatty acid oxidation defects. *Mol Genet Metab*. 2000;71:182–189.
86. Matern D, Hart P, Murtha AP, et al. Acute fatty liver of pregnancy associated with short-chain acyl-coenzyme A dehydrogenase deficiency. *J Pediatr*. 2001;138: 585–588.
87. Nelson J, Lewis B, Walters B. The HELLP syndrome associated with fetal medium-chain acyl-CoA dehydrogenase deficiency. *J Inherit Metab Dis*. 2000;23:518–519.
88. Rakheja D, Bennett MJ, Foster BM, Domiati-Saad R, Rogers BB. Evidence for fatty acid oxidation in human placenta, and the relationship of fatty acid oxidation enzyme activities with gestational age. *Placenta*. 2002;23:447–450.
89. Shekhawat P, Bennett MJ, Sadovsky Y, Nelson DM, Rakheja D, Strauss AW. Human placenta metabolizes fatty acids: implications for fetal fatty acid oxidation disorders and maternal liver diseases. *Am J Physiol Endocrinol Metab*. 2003; 284:E1098–E1105.

Chapter 11

Nutrition Management of Patients with Inherited Disorders of Urea Cycle Enzymes

Rani H. Singh

INTRODUCTION

Urea cycle disorders (UCDs) are a group of inborn errors of protein metabolism caused by a defect in any of six enzymes involved in the synthesis of urea. Patients with these disorders cannot make urea and thus cannot effectively clear excess nitrogen from their bodies. These patients often suffer from mental retardation and other neurological challenges due to the toxic effects of ammonia on the brain. Managing nitrogen (N) metabolism in these patients is a balancing act of nutrition strategies and drug therapy to encourage growth and prevent hyperammonemia. Nutrition strategies include restricting protein intake while providing sufficient energy, vitamins, and minerals to support growth and development. The nutrition management can be enhanced by administering drugs that exploit alternative pathways for N excretion. With proper management, the incidence and duration of hyperammonemic episodes can be lessened, preventing further neurological consequences and maximizing growth potential.

Biochemistry

The metabolism of ingested protein and the turnover of endogenous protein in the body generates an excess of N that is not needed for biological functions. This excess N is incorporated into the water-soluble molecule urea in a series of reactions that are collectively known as the urea cycle. The complete urea cycle is active only in the liver. Each molecule of urea that is synthesized and excreted results in the clearance of two N atoms from circulation, thereby preventing the buildup of the toxic molecule ammonia. The urea cycle is also the biosynthetic pathway for the nonessential amino acid arginine (ARG).

The reactions of the urea cycle are depicted in Figure 11.1. Five enzymes and one producer of a cofactor are involved in the pathway.[1] Flux through the urea cycle is dependent on the production of N-acetylglutamate by N-acetylglutamate synthetase (NAGS; EC.2.3.11). N-acetylglutamate is an allosteric activator of carbamyl phosphate synthetase (CPS1; EC.6.3.4.16) that catalyzes the irreversible synthesis of carbamyl phosphate from bicarbonate and ammonia. Carbamyl phosphate reacts with ornithine (ORN) in a reaction catalyzed by ornithine transcarbamylase (OTC; EC.2.1.3.3) to produce citrulline (CIT). Citrulline is conjugated to aspartate by argininosuccinate synthetase (ASS; EC.6.3.4.5) to create argininosuccinate. Argininosuccinate is then cleaved to ARG by argininosuccinate lyase (ASL; EC.4.3.2.1) with the simultaneous release of fumarate. Arginine is hydrolyzed by arginase (ARG1; EC.3.5.31) to produce urea and ORN. Ornithine reenters the mitochondria as a substrate for OTC and continuation of the urea cycle. Because the reactions of the urea cycle are split between the cytosol and mitochondria, efficient operation of the urea cycle is dependent on two substrate carriers or transporters that permit the transport of substrates across the mitochondrial membrane.[2] The protein, citrin, is responsible for transporting glutamate and aspartate across the mitochondrial membrane, which provides aspartate for the reaction catalyzed by ASS.[3] Ornithine translocase transports ORN into the mitochondria for the synthesis of CIT by OTC.

A defect in any enzyme of the urea cycle except ARG1 leads to a toxic accumulation of ammonia; ARG1 deficiency leads to mild increases in plasma ammonia concentrations. While ammonia accumulation is a common finding in any patient with a urea cycle enzyme defect (UCED), the buildup of the immediate substrate(s) for each urea cycle enzyme and the absence of the product for each enzymatic reaction create a distinct biochemical profile for the corresponding UCD. Patients with CPS1 or NAGS deficiencies have similar biochemical profiles characterized by low plasma CIT concentrations. When OTC is defective, the buildup of carbamyl phosphate leads to increased production and urinary excretion of orotic acid as well as low plasma CIT concentrations. Patients with ASS deficiency, referred to as citrullinemia, are characterized by the accumulation of CIT. Patients with ASL deficiency, called argininosuccinic aciduria, are distinguished by the excretion of argininosuccinate in the urine. And finally, patients with ARG1 deficiency are characterized by the accumulation of ARG in blood.

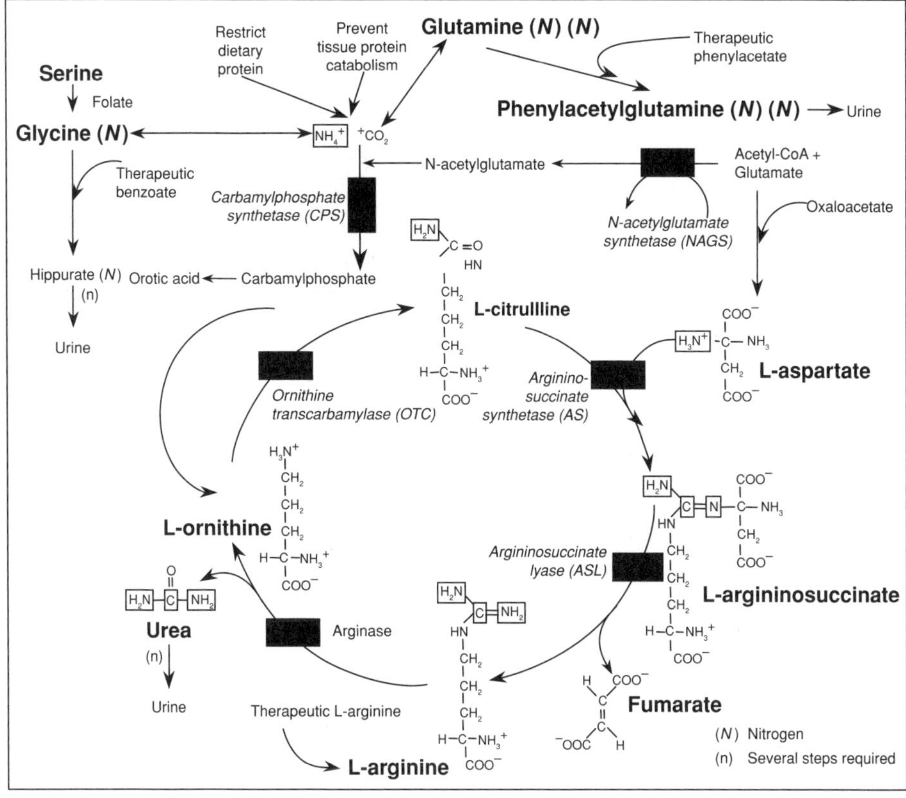

Figure 11.1 *Inherited Metabolic Disorders in the Urea Cycle and Nutrition Approaches to Their Management*

Source: Modified by permission of Elsas LJ, Acosta PB. Inherited metabolic disease: amino acids, organic acids, and galactose. In: Shils ME, Shike M, Olson J, Ross AC, Caballero B, Cousins RJ, eds. *Modern Nutrition in Health and Disease*. 10th ed. Philadelphia, PA: Lippincott Williams & Wilkins; 2005:909–959. Courtesy of Wolters Kluwer Health.

Notes: Ammonia fixation and urea production are metabolically cycled with inherited blocks producing hyperammonemia indicated by black bars.

Important nitrogen molecules and the biochemical origins are outlined in boxes.

Mitochondrial enzymes in urea synthesis are carbamylphosphate synthetase, *N*-acetylglutamate synthetase, and ornithine transcarbamylase.

Use of benzoate, phenylacetate, and phenylbutyrate is indicated to provide alternate pathways for nitrogen excretion.

L-ARG is added to provide urea cycle substrate distal to genetically impaired reactions.

Restriction of protein and addition of energy to prevent protein catabolism are also indicated.

Deficiencies in the transport proteins, citrin or ornithine translocase, cause metabolic disorders that are clinically different from the classic UCDs. Citrin functions as the aspartate–glutamate carrier and is responsible for transporting aspartate out of the mitochondria for urea, protein, and nucleotide synthesis.[4] Deficiencies in citrin can cause adult-onset type II citrullinemia (CTLN2), which is characterized by elevated plasma CIT concentrations and a secondary argininosuccinate deficiency, possibly due to the destabilization of ASS in the absence of cytosolic aspartate. Citrin deficiency can also cause neonatal intrahepatic cholestasis that affects some neonates and is less severe than a deficiency of CTLN2. ORN translocase is responsible for the transport of ORN into the mitochondria. A deficiency in ORN translocase causes hyperornithinemia, hyperammonemia, homocitrullinuria (HHH) syndrome, a very rare disorder that results from high concentrations of orotate and decreased ureagenesis.

Molecular Biology

The genes for all of the enzymes involved in the urea cycle have been identified and many mutations have been characterized.[5] The molecular genetic data are summarized in Table 11.1. The various types of mutations lead to differing amounts of residual enzyme activity, and consequently a wide variability in disease severity.

The most common inherited defects among the urea cycle disorders occur in the gene for ornithine transcarbamylase.[5,6] It is the only defect that has an X-linked inheritance (see Chapter 1). All of the other gene defects for urea cycle enzymes are inherited as autosomal recessive traits. The least common of the UCDs are NAGS and ARG deficiencies. Adult-onset type II citrullinemia is primarily found in the Japanese population with a heterozygote carrier frequency of 1 in 69.[4]

Identification of the genes for these defects has enabled the development of knockout mouse models for each of the UCDs except for NAGS deficiency.[7] These mice can provide models to study the pathogenesis and treatment methods for patients with UCDs.

Newborn Screening

Newborn screening for patients with ASS deficiency, ASL deficiency, and ARG deficiency is available through tandem mass spectrometry (see Chapter 2). The presence of increased analytes (CIT, argininosuccinate, and ARG, respectively) is indicative of a UCD. Screening for these disorders is recommended by the Health Resources and Services Administration of the U.S. Department of Health and Human Services[8] and the American College of Medical Genetics.[9] Both ASS and ASL deficiencies are classified as core metabolic disorders and are currently part of the newborn screening required in all but four states; ARG

Table 11.1 ***Genes Affected in Urea Cycle Disorders***

	Gene	***Symbol***	***Chromosomal Locus***	***Gene Structure***	***Tissue Distribution***
Mitochondrial	N-acetylglutamate synthetase	NAGS	17g21.3	7 exons 4 kb	Liver, intestine, kidney (trace), spleen
	Carbamylphosphate synthetase I	CPS1	2q35	38 exons	Liver, intestine, kidney (trace)
	Ornithine transcarbamylase	OTC	Xp21.1	10 exons 7 kb	Liver, intestine, kidney (trace)
Mitochondrial inner membrane	Citrin	CTLN2	7q21.3	18 exons	Liver, kidney, heart
	Ornithine transcarbamylase	ORNT1	13q14	8 exons	Liver, kidney (trace)
	Argininosuccinate synthetase	ASS	9q34	14 exons 63 kb	Liver, kidney, fibroblasts, brain (trace)
Cytosolic	Argininosuccinate lyase	ASL	7cen-q11.2	17 exons	Liver, kidney, brain, fibroblasts
	Arginase 1	ARG1	6q23	8 exons 11.5 kb	Liver, erythrocytes, kidney, lens, brain (trace)

deficiency is classified as a secondary target and screening is required in only 25 states, but screening is available in many of the others state.[10] CTLN2 is also classified as a secondary target but screening is widely available. Screening for HHH syndrome is currently required in 11 states. Unfortunately, techniques to screen for CPS1, NAGS, and OTC deficiencies are not currently available.

Diagnosis

Diagnosis of patients with a UCD with an unknown or unrecognized family history can occur anytime from a few days after birth to late adulthood. The severity and onset of symptoms are dependent on which enzyme in the urea cycle is affected and the extent of residual enzyme activity. Infants exhibiting symptoms of hyperammonemia within a week after birth are classified as early onset and typically have a more severe disease prognosis than patients with symptoms presenting at a later date. Patients with milder defects or partial enzyme activity may be diagnosed months or years after birth and are classified as late onset.

Newborn infants with a UCD will typically be born full term, have an uneventful birth, and will not display symptoms of hyperammonemia until 24 to 48 hours after birth. These neonates become lethargic and irritable, refuse to suck, and may have vomiting, hypothermia, seizures, respiratory arrest, and progress into coma.[5] All of these symptoms stem from hyperammonemia-induced encephalopathy, and any infant with these symptoms should be suspected of being hyperammonemic and have plasma ammonia concentration determined.

Plasma ammonia concentrations three- to fourfold higher than the normal concentration of 40 μmol/L are considered elevated. Hyperammonemia is a primary finding in patients with a UCD but can also occur in patients with other metabolic disorders. If an infant is premature, the hyperammonemia may be transient.[11] If an infant is full term, further laboratory testing must be performed to determine whether the hyperammonemia is caused by a UCD or another metabolic disorder. The recommended tests include plasma anion gap, pH, CO_2, amino acids, glucose and urine orotic, and organic acids.[12] An elevated anion gap in patients is associated with metabolic acidosis and organic acid disorders as opposed to a UCD. A high plasma CO_2 indicates respiratory alkalosis, which is a common distinguishing finding in patients with a UCD.[13] A plasma amino acid profile that includes a high glutamine concentration is also indicative of a UCD. Plasma glutamine concentrations are highly correlated with plasma ammonia concentrations and hyperglutaminemia often indicates an impending increase in plasma ammonia concentrations.[14,15] As previously mentioned, plasma CIT concentration can be diagnostic of the specific urea cycle defect. Plasma CIT concentration is very low in patients with NAGS, CPS, or OTC deficiency, somewhat elevated in ASL deficiency, and may exceed 1000 μmol/L in those with ASS deficiency. Plasma ARG concentration is low in patients with all UCDs except those with ARG1 deficiency. Urinary orotate elevations are diagnostic of an OTC defect.[5] Hepatomegaly in a patient is another clue to a diagnosis of ASL deficiency. Definitive diagnosis of the specific UCD in a patient can be determined by enzyme assay and mutation analysis.[16-19] Once the symptoms of hyperammonemia are recognized, treatment should begin immediately. Once a patient enters a hyperammonemic coma, brain damage and even death may result if untreated.

Patients who have partial enzyme activity and therefore a detectable amount of urea cycle activity may not be diagnosed with a UCD until faced with a growth spurt, puberty and menarche, a protein load, illness, surgery, or some other stress that induces a catabolic state. These patients are often difficult to diagnose due to nonspecific symptoms, including but not limited to recurrent abnormal neurological symptoms, variable hepatomegaly, poor growth, microcephaly, anorexia, tonic–clonic seizures, and dermatological symptoms of protein insufficiency.[20] The neurologic symptoms may be very similar for NAGS, CPS, OTC, ASS, and ASL defects. One distinguishing characteristic in ASL deficiency is a hair shaft abnormality called trichorrhexis nodosa.[21] It occurs when patients are ARG deficient, which is prominent in ASL deficiency and may also occur in ASS deficiency. Biochemical measures of concentrations of plasma ammonia and amino acids and urinary orotate, as previously mentioned, can provide diagnostic clues to the presence of a UCD in a hard-to-diagnose patient.

Late-onset diagnosis is common in female carriers of OTC deficiency. The disease presentation varies in these females due to random X-inactivation (see Chapter 1) in hepatocytes, and the patients can be asymptomatic or may present with various symptoms that are exacerbated in times of illness or other stressors including menarche and pregnancy. Treatment of seizures in several undiagnosed female carriers of OTC deficiency with the antiseizure drug, valproate, has precipitated hyperammonemic episodes and led to subsequent diagnosis.[22-25]

Late-onset diagnosis is also common in patients with ARG deficiency. Diagnosis usually occurs between ages 2 and 4 years.[26] Arginase deficiency is the least common of the UCDs and typically has its own distinct presentation. The major characteristic of arginase-deficient patients is spastic diplegia or tetraplegia with the lower limbs being most affected. It can also lead to psychomotor retardation, seizure disorders, hyperactivity, and growth failure. Biochemical findings include elevated plasma ARG concentrations and mild hyperammonemia. Neonatal diagnosis is not common unless a sibling is affected or as a result of newborn screening.

Deficiencies in citrin can be diagnosed early, late, or both. Newborns with citrin deficiency can have aminoacidemia, galactosemia, hypoproteinemia, hypoglycemia, and cholestasis and in most cases these symptoms will disappear within a year. Some of the patients will have symptoms of CTLN2 10 or more years later.[27] Adults with CTLN2 are usually diagnosed because of neurological symptoms including erratic behavior, seizures, and coma stemming from underlying hyperammonemia. These patients also have elevated plasma CIT concentrations. Oddly, many of these patients also prefer high-protein foods.

Outcomes if Untreated

Hyperammonemia results in cerebral edema and encephalopathy in patients with a UCD. Without treatment, these patients will enter a hyperammonemic coma resulting in severe brain damage and death. The likelihood of hyperammonemic coma depends on the specific enzyme defect and the extent of residual enzyme activity. Patients with partial enzyme activity who have some urea cycle function have the best prognosis. This includes most of the late-onset patients, females heterozygous for X-linked OTC deficiency, and many ARG1-deficient patients.[28] Although these patients with late-onset disease may experience fewer episodes of hyperammonemia and fewer neurological complications than patients with other UCDs, growth may be below normal.[20] Poor growth is a common finding in ARG1-deficient patients.[29,30]

The poor cognitive outcomes in patients with a UCD are due to the toxic effects of ammonia and glutamine on the brain, but the actual mechanism is not fully understood. The brain swelling has been linked to an ammonia-induced upregulation of glutamine synthetase and an accumulation of glutamine in the astrocytes. This could lead to osmotic compensation, which may result in astrocyte swelling and dysfunction and consequent cerebral edema.[31,32] Another proposed mechanism for the brain edema is that the astrocytes may down regulate the channels that allow ammonia to enter the brain, resulting in water retention and increased extracellular potassium and consequent neuronal dysfunction.[33] Plasma glutamine may also be involved in the increased uptake of tryptophan in the brain, leading to increased production of serotonin.[34] The increase in serotonin may be related to other clinical manifestations in patients with a UCD such as anorexia.[35]

Nutrition Management

Therapy of patients with a urea cycle enzyme defect consists of both nutrition management and drugs. The nutrition management requires administration of L-ARG or L-CIT (except to patients with arginase deficiency), moderate-to-high energy intake, protein restriction, and drug therapy to enhance waste N loss.

Nutrient Requirements

L-Arginine, L-Citrulline

Arginine becomes an essential amino acid in all patients except those with arginase deficiency (see Table 11.2). Supplementation with L-ARG prevents ARG deficiency, allowing ARG to be incorporated into endogenous proteins during anabolism.[36] L-ARG supplementation will also encourage alternative pathways of N excretion as previously mentioned.[37] L-CIT, which is a precursor

Table 11.2 ***Recommended Dietary Intakes (Range) for Patients with Inherited Metabolic Disorders of the Urea Cycle***

Age	*Protein (g/kg)*[a,b]	*Energy (kcal/kg)*[a,b]	*Fluid (mL/kcal)*	*L-Arginine (mg/kg)*[a,c]
Infants, mos				
0 < 1	2.5–1.7	145–120	1.5	100–600
1 < 2	2.1–1.7	140–115	1.5	100–600
2 < 3	2.1–1.6	135–115	1.5	100–600
3 < 4	2.1–1.0	130–110	1.5	100–600
4 < 5	2.0–1.0	125–105	1.5	100–600
5 < 6	1.9–1.0	120–100	1.5	100–600
6 < 9	1.6–1.0	115–95	1.5	100–600
9 < 12	1.6–1.0	110–90	1.5	100–600
Children, yrs		(kcal/day)		
1 < 4	1.8–0.7	900–1800	1.0	100–600
4 < 7	1.3–0.7	1300–2300	1.0	100–600
7 < 11	1.7–0.9	1650–3300	1.0	100–600
Females, yrs				
11 < 15	0.7–0.6	1650–2450	1.0	100–600
15 < 19	0.7–0.6	1500–3000	1.0	100–600
≥ 19	0.7–0.6	1200–3000	1.0	100–600
Males, yrs				
11 < 15	1.4–1.0	2000–3700	1.0	100–600
15 < 19	1.2–0.8	2100–3900	1.0	100–600
≥ 19	1.2–0.8	2300–3300	1.0	100–600
Pregnant[d], yrs				
≥ 19	0.6–1.2	+ 300	1.0	100–600

Sources:

Acosta PB, Yannicelli S. *Nutrition Support Protocols*. 4th ed. Columbus, OH: Ross Products Division, Abbott Laboratories; 2001:418–432.

Acosta PB, Yannicelli S, Ryan AS, et al. Nutritional therapy improves growth and protein status of children with a urea cycle enzyme defect. *Mol Genet Metab*. 2005;86:448–455.

Elsas LJ, Acosta PB. Inherited metabolic disease: amino acids, organic acids, and galactose. In: Shils ME, Shike M, Olson J, Ross AC, Caballero B, Cousins RJ, eds. *Modern Nutrition in Health and Disease*. 10th ed. Philadelphia, PA: Lippincott Williams & Wilkins; 2005:909–959.

Otten JJ, Hellwig JP, Meyers LD. *Dietary Reference Intakes: The Essential Guide to Nutrient Requirements*. Washington, DC: National Academies Press; 2006.

Scaglia F, Carter S, O'Brien WE, Lee B. Effect of alternative pathway therapy on branched chain amino acid metabolism in urea cycle disorder patients. *Mol Genet Metab*. 2004;81(Suppl 1):S79–S85.

Singh RH. *Nutritional Management of Urea Cycle Disorders: A Practical Reference for Clinicians*. Atlanta, GA: Emory University, Department of Human Genetics, Division of Medical Genetics; 2006.

[a]Based on ideal body weight for height and age.
[b]Amount per kilogram body weight declines with age.
[c]Do not administer to patients with arginase deficiency.
[d]Increase slowly beginning at 3 months gestation.

of ARG, can be used instead of or in addition to ARG in patients with CPS1 or OTC deficiency (see Table 11.2). This allows argininosuccinate synthetase to remove two N molecules from circulation by incorporating aspartate N into argininosuccinate (see Figure 11.1, Table 11.2).

Protein

Protein should be provided as a mix of medical foods containing essential and conditionally essential amino acids as well as intact protein[38-42] (see Table 11.2). In infants, optimal growth outcomes have been obtained by supplying an essential amino acid (EAA) mixture at about 50% of protein.[38] As growth slows, the EAA mixture can be reduced and intact protein intake increased. The advantages of providing mixtures high in EAAs are that N intake is reduced from 16 to 14% of protein, and circulating plasma ammonia is preferentially used in the synthesis of nonessential amino acids in vivo, thereby reducing flux through the urea cycle. Furthermore, using medical foods of EAAs that contain high amounts of branched-chain amino acids (BCAAs) is preferred because N-scavenging drugs have been shown to decrease plasma concentrations of BCAAs.[43]

The oral N-scavenging medication phenylbutyrate should be included in any chronic management strategy for patients with a UCD. By maximizing the dose of phenylbutyrate, greater amounts of protein can be tolerated than without its addition, thus providing a diet with improved palatability that in turn will lead to better diet adherence. N-scavenging drugs are usually prescribed to be given three or four times per day. This is optimal assuming protein intake is spread throughout the day. However, if a patient tends to eat the majority of his or her protein allowance at one meal, the dosing of the N-scavenging drugs should be adjusted[44] (see Table 11.2).

Patients with CTLN2 have shown a preference for high-protein foods. While there is not a definitive explanation for this preference, it has been reported that some patients with CTLN2 ingesting a protein-restricted diet become hypertriglyceridemic and that a high-protein, carbohydrate-restricted diet along with L-ARG administration will lower triglycerides in these patients.[45] Because these patients do become hyperammonemic, it is important to administer N-scavenging drugs as well as L-ARG to encourage alternative pathways of N excretion. Each patient should be monitored to determine the appropriate protein-to-carbohydrate ratio.

Fat and Essential Fatty Acids

Dietary reference intakes (DRIs) for fats and the essential fatty acids, linoleic, and α-linolenic are given in Chapter 3, Table 3.1.[39]

Energy and Fluids

In adult patients, the energy needs can be determined by weight based on the recommended 25 to 35 kcal/kg/day or by the Harris–Benedict formula.[46] Actual weight should be used unless the patient is obese or underweight, in which case an ideal body weight for age and height can be used.

Energy intake in patients with a UCD must be sufficient to prevent catabolism without being so great that it causes excess weight gain and obesity. The suggested energy needs of a patient can be found in Table 11.2, which lists the recommended range of intakes based on age.[38-42] By increasing energy intake and maintaining low protein intake, the body will maximize use of amino acids for protein synthesis. If a patient is below the 5th percentile for weight for age (but a higher percentile in height), additional energy will be required for catch-up growth based on the following formula:

$$\text{Energy for catch-up growth} = \frac{\text{kcal/kg/day for age} \times \text{ideal body weight for height (kg)}}{\text{actual weight (kg)}}$$

Fluid intake should be at recommended amounts for age, which are 1.5 mL/kcal in infants under 1 year and 1.0 mL/kcal after 1 year of age through adulthood.[47] Both dehydration, which can trigger hyperammonemia, and overhydration, which is associated with cerebral edema, must be avoided. Constipation is a common complaint, which is another reason to pay close attention to fluid intake.

Minerals and Vitamins

The protein-restricted diets of patients with a UCD can result in low intakes of both macronutrients and micronutrients. Vitamin and mineral intakes in patients should exceed the DRI for age (see Chapter 3, Table 3.1). Additional supplementation of vitamins and minerals is necessary to avoid deficiency, since many minerals, in particular, are poorly absorbed from elemental diets.[48]

Medical Foods

The protein and energy sources for prescribed diets should be a mix of medical foods (see Table 11.3), intact protein, and very-low-protein foods (see Appendix E). Medical foods include amino acid-modified medical foods such as Cyclinex®-1 or -2, WND1 or 2, or Milupa UCD2 (see Table 11.3), as well as energy sources such as ProPhree,® Protein-Free Diet Powder (Product 80056), PFD1, or PFD2 (see Appendix C). Adding flavor such as Hershey's syrup, unsweetened Kool-Aid,® or other N-free agents to these medical foods may encourage diet adherence in children.

Table 11.3 ***Formulation, Selected Nutrient Composition (Per 100 Grams of Powder), and Sources of Medical Foods for Patients with Inherited Disorders of the Urea Cycle***[a]

Medical Foods	Modified Nutrient(s) (mg/100 g)	Protein Equiv[b] (g/100 g, source)	Fat (g/100 g, source)	Carbohydrate (g/100 g, source)	Energy (kcal/100 g/kJ/100 g)	Linoleic Acid/ α-Linolenic Acid (mg/100 g)
			Abbott Nutrition[c]			
Cyclinex®-1	L-carnitine 190, Taurine 40	7.5 Amino acids[d]	24.6 High oleic safflower, coconut, soy oils	57.0 Corn syrup solids	510/2132	3900/375
Cyclinex®-2	L-carnitine 370, Taurine 60	15.0 Amino acids[d]	17.0 High oleic safflower, coconut, soy oils	45.0 Corn syrup solids	440/1839	2800/275
			Mead Johnson Nutritionals[e]			
WND™1	L-carnitine added, Taurine added	6.5 Amino acids[d]	26.0 Palm olein, soy, coconut, high oleic sunflower oils	60.0 Corn syrup solids, sugar, modified corn starch	500/2090	4500/unknown
WND™2	L-carnitine added, Taurine added	8.2 Amino acids[d]	10.2 Soy oil	71.0 Corn syrup solids, sugar, modified corn starch	410/1714	5500/unknown

(continues)

Table 11.3 ***Formulation, Selected Nutrient Composition (Per 100 Grams of Powder), and Sources of Medical Foods for Patients with Inherited Disorders of the Urea Cycle***[a], *Continued*

Medical Foods	***Modified Nutrient(s) (mg/100 g)***	***Protein Equiv***[b] ***(g/100 g, source)***	***Fat (g/100 g, source)***	***Carbohydrate (g/100 g, source)***	***Energy (kcal/100 g/kJ/100 g)***	***Linoleic Acid/ α-Linolenic Acid (mg/100 g)***
			Nutricia North America[f]			
Milupa UCD2	L-carnitine 0, Taurine 0	67.0 Amino acids[d]	0	4.4 Sugar	290/1212	0/0

Sources:
Nutricia Advanced Medical Nutrition Product Reference Guide, Gaithersburg, MD: Nutricia North America; 2008. 800-365-7354.
Pediatric Nutritionals Product Guide. Columbus, OH: Abbott Nutrition, Abbott Laboratories; 2007. 800-551-5838.
Pediatric Products Handbook, Evansville, IN: Mead Johnson Nutritionals; 2004. 800-457-3550.

Notes: ND = no data.
Data supplied by each company. Values listed, although accurate at time of publication, are subject to change. The most current information may be obtained by referring to product labels.
[a]Products without minerals or vitamins are not included for use.
[b]g protein equivalent = g nitrogen × 6.25
[c]Abbott Nutrition, 625 Cleveland Avenue, Columbus, Ohio, 43215. 800-551-5838.
[d]L-amino acids only.
[e]Mead Johnson Nutritionals, 2400 West Lloyd Expressway, Evansville, Indiana 47721. 800-457-3550.
[f]Nutricia North America, PO Box 117, Gaithersburg, Maryland 20884. 800-365-7354

Intact Protein

Infants may receive up to 50% of prescribed protein from proprietary infant formula (see Appendix B) and as tongue thrust disappears, beikost (baby food) is added to the diet. A source for nutrient content of foods may be found at http://www.nal.usda.gov/fnic/foodcomp/search/. Other sources include reference 42 or 49.

Intact protein sources may include fruits, vegetables, and grains as well as very-low-protein substitutes for favorite foods (see Appendix E). Other low-protein foods such as juices can be used to augment energy intake to the prescribed amount.

Patients and their families should be educated to choose acceptable items from menus in school cafeterias and restaurants. Salad bars offer a wide selection of vegetables and fruits that patients may choose to accompany their medical foods. Encouraging intakes of fruits and vegetables that are high in fiber may help alleviate constipation. School nutritionists may also work with patients with a UCD to provide low-protein alternative entrees. By providing foods with a variety of tastes and textures, diet adherence may be achieved.

Initiation of Nutrition Management and During Illness or Following Trauma

While energy is initially administered in an excess amount to suppress catabolism, deletion of protein during the diagnostic period may lead to growth failure if prolonged. Consequently, a diet prescription that supplies all nutrients in adequate amounts should be given. The diet in Table 11.4, which later will require increased protein for growth to proceed, will aid in preventing catabolism and should be administered.

Acute hyperammonemia occurs in neonates shortly after birth and may also occur in older patients during illness, excess protein intake, surgery, or with any stress leading to increased catabolism of endogenous protein. Regardless of the cause of the hyperammonemic episode, the acute management strategies remain the same. Nutrition strategies to reduce plasma ammonia concentration during an acute episode involve an immediate withdrawal of protein with administration of adequate protein-free energy to promote anabolism. This protein-free feed can be administered orally, through a tube, or as parenteral nutrition depending on the mental status of the patient and the functioning of the gastrointestinal (GI) tract.

Oral feeding is preferred for a mentally alert patient with a functional GI tract. If the patient is unable to swallow, tube feeding can be instituted. However, many patients with acute hyperammonemia, especially neonates,

Table 11.4 ***Sample Diet Plan for a 3.3 kg Infant with Argininosuccinate Lyase Deficiency***

Food	***Amount***	***L-ARG (mg)***	***Protein (g)***	***Energy (kcal)***	***Fluid (mL)***
Cyclinex®-1 powder	60 g	0	4.5	306	0
Pro-Phree® powder	55 g	0	0.0	179	0
L-ARG	25 mL[a]	1650	0.0	0	25
Add water to make 651 mL (~22 fl oz)					651
Total/day		500	4.5	485	651
Per kg body weight		152	1.4	148	197

Notes:

A greater protein intake may be required to support normal linear growth, particularly with the administration of phenylbutyrate.

Feed every 2.5 to 3 hours.

[a]66 mg per mL water.

have progressed to a coma with no bowel sounds, and parenteral nutrition should begin immediately. It is essential to provide the protein-free energy as soon as possible, no matter which feeding method is used, to prevent further catabolism.

The first response should be to administer an initial peripheral infusion of a high-energy formula containing dextrose (10%) and Intralipid-20% (Fresenius-Kabi, Schaumburg, Illinois), which should provide provide sufficient energy to prevent catabolism. The infusion rate should be adequate to supply dextrose at 6 to 8 mg/kg/min and lipids at 1 to 2 g/kg/day. If the patient's energy needs are not met through a peripheral line and catabolism is still present, clinicians should consider using a central line to increase dextrose administration to between 10 and 35% to meet increased energy requirements. Insulin may also be administered to promote anabolism.

The protein-free feed may initiate a drop in plasma ammonia concentrations, but typically the reduction of plasma ammonia concentration must also involve administration of the N-scavenging drugs sodium benzoate and phenylacetate. In 1980, the use of sodium benzoate and sodium phenylacetate was first reported in a patient with a UCD.[37] Sodium benzoate reacts with the amino acid glycine to form hippurate, which is excreted in the urine. For every mole of sodium benzoate administered, one mole of N is cleared. Phenylacetate conjugates with the amino acid glutamine to form phenylacetylglutamine, which is also excreted in the urine. Each mole of phenylacetate administered results in the clearance of two moles of N. Phenylbutyrate, which is converted to phenylacetate in vivo, is preferred for oral administration because of the adverse odor of phenylacetate.

Ammonul® (Ucyclyd Pharma, Scottsdale, Arizona) is an intravenous solution containing both sodium benzoate (10%) and phenylacetate (10%), which should be administered along with the protein-free energy in the treatment of acute hyperammonemic episodes. Survival following acute hyperammonemic episodes has been reported to be 96% in patients treated with sodium benzoate and sodium phenylacetate.[50]

Another alternative pathway of waste N excretion is enhanced when the amino acid L-ARG is administered to ASS- or ASL-deficient patients.[51] In these patients, ARG generates ORN for the synthesis of CIT and argininosuccinate, which are excreted in the urine.[52] It is most effective in patients with ASL deficiency because the renal clearance of argininosuccinate is high. The administration of L-ARG is also important for preventing ARG deficiency in all patients with a UCD, except those with ARG1 deficiency, because the endogenous synthesis of ARG does not occur. Therefore, the treatment of acute hyperammonemia should include L-ARG provided at a concentration of 400 mg/kg/day, along with protein-free feed and Ammonul. Administration of the L-ARG base orally is used long term to help prevent the acidosis that occurs with L-ARG HCl.

If plasma ammonia concentrations do not respond to nutrition management and N-scavenging drugs, dialysis is necessary. Dialysis is the most rapid method of plasma ammonia reduction.[5] However, dialysis also removes many other nutrients from circulation, and close monitoring and nutrient support are necessary.[53]

Protein must be reintroduced to patients with a UCD 48 to 72 hours after the initial withdrawal in order to prevent the catabolism of lean muscle mass and avoid further increases in plasma ammonia concentrations. If possible, the protein feeds should be administered enterally and consist of high-quality protein at 50% of prescribed protein intakes (see Table 11.3). L-ARG (400-700 mg/kg/day) should be administered simultaneously with the reintroduction of protein.[54] If the patient is CPS1 or OTC deficient, oral L-CIT administration at 100 to 170 mg/kg/day is preferred; however, it is available only for oral administration. The intake of N-scavenging medication should be continued and the transition to oral phenylbutyrate made if oral feeding is possible.

In treating a patient with an acute episode of hyperammonemia, plasma BCAA concentrations and electrolytes must also be monitored. Fluid intake should be maintained at 1.5 mL/kcal for infants up to 1 year and 1.0 mL/kcal for individuals over 1 year to ensure excretion of waste N in the urine. However, patients must not be overhydrated since it is associated with cerebral edema.[12] The use of N-scavenging drugs is associated with a depletion of plasma BCAAs even with administration of these amino acids.[43] Therefore, medical foods that contain mixtures of essential free amino acids high in BCAAs are necessary. Changes in electrolytes must also be monitored. The anabolic state induced during treatment of hyperammonemia may cause increased cellular uptake of electrolytes. Additionally, potassium excretion in the urine increases as a result of sodium benzoate administration, which contributes to hypokalemia.[44] This can be prevented by administering potassium to meet recommendations in Chapter 3, Table 3.1, or as potassium chloride with the sodium benzoate. Therefore, potassium, phosphate, and magnesium should be monitored and repleted as necessary.[38]

If the patient is known to have NAGS deficiency, the structural analog N-carbamylglutamate has been shown to be effective in activating CPS1 and is approved for use in patients in Europe.[55-57]

Patients should be given a specific "sick-day" regimen to follow during illness or physical trauma and should carry a protein-free medical food (see Appendix C) with them at all times in case of emergency. This regimen should prescribe a decrease in protein intake while maintaining or increasing total energy intake. In addition, phenylbutyrate intake should be continued at or increased to the maximum age-appropriate dose to compensate for increases in plasma ammonia concentration due to the catabolic state. Training caregivers to insert a nasogastric tube is also useful for sick days and has been shown to decrease emergency room visits. The use of antiemetic drugs for nausea and vomiting allows patients to continue feeding, helping prevent further catabolism and avoidance of hospitalization. Instructions to follow up with a pediatrician or emergency room if symptoms persist are part of the sick-day regimen.

Enabling the patient to self-monitor by providing Ketostix® (Bayer, Morristown, New Jersey) can be useful in detecting decompensation due to catabolism or sick days. A Ketostix measures the presence of urinary ketones, which are elevated in catabolic states. Ketones may be elevated in patients with a UCD who become ill and catabolic. If ketones are present in the urine, patients should be instructed to consume energy as carbohydrate to stop the catabolism and should be evaluated by a metabolic clinician. Infants can be tested for catabolism by placing a cotton ball in their diaper to collect urine and then squeezing the urine onto the Ketostix.[36]

Long-Term Nutrition Management

Once a patient is stable and resumes oral feeding, the patient may be discharged with specific instructions for long-term management. After a patient has recovered from an hyperammonemic episode, it is crucial to provide an appropriate diet prescription, ammonia-scavenging medication, emergency or sick-day protocol, and parent or self-monitoring urine ketone reagent strips. Caregivers need to have detailed instructions on how to administer the diet and medication, the importance of adherence to the regimen, how to recognize signs of decompensation, and how to respond if the signs are present. Fear of decompensation often leads patients and their caregivers to over-restrict protein, which can cause a catabolic state. Living with a patient with a UCD presents many challenges to both the patients and the caregivers and appropriate support and education are crucial to successful long-term management.

The primary goal for long-term management is to promote growth and development by meeting the shifting metabolic needs of a patient and to avoid circumstances that would cause plasma ammonia concentrations to increase. This is accomplished by prescribing a protein-restricted diet along with N-scavenging medication.

Chronic management of patients with a UCD requires paying close attention to the energy and protein needs as affected by age, gender, activity levels, pregnancy, and other challenges such as injury or illness. Rapid growth in infants from birth to 6 months necessitates high intakes of energy and EAAs. These needs decrease on a body weight basis when growth slows after 6 months. However, growth rates among children vary and must be constantly monitored to ensure that energy and protein needs are sufficient to support growth, prevent catabolism, and avoid obesity. Another metabolic challenge occurs at puberty, which causes an increase in protein requirements. Adolescent girls may experience decompensation during menarche and menses. Adults have more stable protein requirements than infants, children, and adolescents and can maintain a constant diet. However, pregnancy and childbirth pose another potential risk for decompensation. Finally, depending on the residual activity of the mutated enzyme, protein tolerance can vary significantly among patients with a UCD. Diet prescriptions must anticipate and consider all these factors and temporary or long-term modifications must be made when necessary.

A major consideration for long-term nutrition management is whether to insert a gastrostomy (G) tube in patients to avoid problems with diet adherence. Many children do not have consistent eating patterns, and the insertion of a G-tube will assist parents in ensuring the prescribed diet is consumed and will also be useful for administering N-scavenging medication. Some disadvantages of G-tube insertion include maintenance issues requiring that the G-tube be periodically adjusted for fit and regularly monitored. Furthermore, some patients become overly dependent on the G-tube. Infants can forget how to eat because of the decreased oral intake and may have to undergo occupational therapy to revive oral feeding.

Assessment of Nutrition Management

Assessing the efficacy of treatment in patients with a UCD can be accomplished through anthropometric, biochemical, and neurological testing. These tests should be correlated with the calculation of three-day diet diaries to monitor the adequacy of intake of nutrients and diet adherence (see Table 11.2; Chapter 3, Table 3.1).

Length/height, weight, and head circumference are important indicators of growth and therefore of nutrition status (see Chapter 3). Low height and weight for age should be addressed by providing additional energy and high-quality protein. It is common to see patients with low weight for height because many patients ingest inadequate protein and have protein aversions, often becoming anorexic.

Plasma ammonia, amino acids, and electrolyte concentrations should be determined on a regular basis. Measuring these analytes in blood samples taken after 48 hours of ingesting a specific amount of protein gives the most accurate results of the condition of the patient.[58] Plasma amino acid concentrations should be determined 2 to 4 hours after a feed. Prior studies have recommended that plasma glutamine concentrations be < 1000 μmol/L. BCAA concentrations may be low due to phenylbutyrate supplementation and should be monitored. Blood hemoglobin concentration is a good indicator of long-term protein status, while plasma albumin concentration reflects whether protein intake has been adequate during the previous 1 to 2 months. A serum protein with a short half-life such as transthyretin (pre-albumin) is a good indicator of the adequacy of recent protein and energy intakes (see Chapter 3, Table 3.7). Urinary orotic acid is also an important biochemical marker for CPS1 or OTC deficiencies, with normal concentrations being < 3 μmol/L.

Neurologic testing provides information about the extent of brain damage and the prognosis of patients with a UCD.[59] This testing includes serial electroencephalograms (EEGs) to monitor changes in neurological status and to look for status epilepticus.[60] Other neuroimaging tools, including magnetic resonance imaging, differential tensor imaging, and magnetic resonance spectroscopy, have been suggested as useful for studying the effects of a UCD on brain integrity and function.[59]

Results of Nutrition Management

Rapid diagnosis, the use of N-scavenging drugs, and well-controlled nutrition management have allowed patients with a UCD to survive hyperammonemic coma, albeit with neurodevelopmental delays. According to one retrospective study of patients with an OTC deficiency, survival rates were around 50% in infants who entered a hyperammonemic coma and were treated with varying combinations of protein restriction, sodium benzoate, sodium phenylacetate, L-ARG, peritoneal dialysis, exchange transfusion, or hemodialysis. Among the survivors with documented neurological outcomes, 57% had severe developmental delays.[13] A more recent analysis of patients with CPS, OTC, ASS, or ASL deficiencies seen over a 25-year period found that treatment of hyperammonemic coma with sodium benzoate and sodium phenylacetate and in some cases dialysis (60% of cases) led to survival rates of 65% in neonates up to 30 days of age; older patients were even more likely to survive.[49]

Patients who have survived hyperammonemic episodes have been reported to have varying neurological outcomes including mental retardation, cerebral palsy, seizure disorders, and cortical blindness.[5] Normal neurological outcomes have been reported in patients who have been rescued from hyperammonemic episodes, but most reports have noted moderate to severe cognitive delays in the majority of patients.[61-63] The severity of the delays is highly correlated with the duration of the coma.[62]

Growth in patients with a UCD can be improved by managing nutrition and prescribing appropriate amounts of N-scavenging drugs. In an uncontrolled 6-month study of patients treated with Cyclinex-1 Amino Acid-Modified Medical Food with Iron, the Z-scores for length were positively correlated with protein and energy intakes as a percentage of Food and Agriculture Organization (FAO) recommendations.[41] Batshaw et al. reported normal length/height and weight in 19 of 26 patients with various UCDs treated for 7 to 62 months with L-ARG, sodium benzoate or phenylacetate, and protein restriction.[61] Positive growth outcome has also been reported in a patient with citrullinemia followed for 31 months.[64] However, in a group of patients with ASS deficiency, height-for-age Z-scores were more than 2 SD below the mean when treated with protein restriction and sodium benzoate and/or phenylacetate/phenylbutyrate.[65] The variability in growth outcomes is likely to be related to the protein and energy intakes and can be improved with appropriate titration of N-scavenging drugs.[36]

If diagnosed early, treatment of patients with milder phenotypes of UCDs can result in no symptoms or only mild symptoms. Outcomes in females heterozygous for OTC deficiency are usually good; they are often asymptomatic due to random X-inactivation and may not require treatment. Patients with arginase deficiency may also be asymptomatic with treatment. This may be partially due to the existence of arginase II, a mitochondrial enzyme with a highly conserved active domain, which is upregulated in the kidney in patients with arginase I deficiency.[66]

Brain damage can occur in patients with UCD during the first hyperammonemic episode depending on the severity and duration of the episode and can progressively worsen with subsequent episodes. Prospective treatment of patients identified because of family history improves the cognitive outcome.[67]

Alternative Therapy

Liver transplant has been a successful alternative therapy in some patients with a UCD and is recommended only for patients with extremely severe disease that is difficult to manage, or for patients with progressive liver disease, which is uncommon. At least 59 cases of liver transplant have been documented and the overall survival rate of these patients is 55%.[68] The majority of these transplants occurred in patients with OTC deficiency. Survivors have reported normalized plasma ammonia concentrations within 24 hours, the ability to eat a normal diet, and an improved quality of life. Liver transplantation has been very successful in the treatment of patients with citrin deficiency.[69,70] The procedure is currently used for difficult-to-manage patients with repeated hyperammonemic episodes because of the risks associated with surgery and with sepsis-induced multi-organ failure. Another potential for therapy is gene therapy. However, studies to date have not been successful in humans.[71] The existence of mouse models provides a forum to study other potential therapies.

Maternal UCD

Successful pregnancies have been reported in patients with UCDs. However, postpartum coma due to a hyperammonemic episode is a risk in patients with OTC deficiency.[72] If the patient is known to have a UCD, treatment should be implemented and the patient should be closely monitored. Phenylbutyrate in combination with a protein-restricted diet has been successful in treating a patient with OTC deficiency with no apparent harm to the infant.[73]

CONCLUSION

Early newborn screening, diagnosis, and nutrition management in conjunction with drug therapy have improved outcomes of patients with UCDs. However, infectious illness, problems with diet adherence and other problems may result in hyperammonemia, which is detrimental to the developing brain. Inadequate intake of protein and other nutrients will result in poor growth and other health problems.

REFERENCES

1. Jackson MJ, Beaudet AL, O'Brien WE. Mammalian urea cycle enzymes. *Annu Rev Genet*. 1986;20:431–464.
2. Caldovic L, Tuchman M. N-acetylglutamate and its changing role through evolution. *Biochem J*. 2003;372:279–290.
3. Kobayashi K, Sinasac DS, Iijima M, et al. The gene mutated in adult-onset type II citrullinaemia encodes a putative mitochondrial carrier protein. *Nat Genet*. 1999;22:159–163.
4. Saheki T, Kobayashi K, Iijima M, et al. Adult-onset type II citrullinemia and idiopathic neonatal hepatitis caused by citrin deficiency: involvement of the aspartate glutamate carrier for urea synthesis and maintenance of the urea cycle. *Mol Genet Metab*. 2004;81(Suppl 1):S20–S26.
5. Brusilow S, Horwich A. Urea cycle enzymes. In: Scriver CR, Beaudet AL, Sly WS, Valle D, eds. *The Metabolic and Molecular Bases of Inherited Disease*. 8th ed. New York, NY: McGraw-Hill; 2001:1909–1963.
6. Tuchman M, Lee B, Lichter-Konecki U, et al. Cross-sectional multicenter study of patients with urea cycle disorders in the United States. *Mol Genet Metab*. 2008; 94:397–402.
7. Deignan JL, Cederbaum SD, Grody WW. Contrasting features of urea cycle disorders in human patients and knockout mouse models. *Mol Genet Metab*. 2008;93:7–14.
8. Health Resources and Services Administration and American Academy of Pediatrics. Serving the family from birth to the medical home. A report from the Newborn Screening Task Force convened in Washington DC, May 10-11, 1999. *Pediatrics*. 2000;106:383–427.
9. American College of Medical Genetics. Newborn screening: toward a uniform screening panel and system. *Genet Med*. 2006;8(Suppl 1):1S–252S.
10. National Newborn Screening Information System. Criteria for second screens. Available at: http://www2.uthscsa.edu/nnsis/. Accessed March 14, 2008.
11. Ballard RA, Vinocur B, Reynolds JW, et al. Transient hyperammonemia of the preterm infant. *N Engl J Med*. 1978;299:920–925.
12. Summar M. Current strategies for the management of neonatal urea cycle disorders. *J Pediatr*. 2001;138:S30–S39.
13. Maestri NE, Clissold D, Brusilow SW. Neonatal onset ornithine transcarbamylase deficiency: a retrospective analysis. *J Pediatr*. 1999;134:268–272.
14. Maestri NE, McGowan KD, Brusilow SW. Plasma glutamine concentration: a guide in the management of urea cycle disorders. *J Pediatr*. 1992;121:259–261.
15. Batshaw ML, Brusilow SW. Treatment of hyperammonemic coma caused by inborn errors of urea synthesis. *J Pediatr*. 1980;97:893–900.
16. Gray RG, Black JA, Lyons VH, Pollitt RJ. Ornithine transcarbamylase deficiency: enzyme studies on a further case and a method of diagnosis using plasma enzyme ratios. *Pediatr Res*. 1976;10:918–923.
17. Linnebank M, Tschiedel E, Haberle J, et al. Argininosuccinate lyase (ASL) deficiency: mutation analysis in 27 patients and a completed structure of the human ASL gene. *Hum Genet*. 2002;111:350–359.
18. Haberle J, Koch HG. Genetic approach to prenatal diagnosis in urea cycle defects. *Prenat Diagn*. 2004;24:378–383.
19. Nussbaum RL, Boggs BA, Beaudet AL, Doyle S, Potter JL, O'Brien WE. New mutation and prenatal diagnosis in ornithine transcarbamylase deficiency. *Am J Hum Genet*. 1986;38:149–158.

20. Smith W, Kishnani PS, Lee B, et al. Urea cycle disorders: clinical presentation outside the newborn period. *Crit Care Clin*. 2005;21:S9–17.
21. Fichtel JC, Richards JA, Davis LS. Trichorrhexis nodosa secondary to argininosuccinicaciduria. *Pediatr Dermatol*. 2007;24:25–27.
22. Honeycutt D, Callahan K, Rutledge L, Evans B. Heterozygote ornithine transcarbamylase deficiency presenting as symptomatic hyperammonemia during initiation of valproate therapy. *Neurology*. 1992;42:666–668.
23. Leao M. Valproate as a cause of hyperammonemia in heterozygotes with ornithine-transcarbamylase deficiency. *Neurology*. 1995;45:593–594.
24. Legras A, Labarthe F, Maillot F, Garrigue MA, Kouatchet A, Ogier DB. Late diagnosis of ornithine transcarbamylase defect in three related female patients: polymorphic presentations. *Crit Care Med*. 2002;30:241–244.
25. Oechsner M, Steen C, Sturenburg HJ, Kohlschutter A. Hyperammonaemic encephalopathy after initiation of valproate therapy in unrecognised ornithine transcarbamylase deficiency. *J Neurol Neurosurg Psychiatry*. 1998;64:680–682.
26. Scaglia F, Lee B. Clinical, biochemical, and molecular spectrum of hyperargininemia due to arginase I deficiency. *Am J Med Genet C Semin Med Genet*. 2006;142C: 113–120.
27. Tomomasa T, Kobayashi K, Kaneko H, et al. Possible clinical and histologic manifestations of adult-onset type II citrullinemia in early infancy. *J Pediatr*. 2001;138: 741–743.
28. Cederbaum SD, Yu H, Grody WW, Kern RM, Yoo P, Iyer RK. Arginases I and II: do their functions overlap? *Mol Genet Metab*. 2004;81(Suppl 1):S38–S44.
29. Brockstedt M, Smit LM, de Grauw AJ, van der Klei-van Moorsel JM, Jakobs C. A new case of hyperargininaemia: neurological and biochemical findings prior to and during dietary treatment. *Eur J Pediatr*. 1990;149:341–343.
30. Prasad AN, Breen JC, Ampola MG, Rosman NP. Argininemia: a treatable genetic cause of progressive spastic diplegia simulating cerebral palsy: case reports and literature review. *J Child Neurol*. 1997;12:301–309.
31. Takahashi H, Koehler RC, Brusilow SW, Traystman RJ. Inhibition of brain glutamine accumulation prevents cerebral edema in hyperammonemic rats. *Am J Physiol*. 1991;261:H825–H829.
32. Norenberg MD, Rao KV, Jayakumar AR. Mechanisms of ammonia-induced astrocyte swelling. *Metab Brain Dis*. 2005;20:303–318.
33. Lichter-Konecki U, Mangin JM, Gordish-Dressman H, Hoffman EP, Gallo V. Gene expression profiling of astrocytes from hyperammonemic mice reveals altered pathways for water and potassium homeostasis in vivo. *Glia*. 2008;56:365–377.
34. Bachmann C, Colombo JP. Increased tryptophan uptake into the brain in hyperammonemia. *Life Sci*. 1983;33:2417–2424.
35. Gropman AL, Batshaw ML. Cognitive outcome in urea cycle disorders. *Mol Genet Metab*. 2004;81(Suppl 1):S58–S62.
36. Brusilow SW. Arginine, an indispensable amino acid for patients with inborn errors of urea synthesis. *J Clin Invest*. 1984;74:2144–2148.
37. Brusilow S, Tinker J, Batshaw ML. Amino acid acylation: a mechanism of nitrogen excretion in inborn errors of urea synthesis. *Science*. 1980;207:659–661.
38. Singh RH. *Nutritional Management of Urea Cycle Disorders: A Practical Reference for Clinicians*. Atlanta, GA: Emory University, Department of Human Genetics, Division of Medical Genetics; 2006.
39. Otten JJ, Hellwig JP, Meyers LD. *Dietary Reference Intakes: The Essential Guide to Nutrient Requirements*. Washington, DC: National Academies Press; 2006.

40. Elsas LJ, Acosta PB. Inherited metabolic disease: amino acids, organic acids, and galactose. In: Shils ME, Shike M, Olson J, Ross AC, Caballero B, Cousins RJ, eds. *Modern Nutrition in Health and Disease*. 10th ed. Philadelphia, PA: Lippincott Williams & Wilkins; 2005:909–959.
41. Acosta PB, Yannicelli S, Ryan AS, et al. Nutritional therapy improves growth and protein status of children with a urea cycle enzyme defect. *Mol Genet Metab*. 2005;86:448–455.
42. Acosta PB, Yannicelli S. *Nutrition Support Protocols*. 4th ed. Columbus, OH: Ross Products Division, Abbott Laboratories; 2001:418–432.
43. Scaglia F, Carter S, O'Brien WE, Lee B. Effect of alternative pathway therapy on branched chain amino acid metabolism in urea cycle disorder patients. *Mol Genet Metab*. 2004;81(Suppl 1):S79–S85.
44. Singh RH. Nutritional management of patients with urea cycle disorders. *J Inherit Metab Dis*. 2007;30:880–887.
45. Imamura Y, Kobayashi K, Shibatou T, et al. Effectiveness of carbohydrate-restricted diet and arginine granules therapy for adult-onset type II citrullinemia: a case report of siblings showing homozygous SLC25A13 mutation with and without the disease. *Hepatol Res*. 2003;26:68–72.
46. Harris JA, Benedict FG. A biometric study of human basal metabolism. *Proc Natl Acad Sci USA*. 1918;4:370–373.
47. MacLean W, Graham G. *Pediatric Nutrition in Clinical Practice*. Menlo Park, CA: Addison-Wesley; 1982.
48. Alexander JW, Clayton BE, Delves HT. Mineral and trace-metal balances in children receiving normal and synthetic diets. *Q J Med*. 1974;169:80–111.
49. Singh RH, Lesperance E, Crawford K. *PKUfoodlist*. Atlanta, GA: Division of Medical Genetics, Department of Human Genetics, Emory University School of Medicine; 2006.
50. Enns GM, Berry SA, Berry GT, Rhead WJ, Brusilow SW, Hamosh A. Survival after treatment with phenylacetate and benzoate for urea-cycle disorders. *N Engl J Med*. 2007;356:2282–2292.
51. Brusilow SW, Batshaw ML. Arginine therapy of argininosuccinase deficiency. *Lancet*. 1979;1:124–127.
52. Moser HW, Batshaw ML, Murray C, Braine H, Brusilow SW. Management of heritable disorders of the urea cycle and of Refsum's and Fabry's diseases. *Prog Clin Biol Res*. 1979;34:183–200.
53. Ikizler TA, Pupim LB, Brouillette JR, et al. Hemodialysis stimulates muscle and whole body protein loss and alters substrate oxidation. *Am J Physiol Endocrinol Metab*. 2002;282:E107–E116.
54. Brusilow SW, Danney M, Waber LJ, et al. Treatment of episodic hyperammonemia in children with inborn errors of urea synthesis. *N Engl J Med*. 1984;310:1630–1634.
55. Guffon N, Vianey-Saban C, Bourgeois J, Rabier D, Colombo JP, Guibaud P. A new neonatal case of N-acetylglutamate synthase deficiency treated by carbamylglutamate. *J Inherit Metab Dis*. 1995;18:61–65.
56. Morris AA, Richmond SW, Oddie SJ, Pourfarzam M, Worthington V, Leonard JV. N-acetylglutamate synthetase deficiency: favourable experience with carbamylglutamate. *J Inherit Metab Dis*. 1998;21:867–868.
57. Morizono H, Caldovic L, Shi D, Tuchman M. Mammalian N-acetylglutamate synthase. *Mol Genet Metab*. 2004;81(Suppl 1):S4–11.

58. Lee B, Singh RH, Rhead WJ, Sniderman KL, Smith W, Summar ML. Considerations in the difficult-to-manage urea cycle disorder patient. *Crit Care Clin.* 2005;21: S19–S25.
59. Gropman AL, Summar M, Leonard JV. Neurological implications of urea cycle disorders. *J Inherit Metab Dis.* 2007;30:865–879.
60. Summar ML, Barr F, Dawling S, et al. Unmasked adult-onset urea cycle disorders in the critical care setting. *Crit Care Clin.* 2005;21:S1–S8.
61. Batshaw ML, Brusilow S, Waber L, et al. Treatment of inborn errors of urea synthesis: activation of alternative pathways of waste nitrogen synthesis and excretion. *N Engl J Med.* 1982;306:1387–1392.
62. Msall M, Batshaw ML, Suss R, Brusilow SW, Mellits ED. Neurologic outcome in children with inborn errors of urea synthesis: outcome of urea-cycle enzymopathies. *N Engl J Med.* 1984;310:1500–1505.
63. Uchino T, Endo F, Matsuda I. Neurodevelopmental outcome of long-term therapy of urea cycle disorders in Japan. *J Inherit Metab Dis.* 1998;21(Suppl 1):151–159.
64. Melnyk AR, Matalon R, Henry BW, Zeller WP, Lange C. Prospective management of a child with neonatal citrullinemia. *J Pediatr.* 1993;122:96–98.
65. Maestri NE, Clissold DB, Brusilow SW. Long-term survival of patients with argininosuccinate synthetase deficiency. *J Pediatr.* 1995;127:929–935.
66. Grody WW, Kern RM, Klein D, et al. Arginase deficiency manifesting delayed clinical sequelae and induction of a kidney arginase isozyme. *Hum Genet.* 1993;91:1–5.
67. Maestri NE, Hauser ER, Bartholomew D, Brusilow SW. Prospective treatment of urea cycle disorders. *J Pediatr.* 1991;119:923–928.
68. Leonard JV, McKiernan PJ. The role of liver transplantation in urea cycle disorders. *Mol Genet Metab.* 2004;81(Suppl 1):S74–S78.
69. Yazaki M, Ikeda S, Takei Y, et al. Complete neurological recovery of an adult patient with type II citrullinemia after living related partial liver transplantation. *Transplantation.* 1996;62:1679–1684.
70. Ikeda S, Yazaki M, Takei Y, et al. Type II (adult-onset) citrullinaemia: clinical pictures and the therapeutic effect of liver transplantation. *J Neurol Neurosurg Psychiatry.* 2001;71:663–670.
71. Raper SE, Yudkoff M, Chirmule N, et al. A pilot study of in vivo liver-directed gene transfer with an adenoviral vector in partial ornithine transcarbamylase deficiency. *Hum Gene Ther.* 2002;13:163–175.
72. Arn PH, Hauser ER, Thomas GH, Herman G, Hess D, Brusilow SW. Hyperammonemia in women with a mutation at the ornithine carbamoyltransferase locus: a cause of postpartum coma. *N Engl J Med.* 1990;322:1652–1655.
73. Redonnet-Vernhet I, Rouanet F, Pedespan JM, Hocke C, Parrot F. A successful pregnancy in a heterozygote for OTC deficiency treated with sodium phenylbutyrate. *Neurology.* 2000;54:1008.

Appendices

Appendix A

A. ***Molecular Weights (MW) of Amino Acids and Mathematical Formulas for Interconversion of Plasma Amino Acids Between Micromoles Per Liter and Milligrams Per Deciliter***

Amino Acid	*Molecular Weight*	*Amino Acid*	*Molecular Weight*
Alanine	89.09	Isoleucine	131.17
Arginine	174.20	Leucine	131.17
Asparagine	132.12	Lysine	146.19
Aspartic acid	133.10	Methionine	149.21
Citrulline	175.20	Ornithine	132.16
Cystine	240.30	Phenylalanine	165.19
Glutamic acid	147.13	Proline	115.13
Glutamine	146.15	Serine	105.09
Glycine	75.07	Threonine	119.12
Histidine	155.16	Tryptophan	204.23
Homocystine	268.35	Tyrosine	181.19
Hydroxyproline	131.13	Valine	117.15

$$\mu\text{mol/L} = \frac{\text{mg/dL} \times 10^4}{\text{MW}}$$

$$\text{mg/dL} = \frac{\text{MW} \times \mu\text{mol/L}}{10^4}$$

Where:

MW = molecular weight of amino acid
µmol/L = micromoles per liter
mg/dL = milligrams per deciliter

Sources:

Acosta PB, Yannicelli S. *Nutrition Support Protocols*. 4th ed. Columbus, OH: Ross Products Division, Abbott Laboratories; 2001.

Ajinomoto. *Amino Acids Specifications*. 8th ed. Teaneck, NJ: Ajinomoto; 1997.

Appendix B

B.1 *Selected Nutrients (Approximate) Per 100 Grams Powder of Some Proprietary Infant Formulas by Abbott Nutrition*[a]

Nutrient	Similac® Alimentum®[b]	Similac® Advance® with Iron[c]	Isomil® Advance®[b]
Energy, kcal/kj	507/2119	521/2178	515/2153
Protein, g	13.9	10.8	12.6
Source(s)	Casein hydrolysate	Nonfat milk, whey protein concentrate	Soy protein isolate
Amino acids, mg			
Arginine	775	325	965
Cystine	305	160	155
Glycine	500	220	540
Histidine	540	260	335
Isoleucine	1090	575	580
Leucine	1780	1080	1020
Lysine	1610	895	755
Methionine	540	275	320
Phenylalanine	870	465	675
Threonine	890	585	490
Tryptophan	260	175	165
Tyrosine	290	450	465
Valine	1390	640	580
Other nitrogen-containing compounds, mg			
L-carnitine	Added	Added	Added
Taurine	Added	Added	Added
Carbohydrate, g	51.7	56.3	53.0
Source(s)	Corn maltodextrin, sucrose	Lactose	Corn syrup solids, sucrose

(continues)

B.1 *Selected Nutrients (Approximate) Per 100 Grams Powder of Some Proprietary Infant Formulas by Abbott Nutrition*[a], *Continued*

Nutrient	***Similac® Alimentum®***[b]	***Similac® Advance® with Iron***[c]	***Isomil® Advance®***[b]
Fat, g	28.1	28.1	28.1
Source(s)	Safflower, MCT, soy, C. Cohnii, M. Alpina oils	High oleic safflower, soy, coconut, C. Cohnii, M. Alpina oils	High oleic safflower, soy, coconut, C. Cohnii, M. Alpina oils
Linoleic/α-linolenic acids, mg	9633/Present	5210/Present	5150/Present
ARA/DHA, mg	Present/Present	Present/Present	Present/Present
Minerals/Vitamins[d]	Added/Added	Added/Added	Added/Added

Note: Product information and values listed are subject to change. Refer to product label for the most current information.

[a]Abbott Nutrition, 625 Cleveland Avenue, Columbus, Ohio 43215-1724. 800-227-5767.

[b]One unpacked level scoop = 8.7 g powder.

[c]One unpacked level scoop = 8.6 g powder.

[d]See product label for amounts per 100 kcal.

B.2 *Selected Nutrients (Approximate) Per 100 Grams Powder of Some Proprietary Infant Formulas by Mead Johnson Nutritionals*[a]

Nutrient	*Enfamil® Lipil®*[b]	*ProSobee® Lipil®*[c]	*Nutramigen® Lipil®*[d]
Energy, kcal/kj	470/1965	500/2090	500/2090
Protein, g	9.9	12.5	13.9
Source(s)	Nonfat milk	Soy protein isolate	Casein hydrolysate
Amino acids, mg			
Arginine	240	1000	560
Cystine	129	138	220
Glycine	210	530	340
Histidine	210	340	420
Isoleucine	660	610	830
Leucine	1120	1030	1420
Lysine	750	790	1200
Methionine	210	260	430
Phenylalanine	420	660	670
Threonine	570	460	690
Tryptophan	163	163	220
Tyrosine	490	490	310
Valine	670	640	1050
Other nitrogen-containing compounds, mg			
L-carnitine	9.4	10.0	9.9
Taurine	28.2	30.0	30.0
Carbohydrate, g	51.2	53.0	51.0
Source(s)	Lactose	Corn syrup solids	Corn syrup solids. modified corn starch
Fat, g	24.9	27.0	26.0
Source(s)	Palm olein, soy, coconut, high-oleic sunflower oils	Palm olein, soy, coconut, high-oleic sunflower oils	Palm olein, soy, coconut, high-oleic sunflower oils
Linoleic/α-linolenic acids, mg	4042/ND	4300/430	4300/420
ARA/DHA, mg	160/80	85/170	84/169
Minerals/Vitamins	Added/Added	Added/Added	Added/Added

Notes: Product information and values listed are subject to change. Refer to product label for the most current information.

ND = no data.

[a]Mead Johnson Nutritionals, 2400 West Lloyd Expressway, Evansville, Indiana 47721. 812-429-6399.

[b]One unpacked level scoop = 8.5 g powder.

[c]One unpacked level scoop = 8.8 g powder.

[d]One unpacked level scoop = 9.0 g powder.

B.3 *Selected Nutrients (Approximate) Per 100 Grams Liquid in Human Milk (Mature), Cow's Milk (3.25% Fat), and Skim Milk*

Nutrient	*Human Milk*[a]	*Cow's Milk*[b]	*Skim Milk*[c]
Energy, kcal/kJ	70/291	60/252	37/143
Protein, g	1.03	3.22	3.37
Amino acids, mg			
Arginine	43	75	72
Cystine	19	17	123
Glycine	26	75	50
Histidine	23	75	75
Isoleucine	56	165	150
Leucine	95	265	327
Lysine	68	140	252
Methionine	21	75	62
Phenylalanine	46	147	145
Threonine	46	143	82
Tryptophan	17	46	40
Tyrosine	53	152	148
Valine	63	192	180
Other nitrogen-containing compounds, mg			
L-carnitine	1	1	ND
Taurine	5	5	ND
Carbohydrate, g	6.89	9.78	10.05
Fat, g	3.50	3.25	0.08
Linoleic/α-linolenic acids, mg	374/52	120/75	2/1
ARA/DHA, mg	26/0	0/0	0/0
Minerals/Vitamins	Present/Present	Present/Present	Present/Present

Sources:

Penn D, Dolderer M, Schmidt-Sommerfeld E. Carnitine concentrations in the milk of different species and infant formulas. *Biol Neonate*. 1987;52:70–79.

Picciano MF, McDonald SS. Lactation. In: Shils ME, Shike M, Olson J, Ross AC, Caballero B, Cousins RJ, eds. *Modern Nutrition in Health and Disease*. 10th ed. Philadelphia, PA: Lippincott Williams & Wilkins; 2005:784–796.

United States Department of Agriculture Agricultural Research Service. Nutrient Data Laboratory. Available at: http://www/nal.usda.gov/fnic/foodcomp/search/. Accessed December 30, 2008.

Note: ND = no data.
[a]100 g = 96.0 mL
[b]100 g = 97.0 mL
[c]100 g = 96.6 mL

C. *Energy Sources Free of Protein (Per 100 Grams Powder)*

Medical Food	*Fat (g/100 g, source)*	*Carbohydrate (g/100 g, source)*	*Energy (kcal/100 g/ kJ/100 g)*	*Linoleic acid/ α-Linolenic acid (mg/100 g)*	*Minerals/ Vitamins*
		Abbott Nutrition[a]			
Pro-Phree® powder	28.0 High oleic safflower, coconut, soy oils	65.0 Corn syrup solids	510/2132	4400/400	Yes
Polycose powder	0.0	94.0 Hydrolyzed cornstarch	380/1588	0/0	No
		Applied Nutrition Corp[b]			
Energy Option Protein-Free Bar	25.0 Cocoa butter, coconut oil	25.0 Sucrose	310/1296	348/102	No
		Mead Johnson Nutritionals[c]			
PFD1 powder	32.0 Palm olein, soy, coconut, high oleic sunflower oils	60.0 Corn syrup solids, sugar, modified corn starch	530/2215	5300/450	Yes
PDF2 powder	4.8 Soy oil	88.0 Corn syrup solids, sugar, modified corn starch	400/1672	~1675/125	Yes

(continues)

C. *Energy Sources Free of Protein (Per 100 Grams Powder), Continued*

Medical Food	*Fat (g/100 g, source)*	*Carbohydrate (g/100 g, source)*	*Energy (kcal/100 g/ kJ/100 g)*	*Linoleic acid/ α-Linolenic acid (mg/100 g)*	*Minerals/ Vitamins*
		Nutricia North America[d]			
Super Soluble Duocal powder	22.3 Fractionated coconut, palm kernel, corn, coconut oils	72.7 Sucrose, hydrolyzed corn starch	492/2057	4700/84	No
Polycal powder	96.0	0 Maltodextrin	384/1605	0/0	No

Note: Values listed, although accurate at time of publication, are subject to change. The most current information may be obtained by referring to product labels.
[a]Abbott Nutrition, 625 Cleveland Avenue, Columbus, Ohio 43215. 800-551-5838.
[b]Applied Nutrition Corp, 10 Saddle Road, Cedar Knolls, New Jersey 07927. 800-605-0410.
[c]Mead Johnson Nutritionals, 2400 West Lloyd Expressway, Evansville, Indiana 47721. 800-457-3550.
[d]Nutricia North America, PO Box 117, Gaithersburg, Maryland 20884. 800-365-7354.

Appendix D

D. ***Sources of Total Parenteral Nutrition Services***

Apria Healthcare. Available at: http://apria.com/home/. Click on STATE, enter state name, and submit as directed. Cities in state with telephone number and list of services will appear. Accessed December 18, 2008.

Appendix E

E. *Sources of Very Low-Protein Foods*

Applied Nutrition Corp.
10 Saddle Road
Cedar Knolls, NJ 07927, USA
800-605-0410
http://www.medicalfood.com

Cambrooke Foods
Two Central Street
Framingham, MA 01701, USA
866-456-9775
http://www.cambrookefoods.com

Kingsmill Foods Co, Ltd.
1399 Kennedy Road, Unit 17
Scarborough, Ontario, M1P 2L6, Canada
416-755-1124
http://www.kingsmillfoods.com

Nutricia, NA (United States)
PO Box 117
Gaithersburg, MD 20884, USA
800-365-7354
http://www.shsna.com/pages/products.htm

Ener-G® Foods, Inc.
5960 1st Avenue South
Seattle, WA 98108, USA
206-767-3928
http://www.ener-g.com

Med-Diet® Laboratories, Inc.
3600 Holly Lane North, Suite 80
Plymouth, MN 55477, USA
763-550-2020, 800-633-3438
http://www.med-diet.com/privacy.htm

Nutricia, NA (Canada)
4515 Dobrin Street
St. Laurent, Quebec H4R 2L8, Canada
877-636-2283
http://www.Nutricia-NA.com

Appendix F

F. ***Selected Nutrient Composition of Some Oils Per 100 Grams***

Oil	*Energy (kcal/kJ)*	*Fat (g)*	*Linoleic Acid (g)*	*α-Linolenic Acid (g)*
Canola	825/3448	93	21.00	8.80
Coconut	862/3607	100	1.80	0.00
Corn	884/3699	100	52.23	1.16
Flaxseed	884/3699	100	12.70	53.30
MCT*	830/3471	100	0.00	0.00
Safflower	882/3695	100	14.35	0.40
Soybean	884/3699	100	54.20	7.70
Walnut	884/3699	100	52.90	10.40

Sources:

Novartis Medical Nutrition, MCT Oil™ Medium-Chain Triglycerides. Available at: https://novartisnutrition.com/us/product/detail? Accessed November 11, 2008.

USDA Agricultural Research Service. Nutrient Data Laboratory. Available at: http://www.nal.usda.gov/fnic/foodcomp/search/. Accessed November 11, 2008.

*7.7 kcal/mL or 8.3 kcal/g; 1 Tbsp = 14 mL

Appendix G

G. *Sources of L-Amino Acids*

Fisher Scientific
2000 Park Lane Drive
Pittsburgh, PA 15275
800-766-7000
http://www.fishersci.com
Available in 100-g containers

JoMar Laboratories
583-B Division Street
Campbell, CA 95008
408-374-5920, 800-538-4545
http://www.jomarlabs.com
Available in 150-g and 1-kg containers

Vitaflo USA
123 East Neck Road
Huntington, NY 11743
631-547-5984, 888-848-2356
http://www.vitaflousa.com
L-isoleucine and L-valine available in 50-mg individual packets

Note: Data current as of March, 2008. Check with distributor for most current availability.

Index

References to figures and tables are indicated with f and t following the page number.

C

H

M

U